Aromatherapy Science

Aromatherapy Science

A guide for healthcare professionals

Maria Lis-Balchin

BSc, PhD

Reader in Applied Biochemistry (retired)
Honorary Research Fellow (presently)
School of Applied Science
London South Bank University
London, UK

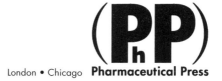

London • Chicago **Pharmaceutical Press**

Published by the Pharmaceutical Press
Publications division of the Royal Pharmaceutical Society of Great Britain

1 Lambeth High Street, London SE1 7JN, UK
100 South Atkinson Road, Suite 206, Grayslake, IL 60030-7820, USA

© Pharmaceutical Press 2006

First edition published 2006

Typeset by Gray Publishing, Tunbridge Wells, Kent
Printed in Great Britain by The Bath Press, Bath

ISBN 0 85369 578 4

A catalogue record for this book is available from the British Library.

Contents

Preface

Aromatherapy has evolved rather as an art than a science. This book has been written by a scientist both for scientifically trained readers and for those wishing to acquire unbiased knowledge on the principles and practice of aromatherapy. It is intended to be a scientific account of essential oil usage in aromatherapy and does not promote the usage of any specific essential oils as therapeutic agents, unless scientific evidence strongly supports it. The book is intended to be in the same general category as *Essential Oil Safety* (Tisserand and Balacs, 1995); it is however rather more broad in its content, encompassing the history, chemistry and functions (both general and physiological, including smell) of aromatherapy, as well as aromatherapeutic practice, clinical studies and safety aspects. Recent research and new legislation on sensitisation is included in this book to supplement the data on toxicology.

Although this book is intended for healthcare professionals it differs from most aromatherapy books in that it does not provide a comprehensive list of aromatherapy usage for every essential oil and for every possible malady. There are so many general activities of essential oils that the concept of specific therapeutic application is grossly undermined (Vickers, 1996). The chemical composition of essential oils differs greatly (Lis-Balchin, 1997, 2002a), but their properties and therapeutic applications are often shown by aromatherapists to be remarkably similar (Ryman, 1991; Lawless, 1992; Rose, 1992a; Price, 1993; Sheppard-Hanger, 1995). These contradictions will be discussed together with the possibility that massage and inhalation of essential oils (Lis-Balchin, 2002b) is responsible for the greater part of their apparent therapeutic value. In the individual essential oil monographs, factual scientific information is given on every aspect of the essential oils normally used by aromatherapists. This is accompanied by some of the attributes for functions and usage made by aromatherapists. A scientific evaluation is given and readers can then make up their own minds.

Maria Lis-Balchin
August 2005

About the author

Maria Lis-Balchin attained a BSc (Hons) in biochemistry/zoology from Queen Elizabeth College, London (now King's) and a PhD in physiology from Westminster Medical School, London whilst working as the hospital biochemist/clinical pathologist and also as toxicologist at BIBRA (British Industrial Biological Research Association), Carshalton.

She took early retirement as Reader in Applied Biochemistry after lecturing at South Bank University (now London South Bank University) for over 30 years in biochemistry, toxicology, nutrition and physiology, and continues research as an Honorary Research Fellow. She lectured to undergraduate and postgraduate degree students and supervised numerous theses for students both at South Bank University, King's College and abroad, including numerous final year pharmacy students from Vienna University.

Maria's research had previously included: neuropsychiatry at the Medical Research Council, Carshalton and brain tumours/cerebral oedema at St George's Hospital (Atkinson Morley's). More recently she has personally researched essential oils for 25 years. Topics included: the biochemistry of essential oils; analysis using gas chromatography and gas chromatography/mass spectroscopy; pharmacological studies on many different animals and their tissues *in vitro*; microbiological assessment of essential oils and also various other fractions of numerous plants, including novel plants; toxicological evaluation of plant extracts including essential oils. She has written or edited three books and published over 100 scientific papers in books, international journals or presented at conferences worldwide. She personally presented five exhibits at the Chelsea Flower Show, London for the South Bank University, which were mainly based on essential oils and medicinal plants.

She has been a guest speaker at aromatherapy conferences in the USA, Australia, New Zealand and Poland and given lectures and workshops at various aromatherapy schools worldwide.

As the University spokesperson for aromatherapy and herbal/alternative medicine, Maria has appeared on numerous television and radio shows and news programmes including Channel 4's *Time Team*, the BBC's *Watchdog* and *Healthcheck*, live broadcasts from Chelsea Flower Show on Radio 4's *You and Yours* and Jazz FM. She has also been quoted in: the *Guardian*, *The Times*, *Daily Mail*, *Daily Telegraph* and *Daily Express*.

Abbreviations

BAN	British Approved Name
BEAM	brain electrical activity mapping
BHA	butylhydroxy anisole
BHT	butylhydroxy toluene
BMA	British Medical Association
b.p.	boiling point
BP	British Pharmacopoeia. Unless otherwise specified, BP references are to the 2002 edition
BPC	British Pharmaceutical Codex
CAM	complementary and alternative medicine
cAMP	cyclic adenosine monophosphate
CAS	Chemical Abstracts Service
cGMP	cyclic guanosine monophosphate
CHIP	Chemicals Hazard Information and Packaging for Supply Regulations 2002
CMA	Chemical Manufacturers Association
CNS	central nervous system
CNV	contingent negative variation
DEP	diethylphthalate
DNA	deoxyribonucleic acid
ECG	electrocardiogram
EEC	European Economic Community, now the European Union
EEG	electroencephalogram
EO	essential oil
ES	electrical stimulation
EU sensitiser total	the maximum levels of fragrance allergens in aromatic natural raw materials: European Parliament and Council Directive 76/768/EEC on Cosmetic Products, 7th Amendment 2002
FAO	Food and Agriculture Organization of the United Nations
FDA	Food and Drug Administration of the USA
FEMA	Flavor and Extract Manufacturers Association of the USA
GC	gas chromatography
GC/MS	gas chromatography with mass spectrometry
GRAS	Generally Recognised As Safe – issued by FEMA
HSE	Health and Safety Executive (UK)
IBS	irritable bowel syndrome
ICR	Institute of Cancer Research
ICR mice	Institute of Cancer Research referring to mice in conflict tests
Ig	immunoglobulin
ISO	International Organization for Standardization (www.iso.org/iso/en/CatalogueDetailPage gives complete set of ISOs)
iu	international unit(s)

kg	kilogram(s)
LD_{50}	a dose lethal to 50% of the specified animals
m	metre(s)
m^2	square metre(s)
MAFF	Ministry of Agriculture, Fisheries and Food (UK)
MAOI	monoamine oxidase inhibitor
max.	maximum
MBC	minimum bactericidal concentration
MCA	Medicines Control Agency (UK)
mEq	milliequivalent(s)
mg	milligram(s)
MIC	minimum inhibitory concentration
min	minute
min.	minimum
mL	millilitre(s)
mm	millimetre(s)
mol. wt	molecular weight
MS	mass spectroscopy
NIH	National Institutes of Health (USA)
NIOSH	National Institute for Occupational Safety and Health
nm	nanometre(s)
PAS	Psychogeriatric Assessment Scales
pH	the negative logarithm of the hydrogen ion concentration
7th Amendment 2002	European Parliament and Council Directive 76/768/EEC on Cosmetic Products
sp.	species (plural spp.)
TENS	transcutaneous electrical nerve stimulators
USAN	US Approved Name
USP	The United States Pharmacopeia 26, 2003 and Supplement 1
UV	ultraviolet
var.	variety
vol.	volume(s)
v/v	volume in volume
v/w	volume in weight
WHO	World Health Organization
w/o	water in oil
wt	weight
wt per mL	weight per millilitre
w/v	weight in volume

1

Introduction

Definitions of aromatherapy

Aromatherapy is one of the fastest growing branches of complementary and alternative medicine. The exact definition of the term 'aromatherapy', however, is in dispute. One definition is: 'the therapeutic use of fragrances or at least of mere volatiles to cure or to mitigate or to prevent disease, infections, and indispositions only by means of inhalation' (Buchbauer, 1996). But this does not mention massage or the absorption of essential oils through the skin and their effect on target organs, which is the mainframe of aromatherapy in the UK, USA and many other countries. There is a general difficulty with the concept of massaging with a volatile solution because, by definition, it volatilises into the air so perhaps a definition more relevant to aromatherapists is: 'use of aromatic plant extracts and essential oils in massage and other treatment' (*Concise Oxford Dictionary*, 1995). However, the term 'aromatherapy', which was coined in the 1930s by René-Maurice Gattefossé in a book entitled *Aromatherapie* first published in 1937 (Gattefossé, 1937/1993), was based on the odour of essential oils and perfumes and their antimicrobial, physiological and cosmetological properties (Gattefossé, 1928, 1952, 1937/1993). 'Pure' essential oils were of no concern in Gattefossé's day and neither was massage, although he used essential oils on the skin as disinfectants for healing wounds.

Nowadays, confusingly, there are apparently almost as many definitions of aromatherapy as there are aromatherapists, a confusion already acknowledged by one of the early authors on the subject in the UK (Tisserand, 1977):

> Aromatherapy is a subject that, at least in England, has so far been steeped in magic and mystery. This may give it a certain amount of appeal, but it also creates a great deal of confusion and misunderstanding, and leaves most people in a state of relative ignorance.

Some definitions encompass the effects on both body and mind. For example, Price (1993) defines aromatherapy as 'the controlled use of essential oils in a positive way to maintain good health and revitalize the body, mind and spirit'. This aspect is emphasised in many recent books (Lawless, 1994; Worwood, 1996, 1998; Hirsch, 1998), as is the link with sexuality (Worwood, 1986; Lawless, 1994; Hirsch, 1998).

Introduction to aromatherapy concepts

The original concept of using essential oils as alternative medicines was based on the assumption that the volatile, fat-soluble essential oil was equivalent in bioactivity to that of the whole plant when inhaled or massaged into the skin. Unfortunately this notion is clearly flawed, as will become evident on closer inspection. In the development of aromatherapy, information about the medicinal and other properties of the plants was often originally taken directly from old English herbals (such as Culpeper, 1653), combined with some more esoteric nuances involving the planets and astrology (e.g. Tisserand, 1977).

The basic limitation of the concept that essential oils exhibit the same properties as the whole plant can be illustrated using the orange as an example. Orange essential oil is extracted from the rind alone – the rest of the orange is not included. Thus the water-soluble vitamins, which include the B vitamins (thiamine, riboflavin and nicotinic acid, etc.) and, of course, vitamins C and A are excluded, as are calcium, iron, proteins, carbohydrates and water. Orange essential oil massaged into the skin would therefore exclude all

1

these components. To give another example, consider whether massaging butter (the fat-soluble component of milk) into the skin of a baby would be equivalent to the baby drinking the whole milk from which it was derived. Would the baby be able to grow and develop simply by having the fat component of milk massaged onto its body, devoid of protein, carbohydrate, water-soluble vitamins, minerals and of course energy? The answer is obviously no. It is therefore impossible to extrapolate the effects of a whole plant or animal produce to that of the essential oil or fat-soluble component.

Recent experiments have also illustrated that different extracts of a plant have different pharmacological properties. When different *Pelargonium* species and cultivars were studied on guinea-pig ileum *in vitro*, substantial differences in bioactivity were found in different fractions. The fractions used included teas (made with boiling water) and methanolic extracts, both of which contained some essential oil, but were mainly water-soluble components, and the essential oil itself (obtained by steam distillation), which contained no water-soluble components. The essential oils of all the plants studied produced a consistent relaxation of the smooth muscle, whereas the other extracts did not (Lis-Balchin, 2002b, ch.12, p.140).

The notion that the birth of modern aromatherapy can be attributed to the Ancient Egyptians is a misinterpretation that has been perpetuated in some aromatherapy texts. There is virtually no evidence that pure essential oils were used by the Egyptians, though some scented plant components were extracted into fat or oil and massaged into the skin; also various resins and herbs were burnt (incense) and some extracts were used for preserving dead bodies in mummification. The plant extracts which were extracted into oil or fat would be equivalent to the present-day herbal infused oils, made with hot or cold oils, and would contain many other components as well as the essential oil. They probably also resembled solvent extracts (e.g. concretes), which are coloured due to the extracted pigments, amongst other components (see Chapter 4). The various resins that were burnt in Ancient Egyptian society included frankincense and myrrh. Clearly the composition of these burnt resins is totally different from that of the pure essential oils produced from the resins.

Botanical misinterpretations are also common in many aromatherapy books. For example, 'geranium oil' bioactivity is widely described using herb Robert,

a hardy *Geranium* species found widely in European hedgerows. However, geranium oil is, in fact, distilled from species of the South African genus *Pelargonium*, which is not related to the genus *Geranium* at all (see Chapter 5). Another example of misinterpretation is the antiviral effect attributed to *Melissa* essential oil; in fact only the water-soluble fraction (containing no essential oil) was found to be active and not the essential oil (Herrman and Kucera, 1967).

What is an aromatherapist?

Just as the term 'aromatherapy' is difficult to define, it is also problematic to define what an 'aromatherapist' is. Anybody can call themselves an 'aromatherapist', even without attending a single lecture or workshop on the subject. There are numerous half-day and one-day aromatherapy courses, which issue 'the student' with a certification in aromatherapy. There are also numerous long Diploma courses run by different aromatherapists in their own 'schools', local technical courses and also universities. In the UK, a unit entitled 'The Science of Essential Oils' was first offered by South Bank University at MSc level in 1988, under the Framework for Continuing Professional Education. This was designed primarily for healthcare professionals interested in aromatherapy. It was later included with an aromatherapy unit in the university degree in complementary therapies (BSc (Hons)/Dip HE Health Studies); the aromatherapy-related units were also acknowledged by the English Nursing Board as well as by aromatherapy organisations. There are now many university courses providing aromatherapy training round the UK, some of which are very costly, although they are usually less expensive than some well-established private courses, which can cost up to £5000. The prospective student should be aware that higher cost does not necessarily imply a higher educational standard (Vickers, 1996).

Aromatherapy, aromatology and aromachology

Aromatherapy is now apparently divided into three sciences: aromatherapy, aromatology and aromachology (or Aroma-Chology). The latter term was coined in 1982 by the president of the Olfactory Research Fund, now the Sense of Smell Institute (SSI) in the USA.

- **Aromachology** is defined by the SSI as: 'a concept based on systematic, scientific data collected under controlled conditions'. Its main aims are to study the interrelationship of psychology and the latest in fragrance technology and to transmit through odour a variety of specific feelings (such as relaxation, exhilaration, sensuality, happiness and achievement) directly to the brain. It also seeks to establish the positive effects of aromas on human behaviour, including feelings and emotions.
- **Aromatherapy** is defined by the SSI as: 'the therapeutic effects of aromas on physical conditions (such as menstrual disorders, digestive problems, etc.) as well as psychological conditions (such as chronic depression)'.

These definitions of aromachology and aromatherapy seem to overlap considerably, as an odour must have an influence via inhalation, whether it is termed under aromatherapy or aromachology. The odour is composed of a mixture of chemicals that are fat-soluble and thus have an effect via inhalation, skin absorption or even directly via the nose on the brain.

Aromatology is concerned with the internal use of oils. This is similar to the use of aromatherapy in most of Europe, excluding the UK; it includes the effect of the chemicals in the essential oils via oral intake, or via the anus, vagina or any other possible opening by medically qualified doctors or at least herbalists, using essential oils as internal medicines (Franchomme and Pénoel, 1990).

Tampons soaked in essential oils are sometimes used for treating '*Candida*' (diagnosed in the UK, Australia and USA by a non-medically qualified, non-herbalist 'clinical aromatherapist', which poses a major safety issue as well as being legally problematical) (see Chapter 7). Aromatology also involves the intensive application of neat oils through the skin, even 3–45 mL a day.

There is a vast difference between the two mainstream aromatherapy procedures, i.e. continental European (and to some extent aromatology) and aromatherapy: the former is 'conventional' whilst the latter is 'alternative'. Alternative medicine is based on 'healing' and healing is largely based on belief (Millenson, 1995; Benson and Stark, 1996). The healing process in aromatherapy, which like conventional therapy involves convincing the patient of the benefits

of the treatment, can be very successful, as aromatherapists are often able to spend more time listening to their clients than are doctors (Lis-Balchin, 1997).

Aromatherapy practice in the UK and USA

Aromatherapy massage is often combined with 'counselling' if a complementary therapist (trained for a day, a week or a year) is involved (see Chapter 3). There are also beauty consultants/therapists using massage skills and a nice odour simply for relaxation; they sometimes include beautifying treatments using the essential oils initiated by Marguerite Maury (1989). Massaging is carried out using very diluted plant essential oils (2–5 drops per 10 mL of carrier oil, like almond oil) into the skin (see Chapter 3).

Many aromatherapists also combine their practice with cosmology, crystals, colours, music, etc. These may also be associated with a commercial sideline in selling 'own trademark' essential oils and associated items, including diffusers, scented candles and scented jewellery.

Aromatherapy has grown into a big business, as exemplified by the high street shops, which sell products supposedly made with 'essential oils' (usually perfumes), such as skin creams, hair shampoos, shower gels, moisturisers, bath salts, lotions, candles, as well as essential oils themselves. All these perfumed products were already previously sold without the 'aromatherapy' label, but the label has increased both the price and the sales. Sadly, this confuses the issue as to what aromatherapy is still further. In many cases it apparently means simply the inclusion of an odour (said to be 'natural', therefore extrabeneficial) in any product, which relaxes and provides a pleasant experience. Many aromatherapy products, like perfumes, are also often linked with sexual attractiveness.

Common uses of essential oils

Many common uses of essential oils are a far cry from aromatherapy (see Appendix 19). Aromatherapy products comprise a minute percentage of the essential oils (and aromachemicals) used in industry, where they are used extensively in foods, cosmetic products, household products and also many other industrial products. The use of essential oils in the food industry (as well as in pharmaceuticals) is based on their odorous properties: they are used to impart the required odour or flavour to the food after processing; in some cases this is accompanied by antimicrobial properties. In cosmetics and perfumery, essential oils are also used for their odour properties, as in the tobacco and textile industries. A large number of products, including veterinary products, make use of the insecticidal/antimicrobial properties of the oils. However, essential oils are also used in the paint industry, which capitalises on the exceptional 'cleaning' properties of certain oils. This, together with their embalming properties, suggest that essential oils are very potent and dangerous chemicals – not the sort of natural products to massage into the skin!

It is difficult to determine, therefore, why essential oils should be of great medicinal value. However, there are numerous miscellaneous functions of different essential oils in everyday life (see Appendices 19 and 20). These range from their use in dentistry (e.g. cinnamon and clove oils), as decongestants (e.g. *Eucalyptus globulus*, camphor, peppermint and cajuput) to their use as mouthwashes (e.g. thyme). There are numerous other functions: external usage as hyperaemics (e.g. rosemary, turpentine and camphor) and anti-inflammatories (e.g. German chamomile and yarrow). Some essential oils are used internally as stimulants of digestion (e.g. anise, peppermint and cinnamon) and as diuretics (e.g. buchu and juniper oils).

In all, therefore, essential oils exhibit pharmacological, physiological, antimicrobial and miscellaneous effects and also psychological ones when acting as odorants (see Chapter 6).

Proven effects of essential oils

Many plant essential oils are extremely potent antimicrobials *in vitro* and can positively affect different bacteria and fungi (Deans and Ritchie, 1987; Bassett *et al.*, 1990; Lis-Balchin, 1995; Lis-Balchin *et al.*, 1996c; Deans, 2001). Many are also strong antioxidant agents, and have recently been shown to stop some of the symptoms of ageing in animals (Dorman *et al.*, 1995a,b). The use of camphor, turpentine oils and their components as rubefacients, causing increased blood flow to a site of pain or swelling when

applied to the skin, is well-known and is the basis of many well-known medicaments such as Vicks VapoRub and Tiger Balm (see Chapter 5). There is also long-standing evidence for the benefits of inhaling certain essential oils to relieve coughs and congestion in the respiratory tract using mixtures of *Eucalyptus globulus*, pine needle and camphor (Martindale, 1993). Some essential oils have also been shown in preliminary studies to alleviate sleeplessness and could apparently save on diazepams and other sleep-inducing drugs (see Chapters 5 and 8). Various oils derived from plants of the Umbelliferae family (e.g. fennel, dill and caraway) are used in remedies for indigestion, flatulence and dyspepsia (as well as peppermint).

Many essential oils have been shown to be active on many different animal tissues *in vitro* (Lis-Balchin *et al.*, 1997b). There is, however, virtually no scientific evidence, as yet, regarding the direct action of essential oils applied through massaging of the skin on specific internal organs rather than through the odour pathway leading into the mid-brain's 'limbic system' and thence through the normal sympathetic and parasympathetic pathways. This is despite some evidence that certain essential oils can be absorbed either through the skin or lungs (Buchbauer *et al.*, 1992; Jager *et al.*, 1992; Fuchs *et al.*, 1997).

Many fragrances have been shown to have an effect on mood (see Chapter 6) and, in general, pleasant odours generate happy memories, more positive feelings and a general sense of well-being (Knasko *et al.*, 1990; Knasko, 1992; Warren and Warrenburg, 1993). Many essential oil vapours have been shown to depress contingent negative variation (CNV) brain waves in human volunteers and these are considered to be sedative (Torii *et al.*, 1988). Others increase CNV and are considered stimulant (Kubota *et al.*, 1992). An interesting single study involving an individual with anosmia (an inability to smell anything) showed that there were changes in cerebral blood flow on inhaling certain essential oils, just as in people able to smell (Buchbauer *et al.*, 1993c). This indicated that the oil had a positive brain effect despite the patient's inability to smell it.

There is some evidence that certain essential oils (e.g. nutmeg) can lower high blood pressure (Warren and Warrenburg, 1993). Some essential oils are already used as orthodox medicines: peppermint oil is used for treating irritable bowel syndrome and some components of essential oils, such as pinene, limonene, camphene and borneol, given orally have been found to be effective against certain internal ailments, such as gallstones (Somerville *et al.*, 1985) and ureteric stones (Engelstein *et al.*, 1992). Externally applied essential oils (e.g. tea tree) can reduce/ eliminate acne (Bassett *et al.*, 1990) and athlete's foot (Tong *et al.*, 1992). This is, however, using conventional chemical effects of essential oils rather than aromatherapy (see Chapter 5).

Most clients seeking out aromatherapy are suffering from some stress-related condition and improvement is largely achieved through relaxation. Future clinical application of aromatherapy will probably be as an adjunct to clinical medicine, especially in hospitals, hospices, geriatric wards and general practice, under the guidance of consultants and senior nursing staff. No miracle cures should be promised, but an alleviation of suffering and possibly pain, mainly through relaxation due to gentle massage and the presence of someone who cares and listens to the patient, will be available. There is a need for this kind of healing contact, and aromatherapy with its added power of odour fits this niche.

Unproven aromatherapeutic virtues

'Aromatherapy' has had very little scientific evaluation to date. As with so many therapies, but especially alternative ones, the placebo effect may provide the largest percentage benefit to the patient (Benson and Stark, 1996). Many aromatherapists have not been greatly interested in scientific research and some have even been antagonistic to any such research (Vickers, 1996; Lis-Balchin, 1997). Animal experiments, whether maze studies using mice or pharmacology using isolated tissues, are considered unacceptable and only essential oils that are 'untested on animals' are acceptable. Unfortunately, all essential oils have already been tested on animals (despite assurances by essential oil suppliers), because this is required by law before they can be used in foods (see Chapter 7).

The actual mode of action of essential oils *in vivo* is still far from clear, and clinical studies to date have been scarce and mostly rather negative (Stevenson 1994; Dunn *et al.*, 1995; Brooker *et al.*, 1997; Anderson *et al.*, 2000). However, the advent of scientific input into the clinical studies, rather than aromatherapist-led studies, has recently yielded some more positive results (Smallwood *et al.*, 2001; Ballard *et al.*, 2002; Burns *et al.*, 2002; Holmes *et al.*, 2002;

Kennedy *et al.*, 2002). Perhaps the main difficulty in clinical studies is that it is virtually impossible to do randomised double-blind studies involving different odours, and therefore impossible to provide an adequate control – a control would have to be either odourless or else of a different odour, neither of which is satisfactory. Secondly, in practice, it appears that there is a variation in the treatment for each client, based on 'holistic' principles, and each person can be treated by an aromatherapist with one to five or more different essential oil mixtures on subsequent visits, involving one to four or more different essential oils in each mixture. Each aromatherapy book lists different essential oils for treating similar ailments, and each therapist likes to show some new applications, based on his or her own experience (see Chapter 3). Thirdly, there is the general assumption amongst alternative medicine practitioners that if the procedure 'works' in one patient, there is no need to study it using scientific double-blind procedures (see Chapter 8).

Scant attention has also been given to the actual chemical composition of the essential oils used and even the exact botanical origin or type of the oil. For example, it is often unclear which of the three main commercial types of chamomile oil or lavender essential oil were used (see Chapter 8). Furthermore, in the main, commercially produced essential oils have been tested, as these are used in the food and cosmetics industries; however large-scale admixing, deterpenation, dilution and adulteration often occurs in these (see Chapter 4).

Conclusion

The main action of essential oils is probably on the primitive, unconscious, limbic system of the brain (Lis-Balchin, 1997), which is not under the control of the cerebrum or higher centres and has a considerable subconscious effect on the person. Mood and behaviour could be influenced by odours, and memories of past odour associations could also be dominant, which is an area that needs to be fully explored before aromatherapy is used by psychologically unqualified people in the treatment of Alzheimer's or other diseases of ageing.

Aromatherapy can, however, be effective in reducing stress and improving mood in terminally ill patients, but only in association with touch and the time to listen to the patient. This is because aroma-therapy, like other alternative medicines, has a placebo effect: the longer the time spent by the therapist with the patient, the stronger the belief imparted by the therapist and the greater the willingness of the patient to believe in the therapy, the greater the effect achieved (Benson and Stark, 1996).

In order to extend the use of aromatherapy, it is clear that more clinical and toxicological research is needed, as well as better teaching. Recent European regulations (the 7th Amendment to the European Cosmetic Directive 76/768/EEC, 2002, see Appendices 27 and 28) have listed 26 sensitisers found in most of the common essential oils used: this could be a problem for aromatherapists as well as clients, both in possibly causing sensitisation and also resulting in legal action regarding such an eventuality in the case of the client. Care must be taken regarding the sensitisation potential of the essential oils, especially when massaging patients with cancer or otherwise sensitive skin. It should also be borne in mind when considering the use of essential oils during childbirth and in other clinical studies (Burns and Blaney, 1994; Burns *et al.*, 2000) that studies in animals have indicated that some oils cause a decrease in uterine contractions (Lis-Balchin and Hart, 1997b).

Future studies, such as those on Alzheimer's syndrome (Perry *et al.*, 1998, 1999), may reveal the individual benefits of different essential oils for different ailments, but in practice this may not be of most importance as aromatherapy (using massage in particular) offers relief from stress and this in itself is of the greatest benefit for most people seeking this type of complementary and alternative medicine.

2

Historical background to aromatherapy

Introduction

The folk medicinal background to the art of 'aromatherapy' has been attributed to both the Ancient Egyptians and Chinese over 4500 years ago. But it is important to note there have been no concrete references to essential oil usage in any herbal, nor in the hieroglyphics of the Ancient Egyptians or other ancient scripts. It is clear that although scented plants and their products were used thousands of years ago in religious practices, as medicines, perfumes, embalming agents (Manniche, 1989, 1999) and to bring out greater sexuality (Schumann Antelme and Rossini, 2001), this does not mean that essential oils as such were used.

In Ancient Egypt, aromatherapy probably referred to the use of crude plant extracts of frankincense, myrrh or galbanum, etc. in an oily vegetable or animal fat which was massaged onto the bodies of workers building the pyramids or the rich proletariat after their baths (Manniche, 1999). The perfumed oils and fats used contained more than just the essential oils, they also contained water-soluble components such as flavonoids and tannins, vitamins, minerals and pigments. In 1922, when King Tutankhamun's tomb was opened, calcite pots filled with spices such as frankincense preserved in fat still gave off a faint odour after 3000 years. It is thought that incense smoke from resinous plant material provided a more sacrosanct atmosphere for making sacrifices, both animal and human, to the gods. The incense was often mixed with narcotics like cannabis to anaesthetise the sacrificial animals, especially when human (Devereux, 1997). Various resins and plant extracts were also used in the very intricate embalming process to preserve the body for its future life. And plant extracts were used extensively for medicinal purposes, as depicted on the walls of many healing temples in Egypt (Manniche, 1999).

Incense: inhalation effects

Incense (Latin *incens*: 'to burn') is composed of resinous or gum-like materials containing volatile essential oils, exuded from cuts in the bark of certain trees. Two of the commonest components of incense, frankincense and myrrh, are both produced from resins that drip down onto the ground from the cuts made in gnarled trees growing in the desert. As the teardrop-shaped drops of gum resin hit the ground they harden. The tears, varying in size according to species and also quality, are ground to a powder and burnt over charcoal in various incensers, like those still used in churches. Nowadays they may be distilled to yield the essential oil.

In Ancient Egypt, the resins were highly prized because they had to be transported across great distances: frankincense was obtained from the land of Punt (probably Somalia) (Atchley and Cuthbert, 1909; Manniche, 1999). The 'in'-famous meeting between Solomon and the Queen of Sheba (Saba) was said to have been primarily about the incense trade (Shawe, 1998).

Scented plants used as incense in Ancient Egypt

Frankincense (*Boswellia carterii; B. thurifera*) (Burseraceae)

The name frankincense originates from the medieval French *franc*, 'free', and the Latin word *incens*. Olibanum, its other name, possibly comes from the Arabic term *al luban*, meaning 'sweet resinous gum', or *liban*, meaning 'milky', which refers to the whitish colour of the resin when new (Manniche, 1999).

Numerous species of *Boswellia* exist, especially in South America, some of which yield a similar resin called copal. The essential oils extracted from the resins differ considerably in odour from that of the corresponding resin. Most have a fresh citrusy odour, whilst the resin, when burnt, has a 'church-like' odour (Arctander, 1960; see also frankincense oil monograph).

Myrrh (*Commiphora myrrha; Balsamodendron myrrha; B. opobalsamum*) (Burseraceae)

The name myrrh probably originates from the old Hebrew and Arabic word *mur*, meaning 'bitter'. The myrrh mentioned in the Bible was possibly a liquid derived from *B. opobalsamum*, balsam of Mecca (Atchley and Cuthbert, 1909). At its thinnest consistency it is called stacte, after the Greek word for 'drops' (Rimmel, 1865). The Egyptians considered stacte to be one of the finest of fragrances, and often mixed it with balanos oil (Manniche, 1999).

Myrrh was also called antiu, which could be 'fresh' from evergreen myrrh trees or 'dry' from deciduous older trees (Manniche, 1999). Myrrh essential oil smells very church-like and dusty and is similar in odour to the burnt resin (Arctander, 1960; see also myrrh oil monograph).

Labdanum (*Cistus ladaniferus*)

A resinous secretion from one or more species of rock rose, labdanum is possibly the same as onycha, one of the legendary magical incenses, as the Hebrew name shechleth was translated as ladana, giving rise to labdanum (Abrahams, 1980). It is slightly liquid but not pourable and is therefore mixed with solvents when sold. The odour is sweet, herbaceous, balsamic and slightly animalic, rich and tenacious (Arctander, 1960).

Galbanum (*Ferula galbaniflua*)

This is a fragrant gum resin, greenish in colour, which exudes from the stems of several species of umbelliferous plants (family Apiaceae) of the genus *Ferula*. It was mentioned in the Bible (Exodus 30:34) as being used for incense. Galbanum may have been the 'green incense' mentioned in Egyptian hieroglyphics (Manniche, 1989). The essential oil has an intensely green, fresh-leafy odour and is very persistent. The resin is intensely rich-green, woody-balsamic with a dry undertone and a typical green-peppers note, which is more pronounced in the essential oil (Arctander, 1960).

Styrax (*Styrax officinalis*) or liquidambar orientalis

The gum resin is the 'storax' of Dioscorides and Pliny (Atchley and Cuthbert, 1909) or Jewish frankincense and red storax (Groom, 1992). The resin has a styrene or gasoline-like odour. The essential oil is very rich, balsamic-sweet, floral, somewhat spicy, reminiscent of lilac, hyacinth etc. but has an unpleasant hydrocarbon top-note (Arctander, 1960).

Balm of Gilhead (*Commiphora opobalsamum*)

This is a resin from amyris, a plant that grew in abundance on the mountains of Gilhead, a ridge running from Mount Lebanon (Rimmel, 1865). It was introduced into Palestine from Yemen during Solomon's time by the Queen of Sheba. Its odour is faintly woody, oily-sweet, balsamic with a peppery top-note reminiscent of cubeb (Arctander, 1960).

Sandalwood (*Santalum album*)

Sandalwood is known as 'chandan' in India, where it has been used since ancient times, mainly for religious purposes. Sandalwood oil from India is scarce and substitutes from other countries such as Indonesia as well as synthetics now flood the market (Chana, 1993, 1994; see also sandalwood oil monograph).

Opoponax (*Opoponax chironium*)

The opoponax resin used in India and China was possibly *Commiphora erythraea* var. *glabrescens*, as used by the Egyptians, and translated as myrrh.

It was known to the Romans as 'scented myrrh' (Groom, 1992). The resinoid is warm, powdery, spicy and oriental. The essential oil is intensely sweet, balsamic, warm but fresh with an 'emptied sherry wineglass' odour (Arctander, 1960).

Uses of incense

The Egyptian term for incense, *senetcher*, is related to *senetcheri*, 'to make divine' (Hoffmeier, 1983). The Ancient Egyptians believed that incense was the odour of the gods, which had come down to Earth as divine perspiration (Stoddart, 1990). Incense was often moulded into small pellets with honey and wine, and burnt in censers. Various concoctions of incense, called kyphi, were burnt three times per day to the sun god Ra: morning, noon and sunset, in order for him to come back. The ingredients were shown on the walls of the laboratory in the temples of Horus at Edfu and Philae. They included raisins, juniper, cinnamon, honey, wine, frankincense, myrrh, burnt resins, cyperus, sweet rust, sweet flag and aspalanthus in a certain, secret proportion (Loret, 1887; Manniche, 1989; Forbes, 1955).

Embalming involved odorous plants like juniper, cassia, cinnamon, cedarwood and myrrh, together with natron to preserve the body and ensure safe passage to the after-life. The bandages in which the mummy was wrapped were also drenched in stacte (oil of myrrh), and sprinkled with other spices.

The Chinese also used an incense, *hsiang*, meaning 'aromatic', made from a variety of plants, with sandalwood being particularly favoured by Buddhists. In India, fragrant flowers including jasmine and the root of spikenard provided incense with a sweet scent. The Hindus obtained cassia from China and were the first to organise trading routes to Arabia where frankincense was exclusively found. The Hebrews traditionally used incense for purification ceremonies. Personal cleansing was accomplished by sitting over pans of burning incense (Atchley and Cuthbert, 1909). Odorants were also used for triumphant occasions: when Alexander the Great conquered Babylon in AD 331, his route was strewn with flowers, and many altars, heaped with incense and perfumes, were erected en route. The production of incense became more elaborate during Herod's time, consisting of about 13 ingredients including myrrh, cassia, spikenard, saffron, costus, mace and cinnamon in addition to the original mix.

The use of incense probably spread to Greece from Egypt around the eighth century BC. Early Greeks preferred to use incense in a powdered form and they discovered that strong fragrances such as myrrh oil became sweeter when mixed with wine, hence the addition of resin to make retsina.

The Christian Church was slow to adopt the use of incense until medieval times, when it was used for funerals, with the body, altar and the burial site being censed. Incense was also used to counteract the smell of musty stone floors and the stench of bodies packed closely together during church services (Genders, 1972). The Reformation reversed the process as it was considered to be of pagan origin. However it still survives in the Roman Catholic Church. The Indians of Mesoamerica used copal, a hard, lustrous resin obtained from pine trees and various other tropical trees by slicing the bark (*Olibanum americanum*). Copal pellets bound to corn-husk tubes would be burnt in hollows on the summits of holy hills and mountains, and these places, blackened by centuries of such usage, are still resorted to by today's Maya in Guatemala (Janson, 1997) and used medicinally to treat diseases of the respiratory system and the skin.

Anointing also involves incense (Unterman, 1991). 'Messiah' is an Anglicised version of the Hebrew word *mashiach*: 'someone who is anointed'. Queen Elizabeth II underwent the ritual in 1953 at her coronation, with a composition of oils originated by Charles I: essential oils of roses, orange blossom, jasmine petals, sesame seeds and cinnamon combined with gum benzoin, musk, civet and ambergris were used (Ellis, 1960). Similarly, musk, sandalwood and other fragrances were used by Hindus to wash the effigies of their gods, and this custom was continued by the early Christians. This probably accounts for the divine odour frequently reported when the tombs of early Christians were opened (Atchley and Cuthbert, 1909).

Aromatic substances were also widely used in magic. Women in labour were often naked except for their amulets and scented cones on the head: the ingestion of fenugreek mixed with honey or a vaginal suppository made of incense, beer and flydung, accompanied by ritualistic chanting and other forms of magic was used to speed up childbirth (Pinch, 1994).

Perfume and cosmetics: precursors of cosmetological aromatherapy

The word 'perfume' is derived from the Latin *per fumare*: 'by smoke'. The preparation of perfumes in Ancient Egypt was done by the priests, who passed on their knowledge to new priests (Manniche, 1989, 1999). Nefertiti and Cleopatra used huge amounts of fragranced materials as unguents, powders and perfumes, often after bathing. The dry desert climate tended to dry the skin so massaging in fragrant oils and ointments helped keep their skin supple and elastic. The workers building the great pyramids even went on strike when they were denied their allocation of 'aromatherapy massage oil' (Manniche, 1999).

Production of perfumed oils

The Egyptians had three methods of producing perfumed oils:

- **Enfleurage** involved steeping the flowers or aromatics in oils or animal fats (usually goat) until the scent from the materials was imparted to the fat. The impregnated fat was often moulded into cosmetic cones and used for perfuming hair wigs, worn on festive occasions, which could last for 3 days; the fat would soften and start melting, spreading the scented grease not only over the wig, but also over the clothes and body – more pleasing than the stench of stale wine, food and excrement (Manniche, 1999).
- **Maceration** was used principally for skin creams and perfumes: flowers, herbs, spices or resins were chopped up and immersed in hot oils. The oil was strained and poured into alabaster (calcite) containers and sealed with wax. These scented fatty extracts were also massaged onto the skin (Manniche, 1999).
- **Expression** involved putting flowers or herbs into bags or presses, which extracted the aromatic oils. Expression is now only used for citrus fruit oils (Lis-Balchin, 1995). Wine was often included in the process and the resulting potent liquid was stored in jars.

Egyptian perfumes often had very complex recipes. For example, lily perfume contained 1000 lilies (*Lilium candidum*), 4.2 litres of balanos oil, 140 g myrrh, 1.5 kg cardamom, 37 g crocus, 2.4 kg sweet flag, 280 g cinnamon, honey, salt and fragrant wine, with some extra cardamoms, and later in the process, best myrrh was used. The honey was used to anoint the hands before mixing in the lilies with the scented oil and the whole process was repeated twice using another 1000 lilies once the first perfume was extracted (Manniche, 1999).

As this is devoid of any synthetics, it could be used in modern aromatherapy: the plant extracts could be said to be almost equivalent to solvent extracts.

Megaleion, an Ancient Greek perfume described by Theophrastus who believed it to be good for wounds, was made of burnt resins, balanos oil, cassia, cinnamon and myrrh. The balanos needed to be boiled for 10 days before the remaining ingredients were added (Groom, 1992). Roses, marjoram, sage, lotus flower and galbanum perfumes were also made. Apart from these, aromatic oils from basil, celery, chamomile, cumin, dill, fenugreek, fir, henna, iris, juniper, lily, lotus, mandrake, marjoram, myrtle, pine, rose, rue and sage were sometimes used in perfumes or as medicines taken internally and externally.

Greek philosophers tended to condemn the growing use of perfumes in their society because it blurred the distinction between freemen and slaves; later, the Romans associated perfume and cosmetics with harlots. Pliny the Elder, in his *Historia Naturalis*, described the use of cosmetics for preserving and improving the complexion.

Dioscorides, in his *De Materia Medica*, discussed the components of perfumes and their medicinal properties, providing detailed perfume formulas.

A more unusual product popular with Roman ladies was a special ointment made of sweat scrapings from the bodies of gladiators. The scrapings were mixed with the oil used to massage the gladiators' bodies. This was sold at a high price as an aphrodisiac called rhypos.

Alexandrian chemists were divided into three schools, one of which was the school of Maria the Jewess, which produced pieces of apparatus for distillation and sublimation, such as the *bain Marie*, useful for extracting the aromatic oils from plant material. Later, perfumes were only used in the church or the court because of their cost, but became more commonly known in medieval Europe as knights returning home from the Crusades (eleventh to thirteenth centuries) brought with them an assortment of musk, floral waters, and a variety of spices.

Medicinal uses: precursors of aromatology or 'clinical' aromatherapy

Modern aromatherapists looking to Ancient Egypt for the origins of their craft can find ancient use of plants, not essential oils, in fragments of Egyptian herbals, thousands of years ago. The names of various plants, their habitats, characteristics and the purposes for which they were used are all included in the following examples: *Veterinary papyrus* (*c.* 2000 BC), *Gynaecological papyrus* (*c.* 2000 BC), *Papyrus Edwin Smith* (an army surgeon's manual, *c.* 1600 BC), *Papyrus Ebers* (includes remedies for health, beauty and the home, *c.* 1600 BC), *Papyrus Hearst* (with prescriptions and spells, *c.* 1400 BC) and *Demotic medical papyri* (second century BC to first century AD).

Magic was often used as part of the treatment and gave the patient the expectation of a cure and provided a placebo effect (Pinch, 1994). The physicians had a systematic method of dealing with patients using a three-phase approach. First, they listened to their patient's symptoms and examined them using their eyes and hands. Secondly, they reached a diagnosis and usually told the patient what it was, and then decided whether the condition was treatable, not to be treated or to be contended with (*Eber's Papyrus*, *Papyrus Edwin Smith*, quoted by Nunn, 1997). Thirdly, the doctor gave the treatment. The term 'placing the hand' appears frequently in a large number of medical papyri: this probably alludes to the manual examination in order to reach a diagnosis but could also imply cure by the 'laying on of hands', or even both (Nunn, 1997). This could be the basis of modern massage (with or without aromatherapy). It is certainly the basis of alternative medicine practised at present (Lis-Balchin, 1997).

Plants were used in numerous ways. For example, acacia leaves, flowers and pods were taken internally for killing worms; as a cough remedy drunk with honey and wine; used as a poultice with honey and ochre for swollen legs; used as a bandage for broken bones with gum and water; used with oil or fat to heal wounds; and mixed with opium for pains to head and eyes. Onions were made into a paste with wine and inserted into the vagina to stop a woman menstruating. Garlic ointment was used to keep away serpents and snakes, heal dog-bites and bruises; raw garlic was given to asthmatics; fresh garlic and coriander in wine was a purgative and an aphrodisiac!

Dill was mixed with alum for a mouthrinse. Juniper mixed with honey and beer was used orally to encourage defecation; it had many other uses. Origanum was boiled with hyssop for a sick ear (Manniche, 1989).

Examples of Egyptian medicinal unguents (external usage) include:

- To soothe the members: cinnamon 1, frankincense 1, dry myrrh 1, ox fat 1, sweet moringa oil 1 – to be used as a poultice for 4 days.
- To cure headache: frankincense 1, cumin 1, juniper berries 1, goose fat 1 – to be boiled and the head anointed with it.
- To cause hair to fall out: lotus leaves boiled and seeped in oil or fat – to be placed on hated woman's head!

Egyptians also practised inhalation. This was administered by using a double-pot arrangement whereby a heated stone was placed in one of the pots and a liquid herbal remedy poured over it. The second pot, with a hole in the bottom through which a straw was inserted, was placed on top of the first pot, allowing the patient to breathe in the steaming remedy (i.e. aromatherapy by inhalation).

Some examples of Egyptian medicinal recipes (internal usage) include:

- To cool the uterus: frankincense and celery were ground in cow's milk, strained through a cloth and administered to the vagina.
- To cool the anus: equal parts of cinnamon, juniper berries, frankincense, ochre, cumin, honey, myrrh and three other unknown ingredients was used as a suppository.
- To cure haemorrhoids: 'Knead with honey some burnt wolf's dung, ground with white pepper: let the patient drink it (but claim your fee first!)'.

It appears that there was a sense of humour attached to some of the prescriptions!

'Mummy liquor' – the 'cure-all'

From around the sixth century, 'Mummy liquor' was prized as a miracle drug (Le Guérer, 1993). The term 'mummy' comes from the Arabic word *mumiyah*, meaning 'pitch', and not only referred to the embalmed bodies of the Ancient Egyptians, but also meant the material that was produced from the embalming. It was this honey-like material, initially obtained from the Egyptian mummies by Arabs who raided the tombs, that was sold to Europeans as an elixir. The idea at that time was that death would bring life, so the fragrant liquid from dead people was treasured above all else. When the supply of Royal mummies ran out, the ordinary mummies replaced the fragrant ones. Later, unscrupulous 'merchants' would raid European graves or steal bodies from scaffolds, treat them with natron and sell it as 'Mummy liquor'. The idea that diseases could be transmitted from the corpses did not occur to the clientele, of course. Incredibly, the popes of the day went along with this form of cannibalism.

The Middle Ages: use of aromatics and quacks

In the twelfth century the Benedictine Abbess Hildegard of Bingen (1098–1179) was authorised by the Church to publish her visions on medicine (*Causae et Curae*), dealing with the causes and remedies for illness (Brunn and Epiney-Birgard, 1989). She was the first person to clearly distinguish between *Lavandula vera* and *Lavandula spica*, the latter being used medicinally.

The foul smell of refuse in European towns in the seventeenth century was thought to be the major cause of disease, including the plague (Classen *et al.*, 1994). Fire was the primary disinfectant to combat the spread of infection, but aromatics were also used for both preventing and in some cases curing disease. Bonfires were set with juniper, rosemary and incense, and herbs such as rosemary were in great demand and sold for exorbitant prices as a prophylactic against the plague (Wilson, 1925). From the mid-1700s rue was used to strew the dock of the central criminal court at the Old Bailey in London to protect the justice against jail fever (Genders, 1972).

People forced to live near victims of the plague would carry some form of olfactory protection with them when they ventured outdoors, like the pomander, which contained a mixture of aromatic plant extracts. Medical practitioners carried a small cassolette or 'perfume box' on the top of their walking sticks which was filled with aromatics when visiting contagious patients (Rimmel, 1865). Some physicians wore a device filled with herbs and spices over their nose when they examined plague patients (Wilson,

1925). These became known as 'beaks' and it is from this that the term 'quack' developed.

Apothecaries were originally wholesale merchants and spice importers and in 1617 the Worshipful Society of Apothecaries was formed, under the control of the London Royal College of Physicians, which produced an 'official' pharmacopoeia specifying the drugs the apothecaries were allowed to dispense. The term 'perfumer' occurs in some places instead of 'apothecary' (Rimmel, 1865).

John Gerard (1545–1612) and Nicholas Culpeper (1616–1654) were two of the better known apothecaries of their time. Nicholas Culpeper, being in the service of the poor, published an English translation of the London Dispensatory from the Latin and also combined healing herbs with astrology as he believed that each plant, like each part of the body and each disease, was governed or under the influence of one of the planets: rosemary was believed to be ruled by the Sun, lavender by Mercury and spearmint by Venus. Culpeper also adhered to the Doctrine of Signatures, introduced by Paracelsus in the sixteenth century, and mythology played a role in many of the descriptive virtues in Culpeper's herbal. For example, he classifies basil as 'an herb of Mars, and under the scorpion . . . called basilicon'. This astrological tradition is carried through by many aromatherapists today, together with other innovations such as ying and yang, crystals and colours.

Culpeper's simple or distilled waters and oils

The simple or distilled waters (equivalent to the present hydrosols) were prepared by the distillation of herbs in water, in a pewter still, and then fractionating them to separate out the essential or 'chymical' oil from the scented plants. The plant waters were the weakest of the herbal preparations and were not regarded as being beneficial. Individual plants like rose or elderflower were used to make the corresponding waters, or else mixtures of herbs were used to make compound waters (Culpeper, 1826/1981; Tobyn, 1997).

Essential oils of single herbs were regarded by Culpeper as too strong to take alone, due to their vehement heat and burning, but had to be mixed with other medicinal preparation. Two or three drops were used in this way at a time. Culpeper mentioned the oils of: wormwood, hyssop, marjoram, the mints, oregano, pennyroyal, rosemary, rue, sage, thyme, chamomile, lavender, orange and lemon. Lavender was spike lavender, not the *L. angustifolia* used in aromatherapy nowadays. Herbs like dried wormwood and rosemary were also steeped in wine and set in the sun for 30–40 days to make a 'physical wine'.

In his *Complete Herbal and English Physician*, Culpeper gave instructions for making ointments, by mixing and pounding bruised herbs with hog's grease, allowing the mixture to stand for a few days, then melting and boiling it, straining out and then adding more herbs and repeating the process several times. This is similar to the process used in Ancient Egypt. Culpeper then instructed the addition of turpentine and wax, as 'grease and oil are offensive to wounds'.

The uses of the oil of caraway includes: good against plague, poison and melancholy, jaundice and dropsy, expels wind, removes obstructions in the liver, spleen and lungs, takes away asthma, good for colds, afflictions of head, nerves, migraine. Dose: 6–10 drops in any convenient liquor. Outwardly, you may anoint with it by mixing with oil of almonds (Culpeper, 1826/1981).

The 'herbal extracts' mentioned in the herbals were mostly water-soluble and at best, alcoholic extracts, none of which are equivalent to essential oils, and which contain many potent chemical components not found in essential oils.

Modern perfumery

In the fourteenth century, alcohol was used for the extraction and preservation of plants, and oleum mirable, an alcoholic extract of rosemary and resins, was later popularised as 'Hungary water', without the resins (Müller *et al.*, 1984).

Animalistic phase

In the sixteenth century perfumes were made using animal extracts, which were the base notes or fixatives, and made the scent last longer (Piesse, 1855). Among these ingredients were ambergris, musk and civet. Each of these on their own have rather obnoxious odours, but when used in small amounts mixed in with other scents they provide a 'bite', a sought-after addition to many perfume creations. Ambergris

is a wax-like substance produced in the digestive tract of the sperm whale (*Physeter catodon*). Musk comes from a gland found in the abdomen of the male musk deer (*Moschus moschiferus*), indigenous to the high mountainous regions of the Himalayas from Afghanistan to China. The musk pod is a sac about the size of a walnut and holds about 1 oz (28 g) of musk in a granular form (Groom, 1992). Civet is a soft, paste-like glandular secretion extracted from a pouch under the tail of both male and female civet cats (*Viverra civetta*) as well as certain other species. Another material derived from animals is castoreum, from the anal glands of the beaver (*Castor fiber*).

Musk and ambergris feature in a number of the *Arabian Nights* tales and civet and musk feature in several of Shakespeare's plays. These animalistic extracts were all pheromonal in odour (see Chapter 6) and were used for attracting the opposite sex as well as masking the person's own more abhorrent body odour.

Perfumes came into general use in England during the reign of Queen Elizabeth (1558–1603), who became fascinated by perfumery after she had been given a pair of perfumed gloves by the Right Honourable Edward de Vere, Earl of Oxford, who had brought them from Italy (Groom, 1992). The Royal Accounts for 1564 showed considerable expenditure on perfumes, notably rosewater and cloves used in the clothes closet; perfumes were also bought for the Banqueting House, Counsel Chamber, the chapel and all the Royal Palaces. Many perfumes, such as rosewater, benzoin and storax, were used for sweetening the heavy ornate robes of the time, which were impossible to wash. Urinals were treated with orris powder, damask rose powder and rosewater. Bags of herbs, musk and civet were used to perfume bath water.

Elizabeth I carried a pomander filled with ambergris, benzoin, civet, damask rose and other perfumes (Rimmel, 1865) and used a multitude of perfumed products in later life. Pomanders, from the French *pomme d'amber* ('ball of ambergris') were originally hung in silver perforated balls from the ceiling to perfume the room. The ingredients, like benzoin, amber, labdanum, storax, musk, civet, rose buds, could be boiled with gum tragacanth and kneaded into balls: the small ones were made into necklaces.

Manuscripts from the sixteenth century record that palaces and rich houses had 'still rooms' where the distillation of fragrant materials took place.

Various recipes were used for preparing aromatic waters, oils and perfumes. Some of these were for perfumes and some undoubtedly for alcoholic beverages, as one of the major ingredients for many concoctions was a bottle or two of wine, which when distilled produced a very alcoholic brew.

Two perfume recipes are as follows:

- **Excellent sweet water for perfume** (1625): Combine a handful each of basil, mints, marjoram, cornflower roots, hyssop, savory, sage, balm, lavender, rosemary. Include ½ oz (14 g) each of cloves, cinnamon and nutmegs. Add 3–4 pinecitrons cut into slices. Infuse with damask rosewater for 3 days, then distil. Add musk, civet, ambergris – a scruple of each in fine cloth and boil with bay leaves, cloves and lemon pills.
- **Damask water by distillation**: Take a handful each of fresh lavender, rosemary, thyme, cypress, cotton lavender, wild thyme, brown holly, bay and walnut leaves and grind together in a mortar and pestle and transfer to the distillation vessel. After the addition of a quart (just over a litre) of white wine and a pint (0.5 L) of rosewater, allow to stand for several days. Distil. Pour the distillate over the same herbs again and re-distil. The next day, sprinkle on top: cloves, cinnamon, dryons, spikenard, amber, maces, nutmegs, saffron, musk and camphor. Stir well and distil. The final product 'pierces the senses'.

Even more elaborate recipes were used for antiplague waters, which often included almost all the medicinal plants available . . . probably for good luck, as the waters did not work.

Pure flowery perfumes

After the indulgence of sexually alluring perfumes a change from animal to vegetable perfumes occurred as a result of women wishing to express their individuality and sensuality with sweet odours rather than those strong violent odours (Dejeans, 1764). Ambergris, musk and civet therefore went out of fashion as the excremental odours could not be reconciled with modesty (Corbin, 1986). The delicate floral perfumes became part of the ritual of bodily hygiene, gave greater variety and allowed Louis XV a different perfume every day. Soaps, powders, waters with floral and fruit scents and even mouthwashes with rosewater and iris toothpaste followed. Cassanova frequently described the washing of the woman's body with rosewater.

Today the sentiment 'Odours are carried in bottles, for fear of annoying those who do not like them' (Dejeans, 1764) is re-emerging as more and more people are becoming sensitive to odours. The use of overbearing perfumes can be very distasteful to people sharing the same building, plane, train, etc. and it can even make people ill, giving them headaches, asthma and migraines.

The Victorians liked simple perfumes made of individual plant extracts. Particular favourites were rose (*Rosa damascena*, *R. gallica* and *R. centifolia*), lavender and violet. These would be steam distilled or extracted with solvents. The simple essential oils produced would often be blended together to produce perfumes, which were incredibly expensive, as 5 tonnes of rose petals produced under a litre of essential oil.

A recipe for eau de Cologne from 1834 is as follows:

- **Eau de Cologne** (1834): Bergamot, 6.2 kg; lemon, 3.1; neroli, 0.8; clove, 1.6; lavender, 1.2; rosemary, 0.8; alcohol 90% to 100 mL.

The first attempt at commercial scent production in the UK was recorded in Mitcham, Surrey, in the seventeenth century, using lavender (Festing, 1989). In 1865, cinnamaldehyde, the first synthetic, was made. The use of synthetics to mimic the scent of many flowers, as well as expensive products such as civet and musk, and to produce new fragrances not known in nature, opened the way for perfumes to be used by the masses owing to the lower cost of production. Adulteration and substitution by the essential oil or component of another plant species became rampant. For example, geraniol, in rose, is cheaper if taken from geranium and palmarosa (see Chapter 4). It is then mixed with other components to produce rose perfume (Groom, 1992), which can also be produced from totally synthetic materials.

Aroma chemicals are synthesised from coal, petroleum by-products and terpenes and are very much cheaper than the equivalent plant products. For example, true vanilla used to be obtained from vanilla pods, which were picked off the vine and dipped into warm water before being packed into barrels, lined with wool (to induce sweating) for a day. They would then be exposed to the sun for a week after which they were spread out on trays in drying sheds for six months. Crystals of the vanilla essential oil would form as a frost on the surfaces of the pods and had to be scraped off (Charabot, 1999). Nowadays, vanillin is synthesised cheaply from cloves; these contain isoeugenol, which is easily converted to vanillin.

Conclusion

The way was now open for the use of scent in the modern era. It seems therefore a retrograde step to use pure essential oils in 'aromatherapy', especially as the 'Father of Aromatherapy', René-Maurice Gattefossé, used scents or deterpenated essential oils (see Chapter 3).

3

Aromatherapy practice

Introduction

The aromatherapy movement in the UK started as a branch of alternative medicine. Tisserand (1977) stated in the first edition of his book, *The Art of Aromatherapy*, that people were becoming increasingly suspicious towards conventional medicines. But what most had forgotten was that many of the conventional medicines were originally derived from plants (e.g. aspirin from willow bark, digitalis from foxgloves and atropine from belladonna) and that later the active principles were obtained from synthetics.

Aromatherapy, using odorous essential oils, is closely aligned with other forms of alternative or holistic medicine. It recognises the need to treat mind, body and soul together. The aromatherapist is therefore often qualified in other forms of alternative therapy, such as meditation, naturopathy, nutrition, reflexology, reiki, shiatsu, yoga and healing.

A 'certified aromatherapist' will often give advice on how to cure all manner of ailments, both physical and psychological, with the use of one or more essential oils. Aromatherapists provide information on how to dilute and administer the essential oils using various methods. They offer their services as a 'professional' and occasionally oils are prescribed for internal usage. Aromatherapists also use essential oils in combination with specific massage techniques. Patients need to be very careful, though, if taking medical advice from aromatherapists as their training in itself does not qualify them to practice medicine and give specific medicinal advice.

Many aromatherapists also have a sideline in selling essential oils and associated items, including diffusers, candles, jewellery and all sorts of products made with essential oils, such as skin creams, shampoos, shower gels, moisturisers, bath salts, lotions, etc. Aromatherapy is indeed big business.

Aromatherapy has almost become synonymous with aromatherapy products. The aromatic oils are often alleged to contain hormones, antibiotics and antiseptics, and to represent the 'life force', 'spirit', or 'soul' of the plant; some proponents even claim that aromatherapy is a complete medical system that can 'revitalise cells', strengthen defence mechanisms, and cure the 'cause of disease'. Caution is advised, however. Although pleasant odours may enhance a person's ability to relax, there is no scientific evidence that they can influence the course of any disease. In addition, some people are allergic to aromatherapy products or find that they irritate the lining of the nose (see Chapter 7).

Aromatherapy basics

The following details are accompanied by remarks regarding the possible legal and other cautions.

Consultation with an aromatherapist

Aromatherapists usually treat their clients (patients) after an initial full consultation, which usually involves taking down a full medical case history. The aromatherapist will then decide what treatment to give, which usually involves massage with three essential oils, often one each chosen from those with top, middle and base perfumery notes, which balances the mixture. Sometimes specific essential oils for the 'disease' will only be used (as taught in a specific aromatherapy school or read in a book, thus perpetuating the art rather than the science) but many aromatherapists ask the client to choose oils from a given selection. Patients are also often advised to use the same essential oil mix in the bath to enhance the treatment (a good selling point for the aromatherapist, who supplies the mixture). Most aromatherapists arrange to see the client 3–5 times and the mixture will often be changed on the next visit, if not on each visit, in order to treat all the possible symptoms presented by the client (holistically), or simply as a substitute when no improvement was initially obtained. Treatment may involve other alternative medicine procedures, including chakras.

Many aromatherapists will offer to treat any illness, feeling that they can help in some way. They will embark on the treatment of endometriosis, infertility, asthma, diabetes and arthritis, convinced of the therapeutic nature of essential oils, but often without the necessary scientific and medical knowledge. 'Psychoneuroimmunology' treatment is the current buzzword for aromatherapeutic treatment. Other phrases, such as 'curing cancer or endometriosis, making a woman fertile and such like' have luckily largely disappeared from the current literature over the years.

Some aromatherapists practise complementary aromatherapy by giving comfort, touch, a pleasant fragrance and verbal support to cancer patients, old people and people in hospital or in a hospice.

Taking down the medical history

The aromatherapy 'treatment' in private practice, i.e. in the aromatherapist's home or in a room in an alternative medicine practice, involves first taking the medical history of the patient, which can run to several pages of intimate detail. This may raise an immediate legal problem of the security regarding these medical notes: what precautions are taken to ensure that they cannot be stolen or passed on to a third person? Although aromatherapists consider themselves professionals, there is no Hippocratic oath involved. The aromatherapist, being non-medically qualified, may not even understand most of the illnesses or symptoms, so there could be a very serious mistake made as potentially serious illnesses could be adversely affected by being 'treated' by a lay-person. Some, but not all, aromatherapists ask the patient to tell their doctor of the aromatherapy treatment.

Counselling

Counselling is greatly recommended by aromatherapy schools. Aromatherapists are not necessarily, however, trained in counselling, and with few exceptions could

do more damage than good, especially when dealing with psychiatric illness, cases of physical or drug abuse, people with learning difficulties, etc., where their 'treatment' should only be complementary and under a doctor's control.

Methods of application of aromatherapy treatment

Various methods are used to apply the treatment in aromatherapy. The most usual methods are the following:

1. A diffuser, usually powered by electricity, giving out a fine mist of the essential oil.
2. A burner, with water added to the fragrance to prevent burning of the essential oil. About 1–4 drops of essential oil are added to about 10 mL water. The burner can be warmed by candles or electricity. The latter would be safer in a hospital or children's room or even a bedroom.
3. Ceramic or metal rings, placed on an electric light bulb with a drop or two of essential oil. This results in a rapid burn-out of the oil and lasts for a very short time due to the rapid volatilisation of the essential oil in the heat.
4. A warm bath with drops of essential oil added. This results in the slow volatilisation of the essential oil, and the odour is inhaled via the mouth and nose. Any effect is not likely to be through the absorption of the essential oil through the skin as stated in aromatherapy books, as the essential oil does not mix with water. Droplets either form on the surface of the water, often coalescing, or else the essential oil sticks to the side of the bath. Pouring in an essential oil mixed with milk serves no useful purpose as the essential oil will still not mix with water, and the premixing of the essential oil in a carrier oil, as for massage, just results in a nasty oily scum around the bath.
5. A bowl of hot water with drops of essential oil, often used for soaking feet or used as a bidet. Again the essential oil will not mix with the water. This is, however, a useful method for inhaling essential oils in respiratory conditions and colds: the essential oil can be breathed in when the head is placed over the container and a towel placed over the head and container. This is an established method of treatment and has been used successfully with Vicks VapoRub, obas oil and *Eucalyptus* oils for many years, so it is not surprising that it works with aromatherapy essential oils!

6. Compresses using essential oil drops on a wet cloth, either hot or cold, to relieve inflammation, treat wounds, etc. Again, the essential oil is not able to mix with the water and can be concentrated in one or two areas, making it a possible health hazard.

7. Massage of hands, feet, back or all over the body using 2–4 drops of essential oil (single essential oil or mixture) diluted in 10 mL carrier oil (fixed, oily), e.g. almond oil or jojoba, grapeseed, wheatgerm oils, etc. The massage applied is usually by gentle effleurage with some petrissage (kneading), with and without some shiatsu, lymph drainage in some cases and is more or less vigorous, according to the aromatherapist's skills and beliefs.

8. Oral intake is more like conventional than 'alternative' usage of essential oils. Although it is practised by a number of aromatherapists, this is not to be condoned unless the aromatherapist is medically qualified. Essential oil drops are 'mixed' in a tumbler of hot water or presented on a sugar cube or 'mixed' with a teaspoonful of honey and taken internally. The inability of the essential oil to mix with aqueous solutions presents a health hazard, as do the other methods, as such strong concentrations of essential oils are involved.

Possible contradictory bioactivity results due to different modes of application of essential oils

Leaving aside the oral route, the application of essential oils via the skin rather than just by vaporisation adds another mode of possible absorption for at least some of the components of essential oils. Not many studies have been attempted to show this possible contradiction in results, but recent studies on sandalwood oil and α-santalol in humans have shown that the results differ widely depending on the method of application. When the oils were applied by inhalation they showed a stimulatory effect, whereas when they were applied by percutaneous absorption following massage, they gave a sedative effect (Hongratanaworskit et al., 2000a,b).

The theme of essential oil absorption is very confused in aromatherapy books. There is no evidence that an essential oil as such is absorbed, because most consist of around 300 components, each of which has its own physicochemical properties that govern its absorption across the many layers of skin (see Chapter 5).

Aromatherapy involves the volatilisation of essential oils, whether massaged into the body or put into the bath or in burners. The actual amount of an essential oil that is volatilised during massage depends on several factors, including the oil's inherent volatility, the temperature and humidity of the room, the temperature and degree of work done by the aromatherapist, the temperature and skin-type of the patient, and the part of the body massaged.

It is reasonable to suggest that the aromatherapist, who is, after all, bending over the patient while massaging, is closer to the volatilised essential oils than the patient. This is especially relevant when the aromatherapist massages the back of the patient, which can amount to half of the total massage time. The amount of essential oil which can be absorbed by the skin as its individual components is probably quite low. Studies have shown that only picograms of components are absorbed (Jager et al., 1992; Jirovetz et al., 1992; see also Appendices 17 and 18). This implies that most components remain unabsorbed through the skin, despite the many contrary statements by aromatherapists. The disappearance of essential oils from the skin may indicate that some of their components are absorbed, but does not indicate that the essential oils are absorbed *per se*.

Substitution

Over 200 essential oils, absolutes, CO_2 extractives and resins may be used in aromatherapy. The cost of having all of these would be prohibitive for the aromatherapist, so most usually only stock and use about 20 different essential oils. There are many sites on the Internet that offer advice for substitution of one essential oil for another. Some of the suggestions can be very bizarre, for example neroli, jasmine and ylang ylang are said to be interchangeable, although they each have a different odour. For 'therapeutic' substitutions, an essential oil with a similar therapeutic effect is recommended, even if its odour is entirely different! Sometimes, substitutions are recommended within the same 'family of plants', which can mean using any of the following in the family Labiatae: rosemary, mints (any), pennyroyal, savory, sages (any), *Melissa*, marjoram, thymes, oregano, lavender (any), patchouli, hyssop and basil.

Great caution must be used in following any advice on the Internet, as it is often totally against any scientific knowledge. Every essential oil has some, often unique, bioactivities and therefore one essential oil can never easily be substituted by another. For example, amongst the lemon-scented essential oils, lemon, lemon verbena, neroli, bergamot and petitgrain have a strong contractile effect on smooth muscle of the guinea-pig (see Appendices 2 and 3), whilst lemongrass, citronella, *Eucalyptus citriodora*, *Litsea cubeba* have a relaxant effect, yet they all smell of lemon.

Massage using essential oils

The most popular method of using aromatherapy is through massage. The first written records referring to massage date back to its practise in China more than 4000 years ago. There is also ample evidence from hieroglyphics and murals in Egypt that it was in use at that time. Hippocrates, the father of modern medicine, wrote, 'the physician must be experienced in many things, but most assuredly in rubbing'.

Massage has been used for centuries in Ayurvedic medicine in India as well as in China, and shiatsu, acupressure, reflexology and many other contemporary techniques have their roots in these sources. Massage was used for conventional therapeutic purposes in hospitals before World War II and is now still used by physiotherapists for various conditions, especially in sports injuries.

Use of massage by original aromatherapists

René-Maurice Gattefossé, credited as being the founding father of modern aromatherapy, never made a connection between essential oils and massage. It was Marguerite Maury who advocated the external use of essential oils combined with carrier oils. 'It is therefore clear that preparations with a basis of essential oils with vegetable oils used as carriers, in other words products taken from the vegetable kingdom, will be of great assistance' (Maury, 1989). She used carefully selected essential oils for cleansing the skin, including that in acne, using a unique blend of oils for each client created specifically for the person's temperament and health situation. Maury

claims never to have found two patients who required the same blend.

Maury's main focus was on rejuvenation: she was convinced that aromas could be used to slow down the ageing process if the correct oils were chosen, the idea being to bring the individual into balance. In view of this it is ironic that recent animal experiments have indicated that oral intake of some antioxidant essential oils can appear to defer ageing, as indicated by the composition of membranes in various tissues (see Chapter 5).

Massage *per se* can be a relaxing experience and can help to alleviate the stresses and strains of daily life. In a review of the literature on massage, Vickers (1996) found that in most studies massage had no psychological effect, in a few studies there was arousal and in an even smaller number there was sedation. It seems that massage may be physiologically stimulating even when psychologically sedating. Vickers also concluded that gentle touch is beneficial for the newborn, some massage has both local and systemic effects on blood flow and possibly on lymph flow and reduction of muscle tension, and there are reductions in anxiety scores in healthy subjects, except where anxiety was low level.

It may be that these variable responses are directly related to the variability of massage techniques, of which there are over 200. Massage can be given over the whole body or limited to the face, neck or just hands, feet, legs – depending on the patient and his or her condition or illness. For example, a hyperactive child would be unable to lie for an hour for a full massage; similarly, patients with learning disabilities and many psychiatric patients are often only able to have limited body contact for a short time.

Massage techniques

Massage is customarily defined as the manual manipulation of the soft tissues of the body for therapeutic purposes, using strokes that include gliding, kneading, pressing, tapping and/or vibrating (Tisserand, 1977; Price and Price, 1999). Massage therapists may also cause movement within the joints, apply heat or cold, use holding techniques, and/or advise clients on exercises to improve muscle tone and range of motion. Some common massage techniques are described below.

Swedish massage

This is the most frequently used technique in aromatherapy. It was developed in the 1820s by a Swedish doctor called Dr Per Henrik Ling, through his study of physiology, gymnastics and massage techniques taken from China, Egypt, Greece and Rome. Swedish massage uses five different strokes: **effleurage** – gliding or long strokes, **petrissage** – kneading (muscles are lightly grabbed and lifted), **friction** – rubbing (thumbs and fingertips work in deep circles into the thickest part of muscles), plus active and passive movements of the joints: **tapotement** – (pounding or chopping, beating, and tapping strokes) and **vibration** – shaking (fingers are pressed or flattened firmly on a muscle, then the area is shaken rapidly for a few seconds).

Swedish massage is said to be effective for most ailments, because massaging the skin, the body's largest organ, sets up a chain reaction that produces a positive effect on all layers and systems of the body; it therefore affects the nerves, muscles, glands and circulation, and promotes health and well-being.

The following massage techniques, described in alphabetical order, are less often used. Many of the methods claim to detect and manipulate subtle 'energies', but none of them has a scientifically plausible rationale or has been shown to favourably influence the course of any physical ailment. Many aromatherapists use a 'hands-above-the-body' type of massage, like therapeutic touch, which saves them considerable energy expenditure but probably has no benefit to the client, unless the aromatherapist has 'healing hands'.

Acupressure

Dating back 5000 years, acupressure is part of traditional Chinese medicine and is often described as 'acupuncture without the needles'. It uses deep finger pressure applied at certain points located along an invisible system of energy channels within the body called meridians. Because these points are said to directly relate to organs and glands of the body, constrictions in the flow of energy at these points supposedly cause disease and discomfort and acupressure stimulates these points to remove blockages, to increase the energy flow, to reduce stress, and to promote health.

Craniosacral therapy

Originally developed in the early 1900s by an osteopath called William G. Sutherland, and later refined and promoted by Dr John Upledger, craniosacral therapy is based on the idea that the bones of the skull are movable and can be manipulated. Some practitioners claim to attune themselves to the patient's 'rhythm' while holding the patient's skull in their hands. Some claim to improve the flow of 'life energy', thereby curing or preventing a wide variety of health problems; some claim to remove blockages to the flow of cerebrospinal fluid or to realign the skull bones. In actuality, the bones of the skull fuse early in life and cannot be moved independently, and considerable research has failed to prove any of the claims made (Kazanjian *et al.*, 1999).

Deep tissue massage

This is designed to reach the deep portions of thick muscles, specifically the individual muscle fibres. Using deep muscle compression and friction along the grain of the muscle, its purpose is apparently to unstick the fibres of the muscles and release both toxins and deeply held patterns of tension.

Infant massage

This is apparently taught to new mothers as a way of bonding with their newborn and of encouraging infant health. It incorporates nurturing touch, massage and reflexology in a loving, fun, one-on-one interaction. Apparently, infants who received 15 minutes of massage a day gained weight 47% faster.

Lymph system massage

Hans Vodder, in the 1930s, noticed the connection between swollen and blocked lymph glands and colds, infections and other ailments. He developed a specific technique that massages the lymph nodes and lymph system using light rhythmic strokes, always with the muscle fibre, as the lymph system runs in that direction.

Polarity therapy

Developed by chiropractor and osteopath Randolph Stone, polarity therapy is a holistic method of treatment incorporating Ayurvedic medicine, Chinese medicine, yoga, acupuncture and shiatsu techniques, which claims to restore health by removing blocks and balancing the flow of 'life energy' between the positive (head) and negative poles (feet) of the body.

Reflexology

Popularized in the United States by physiotherapist Eunice Inghram in the 1930s, this is an acupressure-type technique performed on the hands and feet and is based on the ancient Oriental theory that meridian lines or pathways carry energy throughout the body. Apparently, stimulating reflex points causes stimulation in the natural energy of the related organ. Many practitioners claim foot reflexology can cleanse the body of toxins, increase circulation, assist in weight loss, and improve the health of organs throughout the body and be effective against a large number of serious diseases. Crystalline-type deposits and/or tenderness indicate a dysfunction, and pressure is applied to clear out congestion and restore normal functioning and health.

Reiki

In Japanese, reiki means 'universal life energy'. It was developed by Dr Mikao Usua, a Christian monk in Japan, who came upon ancient manuscripts revealing the healing system in the nineteenth century. Practitioners claim to harness and transmit 'universal life energy' by placing their hands in specific positions on or near the body; or they can visualise special symbols that supposedly enable them to send 'healing energy', even from far away. One form of reiki, 'the Radiance Technique', is claimed to be useful for mental, emotional, physical and spiritual balancing.

Rolfing

Also called structural integration, rolfing was pioneered by American biochemist Dr Ida Rolf in the 1930s, who maintained that when one part of the body is out of balance or misaligned, the rest of the body attempts to compensate until the entire structure is weakened. By manipulating the myofascial tissue in a series of ten sessions, rolfers apparently assist the body to reorganise, lengthen and integrate itself into wholeness.

Shiatsu

This is the most widely known form of acupressure. Shiatsu, literally meaning 'finger pressure' in Japanese, has been practised for more than a thousand years in Japan. It uses rhythmic pressure for from 3 to 10 seconds on specific points along the body's meridians, using the fingers, hands, elbows, knees and sometimes feet to unblock and stimulate the flow of energy. A session may also include gentle stretching and range-of-motion manipulations to treat pain and illness, to relax the body and to maintain general health.

Therapeutic touch

This was developed in the 1970s by Dolores Krieger, a nurse and professor at New York University. Practitioners claim to detect and correct 'energy imbalances' by moving their hands above the patient's body. Healing supposedly results from transfer of 'excess energy' from healer to patient. Neither the forces involved nor the alleged therapeutic benefits have been demonstrated by scientific testing and, in one study, 21 therapeutic touch practitioners were unable to detect the experimenter's 'energy field'.

Benefits and risks of massage

Massage is very basic to everybody: we all rub (massage) any part of the body that hurts. Virtually all cultures used massage for thousands of years: we find reference to it in Ancient Egypt and China, in writings by Hippocrates and also in old medicinal papyri, etc. Nowadays, massage has become not just a relaxant of stiff muscles and tissue, but also a means by which practitioners can focus on the relaxant effect on the whole body. Treatment can be less vigorous and more gentle and flowing to achieve such a total effect. Today's patients are usually treated in clean, comfortable surroundings, which are at the best temperature and provide a peaceful atmosphere.

Massage usually involves the use of a lubricating oil to help the practitioner's hands glide more evenly over the body. The addition of perfumed essential oils further adds to its potential to relax.

In most English-speaking countries, massage is nowadays seen as an alternative or complementary treatment. However, before World War II it was regarded as a conventional treatment (Goldstone, 1999, 2000), as it is now in continental Europe. In Austria, for example, most patients with back pain receive (and are usually reimbursed for) massage treatment (Ernst, 2003a).

Not all massage treatment is free of risk. Too much force can cause fractures of osteoporotic bones, and even rupture of the liver and damage to nerves have been associated with massage (Ernst, 2003b). These events are rarities, however, and massage is relatively safe, provided that well-trained therapists observe the contraindications: phlebitis, deep vein thrombosis, burns, skin infections, eczema, open wounds, bone fractures and advanced osteoporosis (Ernst et al., 2001).

It is not known exactly how massage works, although many theories abound, details of which can be found in Vickers (1996) and Ernst et al. (2001). Some of these theories include the fact that the mechanical action of the hands on cutaneous and subcutaneous structures enhances circulation of blood and lymph, resulting in increased supply of oxygen and removal of waste products or mediators of pain (Goats, 1994). Certain massage techniques have been shown to increase the threshold for pain (Dhondt et al., 1999). Also, most importantly from the standpoint of aromatherapy, a massage can relax the mind and reduce anxiety, which could positively affect the perception of pain (Vickers, 1996; Ernst, 2003a). Many studies have been carried out, most of which are unsatisfactory. It appears that placebo-controlled, double-blind trials may not be possible, yet few randomised clinical trials have been forthcoming.

Different client groups require proper recognition before aromatherapy trials are started or aromatherapy massage is given. For example, for cancer patients the following guidelines must be observed (Wilkinson et al., 1999): special care must be taken for certain conditions such as autoimmune disease (where there are tiny bruises present); low blood cell count, which makes the patient lethargic and needing nothing more than very gentle treatment; and lymphoedema, which should not be treated unless the therapist has special knowledge and where enfleurage towards the lymph nodes should not be used.

Suitable types of massage in most cases of cancer include: acupressure, aromatherapy biodynamic,

manual lymph drainage, polarity therapy, reflexology, gentle shiatsu, Swedish massage and reiki. Deep finger kneading or deep tissue pressure of percussion, rolfing and deep pummelling and hard Swedish massage should be avoided at the cancer site. The aim of the aromatherapist in relation to cancer patients is to improve the quality of life, to alleviate symptoms mainly by aiding relaxation and easing away tension, stress and anxiety, and to provide comfort through the caring touch. The aromatherapist also gives time and empathy and provides a pleasant experience, combining the powerful effects of aroma and touch. There are no known essential oil cancer cures to date, so any remissions should not be regarded as a sign of a successful cure. Remissions occur regularly and patients must never be given false hope.

Recent literature review of the benefits of massage

Individual studies

Recent individual studies to investigate the benefit of massage for certain complaints have shown up variable results. Many are positive, although the standard of the studies has, in general, been poor (Vickers, 1996). The most successful applications of massage or aromatherapy massage have been in cancer care, and about a third of patients with cancer use complementary/alternative medicine during their illness (Ernst and Cassileth, 1998). Massage is commonly provided within UK cancer services (Kohn, 1999), and although only anecdotal and qualitative evidence is available, it is considered by patients to be beneficial. Only a few small-scale studies amongst patients with cancer have identified short-term benefits from a course of massage, mainly in terms of reduced anxiety (Corner et al., 1995; Kite et al., 1998; Wilkinson et al., 1999). These studies have been criticised by scientists, however, as they were either non-randomised, had inadequate control groups or were observational in design (Cooke and Ernst, 2000). Complementary therapy practitioners have criticised medical research for not being sufficiently holistic in approach, focusing on efficacy of treatments in terms of tumour response and survival, rather than quality of life (Wilkinson, 2003).

Scientific surveys

The following studies of massage effects on different physiological/pharmacological systems have been published.

- **Circulatory and respiratory systems:** Massage reduced blood pressure and heart rate (Fakouri and Jones, 1987), systolic and diastolic blood pressure (Cady and Jones, 1997).
- **Psychological/emotional factors:** The effects of slow stroke back massage showed decreases in blood pressure and heart rate, an increase in skin temperature and vital signs indicating relaxation (Meek, 1993). 'Chair massage' reduced anxiety levels for employees (Shulman and Jones, 1996) and back massage, as an alternative or adjunct to pharmacological treatment, is clinically effective for the promotion of sleep (Culpepper-Richards, 1998). Of 113 hospitalised patients receiving one to four massages during their hospital stay, 98% reported increased relaxation and 88% had positive mood changes; over two-thirds of the patients said they had greater energy, greater ease of movement and experienced greater participation in their treatment (Smith et al., 1999).
- **Immune function:** Massage therapy was associated with enhancement of the immune system's cytotoxic capacity (Ironson et al., 1996).
- **Infants and children:** The use of massage showed clinical improvement of infants and children with a variety of medical conditions (Field et al., 1986; Field, 1995). Massage therapy improved weight gain in preterm infants (Scafidi et al., 1993) and reduced anxiety in child and adolescent psychiatric patients (Field et al., 1992).
- **Lymph:** It was shown that extrinsic factors such as massage strongly influence lymph flow (Mortimer et al., 1990); massage increases lymph flow rate by seven to nine times (Elkins et al., 1953). Reduction of lymphoedema occurred with manual lymphatic massage and with uniform-pressure pneumatic massage (Zanolla et al., 1994). The treatment of lymphoedema due to cancer surgery or radiotherapy is no longer treated with diuretics on the whole and the use of mechanical compression devices and/or massage has become more prevalent (Brennan and Weitz, 1992).
- **Musculoskeletal system:** A pilot study involving myofascial release, massage, craniocervical manipulation and physiotherapy showed marked improvements in gait and range of motion (Baumann, 1996). It also demonstrated improvements in measures of spontaneous, muscular contracture and the degree of lumbar extension by massaging with ointment (Ginsburg and Famaey, 1987) and reduced pain, lessened stiffness and fatigue (Sunshine et al., 1996).
- **Pain treatment:** Significant reductions in acute and chronic pain and increased muscle flexibility and tone were noted after using a variety of massage techniques (Weintraub, 1992). Massage also stimulated the brain to produce endorphins, the body's natural pain control chemicals (Kaard and Tostinbo, 1989).
- **Cancer patients:** Therapeutic massage was a beneficial nursing intervention that promoted relaxation and alleviated the perception of pain and anxiety in hospitalised cancer patients (Ferrell-Torry and Glick, 1993). Cancer patient post-test scores on the Rotterdam Symptom Checklist and the State-Trait Anxiety Inventory improved and patients reported that massage reduced anxiety, tension, pain and depression (Wilkinson et al., 1999).
- **Pregnancy:** Massage apparently reduces morning sickness (Dundee et al., 1988) and decreases the need for episiotomy (Avery and Burket, 1986). It also apparently reduces duration of labour, hospital stay and post-partum depression (Field et al., 1997).
- **Sports medicine:** A review of techniques and previous research on effects of massage on blood flow and composition, oedema, connective tissue, muscle and the nervous system demonstrated that the use of massage in sports medicine can be justified (Goats, 1994). Sports massage reduces delayed-onset muscle soreness and creatine kinase when administered 2 hours after the termination of eccentric exercise (Smith et al., 1994).

Systematic reviews

Systematic reviews were not so positive in their overall judgements, due to the fact that the bulk of the literature on massage is methodologically flawed and open to bias, mainly because of a lack of randomisation, blinding and placebo controls. The studies were considered of poor quality and validity.

A general study of the clinical effectiveness of massage

Ernst (1994) used numerous trials, with and without control groups. A variety of control interventions were used in the controlled studies including placebo, analgesics, transcutaneous electrical nerve stimulation (TENS), etc. There were some positive effects of vibrational or manual massage, assessed as improvements in mobility, Doppler flow, expiratory volume and reduced lymphoedema in controlled studies. Improvements in musculoskeletal and phantom limb pain, but not cancer pain, were recorded in controlled studies. Uncontrolled studies were invariably positive. Adverse effects included thrombophlebitis and local inflammation or ulceration of the skin.

Massage for low back pain

The Research Institute for Work and Health has completed a review of studies (randomised or quasi-randomised trials) on the effectiveness of massage for low back pain. Massage was found to be better (in combination with exercises and education) than an inert treatment, but inferior to manipulation and TENS and equal to corsets and exercises. Massage was superior to relaxation therapy, acupuncture and self-care education. There is apparently insufficient evidence to determine whether massage therapy works in the treatment of low back pain, but it is known that massage relaxes the mind and the muscles and is thought to increase the pain threshold (Furlan *et al.*, 2002).

Another systematic review on this topic (Ernst, 1999b) included four trials with 399 patients in total. One trial found massage to be significantly inferior to chiropractic manipulation in uncomplicated chronic/subacute low back pain. The other studies reported no significant difference between massage and the control treatments, except the non-randomised study, which reported massage to be significantly better.

Massage for delayed-onset muscle soreness

In a systematic review by Ernst (1998) seven trials were included with 132 patients in total. One of the randomised trials showed a statistical improvement in pain with daily massage treatment compared with no massage after 48 hours, but no difference at other observations up to 96 hours; another showed no statistically significant difference between massage and control; the other studies showed massage to be more effective than control. In non-randomised studies, two out of three studies reported massage to be more effective than controls but statistical significance was not mentioned in either category.

Effleurage backrub for relaxation

In this systematic review, nine trials were included with a total of 250 patients (Labyak and Metzger, 1997). A 3-minute effleurage produced an 11% decrease in blood pressure and heart rate and a 6% decrease in respiratory rate; a 10-minute effleurage led to an 11% decrease in blood pressure and heart rate and a 25% decrease in respiratory rate. The blood pressure and heart rate of post-coronary artery bypass patients rose. Methodological design, quality or validity of the studies, randomisation or blind study details were omitted.

Aromatherapy blends of essential oils used

Aromatherapists may either choose the essential oils themselves, based on the client's condition which is often as ascertained following a questionnaire in which the client provides medical information, or else they allow the client to choose one or more from a range offered to them. Often, three essential oils are blended, including one of each from the categories of top-note, middle-note and base-note, which balances out the mixture. These are perfumery categories, but seem to go well with holistic thought.

There are numerous suggestions for the use of particular essential oils for treating specific illnesses in books on aromatherapy. However, when collated, each essential oil can treat each illness (Vickers, 1996; compare also individual essential oil monographs).

A few drops of the essential oil or oils chosen are always mixed into a carrier oil before being applied to the skin for an aromatherapy massage. Some of the commonly used carrier oils are grapeseed, almond, light coconut and sesame. The exact dilution of the essential oils in the carrier oil is often controversial and can be anything from 0.5% to 20% and more (see also Chapter 7). Either 5, 10 or 20 mL of carrier oil is first poured into a (usually brown) bottle with a stoppered dropper. The essential oil is then added dropwise into the carrier oil, either as a single essential oil or a mixture of 2–3 different essential oils, and then stoppered.

Volumes of essential oils used for dilutions: controversial advice

The 'dilution' volumes used vary widely in different aromatherapy manuals (see Chapter 5). Some examples are given below to illustrate the potential for confusion:

- 1 drop for every 20 mL of vegetable oil, i.e. 2.5% dilution (Tisserand, 1985)
- 4–6 drops in 10 mL carrier oil; 2–8 drops in 20 mL (Price, 1993)
- 6 drops per oz carrier oil (Jackson, 1987)
- 8 drops in 15 mL (Lunny, 1997)
- 1 drop essential oil to 1 mL carrier oil (Worwood, 1991)
- To get the maximum number of drops of essential oil divide the number of millilitres in the bottle by two. For a 10 mL bottle this means the maximum is 5 drops of essential oil (Westwood, 1991).

The fact that even the size of a 'drop' varies raised the question of possible safety problems (see Chapter 7) and a recent article in a nursing journal makes a request for standardisation of the measurement of the drop size (Ollevant *et al.*, 1999). Appendices 9 and 10 illustrate the variation in the weight of different essential oil drops. The volume and weight of a 'drop' will depend on several factors, including the design of the dropper, the density of the essential oil and the temperature.

Carrier or vegetable fixed oils used for dilution

Many fixed oils are used for dilution, some of which are listed below. Their many aromatherapeutic/cosmetological attributes, as cited in aromatherapy books, journals and websites, are not included here as most of these are neither scientifically validated nor entirely correct. All the fixed oils provide a lubricant, however, and many have a high vitamin E and A content. By moistening the skin, they can assist in a variety of mild skin conditions especially where the skin is rough, cracked or dry (Healy and Aslam, 1996).

The following list gives an idea of the kinds of different fixed oils used and provides some indication as to whether they must be diluted with another oil (usually almond oil) or used as they are.

- Almond, sweet (*Prunus amygdalus* var, dulcis) – cheapest and most commonly used.
- Apricot kernel (*Prunus armeniaca*) – used as a 10–50% additive to main oil.
- Borage seed (*Borago officinalis*) – high in gamma linoleic acid; used as 10% additive.
- Calendula (*Calendula officinalis*) – used as 15–25% additive.
- Coconut oil (*Cocos nucifera*) – unrefined, semi-solid, high in saturated fatty acids; used as 10–50% additive.
- Evening primrose (*Oenothera biennis*) – high in gamma linolenic acid; used as 10% additive.
- Grapeseed (*Vitis vinifera*) – very commonly used, alone or in a mixture.
- Macadamia nut (*Macadamia integrifolia*) – high in unsaturates; used as 10% additive.
- Olive (*Olea europaea*) – virgin pressed; used as 10–50% additive.
- Rose hip seed (*Rosa mosqueta*, etc.) – high in unsaturates; used as 10% additive.
- Soya bean (*Glycine soya*) – cheap; often used alone.
- Sunflower (*Helianthus annuus*) – cheap: often used alone.
- Wheatgerm (*Triticum vulgare*) – expensive, easily rancifies; used as additive to cheaper oils.
- Jojoba (*Simmondsia californica*) – heavy oil; used as 10% additive.

Some aromatherapists have promoted refined oils such as grapeseed and soya on the grounds that they have almost no odour of their own and therefore do not interfere with the aromas of essential oils. Other aromatherapists regard only unrefined oils as adequate for holistic aromatherapy. Many compromise by mixing a refined oil such as grapeseed with a smaller percentage of an unrefined oil such as olive or jojoba. However, there is consensus of opinion regarding mineral oil: it should never be used as a base for essential oils (although it is used as 'baby oil') as it is derived from petroleum. It apparently clogs the pores of the skin, contributing to the development of blackheads and pimples. However, it is still used satisfactorily on a baby's skin!

The latest oil in vogue is emu oil (*Dromiceius novaehol-landiae*), which comes from a thick pad of fat on the bird's back. For centuries, the aborigines of Australia have been applying emu oil to their wounds with excellent results. It is now found in muscle pain relievers, skin care products, and natural soaps.

Mixing techniques for essential oil with fixed oils

The exact method of mixing is controversial, but most aromatherapists are taught not to shake the bottle containing the essential oil(s) and the diluent fixed oils, but to gently mix the contents by turning the bottle in the hand. Differences in the actual odour and thereby presumably benefits of the diluted oils made by different aromatherapists can just be due to the different droppers (see Chapter 7 and Appendices 9 and 10).

Internal usage of essential oils

Oral intake

'True' aromatherapy does not involve the oral ingestion of essential oils, as this produces a chemical effect firstly on the gut and then, after the absorption of the components, on the liver and kidneys. Almost all the other methods of application are based on essential oil volatilisation – the effect of the essential oil is largely on the CNS via the nose and thence the limbic system, which can cause a secondary effect on other parts of the body.

Many aromatherapists consider that essential oils should be limited to external use, as stated by Culpeper (1653).

There is also the safety issue, which is raised by some aromatherapists:

- It is recommended that essential oils taken orally for medicinal purposes are only prescribed by primary care practitioners such as medical doctors or medical herbalists who have intimate knowledge of essential oil toxicology (Tisserand and Balacs, 1995).
- An essence for external use can contain terpenes, but for internal use they must be removed at all cost (Maury, 1989).

Nevertheless, those who practise 'clinical aromatherapy' (as taught mainly by a few French doctors and based on non-scientific books and journals) consider it safe to take certain essential oils internally, as long as they are pure, without offering any scientific proof of effectiveness and safety. They believe that daily ingestion of essential oils guarantees proper balance and functioning of intestines, and fights internal infections (Price, 1983).

It is worth noting that most of us ingest essential oils and their components daily anyway, as they are used in almost all processed foods and drinks, but we are not all healthy.

Information on the dosage and choice of oils for treating particular conditions is also provided by clinical aromatherapists. Maladies treated include: arthritis, bronchitis, rheumatism, chilblains, eczema, high blood pressure and venereal diseases. In clinical aromatherapy there is a real risk of overdosage due to variable droppers on bottles, which can differ by as much as 200% (see Appendices 9 and 10), and this could possibly result in asphyxiation, particularly when peppermint oil is given to children (Bunyan, 1998; see also Chapter 7).

Some components of essential oils are used in prescribed drugs, such as decongestants (menthol), throat drops (thyme), and also in the food industry (see below and Chapter 4). However, there are grave dangers in their usage, especially if adulteration is taken into account.

It is advisable **not** to take any essential oils internally without proper medical advice. It is also unresolved whether non-medically qualified aromatherapists in the UK, even when considered 'qualified', are permitted by law to prescribe essential oils for internal usage to treat a disease(s) diagnosed by themselves. It is possible that they would not be covered by their insurance if there were adverse effects.

Conventional oral use of essential oils

Conventional drugs involving essential oils and their components have been used internally for a long time. Examples include decongestant ointments containing menthol, camphor and pine, and various throat drops containing components from essential oils such as lemon, thyme, peppermint, sage and hyssop.

Essential oils are also used in the food industry, usually in very minute amounts of 10 ppm (parts per million), but even up to 1000 ppm and over in the case of mint confectionery or chewing gum (Fenaroli, 1997). This contrasts greatly with the use of drops of undiluted essential oils on sugar lumps for oral application, or on suppositories in anal or vaginal application. Damage to mucous membranes could result due to the high concentration of the essential oils in certain areas of the applicator.

Essential oils and their components are also incorporated into enterically coated capsules and used for treating irritable bowel syndrome (peppermint in Colpermin), a mixture of monoterpenes for treating gallstones (Rowatol) and ureteric stones (Rowatinex): these are under product licences as medicines

(Somerville *et al.*, 1984; Somerville *et al.*, 1985; Engelstein *et al.*, 1992).

Essential oil use in vaginal, anal and other orifices

Some aromatherapists support the use of essential oils in various venereal conditions. However, it is not recommended that essential oils should be used in any such condition unless medically supervised. Aromatherapists are not qualified to treat venereal disease conditions, nor to make an accurate diagnosis in the first place, unless they are also medically qualified, as diagnosis not only involves inspection of private parts, but also the skills imparted through medical training.

With that proviso, it has been reported that tea tree oil has been used for candidiasis with apparently very encouraging results (Zarno, 1994). Two or three drops of the essential oil were used on a tampon, for internal application, twice a day. *Candida* treatments also include chamomile, lavender, bergamot and thyme (Schnaubelt, 1999). Essential oils used in this way, sometimes for months, often produced extremely painful reactions and putrid discharges. This type of aromatherapy is simply using the essential oils as conventional drugs/chemicals in very sensitive areas.

There is considerable danger in using tampons and suppositories that have been dipped into essential oil 'solutions' or have been treated with drops of essential oil, as there would be concentration differences in different areas of the tampons and suppositories, which could cause severe burns and irritation to the delicate mucosal membranes. There is some doubt whether this practice would be permitted under the present law and whether insurance companies would cover any claims arising from adverse reactions in patients.

Use of pure or synthetic components

Does it really matter whether the essential oil is pure or a synthetic mixture as long as the odour is the same? The perfumers certainly do not see any difference, and even prefer the synthetics as they remain constant, whereas essential oils can change under different conditions. Most chemical components are synthesised from coal and petroleum by-products and there is often a difference in the proportion of different enantiomers of individual components. Different enantiomers (stereoisomers that are mirror images of each other) of a chemical compound often have different odours and different biological properties (Lis-Balchin, 2002a,b). This was not, however, appreciated by Gattefossé (1937/1993) who stated: 'there is no appreciable difference between a pure constituent obtained by analysis and the same constituent reproduced synthetically other than at times, a change in the nature of imperceptible impurities which can taint them and slightly alter their properties'.

Gattefossé, of course, was working with perfumes and not with the 'pure plant essential oils', which form the basis of aromatherapy. Originally employed as a chemist in his family's perfumery business, he studied the antimicrobial and wound healing properties of essential oils on soldiers during World War I (Arnould-Taylor, 1981). In 1906, he published *Formulaires de Parfumerie Gattefossé*, demonstrating that his main interest was perfumery. He later worked in hospitals on the use of perfumes and essential oils as antiseptics and other (unstated) applications and also in dermatology, which led to advances in development of beauty products and treatments and the publication of *Physiological Aesthetics and Beauty Products* in 1936 (Gattefossé, 1992).

It should be remembered that many of the so-called 'pure' essential oils used today are adulterated (Which Report, 2001; Lis-Balchin *et al.*, 1996b, 1998a). Gattefossé promoted the deterpenisation of essential oils because, being a perfumer, he was aware that his products must be stable, have a long shelf-life and not go cloudy when diluted in alcohol. Terpenes had therefore to be eliminated as they are insoluble in aqueous solution of alcohol (as used in the food industry) nor are they very soluble in absolute alcohol. Terpenes also oxidise rapidly, often giving rise to toxic oxidation products (e.g. limonene of citrus essential oils) (see Chapter 7).

In contrast, another recent viewpoint is that terpeneless oils should not be used in aromatherapy. This is because not only is the wholeness or natural synergy of the oil destroyed, but it would also contain a higher percentage of the other components, some of which may be powerful chemicals with which an aromatherapist has to take care (Price, 1993). This view has not been scientifically validated. Bergamot and other citrus essential oils obtained by expression are recommended, despite their phototoxicity, provided the patient is not exposed to sunlight within 2 hours following massage (Price and Price, 1999). However, this may be impossible to adhere to, for example if facial massage is given. Furthermore, the 2 hour limitation of phototoxic effect has not been scientifically validated for all types of skin and people of all ages. The possibility of no adverse effect being produced by citrus essential oils due to their skin application in a fixed oil rather than ethanol, which was used in phototoxic evaluations (Price and Price, 1999), does not pass scientific scrutiny. Numerous essential oils and their components are used as penetration promoters for various drugs and enhance penetration through the horny layer (see Chapter 5). There is no reason why a toxic essential oil should be preferentially used if the non-toxic furanocoumarin-free (FCF) alternative is available. If adverse effects resulted, it is possible that there could be legal implications for the therapist.

Therapeutic claims for the application of essential oils

There are a wide range of properties ascribed to each essential oil in aromatherapy books, without any scientific proof of effectiveness (Vickers, 1996; see also individual monographs). Conflicting instructions for the use of essential oils in treating various illnesses/conditions abound. The following are a few examples:

- Hay fever
  - Lavender, eucalyptus, chamomile and melissa (Davis, 1988)
  - Eucalyptus and thyme (Tisserand, 1977)
  - Hyssop (Valnet, 1982)
  - Chamomile and eucalyptus (Worwood, 1991)
- Diabetes
  - Eucalyptus, geranium and juniper (Tisserand, 1977)
  - Clary sage, eucalyptus, geranium, juniper, lemon, pine, red thyme, sweet thyme, vetiver and ylang ylang (Price, 1993)
  - Eucalyptus, geranium, juniper and onion (Valnet, 1982)
  - Eucalyptus, geranium, cypress, lavender, hyssop and ginger (Worwood, 1991)

- Dandruff
  - West Indian bay, cade, cedarwood (Atlas, Texas and Virginian), eucalyptus, spike lavender, lemon, patchouli, rosemary, sage (clary + Spanish) and tea tree (Lawless, 1992)
  - Chamomile, clary sage, geranium, juniper, lavender, lemon, lemongrass, myrrh, patchouli, rosemary, sage, tea tree and ylang ylang (Keville and Green, 1995)
- Allergies
  - Immortelle, chamomile, balm and rose (Fischer-Rizzi, 1990)
  - Lemon balm, chamomile (German and Roman), helichrysum, true lavender and spikenard (Lawless, 1992)
  - Chamomile, jasmine, neroli and rose (Price, 1983).

There are a number of problems with the lists of essential oils in aromatherapy books, as illustrated above. An obvious omission is that, in most cases, no botanical names are given, even when there are several possible species. No indication is provided as to why these particular essential oils are used and how they are supposed to affect the condition.

Many of the biochemical and physiological statements found in aromatherapy books may sound impressive and scientifically correct to the layman, but are of dubious quality to scientists and professionals in the healthcare sphere. Cure of the condition is often implied but without information about how this is to occur. For example, taking the case of diabetes, where there is a lack of the hormone insulin, it is impossible to say how massage with the given essential oils could cure the condition, as the hormone itself must be replaced in juvenile-type diabetes or some blood glucose-decreasing drugs given in late-onset diabetes.

Unfortunately, constant repetition of a given statement often lends it credence – at least to the layperson, who does not require scientific evidence as to its validity.

False claims challenged in court

The false promotion of products for treating not only medical conditions but also well-being generally is now being challenged in the Law Courts. In 1997, Los Angeles attorney Morsé Mehrban charged that Lafabre and Aroma Vera had violated the California

Business and Professions Code by advertising that their products could promote health and well-being, relax the body, relax the mind, enhance mood, purify the air, are antidotes to air pollution, relieve fatigue, tone the body, nourish the skin, promote circulation, alleviate feminine cramps, and do about 50 other things (Barrett, 2000). The National Council Against Health Fraud served as plaintiff. In September 2000, the case was settled out of court with a $5700 payment to Mehrban and a court-approved stipulation (Stipulation for Judgment) and order prohibiting the defendants from making 57 of the disputed claims in advertising within California (Horowitz, 2000).

Conclusion

Aromatherapy is practised in many different ways and there are often very dubious statements made about the effectiveness of the therapy using different essential oils. As aromatherapy is now being used as a complementary therapy in so many different health centres, many attached to hospitals, hospices and primary healthcare practices, there is a need for the revision of the many claims of the effectiveness of essential oils. Scientific verification should be a prerequisite for any statement made, as there is the possibility of legal redress for false claims as well as a possible ban by the medical profession in future.

4

Chemistry of essential oils

Essential oils: definition

The scientific definition of an essential oil is: 'the volatile oil produced by steam/water distillation'. Essential oils are all fat-soluble and hydrophobic and will completely evaporate from the site of application leaving no visible mark or colour even if the original oil is coloured (e.g. German chamomile oil).

Solvent extracts, like concretes and absolutes, as well as carbon dioxide extractives are not considered to fall into this category, as they contain other products in addition to the essential oil such as plant pigments (which do not evaporate), alkaloids, and some proteins bound up with other components, many of which are water-soluble. However, these extracts are often included as essential oils.

Essential oils are not 'essential' to humans nor to the plants that produce them. The term essential derives from 'essence' which is used in herbal medicine and is normally associated with alcoholic extracts or tinctures and is composed of the more lipophilic components of the plant, including volatiles.

Plants produce essential oils for many possible reasons:

- Simply as a metabolic product.
- As an excretory product.
- As a 'pheromone' to attract specific insects for various purposes. For example, mulberry leaves exude a very characteristic essential oil, the odour of which is attractive to the silkworm. Some flowers produce essential oils to attract pollinating insects (Harborne, 1988).
- As a deterrent to insects. For example bark beetles (Coleoptera: Scolytidae) attack trees by boring through the bark and tunnelling through the phloem and cambium layers surrounding the sapwood. Pines and spruce produce copious amounts of sticky resin

containing monoterpenes to defend against penetration by these beetles (Raffa and Berryman, 1987).
- As a deterrent to other predators. Essential oils are produced in leaves of some *Pelargonium* species, often as sticky exudates, to deter predators from eating them.
- To prevent the growth of other plants in their vicinity.

Essential oil storage organelles

Essential oils are often stored in special glands, especially in plants of the Labiatae, Verbenaceae and Geraniaceae families. These glandular trichomes, which vary in size and shape depending on the actual plant, are located in various places (e.g. leaves, petals and roots) and develop at various stages in the plant's life cycle. In some *Pelargonium* plants they look rather like tiny field mushrooms, with either short or elongated telescopic stems made up of segments varying with the species (Lis-Balchin, 2002a, ch.19; see also below). The essential oil is produced in the plant cells below or nearby and is simply stored in the glands, and liberated when the plant surface is touched. Brushing past lavender bushes creates an instant aroma, and the essential oil is replenished very rapidly in the trichomes.

The Umbelliferae have oil-rich ducts in the fruit and internal secretory cavities known as schizogenous cavities or ducts in their leaves and roots. The latter are also found in the leaves of Myrtaceae, Graminae and Compositae. Other secretory structures occur, called lysigenous canals in the Rutaceae, resin canals in the Coniferae and gum canals in the Cistaceae and Burseraceae.

As the essential oils are stored in trichomes on the leaves of scented pelargoniums, there was a strong possibility that the shape, size and density of trich-omes could be indicative of the resultant odour of each *Pelargonium*, providing a simple means of classification both of odour and also inherent biological properties. However, this was found to be more complex than at first envisaged: a study of 133 species and subspecies of *Pelargonium* trichomes by Oosthuizen (1983) using a dissecting microscope showed numerous classes of indumentum, density and trichome types. The indumentum could be ciliated (thin hairs of equal size), glabrous (without trichomes), glandular (covered with glandular hairs), hirsute (covered with long, stiff, straight hairs), pubescent (covered with short, thin, soft hairs) or could belong to another intermediate category. The density varied from sparse to very dense. The glandular hairs had uniserial stalks of various lengths, and unicellular heads of various shapes. The heads were either globular, bulb-shaped or pear-shaped. Some of the non-glandular trichomes had a short, straight, stiff hair with or without a basal podium, while others were described as soft, with/without podium, etc.

Studies of over 500 species and cultivars of *Pelargonium* using the scanning electron microscope after processing the leaves in glutaraldehyde (to prevent any distortion) and sputter-coating with gold indicated no precise segregation of pelargoniums based on their trichomes (Lis-Balchin, 2002a, ch.19).

Both scented and unscented *Pelargonium* leaves contained both glandular and non-glandular hairs. These varied largely during development of the leaf, more so than differences in different species. Further studies on the essential oil composition of different species and cultivars could not be related to the trichome shapes (Lis-Balchin, 2002a) or to the DNA of the plants (Lis-Balchin, 2002a, ch.15).

Aetiology of essential oil components

Most of the essential oil components arise from acetyl CoA, the most important intermediary product derived from the catabolism of all foods (protein, carbohydrate and fat) in both plants and animals, including humans. Acetyl CoA is also the centre-point of anabolism of the body's own fats, carbohydrates, proteins and other necessary compounds. In humans as well as plants, there is a pathway leading from acetyl CoA resulting in the formation of steroids, including steroid sex hormones and cholesterol. In plants, there is another subsidiary metabolic pathway from the isoprene unit (made up of five carbons) leading via the condensation of two isopentenyl pyrophosphates (IPPs) to geranyl pyrophosphate, containing ten carbons, which leads to the production of monoterpenes (or

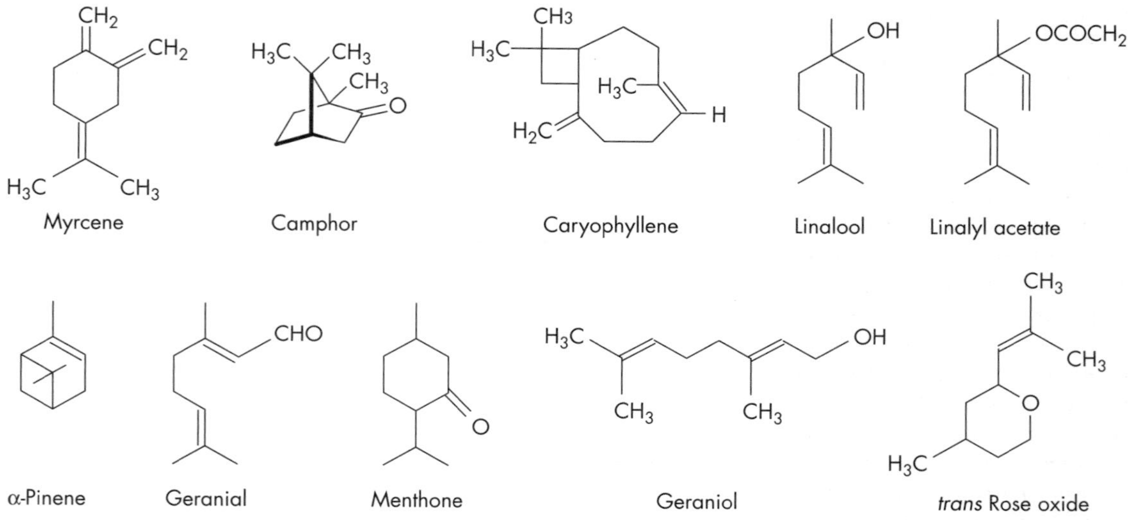

Figure 4.1 Chemical structures of some components found in essential oils.

monoterpenoids), which are the simplest of the essential oil components in plants. Sesquiterpenes contain 15 carbons and are formed by the condensation of three isoprene units. The terpenes can be oxidised either in the plant or during steam distillation to yield the corresponding alcohols, aldehydes, ketones and also form esters (Williams, 1996; and for further information consult any modern biochemistry textbook).

There is very little difference between the molecular weights of terpenes and their oxidation products; the differences lie in their spatial arrangements. Components of essential oils are therefore usually, but not always, drawn in their stereo-format (Figure 4.1). The similarity of many of these structures reflects the difficulty of their chemical detection. There is also the problem of stereoisomerism, whereby one or more groups (alcoholic, methyl, etc.) are arranged in a mirror image style in space compared with its isomer. Here there will be the exact molecular weight for all, making it even more difficult to assess chemically or physicochemically.

Some examples of essential oil components and their sources are given in Table 4.1 (see also Williams, 1996).

Heterogeneity in bioactivity of the chemical groups

In most aromatherapy books too much emphasis is placed on these groupings: different components in all these groups have different odours (e.g. menthone and thujone are both ketones); even the D- and L- forms can differ (e.g. carvone, again in the ketone group). (Note: The D- and L- suffixes denote dextrorotatory or laevorotatory, relating to the optical activity of the chemical.) The individual bioactivity can also vary specifically with an individual component and not the group as a whole. For example, benzaldehyde is less active as an antibacterial than salicylaldehyde; eugenol and thymol are more active than menthol (Friedman et al., 2002). However, there are exceptions: monoterpenes as a whole group are less potent antimicrobials than the oxygenated components; sesquiterpenes are even less active (Lis-Balchin et al., 1998a).

From the point of view of the pharmacological activity, most monoterpenes have a spasmogenic effect on the guinea-pig ileum; sesquiterpenes have a spasmolytic action (Lis-Balchin et al., 1996a; see

Table 4.1 Some essential oil components and their sources

Component	Examples of sources
Monoterpenes	
α- and β-Pinene	Pine needle, galbanum, yarrow, cumin, *Cupressus sempervirens*, frankincense, juniper, rosemary
p-Cymene	Frankincense, thyme, cumin
γ-Terpinene	Tea tree, marjoram, savory
Myrcene	Fennel, lemongrass, cypress
Limonene	Citrus (lemon, orange, grapefruit, lime), dill, celery, caraway, myrtle, pine needle
Sesquiterpenes	
Caryophyllene	Geranium, hops, black pepper
Chamazulene	German chamomile
Patchouline	Patchouli
Cedrene	Cedar
Monoterpenoid aldehydes	
Citronellal	Citronella
Citral (=neral + geranial)	Lemongrass, melissa, *Litsea cubeba*
Anisaldehyde	Anise, star anise
Perillaldehyde	*Perilla frutescens*
Cinnamaldehyde	Cinnamon, cassia
Cuminaldehyde	Cumin, cassia, cinnamon
Salicylaldehyde	Willow
Ketones	
Menthone	Peppermint, geranium, pennyroyal
Isomenthone	Peppermint, geranium, pennyroyal
Fenchone	Fennel
β-Ionone	Rose, osmanthus, boronia
Carvone	(D-) Caraway, dill; (L-) spearmint
Pinocamphone	Hyssop
Pulegone	Pennyroyal, cornmint, buchu, peppermint, spearmint
Thujone	Sage (Dalmatian), tansy, thuja, wormwood
β-Damascenone	Rose
β-Damascone	Rose
Alcohols	
Citronellol	Geranium, rose, citronella
Geraniol	Geranium, rose, palmarosa
Nerol	Rose
Linalool	Lavender, ho wood, rosewood, petitgrain, clary sage, coriander
Borneol	Rosemary, yarrow, pines, lavender, frankincense
Lavandulol	Lavender
Menthol	Peppermint, spearmint

(Continued)

Table 4.1 *(Continued)*

Component	Examples of sources
α-Bisabolol	Roman chamomile
Terpinen-4-ol	Tea tree
Esters	
Geranyl acetate	Palmarosa, ho wood
Geranyl isovalerate	Geranium
Geranyl formate	Geranium
Citronellyl formate	Geranium
Citronellyl tiglate	Geranium
Linalyl acetate	Lavender, bergamot, clary sage
Benzyl acetate	Jasmine, ylang ylang
Benzyl benzoate	Ylang ylang
Butyl angelates	Roman chamomile
Oxides	
1,8-Cineole	Tea tree, rosemary, *Eucalyptus globulus*
Rose oxide	Rose, geranium
Ether oxides	
Myristicine (apiol)	Dill, parsley, nutmeg
Elemicin	Elemi, mace, nutmeg
Phenolics – Some essential oil components are synthesised using the shikimic acid pathway, starting from aromatic amino acids like phenylalanine, e.g.	
Thymol	Thyme, ajowan, oregano
Carvacrol (isothymol)	Thyme, oregano, savory
Eugenol	Cloves, bay, cinnamon leaf, pimento
Phenylethylalcohol	Rose absolute
Safrole	Camphor (brown, yellow), sassafras, cinnamon leaf, star anise, ylang ylang
Anethole	anise, fennel, star anise
Estragole (isoanethole)	Basil, chervil, tarragon
β-Asarone	*Acorus calamus*
Chavicol	Basil, bay (West Indian)
Methyl paracresol	Ylang ylang
Coumarin	Tonka beans
Vanillin	Vanilla
Furananocoumarins (butyl phthalide, menthofuran; bergaptenes: 5-methoxypsoralen, 5-MOP)	Citrus oils, corn mint
Long-chain aliphatic components, e.g. nonanal, hexanal, decanal	
Sulphur and nitrogen components, e.g. allicin (diallyl thiosulphinate)	Garlic or onion essential oils

Appendix 4); some ketones showed both effects, whilst others were spasmolytic (Appendix 4); the oxide 1,8-cineole showed a distinctive rise in tone rather than a spasmogenesis.

It is therefore inadvisable to group chemical components into definitive groups, as shown in several aromatherapy books (Franchomme and Pénoel, 1990; Caddy, 1997). It is also wrong to group components according to their pH (Franchomme and Pénoel, 1990), as there is no measurable pH for hydrophobic components. This mis-statement was eventually corrected by the originator of this theory in a French book but is missed by the majority of aromatherapists (Pénoel, 1991a). The properties of electronegativity and electropositivity attributed to the components is also far-fetched and irrelevant, and could be likened to the allocation of planets (Culpeper, 1653) and colour and ying and yang to essential oils (Tisserand, 1977).

Variation in chemical composition of natural essential oils

The composition of an individual essential oil from a given plant species can change as a result of many factors: stage of maturity, seasonal changes, flowering, amount of rainfall or sunlight, sunlight intensity, altitude, soil composition, external application of fertilisers and also the stability of the species in the formation of, and often the actual variety, of chemotype. This implies that there is no constant composition for a given essential oil from a given plant, although the composition of a given commercial essential oil is often relatively stable. In thyme there is an abundance of natural chemotype formation due to the instability of the genome in this species, which is apparent particularly in the wild. This gives rise to a large variety of thymes with different odours.

Commercial essential oils are usually produced from a certain species (if not subspecies), hybrid, or even a specific variety (or cultivar), or in some cases, clones are used, which may result in similar or variable plants (e.g. tea tree). Different varieties of a species are often used in different parts of the world, due to the growth requirements, local soil/climatic conditions and the commercial needs for a high yield. For example geranium oil produced in Réunion, an island off the coast of South Africa, and in Madagascar is produced from a variety called 'Rosé' (which gives rise to the best quality 'Bourbon' geranium oil). This was probably hybridised in England from *P. capitatum* and *P. radens*. There is a somewhat different variety used in Egypt and Morocco, which produces an essential oil with largely the same odour characteristics but with a different main sesquiterpene in place of the one in the Bourbon oil (Lis-Balchin *et al.*, 1996b).

Different chemical compositions can impart different bioactivities to the essential oils although the name is constant. For example, substantial genetic instability is found in the family of plants from which the 'tea tree' oils from Australia and the New Zealand tea tree oils, manuka and kanuka (Lis-Balchin *et al.*, 2000), come. This gives wide variability in the chemical composition and bioactivity of even closely growing plants. Cloning of the plants and assessment of their chemical composition is imperative.

This natural variability in essential oils accounts for just some of the differences in chemical composition – adulteration can produce even greater differences. Steam distillation and other extraction procedures, such as rectification, can change the essential oil quite dramatically from that of the living plant (analysed by headspace analysis) as various oxidations occur. The 'living aroma' of plants has been used recently to produce 'natural perfumes' using, of course, synthetic ingredients, but following the chemical composition found by headspace analysis. These are known as Living Flower and Living Flavour by IFF (International Flavors & Fragrances Inc.).

There are numerous methods of capturing the odour around a plant or simply round a single flower using odour traps – usually a specially designed glass vessel which is placed over a living flower, leaf or other part of a plant. The air is sucked out of the odour trap by a vacuum pump. A more modern method is solid phase micro extraction (SPME), where the odour is taken up onto a solid absorbent and the odour is then analysed on a gas chromatograph (GC).

Organic essential oils

Farmers in the UK must comply with European Council Regulation (EEC) No. 2092/91, enforced 22 July 1991, regarding organic production and the rules governing the processing and sale of organic products. Land must be put into conversion prior to full-scale organic production and then applications must be made for status with the Soil Association, which inspects the sites. This takes around 3 years and, together with a lower yield due to loss by natural predation, puts up the cost. The premium charged, however, is often treble that of normal produce and reflects the gross over-commercialisation of the produce.

Organic essential oils have not been widely accepted by the main dealers in the food and cosmetics industry and the market is small, reserved mainly for aromatherapists. In France the certification is: ECO-Cert, Qualité France, SOCOTEC, brought in recently to control the expanding organic market. Other countries are following the trend, for example geranium oil is produced in small amounts in South Africa under organic conditions.

There is no difference between the composition of organic essential oils and that of ordinary ones, except for the absence in the organic oils of pesticides; however, these are very difficult to detect, unless one has mega samples for analysis. Many so-called organic essential oils are sold at inflated prices, but may even be obtained from the same commercial distributor as the ordinary essential oils by unscrupulous dealers.

Extraction of essential oils

Steam and water distillation

Steam distillation is the preferred distillation mode for the production of essential oils, but it can be combined with water. Water distillation can also be used (Lawrence, 1995; Williams, 1996; Denny, 2002). The plant material is packed into a glass, or copper or preferably stainless steel distillation flask (used commercially nowadays, as the former was a catalyst for oxidations). The flask is rounded in shape and heated externally to release the volatile oils, which then travel down a vapour pipe exiting from the top, which is bent downwards (the condenser) and leads to a container (receiver) through a tank of cold water. The pipe is often coiled to allow for condensation of the steam to occur more efficiently. The whole apparatus is known as a still. In water distillation, water is introduced into the distillation flask with the plant material. For steam distillation, a separate vessel boils the water, which is then introduced into the flask via a pipe as steam.

The whole complex process of distillation must be carefully controlled (Denny, 2002). The duration of the distillation and the temperature, as well as the actual composition of the vessels determine the composition and thereby the odour of the resulting essential oil. Ylang ylang, for example, is sold in many different grades; the most expensive 'extra' grade results from the shortest distillation time of about 15 minutes, then the progressive grades are those obtained from increasing distillation times. Naturally the yield increases with time so that the best grade has the smallest yield and also the highest proportion of the most volatile components, giving the best odour.

Oils such as nutmeg can change dramatically when the extraction time and temperature are increased. Personal experience has shown that caramelisation occurs after about 30 minutes of extraction using a glass laboratory steam distillation equipment, yielding a very thick oil which solidifies on cooling. This could only be removed from the apparatus by heating the outlet pipe with a hair dryer, and the smell resembled toffee or burnt coffee, rather than the nutmeg odour of the easy-flowing nutmeg oil fraction obtained after the first 10 minutes.

In water distillation, certain very water-soluble components will remain in the distillation water: this gives rise to secondary products like rosewater. However, it is normal to retrieve most of the dissolved components in the case of rose oil, due to the high cost of the essential oil and the small yield. The water containing the dissolved phenylethyl alcohol in the case of rose otto is therefore continuously returned to the distillation flask, a process called cohobation. An alternative method for retrieving the components in the water is by solvent extraction. Cohobation is also used for distilling plants with a high proportion of sesquiterpenes, which take longer to extract than the monoterpenes (e.g. myrrh).

In water distillation especially, the true living 'aroma' chemicals of the plant undergo oxidations and other chemical conversions during distillation, which of course involves high temperatures, the presence of oxygen and a pH which favours transformations. Distillation causes not only oxidations but also hydrolysis of both volatile esters and non-volatile glycosides, releasing volatile components (Williams, 1996). This also happens to a lesser extent in steam distillation. Other hydrolyses, like those of the sulphur-containing proteins in the plant, liberate abnoxious-smelling components, which dissolve in the essential oil, known as

'still notes'. These need to be eliminated by exposure to air. Lastly, the blue of German chamomile is due to chamazulene formed during distillation, which with time changes to a green and then a yellow tinge, a good indication of an ageing oil.

As most of the essential oils produced are for the perfumery and food industries, the actual odour of the oil has been established by the perfumery 'noses' for a long time, and what they want is continuity of the odour, as produced by steam distillation. They will also give the public the 'living' if not artificial odour of the plant.

Fractional distillation is used after the essential oil has been extracted, to remove either terpenes or toxic components like pulegone, etc.

Solvent extraction

This is used for expensive, low-yield plant material like rose, tuberose or jasmine, as the use of solvents gives a higher yield and also keeps the more water-soluble components intact, which would otherwise be lost in distillation. Jasmine flowers are picked by hand early in the morning and extracted as soon as possible by hexane, butane, pentane, petroleum ether, benzene, toluene or other similar solvent. The flowers are delicately distributed onto perforated trays in the extraction vessel and this is then immersed in the solvent. There is an art in the use of the correct number of solvent washes and the time of extraction. The extract is known as a concrete, after removal of the solvent; it is a very coloured, sometimes brownish, waxy mass and is usually viscous. The 'essential oil', or rather the more soluble components contained in this waxy concrete, are extracted by warming it with absolute ethanol at 45–60°C and then by chilling to −5 to −12°C to precipitate out the waxes. The resultant filtrate, separated by filtration, is called 'absolute' after recovery of the ethanol by distillation under reduced pressure. These absolutes are normally coloured as they still contain pigment and often have a proportion of waxes.

Resinous exudates (oleoresins) of myrrh, frankincense, benzoin and labdanum are extracted with solvents after processing to a small particle size and then filtered to remove the unwanted resin, bark, insects, earth, etc. Alternatively the oleoresins are steam distilled, although this yields a different product of a different odour.

Enfleurage

This ancient technique involves the uptake of the volatile oils into a fat layer, and is known to have been used in Ancient Egyptian times. Nowadays it is followed by solvent extraction, although it has largely been superseded due to the high cost of the procedure, low yield and new methods. Enfleurage was only suitable for flowers whose petals stayed alive for a few days after picking (e.g. rose and jasmine). The flowers are removed after a few days and fresh ones are introduced until the fat is saturated with the aroma chemicals.

Carbon dioxide extraction

At 33°C and 200 atm pressure carbon dioxide becomes hypercritical – a state in which it is neither really gas nor liquid, but has qualities of both. This makes it an excellent solvent to use in the extraction of essential oils because of the low temperature required and the fact that the process is near to instantaneous. Furthermore, the carbon dioxide is inert and therefore does not interact chemically with the essence that is being extracted. It is non-toxic, colourless and odourless. To remove the carbon dioxide solvent, you simply need to remove the pressure.

The actual temperature and pressure used is adjusted for different plant materials. To achieve a pressure of 200 atm some heavy-duty stainless steel equipment is required, which explains the high capital investment required for this extraction method. Nevertheless it is the preferred mode of extraction for the food industry (Moyler, 1993).

Expression

The expressed oils from citrus plants can only be very loosely included in the original essential oil definition; although the 'oil' can either just be expressed or obtained from the initial extract by distillation, the two methods yield essential oils with entirely different compositions.

Expression means the squeezing of the rinds of the citrus fruit, formerly done by hand, but now executed mechanically by scarification or compression. The essential oil is washed away with the juice and

pulp to centrifuges, where separation occurs. The citrus oils are unstable and antioxidants are usually added, often the more unpleasant butylhydroxy toluene (BHT) and butylhydroxy anisole (BHA), making the term natural or organic untenable. The expressed oils contain many non-volatile components, including waxes, pigments and, in many species, the phototoxic furanocoumarins. These are normally removed to yield furanocoumarin-free (FCF) oils, which should be used in preference, as there is a danger of sunburn if the skin is exposed to UV light after massaging with untreated citrus oils.

Phytols or hydrosols or distillation waters

The name 'phytonics' was coined by Wilde (1994) for a very energy-efficient process for making phytols, typically using less than 1% of the energy required to process by steam distillation, hydrocarbon extraction, chlorinated solvent extraction and supercritical carbon dioxide extraction. Phytosol solvents such as tetrafluoroethane (e.g. 'Florasol' (R134a)) are non-flammable and non-toxic. They are not ozone depleters and the boiling point of the extraction medium is −26°C inside sealed equipment, therefore continually recycled. The phytols are popular with flavour houses and pharmaceutical companies, as well as perfumery companies selling to customers who do not consume alcohol-containing products.

So-called 'hydrosols' or 'hydrolates' have only been introduced to aromatherapy in recent years, although rosewater and orange flower water have been commercially available for centuries. The vast majority of hydrosols go down the drain as waste-water from the distillation process as the cost of transportation makes them uneconomical to sell. Their production varies enormously depending on distillation techniques and countries of origin. For example in large production plants where distillation is carried out in 'closed' equipment, atmospheric contamination is unlikely; also the heat of distillation will pasteurise the water. The resulting hydrosol is therefore initially safe and uncontaminated with microbes. However, on opening the container, contamination can result immediately and the growth of microbes under conditions of ambient temperature ensures a good supply of potentially dangerous contaminants.

Hydrosols should only contain the water-soluble components of the essential oil being distilled. The more oxygenated components will greatly outnumber the hydrophobic terpenes. However, micro-emulsions and solubilised oil droplets may occur in the hydrosol; moreover, complex micro-emulsion can form and after a few days microbiological and chemical changes may occur to change the hydrosol. Also bear in mind some hydrosols on sale are not true hydrosols, they are essential oils solubilised in water with a surfactant. Obviously the composition of these fake hydrosols bears no relationship to true hydrosols.

As hydrosols can be contaminated by the atmosphere or by the unhygienic conditions in which many smaller stills are located, distillation waters become a microbial soup which can be pasteurised or filtered (as with milk) to make it safe and kept in a sealed bottle. Larger companies add preservatives (which are commonly used in foods), but this is not considered wholesome by some aromatherapists.

Non-genuine hydrosols

A hydrolate, or distillation water, can be home-produced simply by making an infusion of the herb and filtering it. These are sometimes offered for sale as hydrosols. Even freeze-dried herbal extracts reconstituted with water are common. Another way of cheating is to 'dissolve' some essential oil in water using a surfactant for emulsification; even a synthetic perfume compound can be used in this way. The most commonly adulterated hydrosol is rosewater.

Yield and cost of essential oils

The yield largely determines the price of an essential oil, as more plant material is required if the yield is low, thus putting up the price. For example, neroli is often adulterated or simply substituted by petitgrain, as neroli is distilled from the blossom of the *Citrus bigarade* tree and petitgrain from the leaves and branchlets of the same tree, and clearly, a much greater amount in weight of blossom would be required to produce the neroli oil than the petitgrain. This is compounded by the high cost of delicately picking the blossom by hand, compared with machine-picking the leaves and branchlets. Other expensive essential oils include: rose, violet leaf, jasmine, tuberose and other florals. These are mainly extracted with solvents to increase the yield.

Citrus oils

Orange oil is mostly produced as a by-product of the multi-million pound orange juice industry, instead of using cold expression. The residual essential oil is extracted with the juice and is then retrieved from the system by solvent extraction. Deliberate mislabelling, e.g. supplying Florida orange oil as the cheaper Brazilian orange oil at the higher price, is widespread.

The cost of an oil is dependent on its source and market forces due to low yield or lack of raw material. Table 4.2 gives some examples of prices, taking Brazilian orange oil as 1.0 (1993).

In general, the higher the price of an oil, the more likely it is to be adulterated. Adulteration is rampant in the essential oil industry and the purity of the oil is determined largely by the price the buyer is willing to pay. Blending can occur with the true botanical or other botanical or synthetic. Lemon oil, for example, is 10 times more expensive than orange oil, therefore blending can be with orange oil or orange by-products (e.g. terpenes), but still be labelled as natural lemon oil.

The hybridisation of citrus plants is complex and different hybrids are grown in different areas. For example, the sweet orange in Brazil is the Pera variety, in California the Navel; in Florida the Hamlin, Marrs, Parson Brown, Pineapple and Valencia are grown at different times to maximise production in that season. In Israel the Shamouti or Jaffa is grown. There are also 14 different tangerine types.

It is normal practice to graft onto hardy rootstocks. For example, in Italy they graft branches of

Table 4.2 Examples of relative prices for citrus oils (Brazilian is taken to be 1.0)

Sweet Orange	
Brazil	1.0
Florida	1.3
Israel	1.4
Spain	3.0
Lemon	
California	14.0
Italy	15.0
Greece	11.0

lemon onto bitter orange rootstocks, which are more frost-resistant. If the lemon is frost-damaged then more is simply grafted on. The rootstock can impart different characteristics to the essential oil.

Modification of the essential oil

The next variation in essential oils occurs in the hands of the producers and retailers. Once an essential oil is produced, it can be modified by rectification, deterpenation, cutting, substitution, dilution with various organic solvents (e.g. dipropyl glycol or alcohol) and even with petroleum spirits. Many of these adulterations result from necessity; for example the Umbelliferae oils such as fennel, carrot and dill have some unpleasant sulphurous compounds which come off with the fresh distillate and must therefore be removed, otherwise the essential oil would smell of rotten eggs.

Most essential oils have to be diluted in alcohol for perfumery, food additives/flavourings and therefore require some deterpenation to make them more soluble in the alcohol and also prevent tainting or precipitation. The stability of an essential oil is also improved by deterpenation and its shelf-life prolonged. The additional problem of toxicity associated with some essential oil components such as thujone can be undertaken by its removal from Dalmatian sage, etc. by specialised redistilling. The phototoxic furanocoumarins found in expressed citric oils are also removed in this way nowadays, resulting in safer orange, lemon, tangerine and other FCF citrus oils.

The following are all classified as essential oils at times.

1. A natural oil from named fruit and origin (e.g. lemon oil, Sicilian, 100% cold-pressed from *Citrus limonum*, Sicily)
2. A natural oil not from named fruit (e.g. lemon oil from orange oil and lemongrass oil)
3. Nature-identical (NI) oil (e.g. lemon flavouring oil from lemon terpenes, plus 33% synthetic citral, which is chemically identical to natural citral found in lemon)
4. Artificial oil (e.g. lemon artificial, containing only synthetic chemical(s) not found in nature), having the smell of citral-like geranonitrile (used in detergents, scourers, loo cleaners, etc.).

Standardisation

The ISO (International Organization for Standardization) is responsible for setting the standard composition for each essential oil, which has to be adhered to. The ISO may therefore indirectly be responsible for some of the blending, if not adulteration of essential oils in order to keep within their guidelines. Bearing in mind the natural variability of harvests, blending of essential oils from different harvests often occurs, as with wines. There is also the opportunity for the more unscrupulous producers to add some synthetic components or fractions from different plant oils.

Substances used to 'standardise' essential oils include:

- citral (ex *Litsea cubeba* oil or synthetic) to standardise lemon oil
- 1,8-cineole (ex *Eucalyptus globulus* oil) to standardise rosemary oil
- camphor (ex camphor oil) to standardise labiate oils.

Adulteration of essential oils

Adulterations commonly found in commercial essential oils

Adulteration is generally taken to mean the act of lowering the standard or character of a product by the addition of one or more inferior ingredients (BACIS Archives). It involves mainly: standardising, reinforcement, liquidising, reconstitution and commercialising.

- **Reinforcement** is an extension of standardising. When the quality of the natural isolates can be improved, there is always the temptation to add an exaggerated amount of the characteristic compound to improve the quality and to make the end product more 'olfactive value for money'.
- **Liquidising**: Some natural isolates are solids or semi-solids (e.g. gums, oleoresins and certain absolutes). To liquidise these materials a series of solvents are added, including benzyl benzoate, propylene glycol, triethyl citrate, isopropyl myristate, dialkyl phthalates and isononylphenol.
- **Reconstitution**: There are natural isolates, such as rose oil, jasmine oil or orange flower oil, which are too expensive for application in more economic (cheaper) functional perfumery (e.g. perfumes for

soap, detergents or other household products). Therefore these naturals are reconstituted – the natural isolate is rebuilt (compounded) with a mixture of natural or so-called 'nature-identical' chemical compounds; however, only the main components are usually added out of a possible 2–300 found in the natural essential oil.

- **Commercialising** means lowering of the quality of an essential oil in order to make it more profitable for the producer. The 'reconstituted oils' are also examples of 'commercial oils'. Sometimes genuine natural isolates are diluted with reconstituted ones. Sometimes a buyer cannot afford to pay the price of the natural, therefore is willing to buy a commercialised product; but real fraudulent commercialising also exists.

Rose oil can be reconstructed to produce a product very similar to the natural oil (Wabner, 1994). This is not a problem unless it is sold as a natural oil – which aside from being unscrupulous, would attract a rather high profit margin. Synthetic substances such as diethylphthalate (DEP), a plasticiser used in plastics and paints in a great number of industrial processes, has been found in some rose essential oils being sold as 'pure' (Wabner, 1994). Indeed, DEP has been found in many plant extracts due to its use in herbicides and insecticides.

Tolu balsam (*Myroxylon balsamum*) could be a sensitiser itself, but the commercial product in fact consists of benzoin resinoid, styrax resinoids and synthetic chemicals such as benzyl cinnamate, benzyl benzoate, cinnamic acid, benzoic acid, etc. which could account for the sensitisation (Sheppard-Hanger and Burfield, 1999).

Lavender oil is one of the most popular oils used in aromatherapy. However, there is usually much more 'pure' lavender sold in the course of a year than is actually produced. A recent *Which?* Report (2001) showed that out of the numerous 'lavender' oils they had tested several were labelled with the wrong Latin names; the names did not match the essential oil, for example lavandin was labelled as a true lavender *L. angustifolia* in several cases.

The same *Which?* Report found an oil labelled as sandalwood essential oil that was actually a synthetic sandalwood perfume base – santal – used as a sandalwood fragrance in toiletries.

In one study, aromatic drugs reported in the *European Pharmacopoeia*, including absinth, anise, Roman chamomile, German chamomile, cinnamon, fennel, clove, peppermint, sage and thyme, were bought at pharmacies, herbalist's shops, or supermarkets and then subjected to essential oil analysis. The analysed samples were very far from the acceptable qualitative standards, which strongly suggested that they definitely lacked any health benefits (Miraldi *et al.*, 2001).

Note that '100% pure essential oil' on a label does not mean that the contents are unadulterated: pure essential oils of a lesser quality/cost may be added from a different species. Peppermint oil is often adulterated with the cheaper cornmint oil, for example. As the colour test for menthofuran remains the same, this can be difficult to detect even when adulteration is as high as 85% (Lis-Balchin, 1995). In some cases adulteration with a cheaper oil is due to the fact that the more expensive oil is in very short supply. For example, fermented oil from gin manufacture is usually sold as juniper berry oil with components such as the pinenes, camphene and myrcene and lesser priced oils such as juniper wood and juniper twig oil being added (Lis-Balchin, 1995).

In addition to being the most expensive of the various varieties of chamomile essential oil available, German chamomile is easily distinguishable by its deep blue colour. Unfortunately synthetic chamazulene is often added to maintain the colour, thus, in the eyes of most aromatherapists, assuring the quality. Synthetic chamazulene can also be added to a cheap chamomile like Moroccan (which is chemically completely different) and can lull the unsuspecting purchaser into believing they are buying the more expensive oil (Lis-Balchin, 1995; see also Appendix 8).

Detection of adulteration

There are a few visible signs of potential adulteration: a cloudy appearance or an unusual viscosity may sometimes be seen. The smell of the oil can be revealing, but only if the aromatherapist is familiar with the real essential oil odour. There are also a number of laboratory tests that can determine if an essential oil is adulterated, but an aromatherapist who purchases relatively small quantities of oils (with bulk ordering being at least 25 kg per oil) it is very expensive to have the oils independently tested. While it should be up to the supplier to provide paperwork validating the quality of the oil, unless an independent test is done for each batch, there is no guarantee that the oil supplied has the specifications indicated. Customers are often given gas chromatograph traces that are many years old, as new tests for each batch would be very expensive for the supplier; they would also take weeks to be done by specialist university departments or even private companies. The cost of a simple analysis of an essential oil by gas chromatography is around £25 in the UK; a more extensive analysis by gas chromatography/mass spectrometry (GC/MS) costs upwards of £50 (personal experience).

Material Safety Data Sheets

In the UK it is a legal requirement for the supplier to provide an MSDS (Material Safety Data Sheet) for each essential oil. A typical MSDS contains the following in respect of the oil specification:

- Organoleptic description
- Botanical name and origin
- Typical GC/MS profile (major peaks)
- SG (specific gravity)
- RI (refractive index)
- OR (optical rotation)
- FP (flash point).

Some companies will also supply legislative conformity, if it exists: CAS numbers (Chemical Abstracts Service Registry) for each essential oil and component. FEMA (the Flavor and Extract Manufacturers Associations of the USA) is a good source of all information.
    Standards are supplied by:

- BP (British Pharmacopoeia)
- EP (European Pharmacopoeia)
- USP (United States Pharmacopoeia)
- ISO (International Organization for Standardization)
- IFRA (International Fragrance Research Association)
- IFEAT (International Federation of Essential oils and Aroma Trade).

Other information, such as country of origin, method of extraction, and 'best before' date should also be available on request if it is not already indicated on the packaging or paperwork.

Appearance of the oil

This can indicate poor quality. Transparency and colour are a good guide.

Viscosity

This varies from oil to oil with some essential oils, e.g. sandalwood, vetivert and amyris, being very viscous and difficult to get any drops out of the bottle. Orris oil is virtually solid at room temperature and so is attar of roses, if cold, especially when stored in the refrigerator (due to the 20% of stearoptene, a crystalline wax which is part of the distilled rose oil). Such essential oils are best dispensed when warmed up, often just by holding the bottle in the hand. Increased viscosity can indicate oxidation and an 'aged' oil.

Fixed oils

Identification of adulteration using fixed oils is simple: a drop of the sample on blotting paper or a piece of cloth will show a halo of grease on evaporation of the essential oil, usually after a few hours. Pure essential oils evaporate completely.

Other essential oil tests

Testing of specific gravity (SG), refractive index (RI), optical rotation, acid value and ester value will all reveal useful information but these cannot be done by aromatherapists, who have to rely on the supplier.

Gas chromatography and enantiomeric columns

Ordinary gas chromatography can be used to detect solvents such as DPG (dipropyl glycol, a common diluent), when they are used in reasonable quantities, if one knows where to look for them. Gas chromatography, also known as gas–liquid chromatography, originated as paper chromatography which was used for separating coloured pigments of plants. Paper could not be used to separate volatiles such as essential oils, therefore a glass tube, stoppered at one end with glass wool and containing granules of aluminium oxide, moistened with alcohol was devised. The granules formed the 'stationary phase', whilst a solvent, which was poured into the tube, formed the 'moving phase' for separating pigments. The solvent was replaced by a gas, such as hydrogen or helium, for essential oils. In gas–liquid chromatography the original adsorption of pigments onto the aluminium oxide was substituted by a process of partition of the molecules onto the stationary phase.

The original GC columns were very short and relatively wide, and separation of the components travelling through the column was very poor, with many components eluting together. Longer and finer silica columns were therefore introduced, which are from 25 to 100 m in length with an internal diameter (i.d.) of 0.25–0.32 mm. These columns are coiled in order to take up less space in the 'oven', where the temperature can be changed according to a set computer program.

One end of the column is attached to a metal injection device, which has a fine hole to allow the injection of 1 μL of essential oil. Total vaporisation of the essential oil occurs at this point due to the high temperature of the oven or electrically heated injection site. At this point there is an attachment for the gas supply, the carrier gas, which carries the vaporised essential oil through the column. At the end of this is a detector device, which can detect the different components passing out of the column. Detectors can work via ionisation, infra-red (IR) or other means. The components detected cause variations in, for example, the current, and this is amplified to cause a suitable pen recorder to record changes in the current (corresponding to a component appearing) on a sheet of paper. The resulting peak areas are proportional to the concentration of each component emerging.

The distance from the start of each peak (retention time, RT) is an indication of its chemical composition. The RT for each component is determined by using single components injected under the same conditions. Each instrument has to be calibrated for a particular column (its length, i.d., and the particular computerised conditions of elution). It is therefore almost impossible to identify separated components unless all the factors are given. Gas chromatograms presented to buyers of essential oils are therefore usually completely useless unless the person is an expert in the field.

Ordinary gas chromatography can be combined with mass spectrometry (MS) or other identification facilities, such as infra-red (IR), making identification of components more accurate. In mass spectrometry, the eluted component is bombarded by a stream of electrons, which causes the component to lose one of its electrons. This gives positively charged molecular ions of the same molecular weight as the original component. A proportion of these ions break up into positively charged fragments, which are accelerated by an electrostatic field. They are then swept at very high velocity towards a detector in a curved pathway. The lighter the particles, the greater the deflection. The fragmentation patterns of these proportions of ions of different mass give the molecular structure to an expert in the field. The identification of components using this technique is very complex as the purity of the component makes an enormous difference to the results obtained. Any components which were not completely separated by the gas chromatography column will be almost impossible to identify.

GC/MS, even at its best, is still not sophisticated enough to detect most adulterations of essential oils in which fractions of other oils or synthetic components are used. Adulteration with synthetic linalool and/or linalyl acetate can be detected in lavender oil, for example, by the presence of dehydrolinalool, dihydrolinalool, dehydrolinalyl acetate and dihydrolinalyl acetate, which are not normally present (BACIS Archives). Otherwise, normal gas chromatography or GC/MS does not detect the use of synthetics, as these components are chemically identical to the natural ones.

The determination of synthetic adulteration of essential oils was perfected by the use of special enantiomeric or chiral columns, which are used to detect stereochemical isomers (those rotating polarised light either to the right or left) of certain chemical components like the pinenes, limonene, citronellol, etc. which differ in their proportions in different plants (Ravid et al., 1992). These enantiomeric columns are mainly composed of an α-cyclodextrin phase (Lis-Balchin et al., 1998a, 1999). The actual proportion of the right (+) to the left (−) isomer can indicate the degree of adulteration, for example of lemon oil by lemongrass. Synthetic components are usually relatively easy to detect as they are invariably a racemic mixture (i.e. there is 50% of each isomer). Ravid et al. (1992) showed that lavender oil had (3R)-(−)-linalyl acetate of an optical purity of 93% and Mosandl and Schubert (1990) showed that another genuine lavender oil had 100% R-(−)-linalyl acetate. One of the major components, citronellol, occurs in the (−)-form in geranium and rose oils and has a finer rose odour than the (+)-enantiomer, and a sweet, peach-like flavour. The (+)-citronellol enantiomer has been found in citronella oils from Ceylon and Java, *Cymbopogon winterianus*, *Boronia citriodora*, *Eucalyptus citriodora*, Spanish verbena and other essential oils.

The two enantiomers are starting materials for numerous chiral pheromones and flavours (Ravid *et al.*, 1992) and are prepared commercially by partial or total synthesis, sometimes involving particular yeast strains. This abundance of the citronellol lends itself to adulteration on a grand scale. Initial analyses of commercial Egyptian geranium oil yielded almost a racemic mixture of citronellol enantiomers, whilst a true Bourbon oil gave a highly concentrated *S*-(−)-citronellol (Ravid *et al.*, 1992). Recent studies on Australian geranium oils grown from specific *Pelargonium* clones showed that, using ten key chiral components and calculating a so-called 'chiral excess', it was possible to distinguish geographically different and seasonally different essential oils and also adulteration (Doimo *et al.*, 1999).

It is worth noting that chiral columns can also be used by unscrupulous synthetic chemists involved in adulteration of essential oils, as the same type of column can be used to separate out the enantiomers, which could then be added in the correct proportion for a given essential oil!

Differences between essential oil samples using bioactivity criteria as proof of adulteration

Other methods of detecting adulteration involve pharmacological investigations and antimicrobial testing (Lis-Balchin *et al.*, 1996a, 1998a, 1999). The latter tests have been found to be highly sensitive in distinguishing between different commercial geranium oils. Differences in chemical composition between different batches from the same source and/or supplier or different sources were also found for both multiple samples of peppermint (Lis-Balchin *et al.*, 1997c) and geranium oils (Lis-Balchin *et al.*, 1996b). The 14 peppermint samples (of relative low cost) did not vary as much as the 16 samples of geranium oil (high cost), labelled Chinese, Egyptian, Bourbon and Moroccan, where there was a wide range of citronellol and geraniol levels, with the ratio of citronellol:geraniol ranging from 1.7 to 10.9. The antibacterial activity against 25

different bacteria varied between samples of oil, ranging from 8 to 19 inhibited; this was also reflected in a further study (Lis-Balchin *et al.*, 1996b) against 20 different strains of *Listeria monocytogenes*, ranging from 3 to 16. In antifungal studies, the geranium samples varied from 0 to 94% inhibition of *Aspergillus niger*, 12–95% against *A. ochraceus* and 40–86% against *Fusarium culmorum*.

A pure, non-commercial sample of geranium oil obtained directly from the grower/distiller had low bioactivities in general compared with most of the other samples (Lis-Balchin *et al.*, 1996b) whereas the bioactivities of synthetic citronellol and geraniol, used singly or in mixtures, were conversely very high. This suggests that adulteration of most of the samples of commercial geranium oil had occurred using synthetic citronellol and geraniol.

The adulteration of volatile oils with synthetic components may give rise to a different proportion of enantiomers than in a pure botanical sample: this can greatly influence the bioactivity of the subsequent material (Lis-Balchin *et al.*, 1996c, 1999) if used therapeutically.

Conclusion

Pure essential oils are hard to find. Recent European Union legislation (see Chapter 7) has probably arisen due to the gross adulteration of essential oils over the years, which has produced increasing incidences of dermatitis and other sensitisations. The use of the various toxic diluents and synthetic components, which are often accompanied by minute amounts of undesirable and toxic products of the synthetic reactions, has no doubt added to the problem. However, the industries have now devised new formulations in their perfumery/cosmetics range, which exclude the sensitisers but now include new synthetic components to take their place. Doubtless many of these substitutions will become sensitisers in due course.

5

The bioactivity of essential oils

Introduction

Due to the varied uses of 'aromatherapy' the question of the purpose of aromatherapy needs to be answered. Is it to cure illnesses, make one beautiful, kill the 'bad' bugs, or something else? There is probably no common answer, but there are several known bioactivities of essential oils, which may provide some evidence of efficacy in a given field:

- Psychological/physiological effects (see Chapter 6)
- Pharmacological effects
- Antimicrobial effects
- Other miscellaneous effects.

Pharmacological studies on essential oils: *in vivo* and *in vitro*

Aromatherapists use the term 'relaxant (sedative)' and 'stimulant' when using various essential oils in massage. These terms are very general and therefore difficult to define: is the effect simply a psychological one, or a physiological one involving pharmacological effects? Furthermore, if pharmacological, then on what tissues? Can one group all these together? It seems illogical to group the muscles together in view of the fact that the skeletal and smooth muscles are under different hormonal and nerve control systems, as is the heart muscle.

Differences between species in metabolism and percutaneous absorption (Garnett *et al.*, 1994) make comparisons difficult between humans and animals and this is of great relevance in extrapolating studies done mainly in animals. Dogs and cats are especially susceptible to tea tree oil: when rubbed on their backs it acts as a neurotoxin, causing paralysis of the limbs, often quadriplegia, lasting about 12–24 hours

(Villar *et al.*, 1994). This suggests caution when used in humans, especially in young children. Babies should of course be completely excluded.

Comparison of the effects of different essential oils on the guinea-pig ileum with those on the rat ileum shows in many cases a completely opposite effect. For example, angelica root and aniseed both give a contraction in the guinea-pig but a relaxation in the rat (Table 5.1). This shows that there are interspecies differences in the effects of essential oils.

Clearly there is no simple way in which to extrapolate effects accurately between different species such as humans and rodents. Table 5.1 also shows different effects in different tissues of the rat, including the stomach, caecum and vas deferens: the differences in these tissues do not differ too greatly from that of the ileum in the rat, but not the ileum in the guinea-pig. The effect of different essential oils is also often different in skeletal muscle and uterus compared with that of the smooth muscle of the ileum in the guinea-pig *in vitro* (see Appendix 3).

Effects on smooth muscle

Comparative studies in the guinea-pig ileum *in vitro* have shown that many essential oils are either spasmogenic or spasmolytic (see Appendix 2). For example, angelica root, camphor, lemon, nutmeg and orange are spasmogenic, whilst three *Eucalyptus* species, manuka and spike lavender are spasmolytic. Other studies have shown that anise, fennel, caraway and orange were spasmogenic (Hof-Mussler, 1990), plus aloysia and some parsley essential oils (Lis-Balchin *et al.*, 1996a; Lis-Balchin and Hart, 2002).

Many essential oils show both effects: the spasmogenic effect comes first followed by the spasmolytic phase. This suggests that the initial spasmogenic effect in essential oils is apparently shown by components

Table 5.1 The effect of different essential oils on different tissues in the rat compared to that in the ileum of guinea-pig

Essential oil	Ileum		Rat		
	Guinea-pig	Rat	Stomach	Caecum	Vas deferens
Angelica root	***	!!	NA	!!!	!+
Aniseed	**!	!	!	!!! or*	!+
Camphor	***	!	!	!!!	NA
Celery	***	!	!	!!!	!+
Chamomile, blue	!!	!!!	!!!	!!	!!!
Clary sage	***	NA	!	!!!	!
Dill	++!	NA	!!	!!	!+
Fennel	***	!	!!!	!!	!!!
Frankinsence	***	!!!	!!!	!!!	NA
Geranium	!!	NA	!	!!!	!!
Jasmine absolute	!!	NA	!!!	NA	!
Kanuka	**!	!	!!!	!!!	**
Lavender French	!!	NA	!	NA	!!+
Lemon	***	!	nil+	!!!	nil+
Manuka	!!!	NA	NA	!!!	!
Nutmeg	***	!!!	!!	!!!	!!
Orange	***	!!!	!!	!!!	!+
Petitgrain	**	!!!	NA	!	NA
Parsley	**!	NA	!	!!!	!
Peppermint	!!!	NA	NA	!!	NA
Rose absolute	!	NA	!!	NA	!!!
Rosemary	***	!!!	!	!	!
Thyme	!	NA	!!!	!	NA

All diluted ×1000 except when marked +, where diluted ×100.
NA = not assayed.
* Contraction; *** very pronounced contraction; ! relaxation; !!! pronounced relaxation.
From: Lis-Balchin (1997) unpublished data.

with a high volatility. Angelica, basil, bay, bergamot, cajuput, camphor, celery, clary sage, dill, frankinsence, kanuka, lemon, myrtle, nutmeg, petitgrain, pine-needle, rosemary, tea tree and verbena essential oils have an initial strong spasmogenic effect followed by a weaker spasmolytic effect, whilst Roman chamomile has a spasmogenic effect followed by an equal spasmolytic phase (Lis-Balchin *et al.*, 1996d).

The reasons for these differences lie in the chemical composition of the essential oils (see Appendix 4) and the effects of different individual components on the smooth muscle of guinea-pigs. Components that were solely spasmolytic included: azulene, borneol, carvacrol, caryophyllene, citral, citronellal, citronellol, citronellyl formate, eugenol, fenchone, geraniol, guaiadiene, ionone, linalool, linalyl acetate, menthol, methyl eugenol, nerol, perialdehyde, pulegone and thujone; many of these were esters, alcohols, aldehydes and also sesquiterpenes. Components with spasmogenic

properties with/without spasmolysis included 3-carene, 1,8-cineole, *p*-cymene, geranyl acetate, geranyl formate, isomenthone, limonene, linalyl butyrate, menthone, myrcene, α-pinene, β-pinene, α-terpinene, γ-terpinene. The presence of monoterpenes seemed to be a major cause of spasmogenic activity.

Some of the single components also showed a double effect, i.e. a spasmogenic phase followed by a spasmolytic phase: these include many esters and even monoterpenes. The reason for this biphasic effect is unexplained, but could be due to small impurities in the commercial components or some metabolic changes occurring during the experiment.

Other studies showed that spasmolytic essential oils (presented mixed with Arlatone 285 to the small intestine *in vitro*) included: melissa, basil, bitter orange, angelica, chamomile (unknown species), carnation (an absolute), caraway, ginger, clove, pepper, nutmeg, cinnamon, cardamom and the components: eugenol, eugenyl acetate, caryophyllene, caryophyllene oxide, *cis*-citral, *trans*-citral, linalool and citronellal (Brandt, 1988). Emulsions of 1% peppermint, sage (Dalmatian) and rosemary (in Tween at 0.0001% in water) caused spasmolysis (Taddei *et al.*, 1988).

Camphor was reported to be a 'stimulating oil' (Wagner and Sprinkmeyer, 1973), which also stimulates circulation; however, camphor caused a spasmolytic action on smooth muscle *in vitro* (see Appendix 2). Sedative oils and components included: melissa, valerian, lavender and calamus; also citral, limonene, linalool, geraniol, citronellal and citronellol (Wagner and Sprinkmeyer, 1973).

In contrast to the aromatherapists' view of it being relaxant, an initial contraction is often observed with commercial lavender essential oil before the spasmolytic action occurs (Lis-Balchin *et al.*, 1996a) and this is probably due to the presence of 1,8-cineole and α- and β-pinene, which have been shown to contract guinea-pig ileum (see Appendix 2; Lis-Balchin and Hart, 1997b). Clary sage, another relaxant essential oil for aromatherapists, also has an initial spasmogenic action (Appendix 2).

Effects on bronchial muscle

Essential oil actions on bronchial muscle often reflect that on the ileum (Reiter and Brandt, 1985; Brandt, 1988). The actions of several essential oils and their components on tracheal and intestinal smooth muscle were spasmolytic, with intestinal muscle being more sensitive than tracheal. Spasmogenic oils included anise, fennel, sage, cassia, clove and black caraway, at concentrations lower than those causing relaxation, which suggests a solvent effect rather than the essential oils themselves. Components causing relaxation in the trachea included: β-caryophyllene, caryophyllene oxide, cinnamaldehyde, *cis*-citral, *trans*-citral, citronellal, citronellol, eugenol, eugenyl acetate, geraniol, limonene, nerol and linalool and α- and β-pinene. Caryophyllene oxide and anethole caused contractions in the trachea and eugenol was spasmogenic at concentrations lower than those causing relaxation (see also Appendix 2).

Mode of action on smooth muscle

All samples of so-called 'relaxant essential oils' studied by the author (e.g. floral oils like lavender,

geranium and the many types of other *Pelargonium* floral-scented oils, peppermint, manuka and jasmine absolute) have a myogenic action on guinea-pig ileum (Lis-Balchin *et al.*, 1996a; Lis-Balchin and Hart, 1999a,b). They apparently do not affect nerve conduction (local anaesthetic action) or the release of acetylcholine (as seen with opioids such as morphine which act by inhibiting the release of acetylcholine) but act directly on the smooth muscle (Izzo *et al.*, 1996; Lis-Balchin *et al.*, 1996a, 1997a, 1998a,b; Lis-Balchin and Hart, 1999a,b). None of the extracts studied possessed atropine-like activity nor did they appear to contain a chemical which stimulates adrenoceptors. Lavender oil and one of its components, linalool, and other floral essential oils including many species of *Pelargonium* appear to mediate a spasmolytic action on intestinal smooth muscle via a rise in cAMP (Lis-Balchin *et al.*, 1997a; Lis-Balchin and Hart, 1998a) as a result of the stimulation of adenylate cyclase (an enzyme which activates the ATP into its cyclic cAMP form, which now becomes a secondary messenger). The duration of action of the cAMP so produced is limited by its metabolism by phosphodiesterase (this enzyme is decreased by stimulants such as caffeine in coffee). Other essential oils with a more balsamic or medicinal odour do not use this pathway (Lis-Balchin and Hart, 1998b) and the stimulation of guanylate cyclase does not appear to be involved. Potassium channel opening has not been shown to be involved with any essential oil or component in their mode of action (Lis-Balchin and Hart, 1999a,b).

Calcium channel involvement for a number of essential oils has been reviewed (Neuhaus-Carlisle *et al.*, 1993, 1997; Vuorela *et al.*, 1997), but the number of essential oils is small and one cannot generalise that most essential oils use this mode of action and mainly components have been studied so far. For a number of essential oils (Lis-Balchin and Hart, 1999b) calcium channel involvement is apparent only at very high concentrations, except for valerian oil (Lis-Balchin, 2002b, ch.11), which is a very strong sedative, unlike the floral essential oils described before, which use cAMP. Peppermint essential oil and menthol block Ca^{2+} channels in the rat and guinea-pig small intestinal smooth muscle, cardiac muscle and chick neuronal preparations (Hawthorn *et al.*, 1988); peppermint essential oil, however, did not show this ability at lower concentrations in the guinea-pig ileum in another study (Lis-Balchin and Hart, 1999b). The use of different methodologies in different studies and different samples of essential oils can have a great effect on the results. The calcium-blocking activity in rat pituitary GH4C4 cells was best shown by methanolic and chloroform extracts of *Angelica archangelica* root extracts (Harmala *et al.*, 1992a,b), compared with more water-soluble extracts and other solvent extracts. The former extracts could contain some essential oils, but the results cannot be said to mean that essential oils have Ca^{2+}-blocking activity *per se*.

Effects on smooth muscle *in vitro*: the correlation with holistic effects in humans

There is considerable correlation between the effects of different essential oils and mixtures of essential oils on the smooth muscle of the guinea-pig ileum *in vitro* and their chemistry (see Appendices 11 and 12). Simply taking the times of elution of components off an OV1 gas chromatography (GC) column, where the most volatile components come off first, a table was constructed to show the different types of components being eluted at different mean times (Appendix 13). Monoterpenes were eluted at under 10 minutes; mainly oxygenated terpenes (aldehydes, ketones and esters) were grouped into those eluted at mean times of 11–15, 16–20 and 21–30 minutes. Mainly sesquiterpenes were eluted after 30 minutes.

It was found that spasmogenic effects were shown if there was a substantial concentration of the components eluted under 10 minutes (i.e. monoterpenes). The spasmogenic components in the essential oil include the pinenes and other small hydrocarbon monoterpenes, which are the most volatile (and the first to come off an OV1 GC column). The higher the percentage of such monoterpenes, the greater the spasmogenic effect. Oxygenated monoterpenes, such as the aldehydes and ketones etc., come off the GC column later and are associated with a relaxant effect. This is also the case with sesquiterpenes, which come off much later. It follows that the higher the concentration of these relaxant components, the greater overall relaxant effect. The results also indicate that there can be an initial spasmogenic effect followed by relaxation where there is both a considerable quantity of spasmogenic components and also relaxant ones. The use of mixtures of essential oils also showed that the total concentration of the spasmogenic and spasmolytic components gave rise to the final effect (see Appendix 13; Lis-Balchin and Hart, 1997a). If the

total concentration of spasmolytic components grossly outnumbered the spasmogenic components, there was a strong spasmolytic effect.

A correlation is also shown between the predicted effect on the client if the essential oils are massaged into the skin, and both the chemistry and effect on the smooth muscle *in vitro* (see Appendices 11–13; Lis-Balchin and Hart, 1997a). This also applies to mixtures of essential oils. The results indicate that the smooth muscle of the guinea-pig *in vitro* almost reflects the actions of chemicals on the brain and 'whole' person, as first remarked upon by the physiologist WDM Paton (1954), meaning that many of the effects on this 5 cm tissue preparation *in vitro* can be extrapolated to the human body as a whole. This substantiates the relevance of animal experiments to physiological/psychological effects in humans, but will not please those aromatherapists who do not approve of any animal experiments.

Effects on uterine muscle

The effect of different essential oils on the guinea-pig ileum and rat uterus *in vitro* illustrates again that it is impossible to generalise as to the effects of essential oils on different tissues (Appendix 3). All the studied essential oils caused a relaxant effect on the spontaneous contractions of the rat uterus *in vitro*; this effect was also shown by the majority of essential oil components studied (Appendix 4). There is a possibility that the same process could occur in human uterine tissue. It therefore indicates that caution in the usage of essential oils should be paramount, especially for one of the most vulnerable groups, i.e. women during parturition. As the essential oils studied caused a decrease in the force of the contractions, leading to total cessation of the contractions in the rat, they could possibly cause a cessation of the birth process in the human, putting both the fetus/baby and the mother in jeopardy. Experiments during different phases of the rat menstrual cycle showed considerable differences in effect (Lis-Balchin and Hart, 1997b), suggesting that the effects of essential oils could also change during the course of a human pregnancy. There could possibly be a contractile effect on the uterus by some essential oils during pregnancy, which could cause an abortion of the fetus.

The effect of blends of three or more essential oils showed mainly a relaxant effect on uterine muscle

(Appendix 5), but a few cases of an initial contraction followed by spasmolysis were seen.

Note: Research carried out to date suggests that there is possible danger in the use of essential oils during pregnancy and childbirth. For example, lavender oil (which is used frequently) and its components (linalool, linalyl acetate, α- and β-pinene and 1,8-cineole) caused a reduction in uterine activity at concentrations that are spasmolytic on intestinal muscle. The response to French lavender oil depended upon the oestrus state of the rat from which the uterus was removed (Lis-Balchin and Hart, 1997b). In pro-oestrus, lavender reduced spontaneous activity, whilst in oestrus there was a slow increase in the amplitude of the spontaneous activity. There are therefore variabilities occurring during the 3-day oestrus cycle itself and it is not clear as yet what variability could occur during the whole of pregnancy in the rat, let alone the human.

Effects on skeletal muscle

Due to aromatherapy massage being the main form of essential oil administration, the effect on skeletal muscles would be important if the essential oil was absorbed or had a local effect. The actions on skeletal muscle *in vitro* again proved to be different for different essential oils, using the chick biventer cervices or the rat phrenic nerve hemi-diaphragm and either stimulating the phrenic nerve or the muscle directly (Lis-Balchin and Hart, 1997c). A contracture and inhibition of the twitch response to nerve stimulation was produced by clary sage, dill, fennel, frankincense and nutmeg; thyme (thymol high) produced just a contracture, camphor increased the twitch and angelica at the same concentration showed no response (Lis-Balchin and Hart, 1997c). Lavender oil reduced the twitch alone and the action would appear to be myogenic; however, another interpretation was that the essential oil of *Lavandula angustifolia* and its components linalool and linalyl acetate showed local anaesthetic action during pregnancy (Ghelardini *et al.*, 1999). Linalyl acetate caused an increase in the baseline or resting tone, whilst limonene caused a rise in tone, with a decrease in the size of the contractions (Lis-Balchin and Hart, 1997c). A decrease in the twitch when the diaphragm was stimulated directly was obtained using German chamomile, aniseed, manuka, ylang ylang, rose oil, tea tree and geranium.

Using the phrenic nerve–diaphragm preparation (i.e. stimulating the nerve), rosemary increased the twitch, whilst German chamomile, manuka, aniseed, jasmine and ylang ylang decreased the twitch; petitgrain and *Leptospermum citratum* both decreased the twitch and caused a rise in tone, whilst thyme oil caused only a massive increase in tone (Lis-Balchin and Hart, 1997c). These variabilities in essential oil action suggest a complex mechanism of action (Lis-Balchin, 2002b, ch.11).

Absorption of essential oils from skin application

The whole basis of aromatherapy for many aromatherapists is that the essential oils pass into the body from the skin and go to target organs, where they specifically cure illnesses. There is virtually no proof for this. There are, however, a few older studies on the disappearance of essential oils from the skin surface (Appendix 18). Valette (1946–7) studied the 'absorption' of 0.01 mL essential oils from the shaved abdomen of rabbits; the essential oil was covered with a glass which was attached to the skin with a gelatinous substance (Appendix 18). This disappearance, however, does not indicate that the essential oils are absorbed as such. Different components in each essential oil will be absorbed at different times. Some components may never be absorbed. Scientifically, the absorption of a compound is indicated by the appearance of the compound in the blood, not its disappearance from the surface of the skin.

Absorption of chemicals from the skin therefore must first be into the blood and thence to other organs (Appendix 17). The absorption of linalool and linalyl acetate into the blood after percutaneous massage of lavender essential oil was investigated by Jager *et al.* (1992). It had been previously shown that 1,8-cineole appeared in the blood after both oral intake and inhalation of rosemary essential oil (Kovar *et al.*, 1987). The absorption of the sandalwood component α-santalol into the blood after inhalation was shown later (Jirovetz *et al.*, 1992). Components are absorbed into the blood in very small concentrations (nanogram amounts), which could be at the physiological level of application in aromatherapy, and this small concentration is often difficult to estimate using even the most sophisticated equipment. For example, $(-)$-R-carvone, found in large amounts in spearmint leaves, easily passes from skin to blood, attaining maximum plasma concentrations of 25–35 ng/mL in 30 minutes, depending on the different massage techniques used (Fuchs *et al.*, 1997). This experiment was carried out in human volunteers wearing oxygen masks to avoid inhalation. If an occlusion wrap was used, the elimination half-life was significantly higher. There is some doubt whether such low concentrations of components in the blood could influence any organ.

Not much is known about the bioavailability, metabolism and excretion of many essential oils or their components. It is usually assumed that essential oils follow similar patterns to other lipophilic drugs. This is all influenced by an individual's own physiology and metabolism; also there may be the added effect of diet, external factors and also other drugs taken.

The actual absorption is influenced by the temperature, humidity, damage to the skin surface, viscosity of individual essential oils and components, volatility of essential oils (the more volatile the greater the rate of absorption), water, ethanol, skin occlusion, soaps, detergents, etc. There is more information on the effect of essential oils on the absorption of drugs through the skin than on the absorption of essential oils *per se* (see percutaneous absorption enhancers below).

Once the essential oil components are absorbed into the blood they will be distributed according to their physicochemical properties. It is assumed that this follows the pattern of lipid-soluble particles: the brain and other lipid-rich organs and tissues will take up a greater proportion of the more highly fat-soluble components; more water-soluble components will stay longer in the blood and be taken up by organs like the kidneys and skeletal muscle which have a rapid blood flow through them. Biotransformations or detoxifications probably occur in various tissues, especially the liver.

Many compounds bind to plasma albumin in the blood and are therefore sequestered for a time: it is unknown whether essential oil components react in the same way as chemicals with aldehydic, ketonic and carboxylic acid functional groups. Binding of components to plasma proteins can dislodge their natural components and may cause, for example, jaundice. It is unknown whether this does actually occur, but seems unlikely as only minute concentrations of essential oil components have been found in the blood. Phase I and II reactions could presumably occur as with other chemicals and there is some evidence that safrole, citral

and linalool enhance liver enzymes *in vitro* (Roffey *et al.*, 1990). The phase I reactions include redox and hydrolysis and phase II reactions involve conjugation with numerous normal metabolites (e.g. glucuronic acid, glutathione, phosphates, acetyl CoA, etc.). Both these phases increase the water-solubility of the component and enable it to be excreted by the kidney. However, some essential oil components are excreted by the lungs; for example, garlic rubbed on the foot is smelt soon after in the breath.

Studies on some toxicities have revealed that metabolism of at least some essential oil components occurs. D-Pulegone is metabolised in the liver to a very reactive metabolite which binds to components of liver cells and destroys them. And just as liver enzymes can be induced by some components, inhibition can also occur. For example, D-pulegone destroys cytochrome P_{450} *in vitro* (Moorthy, 1991).

Excretion of essential oil components occurs mainly via the kidneys and 70% of components like D-limonene appear in the urine within 72 hours with only 7% in the faeces after oral dosage (Igimi *et al.*, 1974).

There is some evidence to suggest that dermal application of essential oils gives rise to higher concentrations of components in the blood (Tisserand and Balacs, 1995), but this may not be in concentrations high enough to provoke physiological effects directly. Therefore it is unclear exactly how essential oils can have a beneficial physiological effect when applied to the skin surface: the effects are described and discussed under psychological effects (see Chapter 6). The effects of inhalation of essential oils are somewhat more direct and are mostly attributed to the primary effect of odour via the brain, with secondary physiological actions directed from there (see Chapter 6).

Percutaneous absorption enhancers

Many studies have been carried out to investigate the use of essential oils and components (e.g. limonene, L-menthol, (+/−)-linalool and carvacrol) in improving the absorption of drugs (Takayama and Nagai, 1994; Kunta *et al.*, 1997). Percutaneous absorption enhancement of propranolol hydrochloride through pig epidermis by various terpenes was shown *in vitro* (Zhao and Singh, 1999). Pretreatment of epidermal membranes with sesquiterpene oils or solid sesquiter-penes saturated in dimethyl isosorbide increased the rate of absorption of the model hydrophilic permeant 5-fluorouracil (5-FU) (Cornwell and Barry, 1994). Enhancers with polar functional groups were generally more potent than pure hydrocarbons; pretreatment with nerolidol caused the greatest increase. It appears that terpenes with structures suitable for alignment within lipid lamellae were the most potent enhancers. Sesquiterpene enhancers had long durations of action, implying that they did not wash out of the skin easily. Sesquiterpene effects were almost fully maintained for at least 45 days following pretreatment, illustrating poor reversibility. It appeared that an important mechanism of action of the enhancers was to increase the apparent drug diffusivity in the stratum corneum (Cornwell and Barry, 1994).

Permeation experiments performed on excised human epidermal membranes using cyclic terpenes selected from the different chemical classes of hydrocarbons (e.g. α-pinene), alcohols (e.g. α-terpineol), ketones (e.g. carvone) and oxides (e.g. 1,8-cineole, ascaridole) showed various levels of activity (Williams and Barry, 1991). α-Pinene only doubled the permeability coefficient of aqueous 5-FU, whereas 1,8-cineole caused a near 95-fold increase. Essential oils (e.g. chenopodium, which is 70% ascaridole), were less effective than the corresponding isolated terpenes. 5-FU is less soluble in the terpenes than in water, and the terpenes did not exert their action by increasing partitioning of the drug into the membranes as illustrated by stratum corneum water partitioning studies. The principal mode of action of these accelerants may be described by the lipid–protein partitioning theory: the terpenes interacted with intercellular stratum corneum lipids to increase diffusivity, and the accelerant effects were not due to partitioning phenomena (Williams and Barry, 1991). Four terpene enhancers (fenchone, thymol, limonene and nerolidol) produced linear relationships, indicating that they were more effective at enhancing the penetration of hydrophilic drugs rather than lipophilic drugs (El-Kattan *et al.*, 2001). Studies on 26 terpene enhancers on the solubility of 5-FU through human epidermis revealed that terpenes might increase the permeation through the stratum corneum as a result of complex formation and a form of facilitated transport (Moghimi *et al.*, 1998).

Antimicrobial effects

Antibacterial effects

Traditionally, plants and their extracts have been used to extend the shelf-life of foods, beverages and pharmaceutical and cosmetic products through their antimicrobial and antioxidant properties (Jay and Rivers, 1984; Gallardo *et al.*, 1987; Janssen *et al.*, 1988; Péllisier *et al.*, 1994; Cai and Wu, 1996; Baratta *et al.*, 1998a,b; Youdim *et al.*, 1999). The antimicrobial properties of volatile oils and their constituents from a wide variety of plants have been assessed (Appendix 1) and reviewed over the years (Jain and Kar, 1971; Inouye *et al.*, 1983; Janssen *et al.*, 1987; Carson *et al.*, 1995a,b, 1996; Larrondo *et al.*, 1995; Pattnaik *et al.*, 1995a,b, 1996; Nenoff *et al.*, 1996).

It was found that components with phenolic structures, such as carvacrol and thymol, were highly active against test bacteria, despite their low capacity to dissolve in water (Dorman and Deans, 2000). The high activity of the phenolic components may be further explained in terms of the alkyl substitution into the phenolic nucleus, which is known to enhance the antimicrobial activity of phenols (Pelczar *et al.*, 1988). Aldehydes, notably formaldehyde and glutaraldehyde, are known to possess powerful antimicrobial activity. The aldehydes *cis*- and *trans*-citral displayed moderate activity against test bacteria while citronellal was less active. Alcohols are known to possess bactericidal rather than bacteriostatic activity against vegetative bacterial cells. The alcohol terpenoids studied did show some activity against test bacteria, acting as protein denaturing agents, solvents or dehydrating agents.

The ester geranyl acetate demonstrated more activity than the alcohol geraniol. The alcohol terpenoids show some activity against test bacteria, acting as protein-denaturing agents, solvents or dehydrating agents (Lis-Balchin, 2002b, ch.14); also some, but not all, ketones are active agents. Menthone was shown to have modest activity against *Clostridium sporogenes* and *Staphylococcus aureus* (Dorman and Deans, 2000). There is also a complex correlation with the groups (e.g. the inclusion of a double bond increased the activity of limonene relative to *p*-cymene). It was observed that α-isomers are inactive relative to β-isomers and that *cis*-isomers are inactive relative to *trans*-isomers (Lis-Balchin, 2002b, ch.14).

Mode of action of terpenoids on membranes

Investigations into the effects of terpenoids upon isolated bacterial membranes suggest that their activity is a function of the lipophilic properties of the constituent terpenes (Knobloch *et al.*, 1986), the potency of their functional groups and their aqueous solubility (Knobloch *et al.*, 1988). Their site of action appeared to be at the phospholipid bilayer, caused by biochemical mechanisms catalysed by these phosholipid bilayers of the cell. These processes include the inhibition of electron transport, protein translocation, phosphorylation steps and other enzyme-dependent reactions (Knobloch *et al.*, 1986). Their activity in whole cells appears more complex: although a similar water-soluble tendency is observed, specific statements on the action of single terpenoids *in vivo* have to be assessed singularly, taking into account not only the structure of the terpenoid, but also the chemical structure of the cell wall (Knobloch *et al.*, 1988). The plant extracts clearly demonstrate antibacterial properties, although the mechanistic processes are poorly understood.

Chemotherapeutic agents

Such chemicals, used orally or systemically for the treatment of microbial infections of humans and animals, possess varying degrees of selective toxicity. Although the principle of selective toxicity is used in agriculture, pharmacology and diagnostic microbiology, its most dramatic application is the systemic chemotherapy of infectious diseases. The tested plant products appear to be effective against a wide spectrum of microorganisms, both pathogenic and non-pathogenic. Administered orally, these compounds may be able to control a wide range of microbes, but there is also the possibility that they may cause an imbalance in the gut microflora, allowing opportunist pathogenic bacteria, such as coliforms, to become established in the gastrointestinal tract with resultant deleterious effects. This could happen with long-term oral usage of essential oils and/or their components.

However, generalisations as to function versus structure cannot be made with any certainty. This fact is not in evidence in many aromatherapy books (e.g. Franchomme and Pénoel, 1990; Caddy, 1997; Schnaubelt, 1999). Most aromatherapy courses also concentrate on the group names of components rather than the individual function of each component.

There are, however, so many exceptions to the rule that generalisations seem irrelevant. As an example, the monoterpene limonene is used as a paint remover and industrial hand cleanser, but the pinenes and other monoterpenes are not able to perform the same task.

The antimicrobial activity of essential oils is often regarded by aromatherapists as proof of their efficacy in aromatherapy. However, the actual mode of application of such essential oils is far removed from the proper definition of aromatherapy (treatment with odours). Recently, tea tree oil has been lauded as one of the main aromatherapeutic oils. It has great antimicrobial potential (Carson and Riley, 1995b; Lis-Balchin *et al.*, 1998a, 2000). However, its main area of usage is as an antiseptic and antimicrobial applied topically, for athlete's foot, *Candida* and acne (Carson and Riley, 1994), and even internally, using suppositories, for *Candida* and other forms of venereal disease (though it is illegal to treat the latter by non-medically qualified people), and orally for various mouth and throat conditions. The effectiveness of tea tree oil in a massage blend (at a much lower concentration) used all over the body has not been studied in any such medical condition.

Tea tree, lavender, mint, thyme and juniper oils have been assessed against *Staphylococcus aureus* and vancomycin-resistant *Enterococcus faecium* (Nelson, 1997). Not surprisingly, tea tree was the most effective when measured in two different ways using the minimum inhibitory concentration (MIC), which is the lowest concentration inhibiting visible growth in 24 hours, and the minimum bactericidal concentration (MBC), which is the lowest concentration that reduced the original inoculum by more than 99.9% after overnight incubation (i.e. almost complete inhibition of growth). This was followed jointly by lavender, mint and thyme; juniper oil was not found to be very effective. These were, however, *in vitro* tests and when applied in a clinical trial for athlete's foot, tea tree was found to be effective, but did not kill the causative organism (Tong *et al.*, 1992).

Tea tree does not have the ethereal or floral odour associated with 'aroma'-therapy and its use between the toes and in the vagina does not suggest that its application is as an odorant. By the same token, there is no evidence that Vicks VapoRub or similar concoctions act as an odorant, though their benefit as disinfectants and nasal and pulmonary decongestants are obvious. Concoctions similar to Vicks VapoRub have also been used as orally-taken encapsulated products which break down ureteric or gallstones. This is not true aromatherapy, but simply conventional medicine using chemicals. The antiviral activity of tea tree oil was studied *in vivo* against the tobacco mosaic virus (Bishop, 1995) and was found to be effective as a pre-inoculation spray on tobacco plants. The oil gave a significantly decreasing number of lesions for at least 10 days post inoculation. The results do not, however, show destruction of the virus and it seems it is effective only if applied before the infection (but if only we knew when we would be infected before it happened!). Secondly, and most importantly, this is not a human virus and therefore tea tree oil should not be quoted as an antiviral agent based on this research.

Despite its widespread acclaim as an antibacterial agent, studies on manuka honey have not provided scientific evidence of activity. A study in Australia showed that there was virtually no difference in the activity of honeys made by bees from manuka and another plant on several wound-infecting bacteria *in vitro*, though the sensitivity of individual bacteria was slightly different (Willix *et al.*, 1992). Manuka honey is also widely acclaimed as effective against gastric ulcers caused by *Enterobacter pylori*: this, however, has not been proven. The relevance of massaging manuka oil into the skin in a blend to achieve these results is also unproven.

Antibacterial versus antifungal properties of essential oils

There is little differentiation between antibacterial and antifungal activity in aromatherapy books, and yet there is often a directly opposing activity (see Appendices 1 and 7; Lis-Balchin *et al.*, 1998a). In experiments using 25 different bacterial species and three different species of fungi it was found that these activities can be very different in different species (see Appendix 7). Some essential oils are strongly antibacterial but have virtually no antifungal action (e.g. angelica root, frankincense and cajuput); some have very strong antifungal activity and no antibacterial activity (e.g. aniseed); some, despite their reputation for antimicrobial activity, show virtually no activity (e.g. lemon and chamomile (German and Roman), cedarwood (Chinese, Texas, Virginian)). Different *Eucalyptus* species show very different levels of bioactivity. For example, *E. citriodora* has very poor antibacterial activity, whilst *E. globulus*

has strong activity, but this is reversed in the case of antifungal action.

Some essential oils have potent activity against both bacteria and fungi (e.g. bay, tea tree, clove bud and leaf, cassia, cinnamon, cumin, thyme (high thymol/carvacrol)).

Mode of antifungal action

Daferera *et al.* (2000) reported that lavender oil was moderately inhibitory to radial growth and conidial germination of *Penicillium digitatum*, while conidial production was not affected by the oil at concentrations up to 1000 µg/mL. Lavender oil, along with others such as thyme and marjoram, were more effective in the inhibition of conidial germination than of radial growth.

Conidial germination is the first vital step in the sequence of events leading to the establishment of a germ-tube and subsequent hypha. The process begins with hydration followed by the action of lytic enzymes such as chitinase and α- and β-glucanases. This breaks down the thickened conidial cell wall to permit emergence of the germ-tube initial. Once this event takes place, there is a balance between the lytic and synthetic enzyme systems necessary for normal hyphal extension. An imbalance in either enzyme system leads to growth inhibition and/or death (McEwan, 1994). It would appear that these early ontogenic events are highly susceptible to disruption by the component(s) in lavender volatile oil, resulting in lack of successful conidial germination.

Differences in bioactivity between samples of essential oils

Differences between different batches from the same source and/or supplier or different sources were found for both multiple samples of peppermint (Lis-Balchin *et al.*, 1997c) and geranium oils (Lis-Balchin *et al.*, 1996b). The 14 peppermint samples did not vary as much as the 16 samples of geranium (labelled Chinese, Egyptian, Bourbon and Moroccan) bought from different suppliers. There was a wide range of citronellol and geraniol levels in each source category of geranium oil, with the ratio of citronellol:geraniol ranging from 1.7 to 10.9 (which is an enormous range, way out of keeping with the ISO specifications, see Chapter 6).

The antibacterial activity against 25 different bacteria also varied between samples of oil, ranging from 8 to 19 inhibited. The similarity reported between different peppermint samples is probably a reflection of its low price and also the fact that the most active components, like menthol, were always present in roughly the same concentration.

Differences in the inhibition of all the organisms by samples of geranium oil could not be correlated with the chemical composition of the samples. This can be explained by a high degree of blending, if not adulteration, the use of synthetics in the commercial oil industry, and because some of the samples were diluted when sold. Minor components play a substantial role in biological activities.

The study by Lis-Balchin and Deans (1997) indicated considerable variation in the activity of the 'same' geranium oil against different strains of a single bacterium, *Listeria monocytogenes*. This is in agreement with the findings of Aureli *et al.* (1992) and Lis-Balchin *et al.* (1996a). In the latter study, 16 geranium samples were active against 8–18 of the test bacteria; in the former study the number of active oils against *L. monocytogenes* ranged from 3 to 16 out of a set of 20 bacteria.

In antifungal studies, the percentage inhibition reported for geranium samples varied from 0 to 94% against *Aspergillus niger*, 12–95% against *A. ochraceus* and 40–86% against *Fusarium culmorum*. This highlights the wide variation within the group of samples and is rather daunting considering that the samples should be very similar.

If used therapeutically, it is necessary for essential oils to have the same bioactivity in each sample, as in the case of medicines. It is of note that a pure, non-commercial sample of geranium oil, obtained directly from the grower/distiller, had low bioactivities in general compared with most of the other samples. The bioactivities of synthetic citronellol and geraniol, used singly or in mixtures, representing the different proportions in the different geranium samples, were very high. This suggests that adulteration of most of the samples of commercial geranium oil had occurred using synthetic citronellol and geraniol (see also Lis-Balchin *et al.*, 1996b).

The actions of seven different commercial samples of lavender were also tested against the three filamentous fungi mentioned above (Lis-Balchin *et al.*, 1996a). Correlation between chemical composition and antimycotic activity was again not always clear. The test organisms, *Aspergillus niger*, *A. ochraceus* and *Fusarium culmorum*, reacted differently to the oils, with the plant pathogenic *F. culmorum* being less affected, with two exceptions, than the two *Aspergillus* species. The spoilage organism *A. niger* was more inhibited in its growth, again with two exceptions, than the mycotoxigenic *A. ochraceus*.

The adulteration of volatile oils with synthetic components may give rise to a different proportion of enantiomers (see Chapter 6) for some components than is found in a pure botanical sample; this can have a significant influence on the bioactivity of the subsequent material (Lis-Balchin *et al.*, 1996b; 1998a,b). Again this strengthens the adulteration theory of the commercial geranium oils discussed above.

Differences in bioactivity due to mistakes in nomenclature

Different essential oils have different effects due to their composition; this clearly indicates that one cannot just ignore botanical nomenclature, as is often done in aromatherapy books. For example, many of the medicinal properties of geranium oil cited were mistakenly based on geranium species (e.g. *G. robertianum*, which is not a *Pelargonium*) reported in various herbals. These *Geranium* species were useful as an astringent and tonic, in the treatment of diarrhoea, cholera and chronic dysentery (Grieve, 1937/ 1992), but these virtues have not been proven for geranium oil (derived from *Pelargonium* species).

Extracts of *Geranium* species (again, not *Pelargonium*) have been shown to have antibacterial (Ivancheva *et al.*, 1992; Pattnaik *et al.*, 1996a,b), antifungal (Pattnaik *et al.*, 1995a,b, 1996) and antiviral (Zgorniak-Nowosielska *et al.*, 1989; Ivancheva *et al.*, 1992; Serkedjieva, 1995) properties. These are largely due to the water-soluble components (e.g. the polyphenolic complex), some of which have shown activity against herpes simplex virus, vaccinia virus and human immunodeficiency virus type 1 (HIV-1) in cell cultures. Unfortunately, these findings have been erroneously extrapolated to geranium oil, which is a fat-soluble extract from a *Pelargonium* species with a totally different chemical composition to any of the *Geranium* species (see also Chapters 1 and 2).

Another example of misinterpretation occurs in the case of *Eucalyptus* species. Most aromatherapy books do not stipulate which *Eucalyptus* species they are discussing, and this is also unfortunately true of many past scientific papers. There is a distinct difference in activity between species. For example, *E. citriodora* has very little antibacterial activity compared with that of *E. globulus* or *E. radiata*, but the reverse is true in the case of antifungal activity (see Appendix 6).

Antimicrobial activity, MRSA and aromatherapy

To many aromatherapists, 'antimicrobial' means the selective killing of 'bad microbes' leaving the 'good' ones intact, but, in fact essential oils attack the good ones as well as the bad. The observation that some essential oils had an effect on some 'MRSA' (methicillin-resistant *Staphyloccocus aureus*) bacteria at one London Hospital (Buckle, 1994) does not imply that essential oils can kill off MRSA all over the world. This is a very common misconception of essential oil activity against bacteria. In fact, a study conducted at a London hospital on various resistant bacteria, using a few samples of essential oils, including thyme, marjoram and geranium, showed the oils to be effective against only some of the resistant strains (personal unpublished data). There is always the problem of variability in different batches of essential oils and this has been shown to have a profound effect on large numbers of bacteria studied (Lis-Balchin *et al.*, 1998c), as mentioned already.

There is a potential danger involved when unqualified people try to do antibacterial studies, as is sometimes suggested as a legitimate course of action for aromatherapists (Buckle, 1997), or even attempt therapeutics on virulent bacteria. Not only does the person conducting the tests run the risk of becoming infected with virulent strains of bacteria but there is also the danger of spreading the contamination. Microbiological tests in hospital laboratories are done under very strict control conditions, using isolated cabinets in designated areas, with proper airflow out to the outside, special protective garments and equipment. Any microbiological activity by non-experts is not to be encouraged.

Miscellaneous actions

Anti-inflammatory effects

The anti-inflammatory effect of essential oils has been studied in various ways. For example, L-menthol was compared with mint oil in an *in vitro* system using human monocytes. The effect was assessed by measuring leukotriene B4 and prostaglandin E2 as indications of both the lipoxygenase and cyclooxygenase pathways of arachidonic metabolism (Juergens *et al.*, 1998). Production of interleukin-1B (IL-1B) was also analysed. L-Menthol significantly suppressed all three inflammatory mediators by monocytes; the activity was greater than that of the mint oil, containing 44.4% menthol. Using eucalyptol, there was an inhibitory effect on lipopolysaccharide- and IL-1B-stimulated mediator production by human blood monocytes *in vitro*. There was also a significant dose-dependent inhibition in production of tumour necrosis factor α, IL-1B, leukotriene B4 and thromboxane B2 (Juergens *et al.*, 1998). Briefly this implies that there is solid confirmation that an anti-inflammatory effect occurs which is based on the inhibition of prostaglandin synthesis, some of which are directly inhibited by aspirin and non-steroidal anti-inflammatory drugs (NSAIDs) like ibuprofen.

This may not be the only mode of anti-inflammatory action. For example, German chamomile has anti-allergic and anti-inflammatory activities (see German chamomile oil monograph) which are partly due to azulene and probably act by inhibiting histamine release. Chamazulene inhibited the formation of leukotriene B4 in intact cells (by blocking the chemical peroxidation of arachidonic acid) but matricine showed no effect at low concentration, therefore chamazulene may contribute to the anti-inflammatory activity of chamomile extracts by inhibiting the leukotriene synthesis (Safayhi *et al.*, 1994).

Anti-ageing oils

Many antioxidant essential oils have the ability to increase the polyunsaturated fatty acids (PUFAs) in older mice after feeding them for a few weeks at approximately 1 mg oil per day. Young mice have a higher PUFA content than old mice and, as this is reversed by the oil, it is therefore said to be an anti-ageing effect. Effective essential oils include thyme, clove, nutmeg, pepper and lovage (Dorman *et al.*, 1995a; Lis-Balchin, 2002b, ch.14).

It is worth noting that senile dementia, Alzheimer's disease and acute memory loss are also associated with a drop in PUFA levels.

Anticarcinogenic essential oils

There are absolutely no data to support any statement relating to the anticancer properties of any essential oil. There are, however, a small number of papers relating to the delay in appearance of chemically induced cancer in animal studies by some components, but this cannot be equated with anticarcinogenicity in humans. For example, D-limonene did not prevent cancers although it caused a delay (Homburger *et al.*, 1971; Uedo *et al.*, 1999); perillyl alcohol was shown to cause some regression of mammalian carcinomas (Gould *et al.*, 1995; Reddy *et al.*, 1997).

Wound-healing agents in plants

The aerial parts of various plants are prized for their wound-healing properties. This effect may be explained by the presence of tannins. Wound healing by essential oil is, however, affected mainly by their antimicrobial function, as tannins are absent from this fat-soluble fraction.

Neuropharmacological effects

Numerous studies in animals have so far indicated the efficacy of certain essential oils on some aspect of brain function using either intra-peritoneal (i.p.) injection or subcutaneous (s.c.) injection or even oral dosing of the animals (see Chapter 8). Many other studies were *in vitro*. This is not true aromatherapy as it does not involve the odour and should be treated separately. Stimulating effects were shown using i.p. or s.c. or oral dosing of animals with essential oils or components. For example, mice given peppermint essential oil i.p. and i.v. displayed increased movement (Umezu *et al.*, 2001). Antidepressant-like activity was elicited by *Tagetes minuta* given s.c. to rats in forced swimming and maze tests (Martijena *et al.*, 1998); the rats also displayed anxiogenic behaviour.

Sedative effects were produced in rats given *Artemisia annua* i.p. (Perazzo *et al.*, 2003) and mice given *Laurus nobilis* i.p. (Sayyah *et al.*, 2002). Rats given oral *Melissa officinalis* had increased sleep time after small doses of pentobarbital (Coleta *et al.*, 2001). Sedative effects were also shown in mice given species of mint and *Rosa centifolia* i.p. (Umezu *et al.*, 1999, 2000). Sedative and stimulant effects of components are listed in Appendix 15; see also Chapter 6.

Inhibition of binding labelled benzodiazepine to rat and chick membranes of the brain was shown using *Tagetes minuta*; erythrocyte acetylcholinesterase inhibition by Spanish sage, *Salvia lavandulaefolium*, was also observed *in vitro* and *in vivo* (Perry *et al.*, 2000, 2001, 2002, 2003).

Studies of Alzheimer's disease

Ethanolic extracts of various species of sage (*Salvia* species), the related herb lemon balm (*Melissa officinalis*) and wormwood (*Artemisia absinthium*) have been tested for their components' ability to bind to acetylcholine receptors in the human brain *in vitro*. Wormwood contained chemicals that bound strongly to both the nicotinic and the muscarinic acetylcholine receptors; lemon balm bound to either or both, depending on the variety. Pineapple sage (*Salvia elegans*) bound strongly to the muscarinic receptors, but common sage (*S. officinalis*) did not bind strongly to either receptor. The strength of the binding depended on the concentration of the extract, but some samples bound as strongly as carbamylcholine, which resembles acetylcholine.

Caution was expressed, however, against trying to protect mental faculties by drinking absinthe, an especially potent spirit whose main flavouring is wormwood and which also contains lemon balm. It was banned in much of Europe in the nineteenth century because it caused severe mental problems, but has recently become available again in the UK (Perry *et al.*, 1998).

Aromatic inhalations

The use of aromatic inhalations was studied many years ago when Cohen and Dressler (1982) showed that eucalyptus, α-pinene, eucalyptol, camphor and menthol (i.e. the main constituents of common products such as Vicks VapoRub/inhaler, olbas oil and tiger balm) caused significant changes in the forced vital capacity, forced expiratory volume and the slope of the alveolar plateau (i.e. there was a positive and favourable change).

Conclusion

There are diverse functions of essential oils, depending on the mode of application, the actual essential oil, the adulteration of the essential oil, the species of animal to which the essential oil is applied, etc. The pharmacological effect *in vitro* on different tissues in the same and different animals can also vary. It is therefore not possible to generalise about the bio-activity of essential oils on microorganisms or in animal tissues *in vitro*, let alone *in vivo* in humans. Most experimental evidence for essential oil functions is from studies in microbes or animals *in vitro* and there is scant scientific evidence to date about the effects of applying essential oils on the skin or inhaling in animals, including humans. These are discussed in Chapter 6.

6

Science of smell and psychological effects

Aromachology

The term 'aroma' is defined in the dictionary as an odour or scent. Logic dictates that aromatherapy should therefore be defined as 'treatment with odours' (Buchbauer, 1992). However, aromatherapy in the UK mainly involves the application of a very diluted essential oil or mixture of essential oils (1–2%) in a carrier oil, which is then massaged into the skin. The effect of the 'aroma', therefore, is largely ignored and the essential oil is used predominantly as a chemical emollient. However, aromatherapy also includes the addition of drops of essential oil to the bath or a basin of hot water, or into various burners. Here volatilisation of the essential oil(s) by heat occurs and aroma is now the main source with absorption through the nose and lungs. Smell is therefore of the utmost importance.

The other mode of intake (used by medically qualified doctors), involves oral, rectal and vaginal entry points, as used in herbal medicine. In these cases smell is obviously negligible. There are some conventional, medically approved and tested peppermint oil capsules (e.g. Colpermin) on the market, used for treating irritable bowel syndrome, but this could not be called 'aromatherapy' as the aroma is encapsulated when taken orally and therefore cannot be smelt.

Aromachology was defined by the Sense of Smell Institute (SSI) as a science based on the study of the psychological effects of fragrances, especially their hedonistic qualities and behavioural and emotional qualities.

The SSI primarily serves the perfumery industry of course, and so the fragrances are mainly, if not entirely, perfumery products, including synthetic chemicals. The concept does not endear itself to aromatherapists, who only use 'pure' essential oils, mainly bought by their distributors from the same suppliers as those that supply to perfumers (although many believe this to be untrue).

From Aristotle onwards, writers have observed that smell is the most problematic of the five senses. It is deemed to have a double nature, either registering aesthetic delight or pure stench. Both Hippocrates and Galen, following on from earlier Pythagorean tradition, gave smell a particular role in nutrition – smells were believed to be absorbed directly, bypassing the need for digestion. Galen also believed that smell worked in a different way from the other senses. He was the first to associate smell with the brain: he felt that the nose was simply a passage to carry odour (Palmer, 1993). The medical implication was that smells could have a great healing potential because of their ability to penetrate the brain. On the other hand, it was also believed that they could also cause disease. Thus for many centuries it was believed that smells carried the qualities of the substances from which they emanated (Palmer, 1993). This became interpreted to mean that good smells were life supporting and bad smells caused disease (see Chapter 2).

Smell is a basic sense closely linked to emotions. The fundamental difference between an emotional sense and an intellectual sense, such as sight or sound, is that there are no words that can be used to describe the sensation. It is virtually impossible to describe a smell to someone who has not also experienced it. In most cases the only way to define a smell is by comparing it in some way to another smell or perhaps even a mixture of odours. Smell is more 'right brain', and unlike the other senses does not 'cross over' from one brain hemisphere to another (Watson, 1999).

Culpeper and Gerard, the great seventeenth-century herbalists, were the main sources of many aromatherapy legends and although whole herbs were used as teas, alcoholic extracts or in poultices, and these were largely water-soluble and therefore differed greatly from the volatile, odorous, essential oils, some odour was inevitably involved. It is of interest that some of these herbalists also assigned psychological effects and even planets to their herbs. This aspect has been extended by many recent aromatherapists to include associations with ying and yang, energy levels, colour, etc., which may or may not have any bearing on psychological effects afforded by the smell itself.

A particular fragrance can awaken a long-forgotten memory and the emotional pattern associated with it even though the present circumstance in which the smell is produced is totally unrelated. This is exemplified by the 'Madeleine effect' as described by French novelist Marcel Proust in his *Remembrance of Times Past*. When, as an adult, Proust had the occasion to savour a Madeleine cake (made with citrus) with a cup of linden tea, it immediately brought back an array of memories of the small village where he spent his youth. Past events of minute detail filled his consciousness – things that he had not thought about in years. This so intrigued him that he went on to write a seven volume novel dealing largely with his cogitation of things that could be remembered beyond intentional recollection (Proust, 1981).

Scientific research into the psychological effects of essential oils has only recently begun. There is a long tradition in folklore of their use by ordinary people to affect their psychological states. It is important to remember, though, that although this may be suggestive of a real effect, it is always possible that the effect may be due to the placebo effect and expectation rather than some property of the essential oil itself. Kirk-Smith (Lis-Balchin, 2002b, ch. 13) found dozens of quotes on the use of lavender to relieve anxiety and stress in numerous plays and books. For example:

> *The misfortune is, my dear fellow, that I've lost my chapeau bras. . . . Never mind, lean on my arm: we'll retire to my attic; and I've no doubt that a little sal volatile and red lavender will set all to rights again.*
>
> (Charles Dibdin, 1822, in
> *Life in London*)

> *Let us get into the great pot-pourri jar which stands in the corner; there we can lie on rose-leaves and lavender.*
>
> (Hans Christian Andersen, 1872, in
> *The Shepherdess and the Sheep*)

Nowadays, as a result of widespread publicity, lavender is commonly believed to be a soothing and relaxing agent, whilst peppermint is considered to be stimulating. The question is why should some essential oils and their components be calming, whilst others are stimulating, and how do they affect the brain and psychological states?

Introduction to odour and receptors in the brain

When essential oils are breathed in, the molecules rise up the external nares to the top of the nose. Here they meet the olfactory mucous membrane, a yellow patch $1 \, cm^2$ in area, at the top of the palate near the back, under the bridge of the nose, covered in millions of hairy sensory cells (van Toller *et al.*, 1985). Each olfactory neuron is topped by at least 10 hair-like cilia that protrude into a thin bath of mucus at the cell surface. Somewhere on these cilia there are receptor proteins that recognise and bind odorant molecules, thereby stimulating the cell to send signals to the brain. The average life of the cells has been estimated as 28 days. The fact that one odorant molecule interacts with just one receptor site means that structure–activity relationships can be used to study the effects of stimulants.

Humans are capable of registering as many as 10 000 different fragrances, and because both the odorant molecule and the receptor site are chirally active, it is possible to distinguish between different optical isomers (see Chapter 5). The interaction between stimulus and receptor site may be electronic only (for strong polar molecules) or steric (for spherical molecules), but is usually a combination of both. The first interaction (association) is often electronic (dipole interaction, van der Waals' forces, hydrogen bonds), but this is not always necessary (for alkanes and spherical molecules). The electrical impulse (Na^+/K^+ exchange across the cell membrane) is then generated after blocking of the receptor site. The receptors therefore identify the smell and the sensory stimulation is passed on through the olfactory bulb, which is an amplifier, through the olfactory nerve and directly into the limbic system of the brain.

The sense of smell is therefore directly connected with the outside, unlike other senses.

Fibres of the olfactory nerve, which gather up the neuronal processes, run upward from the smell receptors through minute holes in the skull to the paired olfactory lobes. The consequence of this is that any odour almost immediately reflects itself on the brain, as the molecules stimulate the passage of impulses along the olfactory tract to the primitive middle brain. This is in the area of the hypothalamic–hypophysial region, a non-cognitive area forming part of the 'limbic system', a name given to the area due to the formation of a threshold or limbus, around which the higher centres of the brain are built. Different transduction channels probably operate via cAMP or phosphoinositide or arachidonic acid (Dodd, 1991).

The limbic system is the oldest part of the human brain and two important areas of the limbic system are triggered by the nerve impulses – the amygdala and the hippocampus. This is where the centres of memory, sexuality, emotional reactions and creativity are found. The scent is compared with known scents in the memory bank, whilst pictorial representations and feelings from the past (which can include events, people, places and objects) merge with the scent 'information'. We therefore react to an aroma emotionally and physically through our autonomous nervous system (Luck, 1999).

In the limbic system, the nerve impulse is led to the hypothalamus, the control station for the pituitary, which is also the subcentre for the transmission of scent messages to other areas of the brain. As it receives scent data, it conveys chemical messages to the bloodstream. The hypothalamus is also the area of the brain that activates and releases hormones and regulates body functions. The thalamus connects the scent information of the limbic system to the areas of thinking and judgement. This entire, complicated process, from the perception of a smell to the corresponding gland secretion, takes just a few seconds. Recent studies have shown that the blood–brain barrier can be by-passed by several medicinal products when presented via the nose. This has been shown for nerve growth factor in the mouse brain (Frey, 2002) and neuropeptides in the CSF in humans (Born *et al.*, 2002). The extraneuronal pathway can take just minutes using perineural channels, whilst the intraneuronal pathway via the axons takes many hours.

In humans the sense of smell is thousands of times more sensitive than that of taste. Even extremely low concentrations of odour molecules can be detected by the olfactory receptors. Nevertheless, after a short period of time a smell seems to neutralise – we, the perfumed, are no longer consciously aware of it. However, those around us could be very much stimulated by our odour, especially if we have tried a dozen different perfumes in the duty-free shop at the airport and have entered the confines of an aeroplane. Could this array of odours trigger off air-rage perhaps, even if imperceptible to other passengers?

The simple inhalation of an aroma can cause changes in the body and, depending on the information received, can initiate any number of physiological processes. For example the immune system could be activated, blood pressure changed, digestion could be stimulated, etc. This complex reaction of brain and body takes place every time you smell something and can cause us to become calm, lively, euphoric, hungry, satiated, sleepy, active, free from pain, etc.

It is possible that an odour could perhaps stimulate the thalamus into releasing encephalin, a neurochemical that creates a sense of euphoria and simultaneously gives pain relief. Or an odour might stimulate the pituitary gland into releasing other neurochemicals such as endorphins or serotonin, which have a calming effect on fear, stress, aggravation and sleeplessness.

Essential oil molecules which are breathed in are partly exhaled, but some will find their way into the bloodstream via the lungs. Here there is only a one cell obstacle between the outside and the blood. One has also to consider the respiratory system as a two-way organ. The nose and mouth are responsible for excretion of volatiles: if one applies a clove of garlic to the big toe, a few minutes later the garlic odour is apparent from the mouth. Clearly there will have been no psychological effect as the garlic travelled through the blood and then lungs – though a physiological response could be envisaged.

How does the nose distinguish between different odorants?

Odour perception is effected by odorant molecules interacting with specific receptor sites on the olfactory epithelium (Buck, 2000). Different types of receptor site receive different molecular shapes of different odorant molecules and there are a limited number of receptor site types specific for an equal number of 'primary' odorants. Each site specifically recognises certain odorants – translating the chemical 'signature' into an electrical 'signature' from the neurons. Recently, a family of genes coding for the olfactory receptor protein has been identified (Buck and Axel, 1991; Buck, 1992). It appears that there are perhaps over 1000 olfactory receptor types, and they appear to be grouped in subfamilies, possibly for specific odour types (Malnic, 1999, 2004). Different people have different odour perception, and some are unable to sense smell at all (i.e. those with anosmia).

Neurons of the same receptor type are mingled with millions of neurons of different receptor types, so how can the brain interpret all this? How does it 'know' what the nose is smelling? The detail around this is still missing, but we know that the brain distinguishes first between primary odours and then the other groups.

Primary odours, pheromones and behaviour

Primary odours are all produced by the human body: isovaleric acid in vaginal secretions and stale axillary sweat; L-pyrroline in semen and male pubic sweat; trimethylamine in menstrual sweat; 3-methyl-hex-2-enoic acid in human axillary sweat and androstenone in male axillary sweat and stale urine. Musk also appears to be a primary odour.

Human beings are very sensitive to androstenone. Amounts as little as 0.049 μg are detectable and it has been found that women are more sensitive to this male odour than men. The odour of androstenone is perceived predominantly as being similar to urine, perspiration, animalic or amine by 40–50% of the population. Others perceive the odour as musky or floral, i.e. more pleasant (mainly women), and a few cannot detect androstenone at all (Kirk-Smith, 1980).

Humans are highly 'scented', with axillary glands larger and containing more apocrine glands than any other primate, producing musky steroids for which there are matching olfactory receptors (Stoddart, 1990). Pheromonal-like responses to these compounds have been observed. The human axillary 'scent organ' is a secondary sexual characteristic, being under the control of gonadal hormones, and produces these steroids and thus the musky odours at puberty. On the reception side at puberty odour preferences appear to change from sweet and fruity

odours towards these same musky and flowery odours.

The human armpit has three secretory glands: the eccrine (sweat), the apocrine and the sebaceous. The mixing of the watery eccrine secretion with the sticky apocrine secretion and the continuously excreted sebum helps these secretions to spread over the whole of the axillary skin and hair surfaces. The armpits are also highly vascularised with blood vessels, providing heat for evaporation. Axillary hair enhances the diffusion of odour and also provides a very large surface area for bacteria, which, with the combination of heat and humidity of the armpit, allows proliferation of selected bacteria. These break down the glandular secretions and so produce both more odour and the characteristic axillary odour.

Although the function of the human apocrine glands is unknown, their secretion is dependent on endocrine activity, which in turn is sensitive to psychological and social stimuli, e.g. being released in emotional stress (Gower and Ruparelia, 1993). They are also similar in morphology and endocrine dependence to the apocrine glands used for scent marking in other mammals.

Amongst the many odorous compounds present are the 'sweaty' smelling short-chain fatty acids and in particular (E)-3-methyl-hex-2-enoic acid (TMHA), which has recently been identified as having the characteristic odour of the human axillary compounds.

The two odorous steroids present in male axillary sweat, androstenone (5-α-androst-16-en-3-one) and androstenol (5-α-androst-16-en-3-ol) are synthesised in the testes and transported to the axillary glands via the circulatory system. However, their main source is thought to be the breakdown of precursors produced in the apocrine glands by axillary bacteria – which are more common in men than women, and this may explain the presence of these steroids in male axillary sweat. Steroid production is substantially reduced by treating the axillae with a bacteriocide (Stoddart, 1990; Gower and Ruparelia, 1993).

Androstenone is thought to have a predominantly urinous odour and androstenol to have a musky odour, though both androstenone and androstenol are also found in the urine. 'Untrained' women characterise T-shirts bearing a synthetic sweat with an increased concentration of androstenone as more 'male' (Kirk-Smith and Booth, 1980).

These steroids are also active in olfactory communication in the pig. Androstenone and androstenol are concentrated in the submaxillary gland of the boar and enter the saliva. The scent of androstenone in the saliva of boars induces an immobilisation reflex and the adoption of a mating posture in oestrous sows. Interestingly, androstenone is also found in truffles, which explains why sows are used to search for these subterranean delicacies. Finally, androstenol also enhances the onset of puberty in piglets (Gower and Ruparelia, 1993; Kirk-Smith, 1995).

The longevity of odour memory in humans implies that 'odour signatures' may be discriminated for longer periods of time than other phenotypic traits. Human babies may be particularly sensitive to olfactory cues, especially those from lactating women (Engen, 1991). Discrimination of a mother's individual breast odours can be demonstrated in breast-feeding newborns as early as 3 days post partum. Older children of 3–5 years old also prefer their mother's axillary odour rather than other women's odours.

Perfumes: their commercial uses

The memory that an odour evokes can have a non-cognitive effect. For example, the smell of freshly baked bread or cinnamon rolls can unconsciously encourage a willingness to make extra purchases in the supermarket – this is why, of course, such enticing fragrances are installed in shops, usually at the entrance. It is not by accident that perfume counters are always located near the entrance on the ground floor of department stores. This entices the shoppers, without their conscious intent, to spend money on goods in the shop, and because these goods are not necessarily perfumes, the shoppers do not attribute the perfumes to their over-buying.

Scents are often chosen to accentuate a specific environment. For example a hint of essential oil of pine needle dispersed in the air of a shop where pine furniture is sold can have a positive associative effect on the shopper, giving an outdoor, woodland quality to the environment. This can be especially beneficial if a customer is 'shopping around' and so may well be visiting a number of shops in the area that sell pine furniture. When it is decision time, the power of the scent may end up being one of the deciding factors. Another common incentive is to use the 'new car smell' or smell of leather in second-hand cars.

Then there is the old practice of men using axillary odour to sexually arouse women: a young man would carry his handkerchief in his armpit for a time while dancing, and then use it to wipe her perspiring face. A similar tradition existed in Ancient Rome – gladiators' sweat scraped off their armpits was sold in vials to rich ladies!

Sexually alluring odours are usually different in the sexes of a species or, in some cases, only one of the sexes produces them. The scent from the female animal is often produced to guide the male to her, whereas the scent from the male is usually for the purpose of stimulating the female. It is the stimulating scent of the male that can be detected by humans and in most cases it is a pleasing odour (Baker, 1974).

More recently, the search for male olfactory attractants in axillary sweat has centred on the effects of androstenol (musk-scented) and androstenone (urine-smelling), with mixed results across several types of experiments. This discrepancy did not deter entrepreneurs, who make a great business out of selling 'male sex hormones'. In one study, subjects breathing androstenol were asked to assess written descriptions of alleged job applicants. It was found that they rated some candidates differently from controls. In another study, the presence of androstenol at unnoticed levels made women in photographs appear more sexually attractive. Kirk-Smith and Booth (1980) also found that women were attracted to sit on an androstenone-treated seat in a dentist's waiting room, whereas men avoided it. Women exposed to androstenol for a month (placed on their upper lips each morning) rated themselves as more submissive than the placebo group in the middle of their menstrual cycle. In contrast, women exposed to androstenone rated themselves as less sexy than control subjects when judging photographs and descriptions of a stimulus male college student, while men's moods were not affected.

When female job applicants wore fragrance, male interviewers liked them less and rated them lower in intelligence and friendliness, whereas the opposite was true for female interviewers (Engen, 1991). A plausible cognitive interpretation for these findings is that they 'suggest that males were more strongly affected by scent and other extraneous aspects of the applicants' appearance or grooming than females, and were quite aware of this fact. . . . Males may have realised that such scents would interfere with their ability to serve as an effective interviewer. This, in turn, caused them to experience annoyance or resentment towards the applicants and so to downgrade them on several key dependent measures' (Baron, 1983).

These results contrast sharply with those of Kirk-Smith and Booth (1990) that, in the presence of a perfume, both men and women rated photographed men and women as sexier and softer, and rated their mood as becoming more sexy, compared to a no-perfume situation. This shows that odour effects are likely to be both highly variable and unpredictable. This may be because there is an anatomical link between the nose and the pituitary, which is seen during their embryological development; both organs originate from the same patch of cells on the surface of the embryo (Stoddart, 1990). The nose and pituitary also share a common function if one considers that the pituitary samples the chemicals in the blood; the odour perceived by the nose is relayed via hormones produced in the pituitary to the gonads (Stoddart, 1990). Current research being carried out suggests that there are different classes of pheromones which, it is felt, may be processed by segregated groups of sensory neurons lining the vomeronasal organ, a specialised structure at the base of the nasal septum. The input from these sensory neurons seems to remain segregated in the brain and could be sent to different regions of the amygdala and hypothalamus depending on the nature of the message.

Animalistic perfume ingredients

For centuries, mammalian sex attractants from animal secretions, or more recently their synthetic analogues, have been used in perfumes. These include musk extracted from the preputial gland of the Himalayan musk deer, and civet extracted from the anal gland of the civet cat. These animal secretions are considered to be fixatives or 'base-notes' in perfumery, preventing the rapid evaporation of the floral notes of a perfume by acting in a similar way to the wax or resin of a flower or leaf. In high concentrations their odours resemble the musky/urinous odours of androstenol and androstenone and, although they are not steroids, their molecular shapes are remarkably similar.

The use of musk in perfumes has been reliably traced back over 5500 years to China. The first mention of musk in Europe is attributed to St Jerome in about AD 390, and the earliest reference is in a manuscript, now held by the British Museum, dated 1398. Scent formulations made up of 20% musk, 8% civet and 12% storax (a musky smelling plant resin) were common in the past.

Most modern perfumes also incorporate musk or civet analogues; a recent survey showed that 85% of female and 94% of male fragrances contain musk-smelling compounds and 39% and 6% respectively contain civet-smelling compounds. Before the nineteenth century, women used the strongest, most animalistic perfumes to emphasise their body odour as a secondary sexual characteristic. Civet has been used in perfumes since Biblical times. At high concentrations it has a urinous/faecal odour, but in very dilute concentrations civet has a more floral-musky odour than musk. In Shakespeare's *Much Ado about Nothing* Don Pedro says: 'he rubs himself with civet. Can you smell him out by that?' To which Claude replies 'That's as much to say, the sweet youth's in love'.

Like musk, civet was also employed as an aphrodisiac with the power to attract the opposite sex. Other sexy odours abound. An Austrian perfumer asked a number of professional perfumery 'noses' if they could detect which, if any, of the most common incenses had a smell similar to that of body odour, as he hoped he could pinpoint if certain odorants are capable of inducing an unconscious erotic response. The incense resins contained alcohols known as phytosterols which biochemically resemble certain human hormones. The results of the experiment indicated a sort of olfactory simulacra. It was widely agreed that frankincense had a sweet smell that was similar to the armpit odours of people with dark hair. While myrrh, with a somewhat sour smell, more resembled the underarm odour of light-haired people. The experts also felt that laudanum closely matched the smell of head hair in general and styrax had an odour like that of skin. The incense ingredients were then individually blended with a floral eau de Cologne and the experts all agreed that this enhanced the erotic nature of the fragrance in each case (Jellinek, 1954).

Of course, the use of fragrance to encourage erotic impulses has been known to many cultures throughout history. The most famous example of the seductive qualities of perfume is its use by Cleopatra to capture first the attention and then the affection of Mark Anthony (see Chapter 2). Perfume as an amatory lure is even referred to in the Bible in connection with adulterous women. The Romans in particular used perfumes lavishly all over their bodies and garments for such purposes.

Body odour changes with illness and puberty (when it first becomes apparent) and during the menstrual cycle and menopause. The sexual influence of apocrine odours, which are associated with urinary and faecal smells, has already been discussed. That perfumes with these notes are much sought after is not surprising. Hence, the best perfumes contain the animalistic notes of civet, castoreum and musk, which are now, for the most part, of a synthetic nature and are often toxic like the musks (see Chapter 7).

Some societies do not regard body odour as negatively as western society tends to and do not try to camouflage it. Different cultures have different dietary preferences which may contribute towards a particular smell being associated with a particular race of people. In cultures where the diet is mainly made up of fish, for example, a fishy-like smell is often incorporated in a person's body odour. But whatever factors make up the differences in body odour between the various races, because the ability to perceive a smell can disappear as a result of sensory adaptation, an individual is increasingly less able to smell odours they are normally exposed to within their own ethnic group, making the smells of differing ethnic groups more pronounced.

Stage of life is also a factor. Human faeces and sweat smell pleasant to children of 3 or 4 years old, and usually become unpleasant afterwards. Odour is also extremely important in the development of animals, including humans. There is an odour-bonding that occurs between mothers and babies during the first few hours after birth which enables the mother to recognise her young. This bond is so strong in animals, for example, that if a ewe has lost her own lamb, she will actually accept another lamb as her own if the dead lamb's skin is tied on to it. If, as happens with some emergency births in humans, the mother is not given her baby for several hours after the birth, it is possible that this bond may not develop in the same way. In humans, a mother can recognise the blanket that her baby was wrapped in after only 10 minutes initial contact. It takes a baby about 10 days before it can identify the smell of its mother's breasts.

A baby can also acquire associations with artificial odours as well as natural ones – the smell of its mother's perfume, for instance, providing she regularly uses a given fragrance. In contrast to this, the use of a variety of scents might be confusing for a new baby, and may cause the child to suffer from a desensitised sense of smell (Kirk-Smith and Booth, 1987).

The close contact between mother and baby can make their odours similar. In experiments done with T-shirts, people who are unrelated can match a T-shirt belonging to a baby with the one belonging to its mother (Kirk-Smith and Booth, 1987).

The human female's sensitivity to musk-like odours seems to be at its height around the time of ovulation. This has been interpreted by some researchers as proof of the ancestral presence of a musky pheromone in the male. There is also a possibility that androstenol, from male sweat, has an effect on female menstrual cycles and ovulation (Grammer and Jutte, 1997).

To test the hypothesis that women are attracted to the odour of androstenone, a total of 840 patients attending the Birmingham University Dental Health Centre unwittingly took part in an experiment over a period of 12 days. Androstenone had been sprayed onto a seat in a position that had been observed to be previously avoided by women. Three different concentrations were used, with observations being taken at half-hour intervals for 4 days at each level. The results showed that, specifically at the lowest and highest concentrations, significantly more women used the odorised seat. There was also a significant decline in the use of the seat by men when the highest level was used (Kirk-Smith and Booth, 1980). The reasons given by the researchers who designed this experiment as to why women chose the seat that had been sprayed with androstenone were that they were attracted because of positive experiences of its association with men and/or because of a perceived similarity between androstenone and certain components of perfume fragrances which they found pleasing.

In the seventeenth century fear of disease caused the public to be less tolerant of putrid odours, including body odours. Dirt was now seen to obstruct the pores and to favour the decomposition of substances. It was precisely the absence of strong odour, which was evidence of careful hygiene, rather than the use of powerful masking perfumes . . . that cast doubt upon a person's cleanliness! Thus, the harmful effects attributed to putrefaction revolutionised attitudes to bodily products and, in a more general way, to all the animal substances used in perfumery, especially musk and civet, as these were in the products of putrefaction (i.e. faeces and urine). By the mid-nineteenth century, light floral scents such as rose, thyme, violet and rosemary water came to replace animal scents as appropriate for use by women. And lavender and its products represented cleanliness and godliness.

Why are 'perfumes' used nowadays?

Perfumes are generally used for the same purpose as they are marketed, i.e. to enhance sexual attractiveness. This is reflected also in the names chosen (e.g. 'Intimate', 'Sex Appeal', 'L'Aimant' and 'Aphrodisia'). It is also possible that any sexual response to a body odour, albeit unconscious, might be replaced by a more powerful response to synthetic fragrances, perhaps through more frequent pairing in sexual or social sexual situations. Indeed, Kirk-Smith and Booth (1990) found that men and women rated photographed men and women as sexier and softer, and rated their own mood as becoming more sexy in the presence of the perfume 'Shalimar'. These effects were not seen when androstenone was used. In each case, the levels of odour used were unnoticeable.

Manufacturers make sure that their perfume is always the same, in order to obtain the same effect. Odour stimulates emotion: a potent perfume effect (Van Toller and Dodd, 1991). Why is it that each essential oil can vary greatly in composition from batch to batch and supplier to supplier and yet aromatherapists expect the same outcome? Surely, this should affect the results obtained in studies? Yet little notice is taken of this, the naïve assumption being made that they are all pure and natural. Nothing is further from the truth (viz. Gattefosé and his deterpenated lavender oil and the 'perfumes' he used in many other studies). Perfumes are therefore not all bad.

The other assumption made is that all the 'patients' like the smell! A cross-cultural study provided evidence for cultural influence on odour perception. In Germany a woman was found to classify her partner's odour as pleasant, whereas in Japan and Italy it was classed as unpleasant. However, the odour of a 'supposed' partner was classified as pleasant by German and Italian women; but both actual and supposed were rated as unpleasant by Japanese women! This may be due to a strong cultural pressure to suppress obvious body odours in Japan, reflected in the tradition of taking a ritual bath every day.

In a study of 166 German and 88 Japanese subjects, the total number of odours found was 2040 with 3520 associations (Schleidt *et al.*, 1988). The results for both cultures were very similar. Both pleasant and unpleasant odours were remembered to the same extent. Uniformly judged pleasant odours were from plants and unpleasant ones from rotten or decomposed material. Individual likes and dislikes were common to both cultures, as was the small number of differences found between the cultures, which were associated with different habits and values rather than just cultural. Germans mentioned more food smells whilst the Japanese focused more on flower and plant odours.

As pointed out by Buckle (1997): 'For some elderly people, lavender is a much disliked smell, associated with death. This learned memory can be triggered, raising images of dying relatives and friends from times long ago, when the bed-linen smelled strongly of lavender.' In light of this statement it is perhaps surprising that lavender is the most commonly used essential oil for every age group, including the elderly.

It has been established that human responses to odour are a direct result of personal experience (Kirk-Smith and Booth, 1987). Such experiences may have occurred years earlier, very possibly even in early childhood. Memories of the event or circumstance can come flooding back quickly and vividly, particularly when there was an emotional element involved with the initial experience. If a boy in class is continually picked on by his teacher for his lack of ability in front of the entire class, no doubt he will develop a rather negative attitude towards the teacher. And if the teacher always wears the same perfume, this negative attitude will be associated with that particular smell. It is possible that the boy becomes so conditioned by this that in adult life he has a negative response to anyone who happens to wear the same perfume.

If a person dislikes a smell, either subconsciously (more likely) or consciously, then the outcome can be the opposite to that seen as the norm. This could seriously damage any 'therapeutic' action on the patient, and is especially relevant in treating Alzheimer's disease, many geriatric 'illnesses', psychiatric disorders, grief and other stress-related conditions.

Aromachology research

In 1983, a joint programme of aromachology research was initiated between the SSI and Yale University to study the effects of fragrance on mood. Mood changes due to different fragrances in 50 women gave rise to four positive and four negative mood factors (Warren and Warrenburg, 1993). The positive ones were: happiness, sensuality, relaxation and stimulation; the negative ones stress, depression and apathy. This could be shown on a wheel, where the positive mood factors were on the right and negative ones on the left. More physiologically arousing moods such as stress and stimulation were to the top, and the more low-arousal moods like apathy and relaxation to the bottom. When 'living flower' odours were smelled by the subjects, they gave pleasantness ratings with the top to bottom being: muguet, Douglas fir, tuberose, osmanthus and hyacinth. Single note fragrances usually effect a single mood state, while complex fragrances can effect a variety of mood states as people react to the multiple notes in the scent. For example muguet or lily-of-the-valley, a complex fragrance, tended to increase both relaxation and stimulation. This is most unusual, but accounts for a state called 'calm vitality' or in aromatherapy terms, 'balancing'. Douglas fir, on the other hand is a distinctly relaxing fragrance, giving a feeling like a hot bath, which is effective in lowering negative moods. (Heathrow Airport apparently used the scent of pine needles to put travellers at ease and reduce the stress of travel.) Tuberose has a relaxing and sensuous effect and decreases depression and increases happiness and is used to enhance romantic moments. It caused a decrease in depression, reinforcing its positive mood swings. Osmanthus is stimulating and helps to reduce apathy and depression; it is highly coveted in China and Japan, with its floral/fruity smell somewhat like apricot, and showed an increase in happiness, with a decrease in all the negative mood factors. Hyacinth, a very complex fragrance, increases happiness, sensuality, relaxation and stimulation while decreasing all of the negative moods. It may be of note here that one's own favourite fragrance may also make one feel better simply because one takes pleasure in the scent. (It appears that we also like to think that indulgence in perfumes must be accompanied by a high cost for greater pleasure!)

Mid-life mood changes both in men and women were positively affected by pleasant fragrances: their moods were improved using their five popular colognes (Schiffman et al., 1995). Men often experience inner turmoil, altered aspirations, career frustration, confrontation with one's mortality, family and role changes just like women and also have concerns about a decline in sexual potency.

Fragrance can also be used to reduce anxiety during medical procedures (Redd and Manne, 1994), for example, magnetic resonance imaging, which some people find a distressing experience. When exposed to heliotropin, a sweet, vanilla-like scent, patients were found to experience approximately 63% less overall anxiety than a control group of patients.

Taste and smell losses that occur with advancing age can contribute to inadequate nutritional status for the elderly. Flavour and texture enhancements can partially compensate for these losses (Schiffman, 1991, 1992).

Physiological responses to essential oils and psychophysiology

Physiological and psychological responses are often difficult to separate in humans, but animal experiments can show individual effects up to a point. Rats were trained to negotiate a maze to find food and then an assessment made of the effect of exposure to the vapour from essential oils on the time taken to reach the food and the number of errors (Macht and Ting, 1921). Most of these early experiments were on valerian, asafetida tincture (very effective sedative/depressant), lavender tincture, musk tincture and various types of incense. Incense (gums of olibanum and galbanum) were heated to emit fumes and produced depression occasionally; sandalwood incense in small doses had a stimulant action. Diverse effects were shown by alcoholic extract of violets (stimulating sometimes) and attar of roses (sedative only in some experiments). From these results the authors concluded that lavender had a slight sedative action and it was suggested that the vapour from essential oils might be stimulating olfactory sense organs directly.

In another series of studies, lavender essence (L. angustifolia P. Miller) was given orally to mice and changes in activity to electrical stimulation observed. The results were interpreted as showing an anxiolytic (relaxant) effect. In addition, it was shown that lavender essence enhanced the hypnotic action of pentobarbitone (Delaveau et al., 1989).

The sedative action of lavender was confirmed in another study where it was observed that the overall activity of mice decreased when exposed to lavender vapour (L. angustifolia P. Miller); its components linalool and linalyl acetate showed a similar effect

(Buchbauer *et al.*, 1991). Scores in the activity box increased when mice were pretreated with caffeine given by the intraperitoneal route. This increase in activity was very sensitive to inhibition by lavender oil, linalool and linalyl acetate (Buchbauer *et al.*, 1993a). The authors considered that the sedative action is due to the absorption of linalool into the blood and its subsequent transport to the brain by the blood, rather than a direct stimulation of olfactory receptors (Buchbauer, 1992, 1993a,b,c; Jager *et al.*, 1992). A report that linalool produces a dose-dependent inhibition of the binding of glutamate (an excitatory neurotransmitter in the brain) to its receptors on membranes prepared from the cerebral cortex of the rat is a possible explanation for the observed sedative effects (Elisabetsky *et al.*, 1995). More recently this action was related to an anticonvulsant activity of linalool in rats (Elisabetsky *et al.*, 1999).

Other oils with sedative activity were found to be neroli and sandalwood; the active components included citronellal, phenylethyl acetate, linalool, linalyl acetate, benzaldehyde, α-terpineol, isoeugenol (in order of decreasing activity). Stimulant oils included jasmine, patchouli, ylang ylang, basil and rosemary; active components included fenchone, 1,8-cineole, isoborneol and orange terpenes (Appendix 14).

Lavender oil and its component linalool apparently produce a fall in blood pressure in experimental animals, probably due to peripheral vasodilatation (Tisserand and Balacs, 1995). Among the essential oils and components tested, the following showed the highest activity in humans: neroli, nutmeg, mace, valerian and myristicin, isoelemicin and elemicin (Warren *et al.*, 1999), however, reduction of blood pressure only occurred if it was high to begin with. Further physiological effects, mainly due to lavender and its components, have been extensively reviewed recently (Buchbauer, 2002).

There was some considerable similarity in the sedative and stimulant effects of some essential oils studied physiologically (e.g. their effect on smooth muscle of the guinea-pig *in vitro*) and the various psychological assessments, mostly on humans (Appendix 14).

Brain responses to essential oils: scientific studies

In a series of experiments by Buchbauer *et al.* (1993c), two types of reaction times in male and female students breathing either air or vapour from the essential oil of lavender were measured. Reaction times were increased by lavender and it was possible to show that this was not due to a peripheral effect but to central sedation. In the same study, the effects of inhaled essential oils on blood flow through the brain were measured using computerised tomography and, although no changes were found with lavender oil or linalyl acetate, a decrease was observed with 1,8-cineole (Buchbauer *et al.*, 1993c).

Several studies have been carried out on the brain's responses to odour. These have used the changing electrical activity picked up by scalp electrodes in response to lavender odours as a measure of brain activity (EEG) (Van Toller *et al.*, 1993). The most consistent responses to odours were in the theta band (Klemm *et al.*, 1992).

Many essential oil vapours have been shown to depress contingent negative variation (CNV) brain waves (an upward shift in EEG waves that occurs when people are expecting something to happen) in human volunteers (Appendix 14) and these essential oils are considered to be sedative. Others increase CNV and are considered stimulant. The effects of inhaling different essential oils on CNV can also be compared with the effect on mouse motility and the direct effect of the essential oil on smooth muscle *in vitro*. Although these are physiological responses, there is surprisingly frequent agreement in the effect. In CNV studies lavender was found to have a sedative effect on humans (Torii *et al.*, 1988; Kubota *et al.*, 1992; Manley, 1993) and a 'positive' effect on mood, EEG patterns and maths computations (Diego *et al.*, 1998). It also caused reduced motility in mice (Kovar *et al.*, 1987; Ammon, 1989; Buchbauer, 1992, 1993; Jager *et al.*, 1992). However, Karamat *et al.* (1992) found that lavender had a stimulant effect on decision times in human experiments. There was also a good agreement between the effect of individual essential oils (and mixes of three or more) on smooth muscle *in vitro* and the predicted holistic effects on clients, as judged by aromatherapists (Lis-Balchin and Hart, 1997a; see also Chapter 5).

Since the CNV is found to be reduced by sedatives and increased by stimulants, an investigation of the effect of lavender on CNV in trained Japanese perfumers was conducted (Torii *et al.*, 1988). Lavender reduced CNV but, unlike sedatives, had no effect on reaction time or heart rate, possibly due to the low amounts absorbed. These results were later replicated in untrained American subjects (Lorig and Roberts,

1990). The authors commented that this suggests that CNV is robust across cultures. However, they also found that the CNV changed depending on what the subjects thought the real odour was, even though the odour presented was different. High concentrations of lavender were found by subjects to be 'arousing and distracting' and suggest that this may also have led to the lowered CNV. Most subjects hated lavender.

A group breathing lavender showed increased frontal alpha and beta 2 waves in the EEG, suggesting an increase in drowsiness, and this group also rated themselves as more relaxed (Diego *et al.*, 1998). In contrast, Klemm *et al.* (1992) reported that lavender and other odours were associated with a general increase in theta waves, also associated with increased drowsiness, although the typical alpha wave increase during drowsiness was not observed, making these results hard to interpret. EEG responses to the odours varied greatly between subjects. The authors suggest that the differences observed in EEG responses may be due to subjects visualising objects or situations that the odours evoked (i.e. past experiences).

The anxiety-reducing effects of fragrances were also studied using electromyography (King, 1988). The effect of ambient odour compared with no odour in sessions one week apart on creativity, mood and perceived health was studied in 15 men and 15 women (Knasko, 1992). The odours used were lemon, lavender and dimethyl sulphide (DMS, an unpleasant odour). With lemon, fewer health symptoms were reported compared with the non-odour day. Subjects in the DMS group were less happy than those in the lavender group on both odour and non-odour days. The order of giving the odours affected the outcome, which was not very helpful in the study. However, there were no differences in arousal or creativity.

Inhalation studies in a group of 40 staff and students using rosemary oil or lavender oil, and assessing the response with EEG and simple maths computations, showed that lavender increased alpha power, suggesting drowsiness and the subjects stated that they were more relaxed, whilst rosemary instigated decreased frontal alpha and beta power, suggesting increased alertness, and the subjects were faster and more accurate in the maths (Diego *et al.*, 1998). These results suggest that odour has an effect on performance *per se*. However, Knasko *et al.* (1990) used no odour, but lied to their subjects that odour would be given: they also got an improvement in carrying out tasks.

In another study, the effect of ambient odours of lavender and cloves on cognition, memory, affect and mood of 72 volunteers was studied in two sessions separated by a week (Ludvigson and Rottman, 1989). The group was divided into three on each occasion. The experimental report does not really make it clear whether the same odour was given to the same group on the two occasions, or whether the odour given to a specific group was changed. The results showed that lavender adversely influenced arithmetic reasoning in the first session, but not the second session. An obvious cause of this was the high intensity of the odorants, which could have caused a distraction in the first session and decreased performance, which caused annoyance to those in the second session. The subjects' affective reactions to the experiment were favourable, however. Cloves, on the other hand, decreased the willingness of the volunteers to return for another session – the second session's results were very complex, but it became obvious that those who had smelled this odour once did not want to return. Nevertheless, there were no simple effects of odour apparent and the fact that there was no effect on memory was very surprising.

Human attention experiments (Ilmberger *et al.*, 2001) indicated that lavender essential oil was sedative and the stimulant one was jasmine. The effects of peppermint and muguet (lily-of-the-valley) odours on a demanding vigilance task showed that the peppermint was stimulating whilst muguet was relaxing, although both gained similar pleasantness ratings (Warm and Dember, 1999).

A large workplace in Japan has a computer-controlled system to dispense odorised air via the whole building: citrus smells refresh the workers first thing in the morning and after the lunch break. During the course of the morning, floral smells are sent to help them improve their concentration. In the lunch break and during late afternoon, woodland scents are circulated to relax the workers. Increased productivity has resulted (Van Toller and Dodd, 1991). In the United States, by contrast, some states are banning the wearing of perfumes as it encroaches on the space of other people and may make them feel uncomfortable. This follows on from the banning of smoking in public places. It is also possible that the use of a general regime of odorants could have very negative effects on some members of the workforce or on patients on hospital wards, where the use of pleasant odours could mask the usual unpleasant odours (for instance boiled cabbage and urine), which together provide the smell of fear associated with hospitalisation for many people. This illustrates the possibility of negative effects versus positive effects on different people.

An interesting single study involving a patient with anosmia showed that, as in eight neurologically normal people, there were changes in cerebral blood flow (CBF) on inhaling 1,8-cineole, thus showing a positive brain effect to the oil despite the inability to smell it (Nasel *et al.*, 1994). The results showed that in each case there was a global increase in CBF, without preference for a specific area.

Olfaction is different from the other senses in that it adapts – after a while a smell is not perceived. This suggests that its perceptual effect may only last until it has adapted, and that intermittent exposure or varying concentrations might be needed to maintain an effect. This is the reason why we fail to 'smell' the fifth perfume in a row, and the best remedy is to smell your own armpits to neutralise the odours before smelling another odorant.

The conclusion that can be drawn from examples such as these is that it is very difficult to make simple generalisations concerning the effects of any fragrance on psychological responses, which are based on the immediate perceptual effects, rather than the longer term pharmacological effects. This is because the pharmacological effect is likely to affect people similarly, but the additional psychological mechanisms will create complex effects at the individual level. Pleasantness or not is related to the value of an odour in evoking recognition of the source – it may be annoying if given with another task (Lis-Balchin, 2002b, ch. 13). Dosages are also of importance: if the odour is too strong there may be a reaction of distaste and a completely different mood swing than if the odour were at a realistic level. This makes comparisons between different studies very difficult as there are immense differences in the parameters, such as different dosages, tasks, conditions and perceptions.

In real-life circumstances, through repeated use by someone, a characteristic smell, at moderate concentrations may 'signal' the later sedative effects, and thus the smell might acquire, through classical conditioning, a calming effect by itself. This was tried out in a set of preliminary experiments (Betts *et al.*, 1995) on epileptic patients as a complementary therapy, followed up in 100 patients receiving sporadic aromatherapy, hypnosis or both together. Over a third of the patients using aromatherapy with or without hypnosis becoming seizure-free for at least a year. Aromatherapy plus hypnosis seemed to have had the best and most lasting effect (a third of patients were still seizure-free after 2 years), but was the most labour intensive. The author suggested that aromatherapy itself might be best reserved as a short-term treatment for people going through a bad time with their seizures. Although the results were quite good in this uncontrolled and rather non-systematic trial, there is concern that odours could actually provoke more seizures in epileptics, especially if used by non-medically qualified aromatherapists, without expert knowledge of epilepsy.

Clinical studies using essential oils often showed no physiological changes, but some psychological effects were sometimes observed (see Chapter 8). For example, in one study 122 patients in an intensive care unit were randomly allocated to a massage, an aromatherapy massage with 1% lavender oil or a rest period group. Each subject received 1–3 treatment sessions of 15–30 minutes over a 5-day period (Dunn *et al.*, 1995). Physiological data (blood pressure, heart rate and respiratory rate), psychological data (mood and anxiety) and behavioural (motor and facial) measures were taken before and after each session. In the first session the lavender and massage group reported less anxiety than the control group, but no other differences were observed on the other measures. The authors suggest that perhaps a higher concentration of lavender might have shown more effects.

Positive effects of inhaled lavender essential oil (for 10 minutes) in nine healthy females included increased blood flow, decreased galvanic skin conductance and systolic blood pressure, indicating a reduction in sympathetic nervous activity followed by decreased blood pressure (Saeki, 2001). Rosemary decreased blood flow and increased systolic blood pressure immediately after inhalation, indicating its stimulant action on the sympathetic nervous system. Citronella produced changes in the R-R interval on the ECG, decreased blood flow and galvanic conductance. The high-frequency spectral component reflecting parasympathetic activity was significantly increased after both citronella and lavender essential oil inhalation. The authors concluded that relaxant essential oils like lavender produced relaxation in the autonomic nervous system. Citronella had different effects in people and a more complex effect on the autonomic nervous system.

Odours are perceptible even during sleep, as shown in another experiment: college students were tested with fragrances during the night and the day (Badia, 1991). They were presented with either peppermint (an alerting odour) or just room air at intervals to see if they detected the odour during sleep. The students were told to wake up or press a switch if they smelt anything during sleep. The results showed that they were able to detect the odour during sleep, but not as well as during waking. Another test involved all-night presentation of peppermint and jasmine or room air presented continuously. The odours both had a disrupting effect on sleep although jasmine was considered relaxing during waking. Subsequently two more odours were added: the relaxing heliotropin and coumarin. All four were tested against room air during short 30-minute naps during the day. All but heliotropin disrupted sleep, whilst the latter enhanced sleep.

A study to assess the effects of water, lavender or rosemary scent on physiology and mood state following an anxiety-provoking task showed that non-smoking participants, aged 18–30 years, rated the pleasantness of the scent received depending on various external factors (Burnett et al., 2004). When pleasantness ratings of scent were covaried, physiological changes in temperature and heart rate did not differ based on scent exposure, but mood ratings differed by scent condition. Rosemary increased measures of tension–anxiety and confusion–bewilderment relative to the lavender and control conditions. The lavender and control conditions showed higher mean vigour–activity ratings relative to the rosemary group, while both rosemary and lavender scents were associated with lower mean ratings on the fatigue–inertia subscale, relative to the control group. These results suggest that when individual perception of scent pleasantness is controlled, scent has the potential to moderate different aspects of mood following an anxiety-provoking task.

A sex-balanced (13 men and 13 women) randomised crossover design was used to obtain pre- and post-treatment change scores for quantitative sensory ratings of contact heat, pressure and ischaemic pain across separate inhalation treatment conditions using lavender and rosemary essential oils, and distilled water as control (Gedney et al., 2004). Subjective reports of treatment-related changes in pain intensity and pain unpleasantness were obtained for each condition using a visual analogue scale. The results

showed no changes in quantitative pain sensitivity ratings between conditions. However, retrospectively, subjects' global impression of treatment outcome indicated that both pain intensity and pain unpleasantness were reduced after treatment with lavender, and marginally reduced after treatment with rosemary compared with the control condition. These findings may suggest that aromatherapy does not elicit a direct analgesic effect but rather alters affective appraisal of the experience and consequent retrospective evaluation of treatment-related pain.

Brain mapping

EEG measurements using brain electrical activity maps (BEAM) involves computer-generated topographies using FFT (fast Fourier transformations), which generate coloured topographic maps of the brain (Van Toller et al., 1993). A test involving babies showed that different responses were elicited to different food smells (Kendal-Reed, 1990). This could have been emotional, such as liking or disliking foods, which suggests that this is an innate characteristic rather than being learnt over the first few years of life.

An experiment was conducted using six odours against no odour at concentrations that were similar in intensity on 14 students used BEAM techniques (Van Toller et al., 1993). The six odours used were: 5-α-androstan-3-one (urinous and woody or odourless to certain people), chandanol (sandalwood), white sapphire (green floral), linalyl acetate (component of lavender and bergamot), indole (faecal) and smelling salts which include eucalyptus oil. The smelling salts also stimulated the trigeminal (the fifth pair of cranial nerves consisting of motor fibres that fortify the muscles used for chewing and of sensor fibres that conduct impulses from the head and face to the brain) as well as olfactory receptors. All the smells resulted in activity in specific areas of the brain: the first was in the motor and premotor parts of the cortex and corresponded to learned attributes of an odour. The second area was in the sensory part of the cerebral cortex.

Essential oils as psychotherapeutic agents

Various studies have been published in non-peer-reviewed journals on the treatment of psychiatric patients and psycho-aromatherapy in the 1920s and later in 1973 (Tisserand, 1997). These studies by medical doctors unfortunately lacked scientific acumen (Gatti and Cajola, 1923a,b, 1929) but they identified sedative essential oils or essences as: chamomile, melissa, neroli, petitgrain, opoponax, asafoetida and valerian. Stimulants were: angelica, cardamom, lemon, fennel, cinnamon, clove and ylang ylang. Some of these have been confirmed by newer studies (Appendix 14). The odorants were dropped onto cotton wool and applied with masks to the mouth. Similar studies were continued later using sprays of mainly perfumes and mixtures or these were applied to sugar lumps and sucked in the mouth. Green notes were apparently anxiety-relieving for psychiatric patients, but there was little information on their exact illnesses (see also Chapter 8).

Numerous studies in animals have so far indicated the efficacy of certain essential oils on some aspects of brain function. Many of these have, however, been studied using either intraperitoneal injection or subcutaneous injection or even oral dosing of the animals (see Chapter 5). This is not true aromatherapy as it does not involve the odour.

Recent studies showed that lemon essential oil vapour reduced immobility in rats induced by imipramine and had an antidepressant effect using forced swimming tests (Aloisi et al., 2002; see also lemon oil monograph); it also affected the acetylcholinesterase release differently in male and female rats during pain-induced conditions (Ceccarelli et al., 2002). Lemon, tuberose, rose, labdanum, lavender and oakmoss essential oils increased the immune response and thymus weight in mice subjected to stress after three weeks of continuous inhalation of the same essential oils (Komori et al., 1995). Changing the second fragrance to lemon or labdanum after initial pretreatment with tuberose followed by stress increased the immune response. Jasmine vapour also reduced sleeping time induced by pentobarbital administration in mice (Tsuchiya et al., 1991) and male and female rats behaved differently to pain and nociception. This was also shown in another study (Komori et al., 1995) and in contrast to other studies on anosmia, where brain activity was indicted (Nasel et al., 1994), anosmic mice did not react to the jasmine.

Sedative effects were produced by many essential oils and components (see Appendices 15 and 16). Other studies showed antidepressant effects of citral

on imipramine-induced immobility and forced swimming tests in rats (Komori et al., 1995) and the anxiolytic effect of Roman chamomile in mice using plasma adrenocorticotrophin levels (Yamada et al., 1996).

An interesting study showed that there was an increase in the neurogenesis of the adult mouse brain after treatment with enriched odour (Rochefort et al., 2002).

Many aromatherapists have written books on the effect of essential oils on the mind, in which they also give directives for the use of specific plant oils for treating 'the mind'. None of these treatments has been proven and some of the ideas may prove hazardous (see Chapter 7).

Placebo effect of odours?

The placebo effect is an example of a real manifestation of mind over matter. It does not confine itself to alternative therapies, but there is a greater likelihood of the placebo effect accounting for over 90% of the effect in the latter. As Millenson (1995) points out:

> We must distinguish between treatment with essential oils and aromatherapy massage etc. as practised in the UK. The use of pharmacologically-active essential oils as drugs, given internally, or on the skin in places where they are needed or inhaled in considerable concentrations is a therapeutic practice. Contrast that with 'aromatherapy massage' using 1–3% dilutions which hardly have an odour and one has to rely on placebo!
>
> Clearly, the effects of relationship interact synergistically with the effects of active treatment to influence positive patient outcomes. It therefore follows that the practitioner should do everything possible to enhance the relationship effect, otherwise known as placebo.

Reasons for the potency of the placebo effect have been given as: the patient's belief in the method; the practitioner's belief in the method; and the patient and practitioner's belief in each other, i.e. the strength of their relationship (Weil, 1983).

Placebo effects have been shown to relieve postoperative pain, induce sleep or mental awareness, bring about drastic remission in both symptoms and objective signs of chronic diseases, initiate the rejection of warts and other abnormal growths, etc. (Weil, 1983). Placebo affects headaches, seasickness and coughs, as well as having beneficial effects on pathological conditions such as rheumatoid and degenerative arthritis, blood cell count, respiratory rates, vasomotor function, peptic ulcers, hay fever and hypertension (Cousins, 1979).

However, placebo pills or other remedy can elicit undesirable side-effects, such as nausea, headaches, skin rashes, allergic reactions and even addiction, i.e. a nocebo effect. This is almost akin to voodoo death threats or when patients are mistakenly told their illness is hopeless – both are said to cause death soon after. There is sometimes a more complex situation in which the nocebo effect occurs if the patient believes they are receiving a placebo.

No personality type is particularly susceptible to the placebo effect, nor is it correlated with hypnotic suggestibility. If anything, more intelligent people have been shown to have a more enhanced placebo response (Cousins, 1979).

Psychoneuroimmunology

A review of the evidence relating to the effect of discrete lesions in the hypothalamic areas of the brain (anterior-optic, limbic forebrain, brainstem autonomic) and cerebral cortex on specific alterations in immune activity showed that it was either enhanced or depressed (Felten et al., 1987). This effect could be transient or chronic depending on the site of the lesion and its extent.

> This direct evidence for the involvement of CNS circuitry in immune modulation points to an integrated circuitry of the limbic cortex/ limbic forebrain/hypothalamus/brain stem autonomic nuclei that regulates both autonomic outflow and neuroendocrine outflow.
>
> (Felten and Felten, 1987)

There is still little concrete knowledge about the exact mechanism of such regulation. However, there are enough data to suggest that immunology has an effect on behaviour and behaviour has an effect on immunology. Simple herpes virus infection can have an effect on behaviour of mice (Felten et al., 1987). Learning and conditioning can have an effect on immunology. The brain can pick up messages from the immune system directly, so it follows that behavioural

processes can alter immune regulation (Felten et al., 1987).

Odorants and opioids in the brain

Stress-induced analgesia has been reported in rats, possibly due to alteration of the immune function (Shavit, 1987). This is possibly due to the release of opioids. Relaxation can also cause the release of opioids and therefore analgesia. This implies that the immune system as well as analgesia and the release of our own body analgesics or opioids, which are similar to opium, are interconnected. Both opioid agonists and antagonists have also been implicated in cancer development (Shavit, 1987). The general theory that relaxation stops cancer development may therefore not be correct.

Rats were found to have increased levels of opioids in their brains after inhaling certain essential oils. Opioids are a factor in pain relief (Lis-Balchin, 1998b) and can be increased in the body by autosuggestion, relaxation, belief, etc. Pain and anxiety relief is vital in many diseases, especially terminal illnesses like cancer, therefore it is important to verify these results.

The use of aromatherapy for pain relief is best achieved through massage, personal concern and touch of the patient, and also listening to their problems. The extra benefit of 'healers' found amongst some aromatherapists is an added advantage. This is the extra gift of healing, by laying on of hands, or other means, which some people possess.

Alternative or complementary medicine

It appears that aromatherapy is now increasingly being treated more as a complementary rather than alternative medicine. With that in mind, perhaps aromatherapists should forsake some of their more unusual claims in order to be more acceptable to the medical profession. Many claims are made in aromatherapy books regarding essential oils and the metaphysical, which have no scientific collaborative evidence and may only be relevant to a few aromatherapists and some clients. The following statements exemplify some of these claims:

- Myrrh oil – inhale the oil to stimulate the sixth and seventh chakra

- Frankincense works on the sixth chakra and can be mixed with myrrh and balsam tolu as well as lavender
- Orange oil – psychological conditions: selfishness, stubbornness
- Hyssop oil – physical conditions: hypertension, hypotension. Psychological conditions: grief
- Manuka (*Leptospermum scoparium*) – emotional uses: fear, anxiety, stress, low libido and blending all aspects of self. Helps with moulding and shaping emotion and reality. Patience, support, calming, caring and connecting all chakras to the heart chakra
- The aroma of cinnamon increases your ability to tap into your psychic mind and to increase financial prosperity.

It is doubtful whether such statements help aromatherapy to gain a more scientific status.

Conclusion

Although the primary biological mechanism of odour perception is well understood, the final behavioural responses during olfaction by humans are still subjective and often irreproducible. The verbal responses during human olfaction depend on various psychological factors, such as more or less intellectual means, learning processes, mood, mental attitude and physical conditions (sex, age, occupation).

The psychological effects of essential oils and other odorants can have far-reaching effects, which can be pleasant or even unpleasant, depending on the idiosyncratic nature of an individual and past as well as present experiences, which may evoke changes in mood, etc.

Pleasant feelings can usually be achieved by using 'nicely scented' odorants (essential oils), and the general feeling of well-being and relaxation can be greatly enhanced through the concomitant use of massage, a relaxing atmosphere, a friendly person to listen to one's problems and a comfortable and warm bed to lie on. How much of the benefit of such essential oil therapy is due to the essential oils has not been determined, and could be very variable, but a large proportion is probably due to the placebo effect, which is a purely psychological effect. This has been shown to have a profound physiological effect in humans and to be able to help in reversing many clinical conditions, especially those associated with stress. The effect of massage in combination with essential oils in aromatherapy provides a further powerful mechanism for treating stress-related conditions.

7

The safety issue in aromatherapy

Introduction

Many aromatherapists and members of the public consider natural essential oils to be completely safe. This is based on the misconception that all herbs are safe – because they are 'natural'. However, it is dangerous to assume, just because a tea or alcoholic extract of a plant used as a herbal medicine is harmless, that the essential oil derived from that plant is also safe. The dramatic increase in concentration of the essential oil compared with that in the whole plant (often the yield is 0.01%) demonstrates that essential oils are not equivalent to the whole herb. Essential oils are also volatile and fat-soluble and therefore differ from the mainly water-soluble whole herb extracts used in herbal medicine. As suggested in Chapter 1, the comparison is akin to massaging butter into the skin of a baby and believing that this is equivalent to giving the baby whole milk to drink.

The toxicity of essential oils can also be entirely different to that of the herb, not only because of their high concentration, but also because of their ability to pass across membranes very efficiently due to their lipophilicity.

Some aromatherapists believe that aromatherapy is self-correcting, unlike conventional therapy with medicines, and if errors are made in aromatherapy, they may be resolved through discontinuation of the wrongful application of the oil. There is also the belief that if an inflammation follows the use of an irritant oil, it will dissipate as soon as the oil is discontinued without having caused lasting damage. It is said that the occasional mistake is never injurious, but instead provides valuable guidance about how to correctly use the often underestimated power of essential oils (e.g. Schnaubelt, 1999).

This is a very dangerous view due to the considerable amount of evidence of the risks of essential oils.

Essential oil safety has been monitored in a variety of different ways, all of which have been geared to the perfumery, cosmetics and the food industries. The continuous synthesis of new aromachemicals and their widespread usage in 'natural essential oils' together with many diluents, has brought about many problems, the worst being sensitisation. The whole aspect of safety is now being stringently reviewed and new regulations may soon impede the sale and usage of many essential oils and cosmetic products as well as their use in foods.

The toxicity of essential oils does not entirely depend on high concentrations. All essential oils are toxic at very high doses, especially if taken orally. Many essential oils are inherently toxic at very low concentrations due to very toxic components: these are not normally used in aromatherapy (see Appendices 29 and 30). Many essential oils which are considered to be non-toxic can have a toxic effect on some people: this can be influenced by previous sensitisation to a given essential oil, a group of essential oils containing similar components or some adulterant in the essential oil. It can also be influenced by the age of the person: babies and young children are especially vulnerable and so are very old people (who are also more affected by drugs, etc.). The influence of other medicaments, both conventional and herbal, is still in the preliminary stages of being studied. It is possible that these medicaments, and also probably household products, including perfumes and cosmetics, can influence the adverse reactions to essential oils. Very small doses of essential oils taken/used over many months or years could have toxic effects, as shown by many recent studies on sensitisation.

Aromatherapists themselves have also been affected by sensitisation (Crawford *et al.*, 2004): in a 12-month period under study, prevalence of hand dermatitis in a sample of massage therapists was 15%

by self-reported criteria and 23% by a symptom-based method and included use of aromatherapy products in massage oils, lotions or creams. In contrast, the suggestion that aromatherapists have any adverse effects to long-term usage of essential oils was apparently disproved by a non-scientific survey, where adverse reactions to essential oils were blamed on reactions to the clients themselves (Price and Price, 1999). Most aromatherapists apparently experienced only beneficial effects both on the skin and other organs and tissues. This type of survey may be considered unscientific for reasons of bias of the respondents to the survey, notably because aromatherapists who had experienced adverse effects would have left the profession; secondly, most of the respondents had practised for under 4 years and had given fewer than ten treatments per week (as reported by Price and Price, 1999).

The International Organization for Standardization (ISO) has set up standards to make essential oils more consistent (see monographs), but this often encourages adulteration (see Chapter 5). The ISO stipulates that there is a named botanical source, but in commerce the actual plant source is often confused. For example, citrus plants can be grown as scions on a parent plant of a different species. Furthermore hybrids and cultivars are often used, as well as clones obtained by micropropagation (e.g. tea tree).

General guidance for essential oil purchase and storage

Do not buy essential oils from market stalls – these cheap essential oils are often useful only for usage in burners and not for skin application. Many of the essential oils are mixed with considerable volumes of various diluents, which include petroleum spirits. Buy bottles with child-proof caps and efficient droppers. On the other hand do not assume that essential oils sold from high street stores are pure, unadulterated essential oils (see Chapter 5). All essential oils should be sold in brown bottles or platinum containers: do not buy them in clear glass or plastic containers.

Essential oils should always be stored in the refrigerator (preferably in an enclosed plastic container to prevent the odours mingling with stored foods) or in a cool, dark place. Storage areas must be out of reach for children. Do not expose the bottles to light or air for long periods, to prevent oxidation

of the components – as this may make them more toxic. Citrus essential oils are very unstable and may last for only a few months. Many already contain added antioxidants, but one can add vitamin E (squeezed from capsules) to the essential oils as a safe and efficient antioxidant; it also supposedly helps the skin to remain young and healthy.

Toxicity testing in animals

Most aromatherapy suppliers claim to have managed in some way to obtain essential oils, which 'have never been tested on animals', information which they pass on to their clientele. Nearly all the essential oils and extractives commonly used in aromatherapy have however been tested on animals and their monographs are to be found in the journal *Food and Cosmetics Toxicology* from 1973, renamed *Food and Chemical Toxicology* in 1982. This fact is not known by many aromatherapists, who, in their innocence, think they are using only essential oils that have not been tested on animals, sold to them by reputable dealers. This is not only erroneous, but it contravenes the Trades Description Act and also Health and Safety regulations, as only essential oils tested on animals are legally sold and used for foods, perfumes and cosmetics.

Apparently suppliers can get round the legislation using a loophole that involves the issue of certificates stating that 'the essential oils have never been tested on animals if they have not been tested **in the last seven years**'. As most were tested from 1973 to 1992, this seems to be a good ploy by the suppliers. The results of more recent animal tests, published as monographs, include essential oil components and further genotoxicity, mutagenicity and pharmacological evaluations on both essential oils and components. Most cosmetic products are now no longer tested on animals, but all their ingredients have been tested.

As most essential oils were tested over 30 years ago, the toxicity data may now be meaningless, as different essential oils are now used, some of which contain different quantities of synthetic components. There is also the question as to whether all synthetic components are always made in the same way. If not, then there is the possibility of contamination with other chemicals, which changes the composition and therefore the adverse effects, either making them worse or better.

The Living Flavour and Living Flower series (International Flavor & Fragrance Inc.) are produced by trapping the natural odours of the living plant using SPME (solid phase micro extraction) and then assembling them using totally synthetic components. Synthetic products could perhaps account for the increased toxicity of the essential oils bought today, especially in the area of sensitisation.

Published monograph data usually include: LD_{50} (lethal dose for 50% of the test population) and acute symptoms after oral dosing in rats and dermal dosing in rabbits, subacute toxicity data after oral dosing, irritation studies usually after application on the backs of hairless mice or intact/abraded rabbit skin (Appendix 22). Sensitisation tests use a maximisation test on human volunteers at 1–8% in petrolatum, photoxicity on hairless mice/swine and antimicrobial activity. On occasion, carcinogenicity and mutagenicity studies are included, together with other references as to the composition and bioactivities, including pharmacological and insecticidal studies and clinical trials, etc.

Toxicity studies in animals: critique

The major drawbacks of trying to extrapolate toxicity studies in animals to humans concern feelings – from headaches to splitting migraines; feeling sick, vertigo, profound nausea; tinnitus; sadness, melancholia, suicidal thoughts; feelings of hate – which are clearly impossible to measure in animals.

The toxicity of an individual essential oil/component is also tested in isolation in animals and disregards the possibility of modification by other substances, including food components and food additive chemicals, the surrounding atmosphere with gaseous and other components, fragrances used in perfumes, domestic products, in the car, in public transport (including the people), workplace, etc. These could cause modification of the essential oil/component, its bioavailability and possibly the enhancement or loss of its function.

The detoxification processes in the body are all directed to the production of a more polar product(s), which can be excreted mainly by the kidneys regardless of whether this (these) are more toxic or less toxic than the initial substance. Any biotransformation in the body is affected by individual enzymes, which attack certain chemical groups. These include: aromatic,

acyclic and heterocyclic hydroxylation; *N*-, *S*- and *O*-dealkylation; *N*-oxidation and *S*-oxidation; amine oxidation, alcohol and aldehyde oxidation; *N*-hydroxylation; desulphuration and deamination. The process usually occurs through two phases: the primary phase involves these enzymatic biotransformations, the most important being microsomal oxidation using cytochrome P450; this is followed by the secondary phase, involving conjugation. There can be numerous biotransformations following the conjugations as well, giving rise to hundreds of metabolites: the main metabolite(s) vary in different animals, therefore extrapolation from animal to humans becomes difficult if the major metabolite(s) are entirely different. These major metabolites can be influenced by the presence of other components. The latter can also affect the biological half-life, and thereby its activity and accumulation in different tissues in the body.

Dermal absorption and detoxification

Cutaneous enzymes include esterases and other enzymes, including oxidases using cytochrome P450. The activity of these enzymes in the skin is much lower than in the liver, but the large surface area of the skin makes it a significant detoxification process. Any chemicals absorbed will then be dealt with by the liver and other organs/tissues.

Absorption of essential oil components can be quite substantial and is influenced by numerous internal and external factors: idiosyncracy; skin/air temperature, humidity, contact time and concentration, area and site of body as well as the physicochemical nature of each component. There is also the variability introduced by age, follicle number and skin surface status (e.g. undamaged, damaged, shaven, suntanned, protected by creams, etc.) (Hewitt *et al.*, 1993). The more lipophilic molecules are absorbed quickly, but also volatalise more readily; the more hydrophilic components may be very slow in penetrating, if at all, but are also influenced by the presence or absence of occlusion. Coumarin, present in cassia and other oils, is rapidly absorbed to 46% (human unoccluded), β-phenylethanol 64% (rat unoccluded), benzyl acetate 12% (human unoccluded), cinnamaldehyde to 24% (human unoccluded). Some components will accumulate to form a cutaneous reservoir pool (Hewitt *et al.*, 1993) in the lipid-rich stratum corneum. Others components permeate deeper into the skin to be biotransformed by the P450 enzyme systems in the dermis and epidermis, and eventually this mixture of biotransformed and unchanged molecules reaches the systemic circulation via the dermal microvasculature.

Inhalation: absorption and detoxification

Similar enzymes occur in the alveolar cells, modifying any chemicals absorbed through inhalation. There is almost a direct entry into the lung cells for lipophilic molecules in the essential oils as there is only one cell membrane thickness to traverse. This is why the effect of vaporisers or simply breathing in fragrances added to bath water can be substantial. Damage can occur to the lungs due to excessive use of certain chemicals in essential oils, but the actual concentration has not been worked out and very few studies are available (Cooper et al., 1995). The risk of respiratory cancer in workers after 5 years of exposure to industrial terpenes from conifers is greatly increased (Kauppinen et al., 1986). However, in another study, exposure to α-pinene enantiomers for 20 minutes at 10–450 mg/m^3 did not cause acute changes in lung function (Falk et al., 1990). Studies on the absorption of inhaled essential oil components are very rare, but one showed that 1,8-cineole was rapidly absorbed from eucalyptus essential oil, with plasma concentrations at their peak after 18 minutes (Jaeger et al., 1996). The direct entry of lipophilic components from essential oils via the olfactory mucosa is quite substantial and they can act like anaesthetics very rapidly. Entry via the blood–brain barrier can also be substantial, especially in neonates and young children where it is undeveloped.

GRAS status/NOELs

Most essential oils have GRAS (generally recognised as safe) status granted by the Flavor and Extract Manufacturers Association (FEMA) and approved by the US Food and Drug Administration (FDA) for food use, and many appear in the Food Chemical Codex. This was reviewed in 1996 after evaluation by the Expert Panel of the FEMA. The assessment was based on data of exposure, and as most flavour ingredients are used at less than 100 ppm, predictions

regarding their safety can be assessed from data on their structurally related group(s) (Munro et al., 1996). The NOELs (no-observed-adverse-effect levels) are more than 100 000 times their exposure levels from use as flavour ingredients (Adams et al., 1996). Critical to GRAS assessment are data of metabolic fate and chronic studies rather than acute toxicity. Most essential oils and components have an LD$_{50}$ of 1–20 g/kg body weight or roughly 1–20 mL/kg, with a few exceptions as follows:

Boldo leaf oil	0.1/0.9 (oral/dermal)
Calamus	0.8–9/5
Chenopodium	0.2/0.4
Pennyroyal	0.4/4
Savory (summer)	1.4/0.3
Thuja	0.8/4

Teratogenicity studies are infrequent and often deceptive, as they often involve the study of unusual species of plant essential oils. For example, *Salvia lavandulifolia* Vahl or Spanish sage, containing 50% of sabinyl acetate, injected s.c. during pregnancy with 15, 45 and 135 mg/kg essential oil (Pages et al., 1992; see monograph) showed an abortifacient effect, no fetal toxicity but significant maternal toxicity. This amount of sabinyl acetate was similar to that found in *Juniperus sabina* and *Plectranthus fruticosa*, which had a teratogenic effect (neither of these are frequently used, especially in aromatherapy).

Reproductive organ and hormone studies have shown that there are several xenoendocrine disrupters *in vitro* on male reproductive systems; citral has caused enlargement of the prostate gland in animal models and has oestrogenic effects (Nogueira et al., 1995); several fragrances are carcinogenic (e.g. methyl eugenol in mice), whilst others are possible carcinogens (Burkey et al., 2000).

Poisonous chemicals

The National Institute of Occupational Safety and Health (1989) recognised 884 poisonous substances (many synthetics from petrochemicals) from 2983 chemicals used in the fragrance industry. Of these, many cause cancer, birth defects, CNS disorders, allergic respiratory reactions, skin and eye irritation. The Research Institute for Fragrance Materials (RIFM) tests the safety of fragrance materials, but only about 1500 of more than 5000 materials used in fragrances have been tested. This is in contrast to their statement that: 'Over the approximately 30 years since its inception, RIFM has tested virtually all important fragrance materials in common use but it has always been the policy of RIFM that if a material is used by only one company, it is that company's responsibility to see that the material is adequately tested and evaluated' (Frosch *et al.*, 1998). However, patented chemicals are not tested until the patent expires, which may be after 17 years.

The testing done by the RIFM is generally limited to acute oral and dermal toxicity, irritation and dermal sensitisation, and phototoxicity. Testing is limited to individual materials and there is little effort to address synergistic and modifying effects of materials in combination, though the RIFM is aware that they occur. Materials used in combinations often have synergistic and modifying effects and more positive sensitisation reactions occur than when the materials are tested individually (Johansen *et al.*, 1998).

Most chemical data sheets and Material Safety Data Sheet (MSDS) information on fragrance materials clearly state that the chemical, physical and toxicological properties have not been thoroughly investigated. Many materials that were widely used for decades in the past had severe neurotoxic properties and accumulated in body tissues (Spencer *et al.*, 1979; Furuhashi *et al.*, 1994). In spite of this, most fragrance materials have never been tested for neurological effects, despite the fact that olfactory pathways provide a direct route to the brain (Hastings *et al.*, 1991).

Toxicity in humans

Dermatitis and sensitisation

A recent clinical review of the adverse reactions to fragrances has been published (de Groot and Frosch, 1997) and many examples of cutaneous reactions to essential oils have been reported elsewhere (Guin, 1982, 1995). In the USA about six million people have a skin allergy to fragrance. Many of these people reported that this has a major impact on their quality of life. Symptoms include headaches, dizziness, nausea, fatigue, shortness of breath and difficulty concentrating. Fragrance materials are readily absorbed into the body via the respiratory system and once absorbed cause systemic effects. Migraine headaches are frequently triggered by fragrances. Fragrances are known to modify cerebral blood flow and several common fragrance materials are known to have potent sedative effects via inhalation (Buchbauer *et al.*, 1993a). Recent studies in the US by the Institute of Medicine sponsored by the Environmental Protection Agency (EPA) suggest that fragrance materials can act on the same receptors in the brain as alcohol and tobacco, altering mood and function.

Effects on asthmatics

Perfumes and fragrances are recognised as triggers for asthma by the American Lung Association and several other organisations concerned with respiratory health. The vast majority of materials used in fragrances are respiratory irritants and there are a few that are known to be respiratory sensitisers. Most have not been evaluated for their effects on the lungs and the respiratory system.

Respiratory irritants are known to make the airways more susceptible to injury and allergens, as well as to trigger and exacerbate such conditions as asthma, allergies, sinus problems and other respiratory disorders. In view of the recently recorded increase in asthma and other respiratory disorders, reduction in exposures to irritants is essential. In addition, there are a subset of asthmatics that are specifically triggered by fragrances (Shim and Williams, 1986; Bell *et al.*, 1993; Baldwin *et al.*, 1999), which suggests that fragrances not only trigger asthma, they may also cause it in some cases (Millqvist and Lowhagen, 1996). Placebo-controlled studies using perfumes to challenge people with asthma-like symptoms showed that asthma could be elicited with perfumes without the presence of bronchial obstruction and these were not transmitted by the olfactory nerve as the patients were unaware of the smell (Millqvist and Lowhagen, 1996).

People who are sensitive to fragrance often experience great difficulty in obtaining fragrance-free home and personal care products, and suffer health effects as a result of using scented products. Products labelled 'unscented' or 'hypoallergenic' that actually contain fragrance materials are particularly problematical

(HEAL, 2005). Several fragrance chemicals affect the immune response of the skin when inhaled, but the systemic and long-term effects of most fragrance materials are not known.

Adverse reactions to fragrances are difficult or even impossible to link to a particular chemical – often due to secrecy rules of the cosmetic/perfumery companies and the enormous range of synthetic components, constituting about 90% of flavour and fragrance ingredients (Larsen, 1998). The same chemicals are used in foods and cosmetics – there is therefore a greater impact due to the three different modes of entry: oral, inhalation and skin.

Increase in allergic contact dermatitis in recent years

A study of 1600 adults in 1987 showed that 12% reacted adversely to cosmetics and toiletries, 4.3% of which were used for their odour (i.e. they contained high levels of fragrances). Respiratory problems worsened with prolonged fragrance exposure (e.g. at cosmetic/perfumery counters) and even in churches. In another study, 32% of the women tested had adverse reactions and 80% of these had positive skin tests for fragrances (deGroot and Frosch, 1987). Problems with essential oils have also been increasing. For example, contact dermatitis and allergic contact dermatitis caused by tea tree oil has been reported, which was previously considered to be safe (Carson and Riley, 1995a). It is unclear whether eucalyptol was responsible for the allergenic response (Southwell, 1997); out of seven patients sensitised to tea tree oil, six reacted to limonene, five to α-terpinene and aromadendrene, two to terpinen-4-ol and one to p-cymene and α-phellandrene (Knight and Hausen, 1994).

Many studies on allergic contact dermatitis (ACD) have been done in different parts of the world (deGroot and Frosch, 1987):

- Japan (Sugiura et al., 2000): the patch test with lavender oil was found to be positive in increased numbers and above that of other essential oils in 10 years.
- Denmark (Johansen et al., 2000): there was an 11% increase to the patch test in the last year and of 1537 patients, 29% were allergic to scenteds.
- Hungary (Katona and Egyud, 2001): increased sensitivity to balsams and fragrances was noted.

- Switzerland (Kohl et al., 2002): ACD incidence has increased over the years and recently 36% of 819 patch tests were positive to cosmetics.
- Belgium (Kohl et al., 2002): increased incidence of ACD has been noted.

Occupational increases have also been observed. For example, two aromatherapists were reported to have developed ACD: one to citrus, neroli, lavender, frankincense and rosewood and the other to geraniol, ylang ylang and angelica (Keane et al., 2000).

Allergic air-borne contact dermatitis from the essential oils used in aromatherapy was also reported (Schaller and Korting, 1995). Allergic contact dermatitis occurred in an aromatherapist due to French marigold essential oil, *Tagetes* (Bilsland and Strong, 1990). A physiotherapist developed ACD to eugenol, cloves and cinnamon (Sanchez-Perez and Garcia Diez, 1999).

There is also the growing problem that patients with eczema are frequently treated by aromatherapists using massage with essential oils. A possible allergic response to a variety of essential oils was found in children with atopic eczema, who were massaged with or without the oils. At first both massages proved beneficial, though not significantly different; but on re-applying the essential oil massage after a month's break, there was a notable adverse effect on the eczema, which could suggest sensitisation (Anderson et al., 2000).

Photosensitisers

Berlocque dermatitis is frequently caused by bergamot or other citrus oil applications on the skin (often due to their inclusion in eau de Cologne) followed by exposure to UV light. This effect is caused by psolarens or furanocoumarins (Klarmann, 1958). Citrus essential oils labelled furanocoumarin-free (FCF) have no phototoxic effect, but are suspected carcinogens (Young et al., 1990). Other phototoxic essential oils include yarrow and angelica, neroli, petitgrain, cedarwood, rosemary, cassia, calamus, cade, eucalyptus (species not stated), orange, anise, bay, bitter almond, ylang ylang, carrot seed and linaloe (the latter probably due to linalool, which, like citronellol, has a sensitising methylene group exposed) (Guin, 1995). Photosensitiser oils include cumin, rue, dill, sandalwood, lemon (oil and expressed), lime (oil and expressed), opoponax and verbena (the latter being frequently adulterated) (Klarmann, 1958). Even celery soup eaten before UV irradiation has been known to cause severe sunburn (Boffa *et al.*, 1996).

Many of these photosensitisers are now banned or restricted. New International Fragrance Research Association (IFRA) proposals for some phototoxic essential oils include: rue oil to be 0.15% maximum in consumer products, marigold oil and absolute to be 0.01% and petitgrain mandarin oil to be 0.165%.

Commonest allergenic essential oils and components

The most common fragrance components causing allergy are: cinnamic alcohol, hydroxycitronellal, musk ambrette, isoeugenol and geraniol (Scheinman, 1996). These are included in the eight commonest markers used to check for allergic contact dermatitis, usually as a 2% mix. Other components considered allergenic are: benzyl salicylate, sandalwood oil, anisyl alcohol, benzyl alcohol and coumarin.

The IFRA and the Research Institute for Fragrance Materials (RIFM) have forbidden the use of several essential oils and components, including costus root oil, dihydrocoumarin, musk ambrette and balsam of Peru (Ford, 1991; see also Appendices 28 and 29). There is also a concentration limit imposed on the use of isoeugenol, cold-pressed lemon oil, bergamot oil, angelica root oil, cassia oil, cinnamic alcohol, hydroxy-citronellal and oakmoss absolute. Cinnamic aldehyde, citral and carvone oxide can only be used with a quenching agent. Photosensitivity and phototoxicity occurs with some allergens such as musk ambrette and 6-methyl coumarin and has been removed from skin care products. Children were often found to be sensitive to Peru balsam, probably due to the use of baby-care products containing this (e.g. talcum powder used on nappy rash).

As fragrances and foods contain essential oils and components, it is not surprising that fragrance materials have been found to interact with food flavourings. This is of increasing concern. For example, a 'balsam of Peru-free diet' has been devised in cases where cross-reactions are known to occur (Veien *et al.*, 1985). 'Newer' sensitisers include ylang ylang (Romaguera and Vilplana, 2000), sandalwood oil (Sharma *et al.*, 1987) (caution should be considered in accepting this as so much of this essential oil is

adulterated or completely synthetic), Lyral (Frosch *et al.*, 1999; Hendriks *et al.*, 1999) and eucalyptol (Vilaplana and Romaguera, 2000).

Some sensitisers have been shown to interact with other molecules. For example, cinnamaldehyde interacts with proteins (Weibel *et al.*, 1989), which indicates how the immunogenicity occurs.

The international authorities are not satisfied that the cosmetics industry has been vigilant enough in their protection of the public, hence the proposed new EC legislation (7th Amendment), to label cosmetics/perfumes containing sensitisers and reduce or ban them altogether (see Appendices 27–29).

Synthetic musks: a special problem

There have been very few published reports on neurotoxic aromachemicals such as musk ambrette (Spencer *et al.*, 1984), although many synthetic musks took over as perfume ingredients when public opinion turned against the exploitation of animal products. Musk ambrette was found to have neurotoxic properties in orally fed mice in 1967. However, it was in 1985, after studies were again published on its neurotoxic effects, that it was also realised that musk ambrette was readily absorbed through the skin. The IFRA then recommended that musk ambrette should not be used in direct skin contact products, even though it had been used since before the 1920s. In 1991, the FDA still found musk ambrette in skin contact products, proving that the recommendations by the IFRA are not binding.

A similar story occurred with acetylethyltetramethyltetralin (AETT), another synthetic musk, also known as versalide, patented in the early 1950s. During routine tests for irritancy in 1975, it was noted that with repeated applications the skin of the mice turned bluish and they exhibited signs of neurotoxicity. On further application, the internal organs also turned blue and there was severe neurological damage. The myelin sheath was damaged irreversibly in a manner similar to that which occurs with multiple sclerosis. In spite of legitimate concerns, the industry does not demand testing for the neurological and respiratory effects of fragrance materials.

Musk xylene, one of the commonest fragrance materials, is found in blood samples from the general population (Kafferlein *et al.*, 1998) and bound to human haemoglobin (Riedel *et al.*, 1999). Nitro- and non-nitrobenzenoid musk compounds are also found in human adipose tissue (Riedel *et al.*, 1999) and nitro musk metabolites are found in human breast milk (Liebel and Ehrenstorfer, 1993). These musk products have been found to have an effect on the life stages of experimental animals such as the frog, *Xenopus laevis*, and the zebra-fish, *Danio rerio* (Chou and Dietrich, 1999) and the rat (Christian *et al.*, 1999). The effects on animal development have been extended to studies on reproduction and fertility, including hyperplasia of the prostate and testicular effects (Ford *et al.*, 1990; Api *et al.*, 1996). The hepatotoxic effect of musks is under constant study (Steinberg *et al.*, 1999).

Toxicity in young children: a special case

It is clear that there are severe dangers associated with the bad or ill-informed advice given by many aromatherapy books about the treatment of babies and children. For example, one book recommends giving 5–10 drops of 'chamomile oil' three times a day in a little warmed milk to their babies to treat colic. As there is no indication as to which of the three commercially available chamomile oils is to be used and because, depending on the dropper size, the dose could easily approach the oral LD_{50} for the English and German chamomile oils, this could result in a fatality. In the same publication 'syrup of elderflower and peppermint' was recommended for 'fever'. The peppermint could possibly be given by mothers in the form of peppermint oil, which has been known to kill a week-old baby (*Evening Standard*, 1998).

Dosages given in terms of drops can vary widely according to the size of the dropper in an essential oil bottle (see Appendices 9 and 10) and dilutions for massage also vary widely from author to author (e.g. 4–6 drops in 10 mL carrier oil; 1 drop for every 20 mL of vegetable oil). This could make a considerable difference to the toxicity regarding children, especially babies.

Children's cosmetics and toys

Many 'cosmetics' designed for use by children contain fragrance allergens (Rastogi *et al.*, 1999). In Denmark,

samples of children's cosmetics were found to contain geraniol, hydroxycitronellol, isoeugenol and cinnamic alcohol (Rastogi *et al.*, 1999). Children are more susceptible than adults to any chemical, so the increase in childhood asthma reported in recent years could be caused by fragrance components in fast foods (whose consumption is escalating). There is also an increase in fragrance chemicals in everyday products from airfresheners, soaps, cosmetics, bathroom products, 'newcar smells', all of which may interact.

Selected toxicities of certain essential oils and their components

Limonene

This is a common industrial cleaner and is also the main citrus oil component, the latter being often used in aromatherapy in pregnancy and childbirth. D-Limonene is used for degreasing metal before industrial painting; it oxidises to *R*-(–)-carvone, *cis*- and *trans*-isomers of limonene oxide. D-Limonene causes allergic contact dermatitis, particularly when aged (Chang *et al.*, 1997). In one series of studies, 2% of car mechanics with eczema on their hands tested positive to oxidised D-limonene, as did 2% of dermatitis patients (Karlberg *et al.*, 1994a,b).

Allergic contact dermatitis was noted in a histopathology laboratory technician using Parasolve (containing D-limonene) instead of xylene (Wakelin *et al.*, 1998). Pulmonary exposure of human volunteers to D-limonene caused a decrease in the lung vital capacity at highest doses (Falk-Filipsson *et al.*, 1993). The major volatile component of lactating mothers' milk in the USA was found to contain D-limonene and the component is used as a potential skin penetration promoter for drugs such as indometacin, especially when mixed with ethanol (Falk-Filipsson *et al.*, 1993). Lastly, cats and dogs are very susceptible to insecticides and baths containing D-limonene giving rise to neurological symptoms including ataxia, stiffness, apparent severe CNS depression, tremors, coma (von Burg, 1995; see also Beasley, 1999).

In contrast to all the toxicity, D-limonene was shown to have anticarcinogenic properties *in vivo* when applied subcutaneously to mice which were then injected with benzopentaphene. Although the lung tumours took longer to develop and therefore the animals lived longer, it did not prevent the cancer from forming in the first place (Homburger *et al.*, 1971).

Linalool

It has been established that linalool hydroperoxide increases as the linalool decays and the rate of chemical decay is rapid compared with the potential shelf-life and age of oils used in aromatherapy. When linalool was oxidised for just 10 weeks the linalool content fell to 80% and the remaining 20% consisted of a range of breakdown chemicals including linalool hydroperoxide, which was confirmed as a sensitising agent. The fresh linalool was not a sensitiser, therefore the EC regulations which are warning about sensitisation potential are looking for potential harm even on storage (Skoeld *et al.*, 2002).

The sensitising activity of linalool was assessed using a commercial grade of 97% purity, which included linalool hydroperoxide. The sample of commercial linalool was then purified and the only sensitisation reaction was obtained when it was used at 100%; a dramatic reduction in sensitisation occurred when the linalool was 98.6% pure and the dihydrolinalool was below 1.4%. It was suggested that some of the other oxidisation chemicals may also have sensitisation potential apart from linalool hydroperoxide (Basketter *et al.*, 2002).

Safrole

This is the main component of sassafras oil and sweet basil and was used previously in perfumes and food: it is now limited to 1 mg/kg in foods (Council Directive 92/109/EEC, 14 December 1992), except in foods containing mace, nutmeg (15 mg/kg) and alcoholic drinks containing more than 25% of alcohol by volume (5 mg/kg) and other alcoholic drinks (2 mg/kg). Safrole and isosafrole were first studied in 1885 by Heffer, and numerous further studies reported their effects on tumorigenesis in animals and humans (Chen *et al.*, 1999) and the mode of action (Luo and Guenthner, 1996). Safrole and sassafras oil are controlled under the Controlled Drugs Regulations (1993) (Controlled Drugs with subsequent European Directives 3677/90 as amended by Council Regulation 900/92 and Regulation (EC) No 273/2004 of the European Parliament and of the Council of

11 February 2004 on drug precursors) and are listed as category 1 substances, as they are precursors for illicit manufacture of hallucinogenic, narcotic and psychotropic drugs (e.g. ecstasy).

Thujone

In large quantities thujone can cause convulsions associated with lesions of the cerebral cortex (Keith and Starraky, 1935; Opper, 1939) but thujone is permitted at 0.5 mg/kg in foods as α or β or combination (Council Directive, 88/388/EEC, of 21 June 1988) and at 35 mg/kg in bitters.

Wormwood

Wormwood essential oil, obtained via the Internet by a young man who thought it was equivalent to absinthe, caused acute renal failure and rhabdomyolysis when just 10 mL was drunk (Weisboro *et al.*, 1997). In another incident a 2-year-old child survived after drinking 15 mL of the oil. Absinthe was drunk by Van Gogh, together with camphor and turpentine (Bonkovsky *et al.*, 1992), which may explain his style of painting!

Abortifacient and teratogenic oils

Apiol

When apiol (in dill) was studied in animals (Patoir *et al.*, 1936) it was found that the largest doses (not stated) gave rise to bleeding and hepatonephritis as well as abortion (i.e. it was an overall poison). A woman with fatal acute haemolytic anaemia, thrombocytopenic purpura, nephrosis and hepatitis was found to have taken a high dose of a compound containing apiol for amenorrhoea for three months. Other overdose cases of apiol resulted in CNS effects (Lowenstein and Ballew, 1958).

Pennyroyal oil

A large dose of pennyroyal oil taken by a woman in the USA to induce an abortion proved fatal (Gold and

Cates, 1980). Other cases of toxicity of pennyroyal to women who tried unsuccessfully to induce abortion have been described (Tisserand and Balacs, 1995).

Camphorated oil

Taken by mistake instead of castor oil during pregnancy, camphorated oil resulted in one fatality of the baby at birth out of four cases (Weiss and Catalano, 1973). Several cases of accidental poisoning in children are also reported, causing excitation of the CNS resulting in delirium and convulsions followed by depression including uncoordination and coma. Camphor oil was also reported to cause intoxication in 500 people in one year in the USA (Tisserand and Balacs, 1995).

Nutmeg

Nutmeg intoxication during pregnancy (1 tablespoonful of grated nutmeg instead of 1/8th teaspoon in cookies) resulted in acute anticholinergic hyperstimulation, i.e. palpitations, agitation and blurred vision (Lavy, 1987). Treated with morphine and activated charcoal, the expectant mother was well after 24 hours and the baby was born later after slight pre-eclampsia symptoms. Nutmeg oil/grated seed can cause hallucinations and convulsions in large doses; myristicin itself was also shown to produce narcotic effects (Weil, 1965) and in large quantities, nutmeg and mace also showed these effects, which were comparable to alcohol intoxication.

Antifertility oils

β-Myrcene

β-Myrcene above 0.25 g/kg was found to be detrimental to the fertility and progeny number and development in the rat when given during pregnancy by gavage (Delgado et al., 1993).

Phenol methyl ethers

Phenol methyl ethers, in particular anethole, found in fennel and anise are related to the oestrone and oestradiol methyl ethers; however, dill oil is inactive (Zondek and Bergman, 1938; Albert-Puleo, 1980). The activity of anethole was much less than that of oestrone itself, and had a more profound effect on rats than mice, but there may be a remote danger of producing more oestrogens in the body by fennel. trans-Anethole has some minor oestrogenic properties (Zondek and Bergman, 1938).

Genotoxic oils

Dill, peppermint and pine

Genotoxicity of dill, peppermint and pine essential oils has been reported using chromosome aberration and sister-chromatid exchange tests in human lymphocytes in vitro and Drosophila melanogaster somatic mutation and recombination tests in vivo (Lazutka et al., 2001). All these oils were cytotoxic for human lymphocytes. Other cytotoxic and/or genotoxic studies have recently been published on methyl eugenol (Burkey et al., 2000), mint (Franzios et al., 1997), camphor, 1,8-cineole, citral, citronellal, menthol and terpineol (Nogueira et al., 1995; Gomes-Carneiro et al., 1998), oregano essential oils (Karpouhtsis et al., 1998), allyl benzene etheric oils estragole, basil and trans-anethole, D-limonene (Whysner and Williams, 1996). Negative evidence for in vivo DNA-damaging and mutagenic and chromosomal effects of eugenol were also shown (Maura et al., 1989; Abraham, 2001).

Neurotoxic oils

Thuja, sage, cedar, hyssop

The toxicity of Salvia officinalis, thuja, Arbor vitae and cedar Chaemocyparis thyroides, hyssop Hyssopus officinalis (containing pinocamphone and isopinocamphone), as well as thujone-containing Dalmatian sage, were investigated in 65 male and female rats intraperitoneally at progressively increasing doses; the components thujone and pinocamphone were also tested (Millet et al., 1981; see also sage oil monograph). The animals were equipped with four skull electrodes for EEG and convulsions were elicited by all the oils, but varied according to the plant. For hyssop, the dose for no effect was 0.08 g/kg; convulsions were at

0.13 g/kg and it was lethal at 1.25 g/kg. For sage oil it was 0.3, 0.5 and 3.2 g/kg respectively. A daily repeated subclinical dose of hyssop oil (0.02 g/kg) for 15 days precipitated convulsions after just 5 days, but after cessation of injections, the rats returned to normal.

Convulsions were shown for thujone and pinocamphone at lower doses: thujone: at 0.2 g/kg and pinocamphone at 0.05 g/kg. This suggests that small doses every day for a short time could produce convulsions.

Eight cases of poisoning by the four essential oils showed a period of latency of a few minutes to 2 hours, the patients vomited and had convulsions, resembling epileptic fits, sometimes with cyanosis (Millet *et al.*, 1981). In six clinical cases the patients had ingested the oils for therapeutic purposes (e.g. 10 mL thuja oil to be 'in shape', 30 drops of hyssop oil for a common cold). Repetitive intake occurred in an asthmatic 6-year-old girl who had 2–3 drops of hyssop oil per day, but during a dyspnoeic crisis, she received half a teaspoonful of hyssop. Ten drops of hyssop oil was taken 'for flu' during two consecutive days; on the second day the convulsions appeared. A woman with facial acne took 20 drops of undiluted thuja at lunch and dinner for 5 days; after the tenth dose she got convulsions (Millet *et al.*, 1981).

Three case studies associated with the induction of epileptic seizures in normal people, including a child, were reported due to sage and other essential oils. One adult took 'a mouthful' of sage essential oil for hyperlipaemia over several years but after a larger dose she had tonic seizures and became unconscious for an hour, but recovered. Lastly, a baby given five long baths with addition of eucalyptus, pine and thyme over a 4-day period to cure her upper respiratory infection had a fit, followed by two more that day. She was hospitalised and the tests were normal, but she started to have multiple fits with a maximum of 133 in a day and was treated with phenobarbital and phenytoin. Her development was very depressed (Burkhard *et al.*, 1999). Eucalyptus and camphor have been reported to have an effect on the rat cerebral cortex (Steinmetz *et al.*, 1987).

Absolutes and concretes

Absolutes and concretes are potentially dangerous as they have not all been tested on the skin (Lis-Balchin,

1999a). Many solvent extracts are sensitisers (IFRA) and are usually used in lower percentages in all perfumes and cosmetic products. About 4% is the usual recommendation (ISA, 1993): except for neroli, lavender, hyacinth, benzoin (strong sensitiser), myrrh, olibanum at about 8%, also mastic although it is a strong sensitiser and causes irritation. Genet is used at 12% and vanilla at 10%. The absolutes and concretes of verbena are decreased to 2% and tobacco leaf to 1%. Some have not been tested for toxicity dermally, e.g. violet leaf, honeysuckle, orris, narcissus, mimosa, but are used at about 1–2% in perfumes.

Untested common essential oils include: catnip, chamomile (Maroc), *Eucalyptus* oils other than *E. globulus* and *E. citriodora*, *Inula graveolens*, kanuka (*Kunzea ericoides*), manuka (*Leptospermum scoparium*), melissa, naouli, *Ravensara aromatica* and other *Ravensara* species, spikenard, thyme chemotypes, valerian and yarrow.

Phytols

Herbal oils (real phytols or infused oils) are coming into fashion with certain aromatherapists. These include arnica (*Arnica montana*), calendula (*Calendula officinalis*, pot-marigold), centella (*Centella asiatica*, gotu kola or hydrocotyle), comfrey (*Symphytum officinalis*), Devil's claw (*Harpagophytum procumbens*), echinacea (*Echinacea purpurea*), fenugreek (*Trigonella foenumgraecum*), lime blossom (*Tilia* sp.), meadowsweet (*Filipendula ulmaria*) and St John's wort (*Hypericum perforatum*) (Lis-Balchin, 1999a). Most are tea-like or alcoholic extracts, not essential oils, and have no aroma.

All are well known as herbal remedies, usually taken internally or applied to burns or bruises, as poultices or compresses, but many are potentially toxic orally and are sensitisers (Newall *et al.*, 1996; Lis-Balchin, 1999a) and should be given only at the advice of a qualified herbalist – not an aromatherapist. There is no toxicological evaluation for their aromatherapeutic application and their possible dermal irritation or sensitisation is often unknown, therefore their use should be restricted in pregnancy (especially meadowsweet and St John's wort, which are both said to be uteroactive).

Phytol is also the name given to a particular solvent extraction technique, which does not involve the usual benzene or hexane (now considered toxic if not potentially carcinogenic) to produce concretes, which are normally re-extracted with absolute alcohol to give absolutes (Wilde, 1994). The main object of this method was to be able to provide 'absolutes' without the use of alcohol for people who, for religious reasons, cannot drink alcohol or even use perfumes with alcohol. The actual 'phytols' are very similar to the absolutes and CO_2 extracts and none of them has been tested for toxicity, especially on the skin. These phytols contain similar 'plant impurities' to those of absolutes (i.e. the solvent-soluble pigments, alkaloids, etc.) which could cause sensitisation. They could however be useful as food additives, provided safety studies are done, or people accept them as being equivalent to absolutes or CO_2 extracts.

Possible microbiological dangers of hydrolysates or hydrolysats

Many companies are now selling the by-products of essential oil distillation (e.g. rosewater) as alternative, gentle, aromatherapy products. As these products are meant to be pure and wholesome, no preservative is usually added. This means that microbial contamination is very likely, even before leaving the factory, let alone after several months of usage. Many aromatherapists recommend these for treating eye and other infections and spraying the rooms of asthmatics: this could have very serious effects due to possible bacterial contamination. Over a third of samples of bottled water tested contained *Cryptosporidium*, *Giardia* and other cysts (Rose *et al.*, 1993): the same level of contamination can happen to aromatherapy hydrolysates. As many of these waters are used for skin complaints, the addition of microbes could greatly exacerbate the condition – not alleviate it.

Hydrosols from unusual and toxicologically untested plants (e.g. verbenone-type rosemary, ravensara and thyme chemotypes) should be avoided. Statements like: 'They are like homeopathic essential oils' are incorrect as their flower remedies have added alcohol as a preservative. It seems that to date the Food Safety Laws do not apply to hydrosols. This situation should be remedied as they are often drunk as well as applied to the skin. Insurance policies covering aromatherapy practices do not permit therapists to practise herbal medicine (i.e. to treat internally), especially using unknown products.

Some dangerous advice is given in aromatherapy books, such as swabbing down the whole of the lower body with flower water following parturition, including swabbing lightly over stitches and even leaving a clean swab in place. *Helichrysum italicum* and geranium (*Pelargonium graveolens*) waters have also been recommended for the care of open wounds. Other floral waters stated to be useful for wound healing included rose (*Rosa damascena*), myrtle (*Myrtus communis*) and rosemary borneol (*Rosmarinus officinalis* ct. borneol).

Interactions between essential oils and conventional medicines or medical conditions

There is growing evidence that adverse effects are often caused by mixing alternative and conventional therapies. This is shown by reports on herbal medicine interactions, including Chinese herbs (Lis-Balchin, 1999a). A report on the adverse action of a massage with wintergreen oil (containing 98% methyl salicylate) on a patient taking warfarin (given as an anticoagulant), which caused haematomas, is a serious reminder of such dangers (Yeo *et al.*, 1994). Many of the cautions reported were for oral intake of herbal remedies, but where absorption of the active components occurs in large concentrations, essential oils must also come under the same risk category.

Some examples include cautions against the use, via any route, of cornmint or peppermint in cardiac fibrillation (Tisserand and Balacs, 1995) and against the use of annual wormwood, balsamite, camphor, ho leaf, hyssop, cotton lavender in people with epilepsy or patients with fever. All those examples, plus Indian dill, parsley leaf and seed, sage (Spanish) and savin, should not be used in pregnancy and caution is also given for *Lavandula stoechas*, oakmoss, rue and treemoss (Tisserand and Balacs, 1995).

Indian dill, parsley leaf and seed is cautioned against in people with kidney or liver disease and *Backhousia citriodora*, *Eucalyptus stagierana*, lemongrass, may chang and melissa in prostatic hyperplasia (Tisserand and Balacs, 1995). Advice is also given to avoid certain essential oils via dermal administration in certain cases: basil, fennel, ho leaf (camphor/safrole) and nutmeg (East Indian) except at very low concentrations of up to 2% (Tisserand and Balacs,

1995). For cancers and for oestrogen-dependent cancer patients, caution is given against fennel, anise and star anise. For patients with glaucoma, avoidance of *Backhousia citriodora*, lemongrass, may chang and melissa is recommended and in patients with glucose-6-phosphate dehydrogenase (G6PD) deficiency, avoidance of cornmint and peppermint is advised.

Oral intake of certain essential oils is also prohibited (mainly as stated for dermal application before) and caution is advised with bay (West Indian), betel leaf, cinnamon leaf, clove (bud, leaf and stem), garlic, *Ocimum gratissimum*, onion, pimento (berry and leaf) and tejpat leaf, where anticoagulants are used (which include aspirin, heparin and warfarin).

There is considerable reluctance to accept all these cautions as they are probably overexaggerated and the dosage of essential oils is overlooked, however, wormseed (*Chenopodium*) was used to treat intestinal worms and caused poisoning in many children (Mele, 1952) and experiments on monkeys have shown that citral given in small daily doses causes symptoms similar to those of glaucoma (Geldof *et al.*, 1992). Occasionally, completely unfounded contraindications are given in aromatherapy books and it is advisable to cross-reference any such advice with more scientific works (e.g. Tisserand and Balacs, 1995).

The phenomenon of 'quenching': true or false?

Many essential oils do not cause sensitisation even though their main components are very potent sensitisers (Opdyke, 1974). Quenching is the term given to this amelioration or complete stoppage of sensitisation of sensitisers when used in a mixture of components as in essential oils or even perfumes. One should not rely on quenching, however, as most commercial essential oils are commonly adulterated and may contain potent sensitiser chemicals anyway.

Some components like aldehydes (e.g. citral) can quench potent sensitisers in essential oils (Opdyke, 1974). For example, cinnamal was apparently quenched by eugenol not limonene and citral was quenched by limonene.

The latest survey at Unilever Toxicology Unit (2000) pours doubt on the original study as there are no signs of interaction (e.g. Schiff base formations). Studies using modern methods (e.g. murine lymph nodes in mice) have shown no quenching at all. The RIFM produced limited studies that show citral quenched by limonene, but Unilever tests on Opdyke quenchers using guinea-pig models failed to support his work. Ageing perfume mixtures showed no quenching effect either; studies on humans showed no quenching (Basketter and Allenby, 1991). In conclusion, there is no satisfactory physicochemical or immunobiological proof for quenching; it is, at best, a hypothesis, and no 'good components' have been found as yet. Furthermore, as many commercial essential oils are adulterated, potential sensitisers can be added: so it's a no-win situation.

In one instance a high D-limonene-containing (unknown) oil was added to lemongrass (containing citral) by an aromatherapist on the advice of a perfumer, to counteract, by quenching, the sensitising effect on the skin (Price, 1993). One can only wonder if this was a wise move in view of D-limonene's toxicity.

Possible dangers of novel essential oils and plant extracts

There is a trend by some 'clinical aromatherapists' to use uncommon essential oils, often derived from plants which are grown wild and which have a tendency to produce numerous cultivars with different chemical compositions (i.e. chemotypes). These oils are very much more expensive, as they are produced in small amounts; the quality will be variable as well as the yield and composition. The real benefit remains a mystery. The International Federation of Aromatherapists (IFA), which represents well-trained therapists, has published articles in its journal promoting such potentially hazardous oils and even the use of *Verbena* essential oil on the skin (Autumn 1999 edition), stating that this oil 'used sensibly, is safe' despite well-documented evidence proving that this oil should never be applied to the skin due to sensitising and phototoxic potential (IFRA, see Appendix 30).

The vast majority of the commonest essential oils have been well tried and tested and safety levels have been ascertained; however, when an aromatherapist uses novel essential oils, they are using their clients as human guinea-pigs (Lis-Balchin, 1999b). This is also unethical unless the client is told that the safety of such oils is unknown, and legally it could possibly leave the therapist open to court action if the essential oils caused a harmful reaction.

South American and other novel plants and their essential oils, introduced at recent aromatherapy conferences as potential cures for numerous ailments, include muna (*Minthostachys spicata*), a peppermint-smelling herb consisting mainly of pulegone, whose folk usage is as a digestive and spasmolytic when drunk as a tea (Lunny, 1997), and the Bolivian herb *Satureya boliviana*, which also has a high pulegone content. The pulegone-containing European wormwood (*Artemisia absinthium*) must not be used in aromatherapy as aromatherapists believe pulegone to cause abortions. It seems rather odd that *Mentha pulegium* (pennyroyal) is banned, but a new exciting Bolivian herb with a similar composition is thought to be good! Another novel plant, molle (*Schinus molle*), otherwise known as Peruvian mastic, is also suggested as beneficial in aromatherapy (Lunny, 1997), but it is closely related botanically and toxicologically to poison ivy (*Toxicodendron radicans*), one of the most potent dermal irritants and sensitisers known (Lis-Balchin, 1999b).

Dangerous practices of some aromatherapists

A number of particularly dangerous items and suggestions have been published in the many aromatherapy books and journals and presented at aromatherapy conferences. Among them are aromatic perfusion, oral/rectal/vaginal usage, and the use of essential oils during pregnancy and childbirth.

Aromatic perfusion

This practice involves using up to 20 mL of undiluted essential oils directly on the skin for specific conditions (Guba, 2000). Apparently the use of red thyme, ajowan, clove bud oil, oregano at concentrations not exceeding 10% for massage, compared with the use of 90% of non-irritant essential oils (true lavender, *Eucalyptus radiata*, tea tree) and up to 10% of phenolic essential oils is considered to be perfectly acceptable. This treatment could, however, cause severe burns/irritation to the skin, especially if the person is slightly sensitive.

Oral/rectal/vaginal usage

Oral/rectal/vaginal usage of essential oils is advocated by aromatherapists in France and Germany, who are sometimes medically qualified, but also by some medically unqualified aromatherapists in the UK. The use of essential oils in this way is potentially dangerous due to possible damage to the delicate mucosal cells, adulteration of the oils and the use of high dosages. There is also the potential for illegality in the use of untested oils, which are often advocated.

The effects of chemicals, especially cosmetics, are tested on various larger mammals for their potential effects on the sensitive mucous membranes such as in the eyes and mouth. Other specialist products are tested on the membranes of the anus, vagina, and so forth. The animals tested are specially chosen for each type of membrane. For eyes, the rabbit is the only choice due to its large eyes and sensitivity, whilst oral products are tested on the hamster, due to its natural way of storing anything in its food pouches. Dogs or cats are often used for testing penile or vaginal membranes.

Not all essential oils are tested on all membranes, as most are used in cosmetics and foods and are not intended to be used medicinally within the body. However an increasing number of aromatherapists are using these very strong chemicals on tampons inserted into the vagina or anus, and there is a possibility of a patient having a severe reaction to the chemicals on the delicate membranes. This practice is professionally irresponsible, as aromatherapists should not be diagnosing and treating venereal disease unless medically qualified to do so.

Use of essential oils during pregnancy and childbirth

It has been shown that uterine contractions may possibly be decreased or stopped by essential oils (Lis-Balchin and Hart, 1997b). Over 40 essential oils and 20 components studied *in vitro* on the rat uterus had a spasmolytic effect, and at higher doses they completely stopped the spontaneous contractions, following a rapid reduction in their intensity. This could be a dangerous event during childbirth, where strong contractions are so vital. It was also found that during the oestrus cycle, some animals developed irregularity in their uterine spontaneous contractions in response to some essential oils: this suggests their potential danger during pregnancy, as a spontaneous abortion could be initiated. There is also the possibility of anaesthetising the baby in the womb if essential oils are used during parturition, resulting in the baby's inability to display the crying reflex on birth.

Almost all of the claims made in aromatherapy books and journals regarding the use of restricted or banned essential oils during pregnancy are largely based on the traditionally claimed effects of the water-soluble herbal extracts, which were mainly taken internally. Such extracts are totally different from the plant essential oils extracted from them. The common essential oils used in aromatherapy are all used as food flavourings and in perfumery, therefore one would have imagined that the slightest evidence of toxicity of these essential oils to the baby would have restricted their usage by legislation. However, not many teratogenic studies have been conducted on essential oils, although they have been used for years as food additives. The main problem these days is seen as the sensitisation potential of many essential oils, and of course these could also have possible effects on the unborn child.

'Safe' essential oils and their toxicity

The two main essential oils considered by aromatherapists to be safe (and therefore recommended for usage during pregnancy, parturition and on small babies) are lavender and geranium oil, but even these are not without risk. In one case a hairdresser with allergy problems on her hands due to a variety of products reacted most strongly to a lavender shampoo and lavender oil itself (Rudzki et al., 1976). Lavender was said to be a photosensitiser (Brandao, 1986) and patch tests have shown a few allergies due to photosensitisation (Lovell, 1993). Pigmentation has also been reported (Klarmann, 1958).

Most of the references to geranium oil are to contact dermatitis and sensitisation (Romaguera et al., 1986) especially due to one of the main components, geraniol. Although patch tests to geraniol proved negative, dermatitis caused by perfumes containing geranium oil has been observed in a few cases (Klarmann, 1958). Ointments containing geraniol (e.g. Blastoestimulina) have been reported to cause sensitisation

when used in the treatment of chronic leg ulcers (Romaguera et al., 1986; Guerra et al., 1987). Geraniol may be an allergen, as cross-reactions occur with citronella (Keil, 1947), however, the main sensitiser found is citronellal (mainly in palmarosa, *Eucalyptus citriodora* and melissa), with citronellol less reactive; geraniol was even weaker, as was citral. In two cases, strong reactions were obtained with 1% solutions of citronellal and weaker ones with citronellol, geraniol and geranyl acetate (see Appendix 22). In 23/23 cases no response was found using lemon oil, which suggests specificity of the response. However, sensitisation to geraniol using a maximisation test proved negative.

Most cosmetics and perfumes are tested on human 'guinea-pigs' using similar tests to those described for animals. These are demanded by the RIFM as a final test before marketing a product. Further data are accumulated from notifications from disgruntled consumers who report dermatitis, itching or skin discoloration in use. These notifications can result in legal claims, although most cases are probably settled out of court and not reported to the general public.

Possible dangers of using essential oils internally and externally in large doses

Essential oils are used in the food industry usually in very minute amounts of 10 ppm, and even up to 1000 ppm and above in the case of mint confectionery or chewing gum. This does not make it safe to use drops of undiluted essential oils on sugar lumps for oral application or on suppositories for anal or vaginal application. Severe damage to mucous membranes could result from such practices, and the dangers are magnified if cheap, adulterated oils are used.

The Internet has made it possible for a trusting, though often ill-informed, public to purchase a wide range of dubious plant extracts and essential oils. Even illegal essential oils can now be obtained. Furthermore, unqualified people can offer potentially dangerous advice, such as internal usage or the use of undiluted essential oils on the skin for 'mummification', or in order to rid the body of toxic waste. The latter can result in excruciating pain from the burns produced and the subsequent loss of layers of skin.

In one study, aromatherapy trials in high-dose chemotherapy patients were not only unscientific but also very dangerous: essential oils, diluted in water, were given internally or applied externally to very sick patients in a rather haphazard way (reported in Aroma '93). The 'experiments' were conducted by an aromatherapist who probably had little knowledge of essential oil chemistry, function or toxicity. Such studies should not have been passed by the hospital safety committee in the first instance.

In an aromatherapy book steam distillation at home was illustrated by a drawing of a kettle perched on a gas flame over the stove; this was loosely attached to a tube passing through ice in a pan, and the essential oil was then collected into a jamjar close by (Rose, 1992a). From the point of health and safety, this was extremely dangerous.

In another book, readers were advised that a woman in labour can be given jasmine or lemon verbena compresses or massages in the sacral area when suffering pain. Even taking lemon verbena internally was recommended to stimulate uterine contractions (Fischer-Rizzi, 1992). Such advice was very dangerous, especially as no concentrations were given and lemon verbena is a potent allergen. To suggest that it is to be used internally for uterine contractions is totally irresponsible as there has been no scientific verification.

The same book gives a recipe for suntan oil, including bergamot, carrot seed and lemon essential oils (Fischer-Rizzi, 1990). These are all phototoxic essential oils. The author then advises that bergamot oil is added to suntan lotion, to get the bonus of the substance called 'furocumarin', which lessens the skin's sun sensitivity while it helps one to tan quickly. This could cause severe burns.

Elsewhere, sassafras (*Ocotea pretiosa*) was said to be only toxic for rats, due to its metabolism and not dangerous to humans (Pénoel, 1991) and a 10% solution in oil was suggested for treating muscular and joint pain and sports injuries. Safrole (and sassafras oil) is, however, controlled under the Controlled Drugs Regulations (1993) and listed as a category 1 substance, as it is a precursor for the illicit manufacture of hallucinogenic, narcotic and psychotropic drugs like ecstasy (see also nutmeg oil monograph).

French practitioners and other therapists have apparently become 'familiar' with untested oils (Guba, 2000). The use of toxicologically untested Nepalese essential oils, etc. includes lichen resinoids, sugandha kokila oil, jatamansi oil and Nepalese lemongrass (*Cymbopogon flexuosa*), also *Tagetes* oil (Basnyet, 1999).

Melaleuca rosalina (*M. ericifolia*), 1,8-cineole 18–26%, is apparently especially useful for the respiratory system (Pénoel, 1998). Because it is so mild to the skin, 2–3 drops can be applied neat on the side of the neck at the area of the lymphatic nodes when treating infections of the upper respiratory system. This essential oil is untested and could be a sensitiser.

'Nurses warn against rash use of herbal oil treatments' (*The Guardian*, 12 March 1999, p. 9) was the unexpected title of a report from the Royal College of Nursing Congress, as nurses are usually very keen to support aromatherapy. Several dangerous scenarios were mentioned, including the intensive marketing of aromatherapy treatments in a 3-year trial on cancer patients and the danger of non-qualified nurses implementing the treatment. An incident concerning a nurse's daughter, who had been given aromatherapy treatment in a hospital during a 5-day stay, was reported. Apparently no choice, no parental consent and no agreement was given. There was also a warning about the possible use of aromatherapy oils poured over children's heads against headlice by inexperienced parents.

Reporting of adverse effects by aromatherapists

There have been no reports on any adverse effects in the extensive aromatherapy literature, despite the many reports appearing in the scientific literature. There is at present no 'yellow card' scheme or other regarding the thousands of aromatherapists practising in the UK or elsewhere in the world, although this could provide useful data. There seems to be a reluctance by aromatherapists to participate in any scheme which could prove damaging to their profession and thereby jeopardise their income. The few clinical studies on aromatherapy carried out have not only shown no benefits in using essential oils in massage compared with massage alone, but have also yielded no significant data on adverse effects.

The yellow card scheme operates for those few essential oils sold as licensed products, including peppermint oil (e.g. as Colpermin), but these oils are all GRAS and therefore unlikely to be hazardous unless grossly misused.

Safety warnings in the aromatherapy industry

Many aromatherapy suppliers, especially on the Internet, continue to sell dangerous essential oils without adequate warnings. There are also examples of inadequate labelling as to sell by or use by dates, which should always be given especially for essential oils of the citrus and pine families, which develop skin sensitising chemicals on ageing. Shelf-life can be lengthened by the addition of artificial antioxidants; these are disliked by aromatherapists, but vitamin E could be used instead. Warnings should be given that essential oils without antioxidants should not be used on the skin after about six months, but can still be used as fragrances and that storing such oils in optimum conditions, such as in sealed containers in a refrigerator will slow down the chemical changes in the oil.

Legislation: present and future

The Health and Safety at Work Act (1974) together with COSHH (Control of Substances Hazardous to Health) Regulations (1994) and CHIP (Chemical Hazard Information and Packaging) Regulations 1998 now control all chemicals in the UK. The New 7th Amendment: European Parliament 2002: To Annex III – Part 1 (Directive 76/768/EEC) covers the conditions of use and warnings which must be printed on the label.

The following components must be indicated in the list of ingredients and a warning given that they can cause an allergic reaction (see also Appendices 28 and 29):

- Benzyl alcohol
- Cinnamyl alcohol
- Eugenol
- Hydroxycitronellal
- Isoeugenol
- Benzyl salicylate
- Cinnamaldehyde
- Coumarin
- Geraniol
- Anisyl alcohol
- Benzyl cinnamate
- Farnesol
- Linalool
- Benzyl benzoate
- Citronellol
- D-Limonene
- Oakmoss and treemoss extract.

This list is greatly increased by the fragrance industry, which has now produced a *Labelling Manual* (EFFA-IOFI-IFRA, 26.3.2001) for health and environmental effects. The proposals could form the basis of an individual supplier's classification and labelling, and it is recommended that they label their goods within six months of the proposal. Sensitisers are labelled 'Xi (irritant); R43' and it is recommended that a 1% concentration is adhered to. Aspiration hazard is 'Xn (harmful); R65' and is recommended now for all substances with a hydrocarbon greater than 10%. Some chemicals do not require labelling; these include citronella oil (Java type) and farnesol. Citronella oil Ceylon type is however Xn. *Pinus nigra*, terpenes and terpenoids, limonene fraction, turpentine oil are now Xn, N. Most of the other components have an Xi or Xn label, with exceptions like safrole which is T (see Appendices 24–26).

The Medicines and Healthcare Products Regulatory Agency in the UK may bring about changes in aromatherapy practice similar to their threat on herbal remedies. The freedom to describe what the essential oils used in aromatherapy are apparently capable of doing will be restricted. Legislation in the USA has already led to several prosecutions following false claims by aromatherapy distributors (see Chapter 3). Legislation brought in by the Health and Safety Executive (HSE) (R65), which came into force on 20 June 1999, classified 89 essential oils as 'harmful'. The danger of this legislation is that aromatherapists are now using some harmful products in their therapy. This immediately places them at serious risk if there is any untoward reaction to their specific treatment. It virtually means that bottles and containers of essential oils now rank with domestic bleach for labelling purposes. It also means that companies are now obliged to self-classify their essential oils on their labels and place them in suitable containers; this applies both to large distributing companies as well as individual aromatherapists reselling essential oils under their own name.

The EU Biocide Directive, which covers about 40 oils, including lavender, was adopted for implementation on 20 May 2000 but has not yet been implemented. It implies that essential oils cannot be used as biocides, as they are not included in the list.

Finally, new legislation has gone to the Council of Ministers and may imply that only qualified people will be able to use essential oils, and retail outlets for oils will be pharmacies. Their definition of 'qualified' is limited to academic qualifications – doctors or pharmacists.

Conclusion

In the past essential oils have been considered to be relatively safe, with a few exceptions, but with new technological advances in the manufacture of synthetic components and 'designer' essential oils to suit every pocket, there is an increasing danger of toxicity, which can manifest itself as sensitisation. New legislation has now become a reality, and warning consumers of the dangers of essential oils on bottle labels, as well as the labels on other cosmetic products, is imminent. The next stage could be the restriction of sales of concentrated essential oils to pharmacies, under the supervision of pharmacists and medically qualified personnel only.

8

Clinical studies

Introduction

Very few scientific clinical studies on the effectiveness of aromatherapy have been published to date. Perhaps the main reason is that until recently scientists were not involved and people engaging in aromatherapy clinical studies had accepted the aromatherapy doctrine in its entirety, precluding any possibility of a non-biased study. This has been evident in the design and execution of the studies; the main criterion has usually been the use of massage with essential oils and not the effect of the odorant itself. The latter is considered by most aromatherapists as irrelevant to clinical aromatherapy, which implies that it is simply the systemic action of essential oils absorbed through the skin that exerts an effect on specific organs or tissues. Odorant action is considered to be just 'aromachology', despite its enormous psychological and physiological impact (see Chapter 6). In some studies attempts are even made to by-pass the odorant effect entirely by making the subjects wear oxygen masks throughout (Dunn et al., 1995).

The use of particular essential oils for certain medical conditions is also adhered to, despite the wide assortment of supposed functions for each essential oil claimed by different aromatherapy source materials. In many studies it is even unclear exactly which essential oil was used; often the correct nomenclature, chemical composition and exact purity are not given.

Many aromatherapists feel that they know that aromatherapy works as they have enormous numbers of case studies to prove it. But the production of lists of 'positive' results on diverse clients, with diverse ailments, using diverse essential oils in the treatments, and diverse methods of application (which also frequently change from visit to visit for the same client) does not satisfy scientific criteria. Negative results must surely be amongst the positive ones, due to the

change in essential oils during the course of the treatment, which suggests that they did not work, but these are never stated. There are also no controls in case studies and no attempt to control the bias of the individual aromatherapist and clients. Double-blind studies are just not possible in individual case studies. Furthermore, no set criteria for estimating physiological or psychological changes due to the treatment are used and loose phrases such as 'the client felt better' or 'happier' are inappropriate for a scientific study.

These faults in the design and interpretation of results of aromatherapy research have been pointed out by Vickers (1996) and reiterated by other scientists (Kirk-Smith, 1996a; Nelson, 1997; Lis-Balchin, 2002b, Chapter 8). However, the lack of statistically significant results does not prevent many aromatherapists from accepting vaguely positive clinical research results and numerous poor-grade clinical studies are now quoted as factual confirmation that aromatherapy works (see Appendix 32).

Many of the clinical studies have lacked properly diagnosed age-matched and sex-matched patient or control groups taking clinical compatibility into account. In a comparative study, massage, where given, should be provided by one person (if possible) or a small number of people who use exactly the same technique, the same verbal communications and the same environment. It is almost impossible to do a double-blind study using odorants, as the patient and treatment provider would experience the odour differences and would inevitably react knowingly or unknowingly to that factor alone (see Appendix 32). The psychological effect(s) could be very diverse, as recall of odours can bring about very acute reactions in different people, depending on the individual's past experiences, etc. (see Chapter 6). Lastly, there is potential bias as patients receiving aromatherapy treatment could be grateful for the attention given to them and, not wanting to upset the givers of such attention, would state that they were better and happier than before. The proper procedural conditions to be implemented in a clinical study are very diverse and should be strongly adhered to (Kirk-Smith, 1996a,b; Appendix 32).

Note: Purely psychological or psychological/physiological studies have been described in Chapter 6.

Recent clinical studies

Aromatherapy in dementia

A meticulously conducted double-blind study involved 72 dementia patients with clinically significant agitation treated with *Melissa* oil; the patients were from eight National Health Service nursing homes in the UK caring for people with severe dementia (Ballard *et al.*, 2002). Agitation included anxiety and irritability, motor restlessness and abnormal vocalisation – symptoms which often lead to disturbed behaviours such as pacing, wandering, aggression, shouting and night-time disturbance, all characterised by appropriate inventories.

Ten per cent (by weight) melissa oil (active) or sunflower oil (placebo), combined with a base lotion (*Prunus dulcis* oil, glycerine, stearic acid, cetearyl alcohol and tocopheryl acetate), was dispensed in metered doses and applied to the face and both arms twice daily for four weeks by a care assistant, the process taking 1–2 minutes. The patients also received neuroleptic treatment and other conventional treatment where necessary: this was therefore a study of complementary aromatherapy treatment – not an alternative treatment.

The 'Melissa group' showed a higher significant improvement in reducing aggression than the control group by week 4; the total Cohen–Mansfield Agitation Inventory (CMAI) scores had decreased significantly in both groups, from a mean of 68 to 45 (35%; $P < 0.0001$) in the treatment group and from 61 to 53 (11%; $P = 0.005$) in the placebo group. Clinically significant reduction in agitation, defined as a 30% decrease in CMAI score, occurred in 60% of the melissa group compared with 14% of placebo responders ($P < 0.0001$). Neuropsychiatric Inventory (NPI) scores also declined with *Melissa* treatment, and quality of life was improved, with less social isolation and more involvement in activities. The latter was in contrast to the usual neuroleptic treatment effects.

The authors concluded that the *Melissa* treatment was successful, but pointed out that there was also a significant, but lower, improvement in the control group and suggested that a stronger odour should have been used. The effect of the *Melissa* oil was probably on cholinergic receptors as shown by previous *in vitro* studies (Perry *et al.*, 1999; Wake *et al.*, 2000; see also Chapter 5). The authors also concluded that as most people with severe dementia have lost any meaningful sense of smell, a direct placebo effect due to a pleasant-smelling fragrance, although possible, is an unlikely explanation for the positive effects of *Melissa* in this study. Others may disagree with this conclusion as it has been shown that subliminal odours can have an effect (see Chapter 6). Another problem noted by the authors was that the fragrance may have had some impact upon the care staff, and influenced ratings to some degree on the informant schedules.

A further recent study found no support for the use of a purely olfactory form of aromatherapy to decrease agitation in severely demented patients (Snow *et al.*, 2004). Lavender, thyme oil or unscented grapeseed oil was placed every 3 hours on an absorbent fabric sachet pinned near the collarbone of each participant's shirt; following 4 weeks of baseline measurement. Two weeks for each of the five treatment conditions, including the reversal of the lavender and thyme essential oil (10-week total intervention time), was followed by two weeks of postintervention measurement. The authors suggested that cutaneous application of the essential oil may be necessary to achieve the effects reported in previous controlled studies.

Other research (Burns *et al.*, 2002) suggested that aromatherapy and light therapy were more effective and gentler alternatives to the use of neuroleptics in patients with dementia. Three studies were analysed in each category; in the aromatherapy section it included the study above, plus the use of 2% lavender oil via inhalation in a double-blind study for 10 days (Holmes *et al.*, 2002) and a two-week single-blind study using either aromatherapy plus massage, aromatherapy plus conversation or massage alone (Smallwood *et al.*, 2001). All of the interventions in the aromatherapy groups proved significantly beneficial. However, so did the light treatment, where patients sat in front of a light box that beamed out 10 000 lux of artificial light. This therapy adjusts the body's melatonin levels, which affects the body clock, and is used in the treatment of SAD (seasonal affective disorder).

An aqueous cream containing lavender, sweet marjoram, patchouli and vetiver was gently massaged onto the bodies and limbs of 56 patients with dementia (aged 70–92 years) in a care home, five times a day for four weeks. The patients were put into two similar groups who received either massage with the essential oils first followed by massage with just the cream alone or vice versa (Bowles-Dilys *et al.*, 2002). The essential oil therapy significantly decreased the severity of some dementia symptoms but increased resistance to nursing care procedures in one group treated with essential oils, suggesting stimulation by the essential oils. This was not a properly controlled trial and many people were involved in massaging and also collection of data, possibly giving rise to many differences in outcome between patients.

Past clinical studies

In contrast to more recent studies, past clinical trials were often very defective in design and also outcomes. In a recent review, Cooke and Ernst (2000) included only those aromatherapy trials which were randomised and included human patients; they excluded those with no control group or if only local effects (e.g. antiseptic effects of tea tree oil) or preclinical studies on healthy volunteers occurred. The six trials included massage with or without aromatherapy (Buckle, 1993; Stevenson, 1994; Corner *et al.*, 1995; Dunn *et al.*, 1995; Wilkinson, 1995; Wilkinson *et al.*, 1999) and were based on their relaxation outcomes. The authors concluded that the effects of aromatherapy were probably not strong enough for it to be considered for the treatment of anxiety and that the hypothesis that it is effective for any other indication is not supported by the findings of rigorous clinical trials.

A further study included trials with no replicates, and contained six studies. It showed that in five out of six cases the main outcomes were positive; however, these were limited to very specific criteria, such as small airways resistance for common colds (Cohen and Dressler, 1982), prophylaxis of bronchi for bronchitis (Ferley *et al.*, 1989), lessening smoking withdrawal symptoms (Rose and Behm, 1993), relief of anxiety (Morris *et al.*, 1995) and treatment of alopecia areata (Hay *et al.*, 1998). The alleviation of perineal discomfort (Dale and Cornwell, 1994) was not significant.

Psychological effects, which include inhalation of essential oils and behavioural changes, were discussed in Chapter 6.

Critique of selected clinical trials

The following scientific critique illustrates clinical studies which attempted to show that aromatherapy was more efficient than massage alone: they showed mainly negative results, although in some cases the authors clearly emphasised some very small positive result and this was then accepted and reported in aromatherapy journals as a positive trial which supported aromatherapy.

Massage, aromatherapy massage or a period of rest in 122 patients in an intensive care unit (ICU) (Dunn *et al.*, 1995) showed no difference between massage with or without lavender oil and no treatment in the physiological parameters. Although there was a significantly greater improvement in mood and in anxiety levels between the rest group and essential oil massage group after the first session, all other psychological parameters showed no effects throughout. The trial had a large number of parameters: it involved patients in the ICU for about 5 days (age range 2–92 years), who received 1–3 therapy sessions in 24 hours given by six different nurses (only half received all three therapy sessions, less than a quarter received two and the rest just one session). Massage was performed on the back, outside of limbs or scalp for 15–30 minutes with lavender (*L. vera* at 1% in grapeseed oil, which was the only constant parameter). The patients wore oxygen masks but only some of the time. The study was proclaimed by aromatherapists as positive evidence that aromatherapy massage works, despite all the flaws and negative findings.

I had the misfortune to be a patient in an ICU for 5 days and was only semi-conscious most of the time with tubes of every description in almost every orifice and in terrible pain, which was alleviated by morphine i.v. I would not have even felt somebody massage any part of my body and would certainly have been incapable of remembering it, nor able to answer any questions about the treatment or my feelings. I therefore consider this paper as irrelevant, both because of the points raised previously and because of my personal experience in an ICU unit.

Massage with and without Roman chamomile in 51 palliative care patients (Wilkinson, 1995) indicated that both groups experienced the same decrease in symptoms and severity after three full body massages in three weeks. There was, however, a statistically significant difference between the two groups after the first aromatherapy massage and also an improvement in the 'quality of life' from pre- to post-massage. The results seem inexplicable, as massage usually has a positive effect. An important unanswered question is whether the essential oil used was Roman chamomile as stated, as the chemical composition and potential bioactivity given were those for German chamomile.

Aromatherapy with and without massage, and massage alone on disturbed behaviour in four patients with severe dementia (Brooker *et al.*, 1997), was an unusual single-case study evaluating the use of 'true' aromatherapy (using inhaled lavender oil) for ten treatments of each, randomly given to each patient over a three-month period and assessed against ten no-treatment periods. Two patients became more agitated following their treatment sessions and only one patient seemed to have benefited. According to the staff providing the treatment, however, the use of all the treatments seemed to have been beneficial to the patients, suggesting pronounced bias.

An investigation of the psychophysiological effects of aromatherapy massage following cardiac surgery (Stevenson, 1994) showed experimenter bias due to the statement that 'neroli is also especially valuable in the relief of anxiety, it calms palpitations, has an antispasmodic effect and an anti-inflammatory effect . . . it is useful in the treatment of hysteria, as an antidepressant and a gentle sedative'. None of this has been scientifically proven, but as this was not a double-blind study and presumably the author did the massaging, communicating and collating information alone, bias is probable. Statistical significances were not shown, nor the age ranges of the 100 patients and no differences between the aromatherapy-only and massage-only groups were shown, except for an immediate increase in respiratory rate when the two control groups (20 minutes chat or rest) were compared with the aromatherapy massage and massage-only groups.

Atopic eczema in 32 children treated by massage with and without essential oils (Anderson *et al.*, 2000) in a single-case experimental design across subjects showed that this complementary therapy provided no statistically significant differences between the two groups after eight weeks of treatment. This indicated that massage and thereby regular parental

contact and attention showed positive results, which was expected in these children. However, a continuation of the study, following a three-month period of rest, using only the essential oil massage group showed a possible sensitisation effect, as the symptoms worsened. The results indicate the necessity for prolonged studies to investigate a possible sensitisation reaction where essential oils are used. Another area of concern is the use of a large number of different essential oils in this study.

Massage using two different types of lavender oil on post-cardiotomy patients (Buckle, 1993) was proclaimed to be a 'double-blind' study but had no controls and the results by the author did not appear to be assessed correctly (Vickers, 1996). The author attempted to show that the 'real' lavender showed significant benefits in the state of the patients compared with the other oil. However, outcome measures were not described and the chemical composition and botanical names of the 'real' and 'not real' lavender remains a mystery, as three lavenders were described in the text. Although the results were insignificant, this paper is quoted widely as proof that only 'real' essential oils work through aromatherapy massage.

Childbirth: are all essential oils as good?

Aromatherapy trails in childbirth have unfortunately been of dubious design to date and have yielded confusing results (Burns and Blaney, 1994), due mainly to the numerous parameters incorporated. For example, in the study by Burns and Blaney (1994), many different essential oils were used in various uncontrolled ways and assessed during childbirth using possibly biased criteria as to their possible benefits to the mother and midwife. This gave it low scientific merit. The first pilot study used 585 women in a delivery suite over a six-month period using: lavender, clary sage, peppermint, eucalyptus, chamomile, frankincense, jasmine, lemon and mandarin. These oils were either used singly or as part of a mixture where they could be used as the first, second, third or fourth essential oil. The essential oils were applied in many different ways and at different times during parturition, for example, sprayed in a 'solution' of two drops of essential oil to 100 mL of water onto a face flannel, pillow or bean bag; 4–6 drops in a bath; 2–4 drops in a foot bath; a drop onto an absorbent card for inhalation; or two drops in 50 mL almond oil for massage. Peppermint oil was applied as an undiluted drop on the forehead and frankincense onto the palm.

Midwives and mothers were asked to fill in a form as to the effects of the essential oils. This included their relaxant value, effect on nausea and vomiting, analgesic action, mood enhancer action, accelerator or not of labour. The results were inconclusive and there was a bias towards the use of a few oils. For example lavender was stated to be 'oestrogenic and used to calm down uterine tightenings if a woman was exhausted and needed sleep'; clary sage was given to 'encourage the establishment of labour'. This shows complete bias and a belief in unproven clinical attributes by the authors and presumably the perpetrators of the study. There was no attempt to verify which of the lavender, peppermint, eucalyptus, chamomile or frankincense species were used, nor their chemical composition.

The continuation of this study (Burns *et al.*, 2000) on 8058 mothers during childbirth was intended to show that aromatherapy would 'relieve anxiety, pain, nausea and/or vomiting or strengthen contractions'. Data from the unit audit was compared with that of 15 799 mothers not given aromatherapy treatment. The results showed that 50% of the aromatherapy group mothers found the intervention 'helpful' and only 14% 'unhelpful'. The use of pethidine over the year declined from 6% to 0.2% by women in the aromatherapy group. The study also (apparently) showed that aromatherapy may have the potential to augment labour contractions for women in dysfunctional labour, in contrast to scientific data showing that the uterine contractions decrease due to administration of any common essential oils (Lis-Balchin and Hart, 1997a).

It is doubtful whether a woman in her first labour would be able to judge whether the contractions were strengthened or the labour shortened due to aromatherapy. Obviously no control was available. It seems likely that there was some placebo effect (itself a very powerful effector) due to the bias of the experimenters and the 'suggestions' made to the aromatherapy group regarding efficacy of essential oils – which were obviously absent in the case of the control group.

Epilepsy and sleep induction

A neuropsychiatrist (Betts *et al.*, 1995) in a preliminary study showed that out of 30 epileptic patients treated with conventional therapy plus essential oils, nine became free from seizures for some considerable time and another 20 patients were greatly improved. It was interesting to also note that the majority of the patients chose ylang ylang oil from a whole range of different odours. In a follow-up of a trial involving aromatherapy and hypnosis, over a third of the patients using aromatherapy with or without hypnosis became seizure-free for at least a year in an uncontrolled trial. Of the three treatments tried (aromatherapy on its own, aromatherapy plus hypnosis and hypnosis without aromatherapy), aromatherapy plus hypnosis seemed to have had the best and most lasting effect (a third of patients still seizure free at 2 years), but was the most labour intensive and needed medical therapist input (Betts, 2003).

Aromatherapy itself was considered by the author to be best reserved as a short-term treatment for people going through a bad time with their seizures. These studies are very often quoted as an example of 'alternative' medicine, but the essential oils were used as complementary to conventional treatment. Many aromatherapists unfortunately believe that they can cure epilepsy with essential oils, especially ylang ylang, but the possibility of inducing convulsions by odour use is more probable, especially when used by non-medically qualified people.

Lavender oil (volatalised from a burner during the night in their hospital room) has been successful in replacing medication to induce sleep in three out of four geriatrics (Hardy *et al.*, 1995). There was a general deterioration in the sleep patterns when the medication was withdrawn, but lavender oil seemed to be as good as the original medication. However, the deterioration in the sleep patterns on withdrawal of the sedatives could have been due to 'rebound insomnia' and the apparent beneficial results in the use of lavender oil in place of sedatives may simply have been due to recovery of normal sleep patterns (Vickers, 1996).

Depression

After treatment of depressed patients with a continuous application of a citrus fragrance for 4–11 weeks there was a significant reduction in the Hamilton rating scale for depression (as with antidepressant therapy) and the use of antidepressants was greatly reduced (Komori *et al.*, 1995).

Nausea

The efficacy of peppermint oil was studied on post-operative nausea in 18 women after gynaecological operations (Tate, 1997) using a control, 'placebo' (smelling peppermint essence) and test group (smelling peppermint oil from a 5 mL bottle). On the day of the operation a statistically significant difference was found between the controls and the test group and between the latter and the placebo group. The test group required less antiemetics and received less opioid analgesia. The authors concluded that peppermint was a useful adjunct for nausea. However, the use of a peppermint essence as a placebo seems rather like having two test groups as inhalation was used and therefore a similar smell was apparent.

Anxiety before or during medical procedures

A group of 313 patients undergoing radiotherapy were randomly assigned to receive either carrier oil with fractionated oils, carrier oil only, or pure essential oils of lavender, bergamot and cedarwood administered by inhalation concurrently with radiation treatment. There were no significant differences in HADS (Hospital Anxiety and Depression Score) and other scores between the randomly assigned groups. However, HADS scores were significantly lower at treatment completion in the carrier oil-only group compared with either of the fragrant arms ($P \geqslant 0.04$). Aromatherapy, as administered in this study, was not found to be beneficial (Graham *et al.*, 2003).

Heliotropin, a sweet, vanilla-like scent, reduced anxiety during magnetic resonance imaging (Redd and Manne, 1991), which causes distress to many patients as they are enclosed in a 'coffin'-like apparatus. Patients experienced approximately 63% less overall anxiety than a control group of patients.

A double-blind randomised trial was conducted on 66 women undergoing abortions (Wiebe, 2000). Ten minutes was spent sniffing a numbered container with either a mixture of the essential oils (vetivert, bergamot and geranium) or a hair conditioner (placebo). Outcome measures for anxiety measured before and after the intervention (using a verbal anxiety scale from 0 to 10) showed that the score was reduced by 1.0 point (5.0–4.0) in the aromatherapy group and by 1.1 points (6.1–5.0) in the placebo group ($P = 0.71$, therefore insignificant). The author concluded that aromatherapy involving essential oils is no more effective than having patients sniff other pleasant odours in reducing pre-operative anxiety.

Cancer patients

An audit into the effects of aromatherapy in palliative care (Evans, 1995) showed that the most frequently used oils were lavender, marjoram and chamomile. These were applied over a period of six months by a therapist available for 4 hours on a weekly basis on the ward. Relaxing music was played throughout each session to allay fears of the hands-on massage. The results revealed that 81% of the patients stated that they either felt 'better' or 'very relaxed' after the treatment; 62% reported that the benefits lasted for several hours and a further 25% stated that the benefits lasted for more than a day. Most appreciated the music greatly. The researchers themselves confessed that it is uncertain whether the benefits were the result of the patient being given individual attention, talking with the therapist, the effects of touch and massage, the effects of the aromatherapy essential oils or the effects of the relaxation music.

The responses of 17 cancer hospice patients to humidified essential lavender oil aromatherapy for 30 minutes was studied against a no treatment (control) and a water humidification (control) given to all on different days. Vital signs as well as levels of pain, anxiety, depression and sense of well-being were measured (using an 11-point verbal analogue scale). The results showed a positive, yet small, change in blood pressure and pulse, pain, anxiety, depression and sense of well-being after both the humidified water treatment and the lavender treatment. However, after the no treatment session, there was also slight improvement in vital signs, depression and sense of well-being, but not in pain or anxiety levels (Kowalski, 2002).

Aromatherapy massage studied in eight cancer patients did not show any psychological benefit. However, there was a statistically significant reduction in all four physical parameters, which suggests that aromatherapy massage affects the autonomic nervous system, inducing relaxation. This finding was supported by the patients themselves, all of whom stated during interview that they felt 'relaxed' after aromatherapy massage (Hadfield, 2001).

Forty-two cancer patients were randomly allocated to receive weekly massages with lavender essential oil with an inert carrier oil (aromatherapy group), an inert carrier oil only (massage group) or no intervention for four weeks (Soden *et al.*, 2004). Outcome measures included a visual analogue scale (VAS) of pain intensity, the Verran and Snyder-Halpern Sleep Scale (VSH), the Hospital Anxiety and Depression Scale (HADS) and the Rotterdam Symptom Checklist (RSCL). No significant long-term benefits of aromatherapy or massage in terms of improving pain control, anxiety or quality of life were shown. However, sleep scores improved significantly in both the massage and the combined massage (aromatherapy and massage) groups. There were also statistically significant reductions in depression scores in the massage group. In this study of patients with advanced cancer, the addition of lavender essential oil did not appear to increase the beneficial effects of massage.

A randomised controlled pilot study was carried out to examine the effects of adjunctive aromatherapy massage on mood, quality of life and physical symptoms in patients with cancer attending a specialist unit (Wilcock *et al.*, 2003). Patients were randomised to conventional day care alone, or day care plus weekly aromatherapy massage using a standardised blend of oils for four weeks. At baseline and at weekly intervals, patients rated their mood, quality of life and the intensity and bother of two symptoms most important to them. Although 46 patients were recruited to the study, only 11 of 23 (48%) patients in the aromatherapy group and 18 of 23 (78%) in the control group completed all four weeks. Mood, physical symptoms and quality of life improved in both groups but there was no statistically significant difference between groups. Despite a lack of measurable benefit, all patients were satisfied with the aromatherapy and wished to continue it.

Physically or mentally challenged patients

Aromatherapy sessions in deaf and deaf-blind people became an accepted, enjoyable and therapeutic part of the residents' lifestyle in an uncontrolled series of case studies. It appeared that this gentle, non-invasive therapy could benefit deaf and deaf-blind people, especially as their intact senses can be heightened (Armstrong and Heidingsfeld, 2000).

The effects of four frequently used therapies (Snoezelen, active therapy, relaxation and aromatherapy/hand massage) on the communication of eight people with profound intellectual disabilities was assessed in another study (controls were absent); each received all four of the therapeutic procedures in a counterbalanced design: both Snoezelen and relaxation increased the level of positive communication and had some effect on decreasing negative communication. However, active therapy and aromatherapy/hand massage had little or no effect on communication (Lindsay *et al.*, 2001).

In all the trials above there was a more positive outcome for aromatherapy if there were no stringent scientific double-blind and randomised control measures, suggesting that in the latter case, bias is removed (see Appendix 32).

Studies published in non-scientific journals or presented at aromatherapy conferences only

The following studies all incorporated obvious major faults, which make them scientifically unacceptable.

A study of the effect of aromatherapy on endometriosis (Worwood, 1996) involved 22 aromatherapists who treated a total of 17 women in two groups, over 24 weeks. One group was initially given massage with essential oils and then not 'touched' for the second period, whilst the second group had the two treatments reversed. Amongst the many parameters measured were constipation, vaginal discharge, fluid retention, abdominal and pelvic pain, degree of feeling well, renewed vigour, depression and tiredness. The data were presented as means (or averages, possibly, as this was not stated) but without standard errors of mean (SEM).

The study of was well intended, but the data lacked any basic statistical analyses. Furthermore, the values for the parameters measured 'without' treatment in the two groups showed disparate values and therefore no conclusions could ever be made, with such discrepancies. The authors concluded that there was a large increase in the 'feel-good' factor of renewed vigour in the group that had massage following non-intervention for 12 weeks, but ignored the fact that it did not show any great change in the other group. Unfortunately the study has been accepted by many aromatherapists as being conclusive proof of the value in treating endometriosis using aromatherapy.

Studies of the use of essential oils in 'depression' (Rovesti and Colombo, 1973) have offered very little in the way of scientific evidence on their efficacy, as perfumes were mainly used in an atomiser. The various scents were squirted at 'depressed' patients or poured onto cotton wool pads which the patients then smelt (for an unknown period of time, at unknown intervals). Some chemical formulations of these 'antidepressant perfumes' were provided in the text, but there was no mention of controls, nor the precise diagnosis of the patients, their symptoms, and which of these symptoms were relieved, the number of patients involved and the statistical significance or otherwise of the results. Under such circumstances the evidence is at best anecdotal.

Note: Scientific studies on essential oils and perfumes and their psychological and physiological effects are described in Chapter 6.

Use of essential oils mainly as chemical agents

Peppermint and caraway oil

The efficacy and safety of capsules containing peppermint oil (90 mg) and caraway oil (50 mg), when studied in a double-blind, placebo-controlled, multicentre trial in patients with non-ulcer dyspepsia was shown by May et al. (1996). After four weeks of treatment, intensity of pain was significantly improved for the experimental group compared with the placebo group. Before the start of treatment all patients in the test preparation group reported moderate to severe pain, while by the end of the study 63.2% of these patients were free from pain. The pain symptoms had improved in a total of 89.5% of the patients in the active treatment group.

Perineal repair

Six drops of pure lavender oil included in the bath water for 10 days following childbirth was assessed against 'synthetic' lavender oil and a placebo (distilled water containing an unknown GRAS additive) (Cornwell and Dale, 1995). No significant differences between groups were found for discomfort, but lower scores in discomfort means for days 3 and 5 for the lavender group were seen. This was very unsatisfactory as a scientific study, mainly because essential oils do not mix with water and there was no proof

whether the lavender oil itself was pure. Finally, the results were inconclusive.

Alopecia areata

Alopecia areata was treated in a randomised trial using 'aromatherapy' carried out over seven months. The test group massaged a mixture of two drops of *Thymus vulgaris*, three drops *Lavandula angustifolia*, three drops *Rosmarinus officinalis* and two drops of *Cedrus atlantica* in 3 mL of jojoba and 20 mL grapeseed oil into the scalp for 2 minutes minimum every night. The control group massaged in the carrier oils alone (Hay et al., 1998). There was a significant improvement in the test group 44% (19/45 patients) compared with the control group of 15% (6/41). The smell of the essential oils (psychological/physiological) and/or their chemical nature on the scalp may have achieved these long-term results. On the other hand, the scalp may have healed naturally anyway.

Ureterolithiasis

Rowatinex, a mixture of mainly terpenes that smells rather like Vicks VapoRub, was tested orally against ureteric stones in 43 patients against a control group treated with a placebo. The overall expulsion rate of the stones was greater in the Rowatinex group (Engelstein et al., 1992). Similar mixes have shown both positive and negative results on gallstones over the years (see Chapter 5). This is definitely an internal usage of chemicals as medicines as odour does not affect internal organs.

Headaches

In a double-blind, placebo-controlled, randomised crossover study involving 332 healthy subjects, four different preparations were used to treat headaches (Gobel et al., 1994). Peppermint oil, eucalyptus oil (species not stated) and ethanol were applied to large areas of the forehead and temples. A combination of the three increased cognitive performance, muscle relaxation and mental relaxation, but had no influence on pain. Peppermint oil and ethanol decreased the headache. The reason for the success could have been the intense coldness caused by the application of the latter mixture, which was followed by a warming up as the peppermint oil caused counterirritation on the skin; the essential oils were also inhaled.

Acne

A clinical trial on 124 patients with acne, randomly distributed to a group treated with 5% tea tree oil gel or a 5% benzoyl peroxide lotion group (Bassett *et al.*, 1990), showed improvement in both groups and fewer side-effects in the tea tree oil group. The use of tea tree has, however, had detrimental effects in some people (see Chapter 7).

Athlete's foot

A 10% tea tree oil was used on 104 patients with athlete's foot (tinea pedis) in a randomised double-blind study against 1% tolnaflate and placebo creams. The tolnaflate group showed a better effect; tea tree oil was as effective in improving the condition, but was no better than the placebo at curing it (Tong *et al.*, 1992). Surprisingly, tea tree oil is sold, and bought, as a cure for athlete's foot.

Single-case studies

In the past few years the theme of the case studies (reported mainly in aromatherapy journals) has started to change and most of the aromatherapists are no longer saying that they are 'curing' cancer and other serious diseases. Emphasis has swung towards real complementary treatment, often in the area of palliative care. However, the so-called 'clinical aromatherapists' persist in attempting to cure various medical conditions using high doses of oils mainly by mouth, vagina, anus or on the skin. Many believe that healing wounds using essential oils is also classed as aromatherapy (Guba, 2000) despite the evidence that odour does not kill germs and any effect is due to the chemical activity alone.

Because of the lack of scientific evidence in many studies, we could assume that aromatherapy is mainly based on faith: it works because the aromatherapist believes in the treatment and because the patient believes in the supposed action of essential oils. In fact they may actually work, but probably only as the result of the placebo effect.

Decreasing smoking withdrawal symptoms

In one study the effect on 48 cigarette smokers of either black pepper oil puffed out of a special instrument for 3 hours after an overnight cigarette deprivation or mint/menthol or nothing was studied (Rose and Behm, 1994). Craving for cigarettes was significantly decreased by the black pepper, as were negative feelings.

Chronic respiratory infection treated by aromatherapy (but with proprietary medicines used as well)

A woman with chronic respiratory infection was massaged with tea tree, rosemary and bergamot oils whilst on her second course of antibiotics and taking a proprietary cough medicine. She also used lavender and rosemary oils in her bath, a drop of eucalyptus oil and lavender oil on her tissue near the pillow at night, three drops of eucalyptus and ginger for inhalations daily and reduced her dairy products and starches. In a week, her cough was better and by three weeks it had gone (Laffan, 1992). It is unclear which treatment actually helped the patient, and as it took a long time, the infection may well have gone away by then without any medicinal aid.

Combating infertility with essential oils

After just one treatment of aromatherapy massage using rose oil, bergamot and lavender at 2.5% in almond oil, a 36-year-old woman managed to get pregnant after being told she was possibly infertile following the removal of her right fallopian tube (Rippon, 1993).

Multiple sclerosis and aromatherapy

Aromatherapy can apparently help patients with multiple sclerosis, especially for relaxation, in association with many other changes in the diet and also use of conventional medicines (Barker, 1994). French basil, black pepper and true lavender in evening primrose oil with borage oil was used to counteract stiffness and also to stimulate; this mixture was later changed to include relaxing and sedative oils like Roman chamomile, ylang ylang and melissa.

Aromatherapy and dementia

Specific improvements in clients given aromatherapy treatment in dementia include increased alertness, self-hygiene, contentment, initiation of toileting, sleeping at night and reduced levels of agitation, withdrawal and wandering. Family carers reported less distress, improved sleeping patterns and feelings of calm (Kilstoff and Chenoweth, 1998). Other patients with dementia were monitored over a period of two months, and then for a further two months during which they received aromatherapy treatments in a clinical trial; they showed a significant improvement in motivational behaviour during the period of aromatherapy treatment (MacMahon and Kermode, 1998).

Problems arising in aromatherapy studies

Scant attention has been given to the actual chemical composition of the essential oils used or even the exact botanical origin type of the oil. For example, there are many main commercial types of 'lavender oil', all differing in both genus and composition. There are also a large number of chemotypes of *Lavandula* essential oils, and of these, often vague chemotypes are preferentially used by some aromatherapists (Lis-Balchin, 1999). The danger here is that little is known about the different chemotypes, the composition is very variable and no toxicity tests have been carried out on most of them. Large-scale admixing, deterpenation, dilution and adulteration also occurs, giving rise to a multitude of different lavender oils.

Reactions of aromatherapists to research

Although the *International Journal of Aromatherapy* is supposed to promote research, this excludes anything that involves animals, except for bacteria and viruses. Pharmacological studies, which are of more consequence to aromatherapy than the action of essential oils on some bacterial or viral populations, are disregarded. No scientific talks that involve pharmacological research on isolated tissues of animals are acceptable at aromatherapy conferences. An exception was given regarding mice subjected to essential oil odours (Buchbauer *et al.*, 1992), which involved the mice running up and down corridors or being observed in a cage. Experiments on humans, as used by the Fragrance Foundation for Perfumery, were tolerated.

Scientific methodology acceptance by aromatherapists

A recent letter in an aromatherapy journal (Minski and Bowles, 2002) indicates that aromatherapists are at last adapting to scientific methodology (Kirk-Smith, 1996a) and even questioning their own past results. In this case, marjoram oil was applied by massage or inhalation and reduced blood pressure, but as no control group was used the authors belatedly realised that the results were impossible to allocate to the effects of just the essential oil. This perhaps shows that scientists have been correct in their critique in the past.

Conclusion

Aromatherapy, using essential oils as an odorant by inhalation or massage onto the skin, has not been shown to work better than massage alone or a control. However, many patients have been pleased with aromatherapy treatment, as indicated by the many books written by aromatherapists and articles in aromatherapy journals. There has not been any great outcry about its failures. However, one has to consider whether the patients were getting better or just feeling better. Many patients feel better, even if their disease is getting worse, due to their belief in an alternative therapist. This is perhaps a good example of 'mind over matter', i.e. the placebo effect. This effect has been recommended by some members of the House of Lords Select Committee on Science and Technology, Sixth Report (2000), as a good basis for retaining complementary and alternative medicine, but other members argued that scientific proof of effects is necessary.

It is hoped that aromatherapists do not try to convince their patients of a cure, especially in the case of serious ailments such as cancer, which often recede naturally for a time on their own. Conventional treatment should always be advised in the first instance and retained during aromatherapy treatment with the consent of the patient's primary healthcare physician or consultant. Books on the value of alternative medicine for curing cancer must acknowledge when conventional treatment was also used and should not suggest that the alternative therapy had a sole, positive effect when in fact it was complementary.

Aromatherapy can provide a useful complementary medical service both in healthcare settings and in private practice and should not be allowed to become listed as a bogus cure in alternative medicine.

Introduction to the monographs

The information given in the monograph profiles attempts to give a full scientific account of the essential oil. The headings that appear in each monograph are explained more fully below.

Name of essential oil/absolute

CAS numbers: USA and European. These are for the identification of each essential oil/absolute and are different in the USA and Europe.

Species/Botanical name

The botanical name of the plant from which the essential oil is mainly derived is provided together with the synonyms that are commonly used. The common name(s) are also included. In some cases, e.g. sage oil – the two main types, Dalmatian and Spanish, are discussed together, while the completely different clary sage has its own monograph.

Note: The botanical names used in the essential oil industry are often different to those used in botanical books. There are many varieties, clones, cultivars, subspecies and chemotypes for a number of the oils. In some cases even more confusion arises as a result of cultivation practices. For citrus, for example, a species may be cloned on to a sturdy rootstock of another species and it is then unclear which of the botanical names should apply. This also happens with other trees and shrubs.

Safety

This is a quick survey of relevant safety data:

CHIP details

CHIP is the Chemicals Hazard Information and Packaging for Supply Regulations 2002: Physicochemical letters; Health; Risk phrases; Safety phrases (see Appendix 26).

RIFM recommended safety of use limits

A percentage figure is given (see Appendix 23).

EU sensitiser total

These are the maximum levels of fragrance allergens in aromatic natural raw materials: European Parliament and Council Directive 76/768/EEC on Cosmetic Products, 7th Amendment 2002: The presence of the substances must be indicated in the list of ingredients when its concentration exceeds 0.001% in leave-on products and 0.01% in rinse-off products (see Appendices 27 and 28; see also sensitisation under toxicity heading).

GRAS status

GRAS (generally recognised as safe) is a safety term used by the food industry to denote that the product has been tested for human consumption and has been shown to be safe; another status in the food category is provided if no GRAS status has been afforded. The fact that GRAS status has been given does not imply that the essential oil is safe to use on the skin, etc.

Extraction, source, appearance and odour

Extraction

The part of the plant used for the essential oil is given with details of special distillation or other extraction techniques.

Source

The major countries producing the essential oil at present are given; these are obtained from current essential oil production data on the Internet. These origins can change with time as economic or environmental factors come into force. France, for example, has ceased to be a major producer of essential oils and acts mainly as a 'middleman', thus much of the past literature can give the wrong source information. For example, Guenther (1948–1952) should be viewed as a historical book and is not entirely relevant to modern industrial production.

There is often no difference in the chemical composition of essential oils from different sources due to blending and adulteration.

Appearance and odour

The data are taken from the Perfumer's 'bible': Arctander (1960). However, different data are often given in the many aromatherapy books published and it is of note that this could be a subjective area, as different people have a different appreciation of odour.

Aromatherapy uses

The main source of any aromatherapy use of essential oils is the herbal usage of the relevant plant; the usages given by aromatherapists are therefore invariably unproven scientifically and include an extensive list of almost identical uses for each essential oil (Ryman, 1991; Lawless, 1992; Rose, 1992a,b; Price, 1993; Sheppard-Hanger, 1995; Price and Price, 1999). The extrapolation from herbal use is equivalent to assuming that drinking whole milk has exactly the same pharmacological, psychological, antimicrobial and toxicological effects as massaging the skin with butter (see Chapter 1).

Scientific comment

This is to provide a balanced view on the possibility of essential oil action; both aromatherapy massage and the use of the odour (fragrance) is considered in conjunction with scientific data.

Note: Definition of fragrance use: the fragrance is simply the odour of the essential oil, which can be volatalised in burners or heated rings or added to warm/hot water – but not applied to the skin as a perfume. Its effect will be initially as an inhalant and therefore largely psychological, with the possibility of physiological effects later. In the case of some essential oils, such as *Eucalyptus globulus*, there can be a physiological effect on the respiratory system directly.

Herbal uses

Data about any relevant herbal usage of the essential oil in the past and at present are provided, together with those about any relevant essential oil-containing extracts or the herb itself.

Conventional uses

Pharmacopoeias: Uses described in European or US pharmacopoeias.

Food and perfumery uses

The Flavor and Extract Manufacturers Association of the United States (FEMA) numbers are given for the essential oil with an indication of its usage in foods and beverages. The list is often very large and includes: baked goods, dairy products, candy, puddings, non-alcoholic and alcoholic beverages and chewing gum (the latter has often the highest percentage of the essential oil added). In the case of herbs the usage includes meat products, gravies, condiments, fats and oils (Fenaroli, 1997).

The main perfumery uses are given based mainly on data in Arctander (1960).

Chemistry

Only a few of the major components are given, plus any minor ones thought to contribute to the bioactivity of the essential oil (e.g. odour or toxicity). Commercial essential oil values are provided, which means there is often a wide range. The values have been taken from numerous monographs by Lawrence (1976–1978; 1979–1980; 1981–1987; 1988–1991; 1994–1995) which are reprints from *Perfumer and Flavorist*.

Sensitising components are indicated in the composition, where applicable.

Adulteration

This is of immense importance as there is a general opinion by those practising aromatherapy that only pure essential oils can be active. This is not always adhered to, as Gattefossé used deterpenated essential oils. Synthetic components and fractions of other essential oils which are often added make a difference to the bioactivity. The higher the price of a given essential oil, the more likely it is for adulteration to have occurred. The most frequently asked question by newly qualified aromatherapists and lay people is: 'which is the best supplier?'. The most frequent reply is: 'how much do you want to pay?' The highest price, however, does not always indicate purity, as there is the factor of greed in the retail industry. There is also the problem of the 'best odour for perfumery' to contend with, meaning that essential oils are geared to the 'Noses' in the perfumery industry – there, the actual odour counts and adulteration is not considered a great problem.

Organic, wild-crafted and other terminology depicting the origin of essential oils does not necessarily imply naturalness and often means that the essential oils have very different chemical compositions compared with the norm, and thereby have different odours; they can also have different biological effects *per se*.

Toxicity

The acute toxicity studied in animals is given for each essential oil (where it is available). This is provided by the relevant RIFM monographs, which are listed alphabetically in Appendix 22.

The LD_{50} is a relative measure of toxicity and is not a very good indicator of toxicity in essential oils as the value is almost identical in each case; the toxicity is also relatively low, as the essential oils would otherwise be banned.

Subacute toxicity is also provided where available from the RIFM monographs (see Appendix 22).

Irritation and sensitisation

Sensitisation is the toxic effect after multiple applications of the essential oil, not an initial reaction after a single application. The effects can take days or even years to become apparent. There is a strong possibility that essential oils with similar chemical components will cause sensitisation once it has been established by one essential oil; it is therefore essential to determine the component causing the effect in order to avoid problems of such cross-sensitisation.

Symptoms of sensitisation can be dermal or internal. For example, they may affect the lungs, causing asthma or breathlessness, or other organs or tissues, causing headaches, migraines, panic attacks, vertigo, nausea and stomach ache (see also Chapters 5 and 7).

Relevant data are given regarding sensitisation, both in animals and humans: sensitisation through skin application of essential oils has been studied for many years in humans by the cosmetics industry. These findings are therefore very relevant to aromatherapy. Other studies of toxicity are often in sensitive animals, but can be extrapolated to humans.

Phototoxicity

This information is provided, where applicable, usually from the RIFM monographs (see Appendix 22), unless otherwise stated. Phototoxicity involves the effect of UV light in sunlight, light used during irradiation on sunbeds and also UV light used in the treatment of skin conditions like psoriasis. Oral intake of an essential oil-containing herb (parsley) has even shown an effect on the skin – the symptoms being equivalent to sunburn (see also Chapter 7).

Drug interactions

The interaction of herbal medicines and conventional drugs is becoming increasingly reported, but not much information is as yet available for the essential oils. Data concerning drug interactions with the essential oil, its components or also those of related species are provided, where available.

Bioactivities

The bioactivity of the essential oil and its components is a measure of the authenticity of its folk medicinal status. Some information is given regarding herbal usage where the extract has at least some essential oil content (i.e. it is an alcoholic extract or even a hot tea), but this does not generally include cold water-soluble extracts. Consideration is also given in some cases to different but related species of the plant in question, although there is often a large difference in their chemical composition. Essential oils from such related species are sometimes found on the market, but it must be pointed out that these 'novel' essential oils have not usually been toxicologically evaluated, nor have chemotypes.

Pharmacological activities *in vitro* and *in vivo*

Smooth muscle The pharmacological activities, even in animal models, are a strong indicator of the essential oil activity in humans, either in the same organ/tissue or even in the truly holistic sense. Studies on the activity of essential oils alone and in mixtures on the smooth muscle of the guinea-pig ileum *in vitro* showed very similar activities compared with their probable holistic action (suggested by aromatherapists). Spasmolytic (sedative) essential oils had a relaxant holistic effect in humans, while contractile oils (stimulant) oils had the opposite affect (see Chapter 5 and Appendices 11–13). Mixtures of two to four essential oils, as used in aromatherapy, produced an effect which was based on their additive chemical composition; this showed that a high proportion of monoterpenes would produce a stimulant effect on humans, whilst producing a contractile effect on the guinea-pig ileum. This is exemplified by the fact that citrusy perfumes (containing a high concentration of monoterpenes) are stimulating.

The comparative effect of the essential oil on smooth muscle is initially given in each case, unless unavailable and is shown in alphabetical order for essential oils in Appendix 2. Other published data are then given.

Uterus The effect of essential oils on the uterus has not been studied to any great degree, certainly not *in vivo*. *In vitro* studies on the uterine muscle of the rat show that all the essential oils and most of the components have been relaxant (see Appendix 3). There is therefore some contraindication for their use in childbirth, where contractions are of great importance. Their effect during pregnancy may also be hazardous if used at high concentration, but virtually no scientific studies are available.

Other activities Other pharmacological, physiological and miscellaneous effects are indicated, sometimes including herbal extracts, to throw some light on the probable function of essential oils in humans.

Psychological studies of essential oils are of special interest in aromatherapy, as the odour effect is one of the most important aspects of this example of complementary and alternative medicine. There is sometimes a correlation between the psychological and physiological effect of an essential oil or mixture that can also be extended to the holistic effect in humans (see Appendix 14).

Antimicrobial activities

Most essential oils have antimicrobial activities. Some are active towards both bacteria and fungi, while others are active against one and not the other. The relative data are given for comparison of activities (see Appendices 1 and 7) as well as data from other published literature. There is no definitive proof that essential oils are viricidal as yet, other than for a few *in vitro* studies, although many of the more water-soluble herbal extracts have this effect. Antioxidant activity *in vitro* is indicated where appropriate.

Clinical studies

Data are given for the essential oil or its main components where available.

Use in pregnancy and lactation: contraindications

Cautions are given for individual essential oils regarding their use during these periods. Very few scientific data are available regarding the effects on the uterus, and clinical studies during parturition have not approached this problem scientifically. There are many references for some essential oils on the effects of oral intake of the herb, rather than the essential oil, but as the herb contains the essential oil in hot teas or alcoholic preparations, some of that data will be included. Advice is given on the use of essential oils in aromatherapy massage as well as the use of the essential oil as an odorant (fragrance), which is not applied to the skin.

Pharmaceutical guidance

This summarises the data in the scientific literature and an attempt is made to provide an assessment as to whether the essential oil should be used safely in aromatherapy as a fragrance (inhaled) or massaged into the skin; however, as the data are often abstracted from oral studies of the herb rather than the essential oil, in both animals and humans, it may not always be relevant. There is therefore some difficulty in the interpretation of the combined data. The new European guidelines and cautions regarding sensitisation are also included. The advice is therefore often more cautionary than is warranted by the long-term usage of certain well-known essential oils.

Use in babies and young children

It is advisable not to use essential oils on the skin of babies and young children, nor to allow high concentrations of the essential oil near them.

Tisserand and Balacs (1995) recommend a reduction in the oral dosage of essential oils for children of 3–6 drops per 24 hours for a body weight of 20 kg (adult dose approximately 60 mL maximum) and oral dosing is not recommended for children under this body weight. Furthermore, oral dosing must be under medical supervision only. The use of many essential oils in babies and young children under 2 years is not recommended by Tisserand and Balacs (1995) and they state that it is easier to list unsafe essential oils than to list safe ones. For this reason, as well as due to consideration of the immaturity of the skin and the delicate nature of this thinner skin, it is inadvisable for essential oils to be used. This is also a necessary precaution due to the risk of sensitisation of the children at this young age (see Chapters 5 and 7).

Instillation or administration of essential oils near the baby or young child's nose is not only not recommended, but distinctly inadvisable as there have been numerous cases reported of severe toxicity and even death from such applications (Tisserand and Balacs, 1995; see also Chapter 7).

Angelica Oil

CAS numbers

USA: 8015-64-3; EINECS: 84775-71-7

Species/Botanical name

Angelica archangelica L. (Apiaceae/Umbelliferae)

Synonyms

Angelica officinalis Moench and Hoffm., root of the Holy Ghost

Safety

CHIP details

Xn; R10, 65; 95%; S62 (A26)

RIFM recommended safety of use limits

0.78% (phototoxic) for root and seed oils (A23)

EU sensitiser total

18.3 (based on limonene and linalool) (A27)

GRAS status

Granted (Fenaroli, 1997).

Extraction, source, appearance and odour

Extraction

Both root and seed essential oils are obtained by steam distillation. Roots take 12–24 hours to distil (Arctander, 1960).

Source

Both oils are obtained mainly from Hungary, Holland, Belgium, Germany, France and India.

Appearance and odour

Seed oil is a pale-yellow liquid with a strong, fresh, light peppery odour; the top-note is terpentine-like and there is a sweet, anisic undertone (Arctander, 1960). It has less tenacity than the root oil. The main component, phellandrene, is liable to polymerise and resinify if the essential oil is incorrectly stored or aged. There is wide variation in the quality of the essential oil dependent on source, storage conditions and age (Arctander, 1960).

Root oil is pale-yellow to deep amber with warm, pungent, musky-animalistic/earthy odour, due to the various lactones and a fresh peppery top-note, due to phellandrene (Arctander, 1960).

Angelica root absolute is also produced. It is a viscous, yellow-brown liquid. There is little or no phellandrene and the odour is intensely musky-woody, somewhat spicy with resemblance to *Pimpinella* root (Arctander, 1960).

Aromatherapy uses

Very few aromatherapy books include angelica oil and those that do often treat the herb and essential oil as being equivalent and oral usage is often implied. Uses include: rheumatism, indigestion, colic, premenstrual tension, menopause, bruises, scars, psoriasis, coughs, bronchitis, water retention, anaemia, anorexia, migraine, nervous tension and stress disorders. Angelica root oil added to bath water is said to remove toxins and the fragrance also apparently stimulates appetite (Ryman, 1991; Lawless, 1992; Rose, 1992a).

Scientific comment

Angelica root essential oil has a rather pervasive, unpleasant odour and does not lend itself to use as a fragrance; massage itself can alleviate many stress conditions and there is no proof that including the essential oil has any benefits at all for any of the uses listed above; it is also likely to cause photosensitisation, so is best avoided.

Herbal uses

No traditional angelica essential oil uses have been documented; most of the data are for whole herbal extracts (Wren, 1988; Blumenthal *et al.*, 2000; Barnes *et al.*, 2002). Angelica can be used for lack of appetite and dyspeptic complaints such as mild stomach cramps and flatulence (Blumenthal *et al.*, 2000). Many related species, including *A. sinensis* (dong quai), are traditionally used in Chinese medicine (Barnes *et al.*, 2002) and the latter occurs in about 70% of all traditional Chinese medicine prescriptions to treat dysmenorrhoea, but no proof has been provided as to its effectiveness.

Food and perfumery uses

Food Root oil (FEMA 2088) and seed oil (FEMA 2090) are used in baked goods, beverages and candy (Fenaroli, 1997).

Perfumery Seed essential oil is used in chypres and fougeres, but the root oil is preferred in perfumery (Arctander, 1960). Root essential oil is used in various perfumes like heavy chypres, oriental bases, fougeres and citrus colognes. In food flavours it is used in Cointreau-type liqueurs. Root absolute is used in perfumery for its tenacity; the odour threshold is about 0.005 mg%, making it one of the most powerful flavour materials of plant origin (Arctander, 1960).

Chemistry

Major components

Major components	% (Lawrence, 1976–2001)
α-Phellandrene	0.2–15
β-Phellandrene	trace–28
α-Pinene	20–32
β-Pinene	>1–2
Limonene	1–10
Linalool	trace–2

Similar composition is reported for both the root and seed oils; both show variable data.

Minor components

Other monoterpenes including sabinene, α-thujene, borneol (Lawrence, 1976–2001) make up to 80–90%; also four macrocyclic lactones and many sesquiterpenes. Over 20 furanocoumarins, including angelicin, archangelicin and bergapten, have been found in the root (Blumenthal *et al.*, 2000; Barnes *et al.*, 2002).

Adulteration

Angelica root oil is one of the most expensive oils due to its low yield and the fact that the roots are best at 2 years and the seed takes 3 years to be produced. Roots from the 3-year-old plants give an even lower yield and the odour is very different. Angelica seed oil is often used for cutting the root oil. Both the essential oils can be adulterated with synthetic monoterpenes (A8; Arctander, 1960; see also Chapter 4).

Toxicity

Acute toxicity (A22)

Oral LD_{50} Root oil 2.2 g/kg body weight (mouse) and 11.2 g/kg (rat); root oil and seed oil >5 g/kg (rat).

Liver and kidney damage was cause of death in the acute studies, however damage was reversible in animals surviving for 3 days.

Dermal LD_{50} Root oil >5 g/kg (rabbit); seed oil >5 g/kg.

Subacute toxicity The tolerated dose in the rat was 1.5 g/kg for root oil; seed oil was non-toxic at 5 g/kg.

Irritation and sensitisation (A22)

The root at 1% and seed oils at 2% are non-irritant and non-sensitising on animals and humans but contain potential sensitisers.

Phototoxicity

Extreme photosensitisation occurs if skin is exposed to sunlight or UV light following application of the root oil to the skin. A top 0.78% is advised by the International Fragrance Association (IFRA) in any products, as over that level phototoxicity can occur and is dose-dependent. There is also a possible carcinogenic risk due to the bergapten (5-methoxypsoralen) (A22; Barnes *et al.*, 2002).

New IFRA regulations: Natural extracts containing furocoumarin-like substances may be used in cosmetic products, provided that the total concentration of furocoumarin-like substances in the finished cosmetic product do not exceed 1 ppm. These extracts include angelica root oil (*Angelica archangelica* L.), bergamot oil and all citrus-expressed oils.

Drug interaction

No data are available for the essential oils. An extract of a related species, dong quai, given subcutaneously to rabbits affected prothrombin time after a single dose of warfarin (Leung, 1980). Increase in prothrombin time was found in a patient previously stabilised on warfarin after taking dong quai (Lo *et al.*, 1995). This could be a serious problem if skin application of the angelica oil resulted in a similar effect.

Bioactivities

Pharmacological activities *in vitro* and *in vivo*

Smooth muscle   There was a strong spasmogenic action by angelica essential oil on smooth muscle of the guinea-pig *in vitro* (A2; Lis-Balchin *et al.*, 1996a) and this reaction was also found on tracheal muscle as well as ileum (Zobel and Brown, 1991). A methanolic extract of *A. archangelica* root showed antispasmodic activity against spontaneous contractions of circular smooth muscle and inhibited acetylcholine- and barium chloride-induced contractions of longitudinal smooth muscle (Reiter and Brandt, 1985). Extracts of *A. archangelica* root exhibit calcium channel-blocking activity (Izzo *et al.*, 1996), and some of its coumarins showed calcium channel antagonist activity (Harmala *et al.*, 1992b).

Uterus   Angelica root oil and some of its components caused a decrease in the spontaneous contractions of rat uterus (A3; A4; Lis-Balchin, Hart, 1997b). In rabbits, a uterotonic action was shown after intraduodenal administration of a methanolic extract of the related angelica root, *A. sinensis* (Harada *et al.*, 1984), and this species has also induced both uterine contraction and relaxation (Lis-Balchin and Hart, 1997b).

Antimicrobial activities

Antibacterial activity
Relative data: 23/25 different bacteria and 20/20 *Listeria monocytogenes* varieties (A1; Lis-Balchin and Deans, 1997; Lis-Balchin *et al.*, 1998a).

Antifungal activity
Relative data (% inhibition): *Aspergillus niger* 0%, *A. ochraceus* 16%, *Fusarium culmorum* −18% (A1). Antifungal activity was reported for 14 of 15 fungi tested (Maruzella and Liguori, 1958).

Clinical studies

No clinical studies have been documented for angelica oil (*A. archangelica*). Bergapten has shown severe burning potential when used in the treatment of psoriasis using PUVA (psoralen (P) and high-intensity long-wavelength UV irradiation treatment) (Martindale, 1996). Bergapten used to be used as an ingredient in suntan preparations and cosmetics due to its 'tanning' potential. However, due to occasional sunburn and concern regarding the risk of skin cancer, its use is not advised (Martindale, 1996).

Use in pregnancy and lactation: contraindications

There is a loss of spontaneous contractions in the uterus when the root essential oil is applied *in vitro* to the rat. Angelica root is also reputed to be an abortifacient and to affect the menstrual cycle. Due to these possible effects and the photosensitising constituents, angelica root oil should not be used on the body during pregnancy and lactation; angelica seed oil could possibly be used sparingly on the body provided it has been obtained by steam distillation of the seed alone and is not adulterated with the root oil.

Pharmaceutical guidance

There is scant pharmacological information available for *A. archangelica* essential oils to justify their aromatherapy uses. The photosensitising bergaptens, which may be carcinogenic in angelica root oil, do not recommend its usage in aromatherapy massage, especially above the IFRA recommended maximum dose of 0.78% if the skin is then exposed to sunshine, but it could be used as a fragrance at low doses. In addition, excessive doses may interfere with anticoagulant therapy because of the coumarin constituents. Angelica root oil should not be used on babies and children. The use of the seed oil shows little apparent hazard but it has not been used by aromatherapists.

Use in babies and young children

Due to the immaturity and the delicate nature of the skin of babies and young children, it is inadvisable for any essential oils to be used in massage however much the essential oil has been diluted in the carrier oil. This is also a necessary precaution due to the possibilities of sensitisation of the children at this young age through skin or air-borne odorant effects (see Chapters 5 and 7).

Instillation or administration of essential oils near the baby or young child's nose is not only not recommended, but distinctly inadvisable, as there have been numerous cases reported of severe toxicity and even death from such applications (see Chapter 7).

Aniseed and Star Anise

CAS numbers

USA: 8007-70-3; EINECS: 84650-59-9

Species/Botanical name

Pimpinella anisum L. (Apiaceae/Umbelliferae)

Synonyms

Aniseed oil, esencia de anís, essence d'anis, oleum anisi

Pharmacopoeias

In Chinese, European and Polish Pharmacopoeias. Also in United States National Formulary.

Other species

Illicium verum L. (star anise)

Safety

CHIP details
None

RIFM recommended safety of use limits
Aniseed (*Pimpinella anisum*) and star anise (*Illicium verum*): 2% (A23)

EU sensitiser total
4 (A27)

GRAS status
Granted (Fenaroli, 1997).

Extraction, source, appearance and odour

Extraction
Aniseed oil and star anise oil are produced by steam distillation of the fruit. Yield of essential oils: 2–6%.

Source
Argentina, Bulgaria, Chile, China, Germany, Hungary and Poland.

Appearance and odour
Aniseed oil is a clear to pale yellow liquid with iridescent sheen and a sweet characteristic odour reminiscent of anethole (licorice) (Arctander, 1960).

Aromatherapy uses

Aromatherapists list: as treatment for lumbago, palpitations, abdominal cramps, flatulence, indigestion, menopause, lack of periods, painful periods, frigidity, impotence, migraine, nervous exhaustion and stress-related disease, dull congested skin, psoriasis, accumulation of toxins, arthritis, gout, rheumatism, water retention, bronchitis, coughs, anaemia and anorexia (Ryman, 1991; Lawless, 1992; Rose, 1992a,b; Price, 1993; Sheppard-Hanger, 1995).

Scientific comment

It is unlikely that the concentration of essential oil used in the usual dilution for massage could provide the dosage required for most of the uses given, which are unsupported by any scientific data. The volatalised essential oil may possibly provide some relief from coughs and have antifungal benefits. Massage alone could alleviate some of the stress conditions, including skeletal muscle pain, but due to the possible carcinogenic, irritant and sensitisation potential, aniseed essential oil is likely to cause more harm than good.

Herbal uses

Aniseed apparently has expectorant, antispasmodic, carminative and parasiticidal properties. Its uses include treatment for bronchial catarrh, tracheitis with persistent cough, pertussis, spasmodic cough, flatulent colic (British Herbal Medicine Association, 1983; Wren, 1988; Wichtl, 1994; Barnes *et al.*, 2002), also topically for pediculosis and scabies. Aniseed has been used as an oestrogenic agent (Albert-Puleo, 1980) and is said to increase milk secretion, promote menstruation, facilitate birth, alleviate symptoms of the male climacteric and increase libido. Anethole is used as a carminative and is a mild expectorant and a common ingredient in cough mixtures and lozenges.

Conventional uses

Anise oil is carminative and mildly expectorant and is a common ingredient of cough preparations

(Martindale, 2004). Pharmacopoeial preparations include camphorated opium tincture, compound orange spirit, concentrated anise water, concentrated camphorated opium tincture (BP 2003) and compound orange spirit (USNF 22).

Food and perfumery uses

Food Anise (FEMA 2094) is used in baked goods, candies, beverages and chewing gum; *trans*-anethole is used mainly in food flavouring. The essential oil is used extensively in alcoholic drinks such as raki, anisette, etc. The cheaper anethole is normally used rather than the essential oil (Fenaroli, 1997).

Perfumery Anise masks off-notes like hydrogen sulphide. It is not used extensively due to the cost, as anethole is cheaper. Anethole is used particularly for dentifrices (Arctander, 1960).

Chemistry

Major components

Major components	% (Lawrence, 1976–2001)
trans-Anethole	80–95
Estragole (methyl chavicol)	trace–5
Anisaldehyde	trace–1

Minor components

These usually account for just a small proportion and include the oxidation products of anethole (anise ketone (*p*-methoxyphenylacetone) and anisic acid), linalool, limonene, α-pinene, pseudoisoeugenol-2-methyl butyrate, acetaldehyde, *p*-cresol, cresol, hydroquinone, the sesquiterpenes (β-caryophyllene, β-farnesene, α-, β- and γ-himachalene, bisabolene, *d*-elemene, ar-curcumene) and myristicin (Lawrence, 1976–2001; Burkhardt *et al.*, 1986). Bergapten (furanocoumarin) also occurs in minute concentrations.

Anise oil, anisi aetheroleum (Ph. Eur. 4.8) is an essential oil obtained by steam distillation from the dry ripe fruits of *Pimpinella anisum*. It contains less than 1.5% linalol, 0.5–5.0% estragole, less than 1.2% α-terpineol, 0.1–0.4% *cis*-anethole, 87–94% *trans*-anethole, 0.1–1.4% anisaldehyde and 0.3–2.0% pseudoisoeugenyl-2-methyl butyrate. Star anise oil, anisi stellati aetheroleum (Ph. Eur. 4.8) is an essential oil obtained by steam distillation from the dry ripe fruits of *Illicium verum*. It contains 0.2–2.5% linalol, 0.5–6.0% estragole,

less than 0.3% α-terpineol, 0.1–0.5% *cis*-anethole, 86–93% *trans*-anethole, 0.1–0.5% anisaldehyde and 0.1–3.0% foeniculin.

Adulteration

Star anise is often fraudulently substituted for the oil of anise. There has reputedly been a fatality of a child in Spain who consumed a herbal drink infusion containing 'aniseed' spice, which was probably star anise or Japanese anise, containing safrole (FDA Star Anise Tea Advisory posted on 09/11/2003).

Most of the oil of commerce is of the star anise *Illicium verum* type from China and Vietnam. Smaller amounts of anise oil *Anisum pimpanellum* is also available. Both have *trans*-anethole as their major component at ~90% and no more than traces of safrole isomers. Neither should be confused with the so-called Japanese aniseed *Illicium religiosum* (*Illicium anisatum*), which has isosafrole as its major component, instead of *trans*-anethole. The essential oil from this plant is not thought to be produced or traded in commercial quantities. Safrole and isosafrole are known to be toxic and sassafras oil *Sassafras albidum* (90% + safrole) has a CHIP guidance label as T = Toxic.

Toxicity

Acute toxicity (A22)

Oral LD$_{50}$ Anise oil 2.3 g/kg body weight (rat); star anise oil >2.6 g/kg (rat); *trans*-anethole 2–3 g/kg.

Dermal LD$_{50}$ Anise oil >5 g/kg (rabbit); star anise oil >5 g/kg.

Irritation and sensitisation

The anise essential oil and anethole are both irritant and sensitising (Mitchell and Rook, 1979; Fetrow and Avila, 1999). Star anise oil at 2% and 1% causes sensitisation in 5% of people, and positive patch tests in a third of dermatitis patients. Sensitive people are frequently positive to anethole and also α-pinene, limonene and safrole (Rudzki *et al.*, 1976). Contact dermatitis reactions to aniseed oil have been attributed to anethole (Mitchell and Rook, 1979; British Herbal Medicine Association, 1983; Fetrow and Avila, 1999), including creams and toothpastes flavoured with aniseed oil (Mitchell and Rook, 1979). Two female workers in a cake factory developed severe dermatitis, and patch tests indicated sensitivity to anise oil and to anethole (British Herbal Medicine Association, 1990).

Phototoxicity

Bergapten causes photosensitivity and there is also a possible carcinogenic risk (Martindale, 1989).

Other toxicities

Oesophageal cancer in France is strongly associated with aniseed aperitif, warm spirits and beer (Gignoux and Launoy, 1999). In the case of larynx supraglottis cancers, more drinkers of aniseed spirit were found than expected. The link between the risk of oesophageal cancer and alcohol varies greatly according to the type of alcoholic beverage, with aniseed aperitifs, hot spirits (especially hot Calvados) and beer carrying the highest risk (Launoy et al., 1997). Malignant arterial hypertension induced by the ingestion of 'alcohol-free aniseed drink' (Toulon et al., 1983) and a case of hypertension and quadriparesis from a non-alcoholic pastis (an anise-based aperitif) containing glycyrrhizinic acid have been described (Trono et al., 1983). Moderate genotoxic effects were found with anise (Balachandran et al., 1991).

trans-Anethole oxide is mutagenic for Salmonella and carcinogenic in the induction of hepatomas in B6C3F1 mice and skin papillomas in CD-1 mice (Kim and Cho, 1999).

There seems to be a discrepancy between the many warnings to: 'Avoid during pregnancy' and 'Do not use on children under 5 years' in aromatherapy books and the status of anise and star anise oils as permitted as common food flavourings in sweets and biscuits, etc. that are regularly consumed by children and adults.

The US Food and Drug Administration (FDA) released an advisory warning to consumers against drinking teas with star anise which probably contained the toxic Japanese variety (*Illicium anisatum*) (FDA Star Anise Tea Advisory posted on 09/11/2003). These have caused illness in approximately 40 individuals, including 15 infants. Symptoms ranged from seizures and vomiting to jitteriness and rapid eye movement.

Ingestion of as little as 1–5 mL of anise oil can result in nausea, vomiting, seizures and pulmonary oedema (Chandler and Hawkes, 1984). There was a case of an asthma patient with high levels of specific anti-aniseed IgE antibodies (Fraj, 1996). The leukotriene C4 release test showed a good correlation with clinical history for four patients sensitised to wheat flour, oyster, lobster and anise, whereas specific IgE determinations were less sensitive (Sainte-Laudy, 1997).

Anethole is the main cause of anise oil toxicity when given orally (see also fennel oil), resulting in liver lesions in short-term oral tests (Albert-Puleo, 1980) in rats fed 1% of their daily diet for 15 weeks (Duke, 1985) and rats fed with 0.1% trans-anethole for 90 days. Lower, more therapeutic doses, apparently cause minimal hepatotoxicity (Duke, 1985). Oral trans-anethole in rats resulted in dose-dependent anti-implantation activity and significant oestrogenic activity; however, anti-oestrogenic, progestational, antiprogestational, androgenic or antiandrogenic activity was not shown (Dhar, 1995). trans-Anethole poses no significant carcinogenic risk to humans due to a different detoxification mechanism to that in animals. Cross-reactivity is the cause of many reactions with anise, carrot, parsley, fennel and caraway (Wuthrich and Dietschi, 1985). Positive scratch tests in 70 patients with positive skin tests to birch and/or mugwort pollens and celery were found with aniseed, fennel, coriander and cumin – all from the same botanical family (Apiaceae) as celery – in more than 24 patients (Stager et al., 1991). It is unclear whether these cross-reactions occur with essential oils or components.

Bioactivities

Pharmacological activities *in vitro* and *in vivo*

Smooth muscle A strong spasmogenic action followed by a lesser spasmolytic action on electrically stimulated smooth muscle of the guinea-pig *in vitro* has been reported (A2; Lis-Balchin et al., 1996a). Relaxation of tracheal smooth muscle was found with the volatile oils of 22 plants but anise and fennel oil increased phasic contractions of ileal muscle cells (Reiter and Brandt, 1985). A strong contraction was also reported in tracheal muscle (Reiter and Brandt, 1985). Anise oil (200 mg/L) has been shown to antagonise carbachol-induced spasms in a guinea-pig tracheal muscle preparation (ESCOP, 1996–1999). The bronchodilatory effects of the essential oil (and aqueous and ethanol extracts) on methacholine precontracted isolated tracheal chains of the guinea-pig showed significant relaxant effects compared with those of controls. The results apparently showed that the relaxant effect is not due to an inhibitory effect of histamine (H1) or the stimulatory effect of beta-2-adrenergic receptors, but due to inhibitory effects on muscarinic receptors (Boskabady et al., 2001).

Uterus Anise essential oil caused a decrease in the spontaneous contractions of rat uterus (A3; A4; Lis-Balchin and Hart, 1997b).

Other activities Anise oil increased respiratory tract fluid in anaesthetised guinea-pigs, rats and cats and a similar action was observed in anaesthetised rabbits inhaling anise oil (ESCOP, 1996–1999). The 'lactogogic' action of anise has been attributed to anethole, which exerts a competitive antagonism at dopamine receptor sites, as it is structurally related to the catecholamines adrenaline, noradrenaline and dopamine (dopamine inhibits prolactin secretion), and to the action of polymerised anethole, which is structurally related to the oestrogenic compounds stilbene and stilboestrol (Albert-Puleo, 1980). It appears that the *P. anisum* essential oil may reduce the effects of morphine via a GABAergic mechanism in mice (Sahraei *et al.*, 2002).

Anise oil given intraperitoneally to mice increased the dose of pentylenetetrazole needed to induce clonic and tonic seizures in a dose-dependent manner and also those due to maximal electric shock (Pourgholami *et al.*, 1999). Motor impairment was observed at higher doses. Pentobarbital-induced sleeping time was prolonged by intraperitoneal administration of anise oil (50 mg/kg) to mice (ESCOP, 1996–1999).

Aniseed has been found to slightly elevate gamma-aminobutyric acid (GABA) concentrations in brain tissue (Barnes *et al.*, 2002).

Behaviour-conditioning experiments with odours of anise have been carried out (Lucas and Sclafani, 1995). The alleged psychoactivity of guarana essential oil is presumably due to its estragole and anethole content (Benoni *et al.*, 1996).

A hair growth promoter consisting of fennel, anise, caraway, etc. has been patented (US Patent 5,422,100) and an insect repellent composed of oils of *Hedeoma pulegioides*, *Pimpinella anisum* and *Chrysanthemum* (US Patent 5,208,029).

Antimicrobial activity

Antibacterial activity
Relative data: Aniseed essential oil was very inactive: there was minimal activity against only 6/25 different bacteria and 0/20 *Listeria monocytogenes* varieties (A1; Lis-Balchin amd Deans, 1997; Lis-Balchin *et al.*, 1998a). Both the essential oils were active against several bacteria (Friedman *et al.*, 2002); there was some activity against 4/5 different bacteria (Maruzella and Sicurela, 1960; Aureli *et al.*, 1992). *Salmonella enteritidis* was particularly sensitive to inhibition by a combination of oil of anise, fennel or basil with methyl paraben; *Listeria monocytogenes* was less sensitive (Fyfe *et al.*, 1997).

Antifungal activity
Relative data (% inhibition): Aniseed oil displayed considerable activity: *Aspergillus niger* 83%, *A. ochraceus* 82%, *Fusarium culmorum* 69% (A1).

Other activities
Anethole, anisaldehyde and myristicin have shown mild insecticidal properties (Leung, 1980). Insecticidal, acaricidal and plant inhibition activities of rare phenylpropanoids from *Pimpinella* have been reported (Reichling *et al.*, 1991).

Clinical studies

Flight controllers were less tired after a shift when volatile phytoncides of brandy mint, lavender and anise were used (Leshchinskaia *et al.*, 1983). Headlice treatment using essential oils of aniseed, cinnamon leaf, red thyme, tea tree, peppermint and nutmeg showed good results (Veal, 1996).

Use in pregnancy and lactation: contraindications

Traditionally, aniseed is considered to be an abortifacient (Duke, 1985) and also to promote lactation. It also caused a relaxation in the spontaneous contractions of the rat uterus *in vitro*. The safety of aniseed taken during pregnancy, parturition and lactation in the human has not been established and therefore the use of the essential oil should be curtailed during those times.

Pharmaceutical guidance

Aniseed is used extensively as a spice and is widely used in conventional pharmaceuticals for its carminative, expectorant and flavouring properties. Aniseed contains anethole and estragol, which are structurally related to safrole, a known hepatotoxin and carcinogen. Aniseed may cause an allergic reaction. It is recommended that the use of aniseed oil should be avoided in dermatitis, and inflammatory or allergic skin conditions (Tisserand and Balacs, 1995; Fetrow and Avila, 1999). Avoidance of the aniseed essential oil in cases of cancer and hepatic disease has been suggested (Tisserand and Balacs, 1995); also avoidance of anethole-high oils in general (Zondek, 1938; Albert-Puelo, 1980). Aniseed should be avoided by people with known sensitivity to anethole (ESCOP, 1996–1999). Bergapten may cause photosensitivity in sensitive individuals. The potential oestrogenic activity of anethole and its dimers may affect existing hormone therapy, including the oral contraceptive pill and hormone replacement therapy, if excessive concentrations are used. Neurological effects similar to those documented for nutmeg could be envisaged, as in consumption of large amounts of aniseed. Its use in aromatherapy massage therefore cannot be justified.

Use in babies and young children

Due to the immaturity and the delicate nature of the skin of babies and young children, it is inadvisable for any essential oils to be used in massage, however much the essential oil has been diluted in the carrier oils. This is also a necessary precaution due to the possibilities of sensitisation of the children at this young age through skin or air-borne odorant effects (see Chapters 5 and 7).

Instillation or administration of essential oils near the baby or young child's nose is not only not recommended, but distinctly inadvisable, as there have been numerous cases reported of severe toxicity and even death from such applications (see Chapter 7).

Note: PVC bottles softened and distorted fairly rapidly in the presence of anise oil. It should not be stored or dispensed in such bottles (Martindale, 2004).

Basil Oil

CAS numbers

Linalool type: USA: 8015-73-4; EINECS: 84775-71-3

Methyl chavicol type: USA: 8015-73-4; EINECS: 84775-71-3

Species/Botanical name

Ocimum basilicum L. (Labiatae)

Synonyms

Sweet basil oil, French basil (linalool type); exotic, Reunion type (camphor-methyl chavicol (estragole) type or linalool type); methyl cinnamate type. Many more chemotypes are found.

Safety

CHIP details
Xn; R22 (A26)

RIFM recommended safety of use limits
4% (A23)

EU sensitiser total
Sweet basil: 78 (based on eugenol, geraniol, limonene and linalool); methyl chavicol type: 2.4 (based on eugenol, limonene and linalool) (A27)

GRAS status
Granted for sweet basil (Fenaroli, 1997).

Extraction, source, appearance and odour

Extraction
Essential oils are obtained by steam distillation of the flowering plant (Arctander, 1960).

Source
Essential oils are obtained mainly from Hungary, Holland, Belgium, Germany, France, India; also Egypt, Italy, USA, Comoro Islands, Seychelles and Madagascar.

Appearance and odour
Sweet basil oil is a pale yellow to amber essential oil with a sweet, greenish, faint balsamic odour (Arctander, 1960).

Exotic is a yellow or greenish-yellow to pale green essential oil; sweet, anisic top-note, then harsh camphoraceous/spicy note with the chavicol note very prominent (Arctander, 1960).

The methyl cinnamate type, produced in East and West Africa, India and the West Indies is yellow with a sweeter odour than exotic and a more fruity odour compared with the sweet basil (Arctander, 1960).

Aromatherapy uses

Uses include: tonic for nerves, focusing concentration, calming hysteria and lightening depression; headaches and migraines; sinus congestion, asthma, bronchitis, emphysema, influenza, restoring sense of smell due to catarrh; digestive disorders, vomiting, gastric spasm, nausea, and dyspepsia; scanty periods, engorgement of breasts and expulsion of afterbirth; useful with deep massage to ease muscular pain and spasm, to stimulate blood flow; tonic to congested skin; may control acne (Ryman, 1991; Lawless, 1992; Rose, 1992a; Price, 1993; Sheppard-Hanger, 1995).

Scientific comment

The 1,8-cineole content of sweet basil essential oil could perhaps be useful for clearing sinuses and ameliorating catarrh, as in the case of *Eucalyptus globulus* essential oil, which is also supported by its good antimicrobial activity *in vitro*. The high linalool content provides a relaxing odour which has also been shown to relax smooth muscles *in vitro* and could at high concentrations be also beneficial *in vivo*. Massage itself can alleviate various stress-related and muscular conditions (see Chapter 3). There is no evidence for the usefulness of basil essential oil in childbirth and other female problems nor for digestive disorders or skin complaints. Basil has, however been found to be a stimulant in human brain studies (A14) and the odour could be useful as such when used as a fragrance. This would be in contradiction to the soothing action of massage, however, if used together.

Herbal uses

No traditional basil essential oil uses have been documented; most of the data is for whole herbal extracts. The herb is aromatic, carminative, vermifuge, antibacterial and analgesic. Uses include: diseases of kidney and as a confirmed anti-acne and vermicidal agent (Wren, 1988; Blumenthal *et al.*, 2000; Barnes *et al.*, 2002).

Food and perfumery uses

Food   Basil (FEMA 2119) is used in baked goods, meat, vegetables, sweets, soups, beverages, chewing gum (Fenaroli, 1997) and also used in dental and oral products.

Perfumery   They are all used in some perfumes (Arctander, 1960).

Chemistry

Major components

	% (Lawrence, 1976–2001)		
	Sweet	*Exotic*	*Met-cinnamate*
1,8-Cineole	3–27	3–7	0.5–6
Methyl chavicol	0–32	68–87	1–2
Methyl eugenol	0–7	0.5–2.5	0
Eugenol	0–7	trace	0
Z-Methyl cinnamate	0	0	1–5
E-Methyl cinnamate	0	0	40–52
Linalool	44–69	0.3–2.2	20–42
β-Caryophyllene	0.5–14.5	0	0

The European basil oils, considered to be the highest quality, contain methyl chavicol, D-linalool and to a lesser extent 1,8-cineole, plus many other compounds (Simon *et al.*, 1984; Guenther, 1985). Egyptian basil oil is similar to the European, except that the concentration of D-linalool is lower and methyl chavicol is higher. Reunion or Comoro essential oil contains little D-linalool, but has a very high concentration of methyl chavicol (Lawrence *et al.*, 1976–2001; Simon *et al.*, 1984). Bulgarian basil oil is rich in methyl cinnamate and Java basil oil is rich in eugenol (Heath, 1981). From an evaluation of the entire USDA collection plus other commercial and wild sources, a wide range of chemical variation within *O. basilicum* and other species (*O. canum*, *O. sanctum*, *O. gratissimum* and

O. kilimandscharicum) was observed (Simon, 1999).

Adulteration

Many different types of basil oil are available and many are 'doctored' with synthetic components. The exotic basil has synthetic linalool added (about 60%), and is then sold as French basil. The flavour properties of the sweet basil oil are lowered by the adulteration. The methyl cinnamate type is often produced by the addition of the synthetic component to any of the other basil essential oils (A8; see also Chapter 4).

Toxicity

Acute toxicity (A22)

Oral LD_{50}   Sweet basil oil 1.4–<3.5 g/kg body weight (rat).

Dermal LD_{50}   >1.5 g/kg (rabbit).

Irritation and sensitisation

No irritation or sensitisation at 4% (human). Note: methyl chavicol is a sensitiser, therefore the more exotic basil oils may cause sensitisation in some people. The other chemotypes have not been tested (A22).

Phototoxicity

None reported.

Other toxicities

Methyl chavicol (=estragole) occurs as a major component (95%) in Mexican avocado leaf oil, basil and tarragon oils and fennel oils. It has also been shown to produce hepatocellular carcinomas in mice (Drinkwater *et al.*, 1976), but investigations of genotoxicity of two basil oils and one tarragon oil (Tateo, 1989), whilst showing tarragon to be genotoxic, did not the show basil oils to be genotoxic at all. Highly purified methyl chavicol was found to be free from mutagenic effects to *Salmonella* T100, whereas 96% was positive to *Salmonella* TA100 TA 1535, TA98 and TA1537 in the Ames test (Sekizawa and Shibamoto, 1982).

Bioactivities

Pharmacological activities *in vitro* and *in vivo*

Smooth muscle   There was an initial spasmogenic action followed by a spasmolytic action on electrically stimulated smooth muscle of the guinea-pig *in vitro* (sweet basil) (A2; Lis-Balchin *et al.*, 1996a). An unknown basil caused a spasmolytic action in smooth muscle (Brandt, 1988) and tracheal muscle of guinea-pig (Reiter and Brandt, 1985).

Uterus Sweet basil oil and some of its components caused a decrease in the spontaneous contractions of rat uterus (A3; A4; Lis-Balchin, Hart, 1997b).

Other activities Basil is a stimulating oil according to contingent negative variation data (A14). Experimental studies on albino rats reported that a leaf extract of *Ocimum sanctum* and *Ocimum album* (holy basil) had a hypoglycaemic effect (Agrawal *et al.*, 1996).

Antimicrobial activities

Antibacterial activity
Relative data: Basil: 15/25 different bacteria; methyl chavicol type 15/25; basil: 20/20 *Listeria monocytogenes* varieties (A1).

Basil oil limited the growth of 5/5 *Listeria* varieties (Aureli *et al.*, 1992). Sweet basil oil vapour had an effect on 1/5 bacteria (Maruzelli and Sicurela, 1960). *Listeria monocytogenes* and *Salmonella enteritidis* inhibition was shown by a synergistic mixture of essential oils of anise, fennel and/or basil with methyl paraben (Fyfe *et al.*, 1997). Sweet basil was mainly poorly active against 20/25 different bacteria (Baratta *et al.*, 1998b).

Antifungal activity
Relative data (% inhibition): Methyl chavicol-rich basil showed good activity: *Aspergillus niger* 94%, *A. ochraceus* 76%, *Fusarium culmorum* 71% (A1). Sweet basil was moderately to very active against 5/5 fungi (Maruzella, 1960). The effect of basil oils, both sweet linalool type and methyl chavicol type were studied against a wide range of bacteria, yeasts and moulds *in vitro* and were found to have poor activity except against *Mucor piriformis* and *Penicillium candidum* (Wan *et al.*, 1998). Sweet basil was very active against *Aspergillus niger* (Baratta *et al.*, 1998b). Basil essential oil was active against *Aspergillus flavus*, *A. parasiticus*, *A. ochraceus* and *Fusarium moniliforme* at a very high concentration (3000 ppm) (Soliman and Badeaa, 2002). Sweet basil had very poor antioxidant activity (Baratta *et al.*, 1998b).

Clinical trials

Lowering of plasma levels of dienic conjugates and ketones, and activation of catalase in red cells characteristic of antioxidant effect were observed in exposure of 150 bronchitis patients to essential oils of rosemary, basil, fir and eucalyptus (Siurin, 1997). Fasting blood glucose fell by 21.0 mg/dL, postprandial blood glucose fell by 15.8 mg/dL, and cholesterol levels had mild reduction in a placebo-controlled crossover human trial. Urine glucose levels showed a similar trend (Agrawal *et al.*, 1996).

Use in pregnancy and lactation: contraindications

There is a loss of spontaneous contractions in the uterus when the essential oil of sweet basil is applied to the rat uterus *in vitro* and therefore caution is advised during any time of pregnancy and parturition. The possible carcinogenic action of methyl chavicol suggests that it should also be avoided during lactation.

Pharmaceutical guidance

There is scant pharmacological information available for basil oils. The high concentration of methyl chavicol in the sweet and exotic basil oils and unknown effects of these and other basil oils suggests caution in their usage. It has been suggested that the essential oil should be avoided in cases of cancer (Tisserand and Balacs, 1995) also in hepatic disease. There are not enough data to predict the carcinogenic effects of methyl chavicol in basil oil reliably, therefore basil essential oils are not recommended for aromatherapy use in massage, especially on babies and children, but can be useful as a fragrance in small doses as the odour has been found to have stimulant effects on the human brain (A14).

Use in babies and young children

Due to the immaturity and the delicate nature of the skin of babies and young children, it is inadvisable for any essential oils to be used in massage, however much the essential oil has been diluted in the carrier oils. This is also a necessary precaution due to the possibilities of sensitisation of the children at this young age through skin or air-borne odorant effects (see Chapters 5 and 7).

Instillation or administration of essential oils near the baby or young child's nose is not only not recommended, but distinctly inadvisable, as there have been numerous cases reported of severe toxicity and even death from such applications (see Chapter 7).

Bay Oils: Laurel and Pimenta

CAS numbers

Laurel leaf: USA: 8002-41-3 (8007-48-5); EINECS: 84603-73-6 (283-272-5)
Pimenta: USA: 8006-78-8; EINECS: 85085-61-6

Species/Botanical name

Laurus nobilis (Lauraceae)

Synonyms

Laurel leaf oil, sweet bay, true bay, Roman laurel, noble laurel

Other species

Pimenta racemosa (Miller) J.W. Moore (Myrtaceae), bay rum, bayberry, wild cinnamon; myrcia oil, oleum myrciae, *P. officinalis*, *P. acris* Kostel; West Indian bay

Safety
CHIP details
Laurel: Xn; R10, 22, 65; 30%; S62 (A26)
Pimenta: Xn; R10, 65; 30%; S62 (A26)

RIFM recommended safety of use limits
2% (both)

EU sensitiser total
Pimenta: 55 (based on eugenol, 50%, limonene, 3% and linalool, 2%)
Laurel: 14.8 (based on eugenol, 1.5%, geraniol, 0.3%, limonene, 2% and linalool, 11%) (A27)

GRAS status
Granted (Fenaroli, 1997).

Extraction, source, appearance and odour
Extraction
Bay leaf oil is the essential oil obtained by steam distillation of laurel/*Pimenta racemosa* leaves and branchlets (Arctander, 1960).

Source
Laurel leaf comes from Morocco, Italy, Yugoslavia, Turkey and China. Pimenta comes from Spain, Morocco, USA and the West Indies.

Appearance and odour
Pimenta (West Indian bay) is a yellow to dark brown essential oil, tending to darken with time and has a spicy, medicinal, clove-like odour and a sweet balsamic undertone, which may be obnoxious to some people, but is fresh and pleasant to others. A terpeneless bay leaf oil (pimenta) is also produced and this removes most of the terpenes and some oxygenated components (called topping-off); this leaves the sesquiterpenes (Arctander, 1960). It is an intensely sweet deep and mellow scented essential oil of a spicy balsamic type with a lemony top-note.

Laurel leaf oil is pale yellow to very pale olive green and even colourless, with a fresh, strong but sweet, aromatic-camphoraceous, somewhat spicy-medicinal odour. The dry-out notes are sweet, pleasant and slightly spicy, unlike the essential oils of *Eucalyptus globulus*, cajuput and myrtle (Arctander, 1960).

Aromatherapy uses

Laurel is apparently known for its strong effects on the nervous system and is mildly narcotic. Uses include: neuritis, depression, anxiety, fear, psychosis, bringing awareness, courage, confidence; sinus infection, headaches, pneumonia, bronchitis, asthma; muscular aches, pains, sprains, arthritis, rheumatism, arthrosis, sclerosis, atherosclerosis, angina, hypertension; colds, flu, tonsillitis, dental infection, diarrhoea; tonic to the kidneys and reproductive system; scars, acne, pimples, boils, scabies; a tonic to the hair and scalp stimulating hair growth and aiding dandruff (Ryman, 1991; Lawless, 1992; Rose, 1992a,b; Price, 1993; Sheppard-Hanger, 1995).

Bay laurel is used for infections of the respiratory system (Schnaubelt, 1999). It is a bactericide and fungicide, particularly for chronic pathologies (Mailhebiau, 1995) and an expectorant with mucolytic properties. In cases of chronic bronchitis and emphysema, blending bay laurel with other pulmonary regenerators such as *Eucalyptus globulus* for its expectorant and mucolytic properties is recommended. It is also used as an antidepressant for people who are unable to verbalise and give concrete expression to their abilities. It may be of note that both Schnaubelt (1999) and Mailhebiau (1995) use the essential oil orally or in high concentrations locally.

The oil is apparently ideal for writers, poets, painters, musicians and creative artists of all types, especially those who depend on intuition and inspiration for their work (Lawless, 1994) and encourages the gift of prophecy and creativity (Worwood, 1998).

Scientific comment

Although the essential oils are very strong antimicrobial agents, their use in massage at the usual low concentrations for aromatherapy may not bring about the desired effects on various infections internally, although some benefit for respiratory conditions can be envisaged if they are inhaled from bowls of hot water. The effect on any other of the medical, physiological and psychological conditions have not been proven and the aromatherapy uses are based solely on internal usage (orally) or external local uses at high concentration.

Herbal uses

The 'ancients' apparently valued bay leaves and laurel berries, using them as astringents, stimulants and stomachics: the root-bark was used as a remedy in dropsies and disorders of the urinary tract; the leaves and fruit were applied locally to insect bites and stings, scalp eruptions, and in leucorrhoea when accompanied by lax vaginal walls (Felter and Lloyd, 1898). It is said to be a coronary dilator, blood thinner, cholagogue, diaphoretic, digestive, diuretic, emmenagogue, expectorant, febrifuge, fungicide, hepatic, hypotensive, immunostimulant, insecticide, mucolytic, parturient, sedative, sudorific, tonic (neurotonic – regulates sympathetic nervous system and parasympathetic nervous system), but no references are provided (Sheppard-Hanger, 1995).

Food and perfumery uses

Food   Pimenta (West Indian bay) (FEMA 2122) is used in baked goods, frozen diary, meat and vegetables, candies and beverages. Laurel leaf oil (FEMA 2613) has a similar function (Fenaroli, 1997).

Perfumery   Pimenta is used in lower grade cosmetic preparations and perfumes, especially men's perfumery and cosmetic products (Arctander, 1960).

Chemistry

Major components

	% (Lawrence, 1976–2001)	
	Pimenta	*Laurel*
α-Pinene	1–5.4	7
β-Pinene	1–4.4	4
1,8-Cineole	25.5–43	40
Linalool	4–23*	10–12
α-Terpinyl acetate	9.5–18	9
Methyl eugenol	4.7–9	1–5
Eugenol	1.4–55	1–5
Limonene	trace–2*	trace–3
Costunolide		tr

*Sensitisers.

Adulteration

Pimenta oil is commonly adulterated with clove leaf oil, bois de rose terpenes, lime oil terpenes, synthetic myrcene and other terpenes and therefore has variable qualities. Terpenes from the production of terpeneless bay leaf oil are also used (A8; see also Chapter 4). Laurel leaf oil is often adulterated with *Eucalyptus globulus*, cajuput and the synthetic monoterpenoids (A8; see also Chapter 4).

Toxicity

Acute toxicity (A22)

Oral LD$_{50}$ Pimenta >3.6 g/kg (rat); laurel >3.5/4 g/kg (rat).

Dermal LD$_{50}$ Pimenta >2.8 g/kg (rabbit); laurel >4–5 g/kg (rabbit).

Irritation and sensitisation

No irritation or sensitisation reported for laurel at 2–10% in healthy volunteers; however, contact allergy has been experienced by many people in European countries, causing hyperaemia and severe inflammation, caused by an unsaturated ketone, therefore one should reduce the concentration to less than 0.1% in sensitive people.

Phototoxicity

None reported.

Bioactivities

Pharmacological activities *in vitro* and *in vivo*

Smooth muscle Bay essential oil had an initial spasmogenic effect followed by a strong spasmolytic effect on guinea-pig ileum *in vitro* (A2; Lis-Balchin *et al.*, 1996a).

Uterus There was a decrease in the spontaneous contractions in the rat uterus for laurel oil and some of the other components (A3; A4; Lis-Balchin and Hart, 1997b).

Other activities Bay leaves were distilled with rum and used as hair tonic and for muscular pains and colds. A study of the inhibitory mechanism of costunolide, a sesquiterpene lactone isolated from *Laurus nobilis*, on blood ethanol elevation in rats showed its involvement in the inhibition of gastric emptying and increase in gastric juice secretion (Matsuda *et al.*, 2000). Evaluation of the gastroprotective effect of *Laurus nobilis* seeds on ethanol-induced gastric ulcer in rats showed good results for the essential oil fraction as well as the water-soluble one (Afifi *et al.*, 1997).

Antimicrobial activities

Antibacterial activity

Relative data: Bay essential oil had very strong activity against 25/25 different bacterial species and 20/20 *Listeria monocytogenes* varieties (A1; Lis-Balchin *et al.*, 1998a, Lis-Balchin and Deans, 1997). Similar results for bay essential oil were obtained with the same bacterial species as above (Deans and Ritchie, 1987). Bay inhibited all organisms studied at concentrations below 2% v/v (Hammer *et al.*, 1999a; Smith-Palmer *et al.*, 2004) and was also very active against four bacteria (Friedman *et al.*, 2002).

Oils of bay (as well as cinnamon, clove and thyme) were the most antimicrobial against *Campylobacter*, *Salmonella*, *E. coli*, *Staphylococcus aureus* and *Listeria* (Smith-Palmer *et al.*, 1998). Laurel leaf inhibited 5/5 strains of bacteria (Raharivelomanana *et al.*, 1989).

Antifungal activity

Relative data (% inhibition): *Aspergillus niger* 95%, *A. ochraceus* 80%, *Fusarium culmorum* 69% (A1).

Use in pregnancy and lactation: contraindications

Due to the lack of scientific information as to their biological effects during pregnancy and lactation and the possibility of a spasmolytic action on the uterus as shown in animal studies *in vitro*, together with a possible sensitisation effect, pimenta and laurel oils are not recommended during pregnancy, parturition and lactation.

Pharmaceutical guidance

Both pimenta and laurel bay oils contain eugenol, which is a known sensitiser (higher in pimenta which also has methyl eugenol), so there is a risk of a sensitisation reaction, especially in sensitive people. Other than that there is little documentary evidence of their biological activities except for *in vitro* animal studies; they show relatively non-toxic effects based on their LD_{50} and they are very potent antimicrobial agents. However, care should be taken in their usage. The essential oils should be avoided in hepatic disease, renal disease, cancer and should not be used on damaged skin (Tisserand and Balacs, 1995).

Use in babies and young children

Due to the immaturity and the delicate nature of the skin of babies and young children, it is inadvisable for any essential oils to be used in massage, however much the essential oil has been diluted in the carrier oils. This is also a necessary precaution due to the possibilities of sensitisation of the children at this young age through skin or air-borne odorant effects (see Chapters 5 and 7).

Instillation or administration of essential oils near the baby or young child's nose is not only not recommended, but distinctly inadvisable, as there have been numerous cases reported of severe toxicity and even death from such applications (see Chapter 7).

Benzoin Tinctures and Resinoids

CAS numbers

USA: 9000-05-9; EINECS: 9000-72-0

Species/Botanical names

Sumatran: *Styrax benzoin* Dryand (Styracaceae),
S. paralleloneurus Perkins
Siam: *Styrax tonkinensis* Pierre, *S. mycrothyrsus* P.

Synonyms

Sumatra benzoin: Benzoin, benzoim, gum benzoin,
gum benjamin, benzoë
Siam benzoin: Benjoin du Laos, benzoe tonkinensis

Pharmacopoeias

Sumatra benzoin: In British and Japanese Pharma-
copoeias. Note: US Pharmacopoeia allows both
Siam benzoin and Sumatra benzoin under the title
benzoin.
Siam benzoin: In Chinese, French, Italian and Swiss
Pharmacopoeias.

Safety

CHIP details
None

EU sensitiser total
1 (based on benzyl benzoate and benzyl cinnamate) (A27)

GRAS status
Granted (Fenaroli, 1997).

Extraction, source, appearance and odour

Extraction
Benzoin tinctures are produced by extraction of
the tears or lumps (produced as a result of incisions
in the trees) of 20 parts by weight of Siam benzoin
with 90–96% ethanol. There is usually a good yield
of 95% plus even for the benzoin resinoids produced from either source, using benzene and then
distilling off the solvent or cold-alcohol extraction
instead of or after to give the absolute. Sumatran
benzoin can vary from whitish lumps to large, black
masses weighing over 0.5 kg (Arctander, 1960).

Source
Siam, Sumatra, Java and Borneo.

Appearance and odour
Benzoin tincture is amber-coloured, with a sweet
balsamic vanilla-like odour. It is used as a fixative
in fine perfumery, colognes, etc. Benzoin resinoids
are amber-coloured resinoids with a balsamic fragrance and are used in perfumed products of lower
grade and Friar's balsam (Arctander, 1960; Evans,
1996).

Aromatherapy uses

Uses of benzoin oil include: bronchitis, coughs,
colds, wounds, acne, eczema, psoriasis, rheumatism, arthritis, scar tissue, circulation, nervous tension, stress, muscle pains, chilblains, rashes and
mouth ulcers. It has a calming effect on the nervous
and digestive systems, a warming effect on circulation problems and a toning effect on the respiratory
tract. In vapour therapy, benzoin oil is used for:
nervous system, calming and bringing comfort to
the depressed and emotionally exhausted. Benzoin
oil can be diluted in the bath to assist with general
aches and pains; arthritis, rheumatism, chronic
bronchitis, coughing, poor circulation can also
benefit as well as stiff muscles (Lawless, 1992;
Sheppard-Hanger, 1995).

Scientific comment
Massaging with benzoin is not advisable due to
the strong sensitisation potential. The use of massage alone can alleviate many stress and muscular
symptoms and the fragrance of benzoin could add
to the therapy.

Herbal uses

The effects of benzoin are much the same as those
of benzoic acid, its most abundant constituent,
modified by the resin and essential oil (Nair, 2001b).

Benzoin exerts a stimulating influence on the mucous tissues, and has been used to promote expectoration in chronic diseases of the air passages. It is also stated to stimulate the sexual organs. It is a constituent of many balsams that exert a salutary influence in healing wounds; the fumes or vapour inhaled into the lungs have been strongly recommended in chronic pulmonary catarrhs and old laryngeal inflammations. The tincture is protective as a dressing for fresh wounds (Felter and Lloyd, 1898).

Food and perfumery uses

Food   Benzoin (FEMA 2132) and benzoin resin (FEMA 2133) are used in a wide variety of foods, and alcoholic and non-alcoholic beverages (Fenaroli, 1997). Siam benzoin has also been used as a preservative and was formerly used in the preparation of benzoinated lard (Martindale, 2004).

Perfumery   The Siam benzoin resinoid, absolute, etc. are used in high-quality perfumes, while the harsher Sumatran benzoin is used for cheaper products; they are not interchangeable (Arctander, 1960).

Chemistry

Major components

Sumatran benzoin contains esters of benzoic and cinnamic acids as well as the acids (20% on average) (Lawrence, 1976–2001; Evans, 1996); free cinnamic acid is usually twice as concentrated as the benzoic acid, totalling 20% (Evans, 1996). Vanillin is also present. Siamese benzoin contains less cinnamic acid and does not give off fumes of benzaldehyde when warmed. The major constituent is said to be the ester coniferyl benzoate (up to 75%) (Evans, 1996).

	% (Lawrence, 2004)	
	Siam	Sumatran
Benzyl benzoate	80	76
Benzylaldehyde	0.4	0.9
Methyl benzoate	1.5	0.5
Benzoic acid	12.5	1.7
Ethyl benzoate	1.1	0.2
Allyl benzoate	1.5	0.9
Cinnamic acid	0	3.5
Allyl cinnamate	0	0.5
Isobutyl cinnamate	0	0.1
Cinnamyl benzoate	0	1.4
Cinnamyl cinnamate	0	0.9

Adulteration

Siam benzoin is the most sought after and is more expensive, therefore is often adulterated with the Sumatran benzoins. Many solvents are used in diluting the product and this makes it runnier and easier to dispense (A8; see also Chapter 4).

Toxicity

Acute toxicity

Oral LD_{50} >10 g/kg (rat) (Margolin, 1970).

Dermal LD_{50} >8.87 (3.98–19.75) g/kg (rabbit) (Margolin, 1970).

Irritation and sensitisation

No irritation reported at 8% (human) (Kligman, 1966a). Eczema has occurred (cross-sensitisation to balsam of Peru) (Spott and Shelley, 1970). Compound tincture, containing tolu, Peru and styrax balsams caused sensitisation in some people (A22).

There have been fewer than 30 reported cases of contact allergy from compound tincture of benzoin, and none in the last decade. However, the results of patch testing to a compound tincture of benzoin in 477 patients performed at the Contact Dermatitis Clinic at the Skin and Cancer Foundation in Melbourne, Australia during 1999 showed 45 out of the 477 patients had a positive reaction. This was the third most common allergen in the series. Twenty-eight of these patients had cross-reactions to similar allergens (fragrance mix, balsam of Peru, colophony and tea tree oil). Of the 14 patients with a strong positive reaction to compound tincture of benzoin, 11 had at least one other positive cross-reaction to the above allergens. This may explain the high frequency of reaction to compound tincture of benzoin found in this study (Scardamaglia *et al.*, 2003).

Benzoic acid is used in a wide variety of cosmetics as a pH adjuster and preservative. Benzyl alcohol is metabolised to benzoic acid, which reacts with glycine and is excreted as hippuric acid in the human body. Acceptable daily intakes have been established by the World Health Organization at 5 mg/kg for benzyl alcohol, benzoic acid and sodium benzoate. Benzoic acid and sodium benzoate are generally recognised as safe in foods according to the US Food and Drug Administration. No adverse effects of benzyl alcohol were seen in chronic exposure animal studies using rats and mice. Effects of benzoic acid and sodium benzoate in chronic exposure animal studies were limited to reduced feed intake and reduced growth.

Some differences between control and benzyl alcohol-treated populations were noted in one reproductive toxicity study using mice, but these were limited to lower maternal body weights and decreased mean litter weights. Another study also noted that fetal weight was decreased compared with controls, but a third study showed no differences between control and benzyl alcohol-treated groups. Benzoic acid was associated with an increased number of resorptions and malformations in hamsters, but there were no reproductive or developmental toxicity findings in studies using mice and rats exposed to sodium benzoate, and, likewise, benzoic acid was negative in two rat studies. Genotoxicity tests for these ingredients were mostly negative, but there were some assays that were positive. Carcinogenicity studies, however, were negative.

Clinical data indicated that these ingredients can produce non-immunologic contact urticaria and non-immunologic immediate contact reactions, characterised by the appearance of wheals, erythema and pruritus. In one study, 5% benzyl alcohol elicited a reaction, and in another study, 2% benzoic acid did likewise. Benzyl alcohol, however, was not a sensitiser at 10%, nor was benzoic acid a sensitiser at 2%. Recognising that the non-immunologic reactions are strictly cutaneous, likely involving a cholinergic mechanism, it was concluded that these ingredients could be used safely at concentrations up to 5%, but that manufacturers should consider the non-immunologic phenomena when using these ingredients in cosmetic formulations designed for infants and children. Additionally, benzyl alcohol was considered safe up to 10% for use in hair dyes. The limited body exposure, the duration of use and the frequency of use were considered in concluding that the non-immunologic reactions would not be a concern.

Because of the wide variety of product types in which these ingredients may be used, it is likely that inhalation may be a route of exposure. The available safety tests are not considered sufficient to support the safety of these ingredients in formulations where inhalation is a route of exposure. Inhalation toxicity data are needed to complete the safety assessment of these ingredients where inhalation can occur (Nair, 2001b).

Bioactivities

Pharmacological activities *in vitro* and *in vivo*

Smooth muscle No data found.

Antimicrobial activities

Antibacterial activity

There was low antibacterial activity against 5/5 different bacteria (Friedman *et al.*, 2002).

Antifungal activity

No data found.

Use in pregnancy and lactation: contraindications

Due to the numerous cases of contact allergy and the danger of cross-reaction to similar allergens, benzoin is not recommended for aromatherapy massage. Its use as a fragrance poses little threat.

Pharmaceutical guidance

Benzoin has been used for a number of years in food, perfumery and medicines and has a negligible sensitisation potential. However, there are increasing numbers of dermal contact allergic responses and cross-sensitisations to similar fragrance materials. Benzoin resinoid and oil are well-documented sensitisers and the RIFM recommend that only grades processed to remove the allergens should be used in consumer products. These grades are not generally available via aromatherapy suppliers. In addition, there is no such thing as benzoin oil – it is always a resin dissolved in a solvent, which is often synthetic. The use of benzoin on the skin is therefore not recommended, although its use as a fragrance and food additive is not banned or restricted.

Use in babies and young children

Due to the immaturity and the delicate nature of the skin of babies and young children, it is inadvisable for any essential oils to be used in massage, however much the essential oil has been diluted in the carrier oils. This is also a necessary precaution due to the possibilities of sensitisation of the children at this young age through skin or air-borne odorant effects (see Chapters 5 and 7).

Instillation or administration of essential oils near the baby or young child's nose is not only not recommended, but distinctly inadvisable, as there have been numerous cases reported of severe toxicity and even death from such applications (see Chapter 7).

Bergamot Oil

CAS numbers

USA: 8007-75-8; EINECS: 89957-91-5 (expressed oil)

Species/Botanical name

Citrus bergamia Risso

Synonyms

Citrus aurantium L. subsp. *bergamia* Wright & Arn., bergamot essence, oleum bergamottae

Pharmacopoeias

In French and Italian Pharmacopoeias:
   Note: Confusion with Bergamot herb frequent: Bergamot Leaf, Wild, C/S (*Monarda didyma*); Oswego tea; bee balm

Safety

CHIP details
Xn; R10, 65; 95%; S62 (A26)

RIFM recommended safety of use limits
0.4% phototoxic (expressed) 20% rectified (A23)

EU sensitiser total
57.5 (based on limonene and linalool mainly) (A27)

GRAS status
Granted (Fenaroli, 1997).

Extraction, source, appearance and odour

Extraction
Expressed oil is obtained from the orangey rind of the fruit of the bitter orange tree. Rectification by steam distillation is frequently used to remove toxic furocoumarins and to give FCF (furanocoumarin-free) oil (Arctander, 1960). This is not a true essential oil.

Source
Italy, France, Germany and South America.

Appearance and odour
Colourless to yellow, greenish, even brownish, depending whether or not FCF. FCF fades to a light yellow with age; expressed bergamot darkens. It has a sweet to bitter, sweet-fruity, citrusy odour followed by a characteristic oily-herbaceous, balsamic dry-out (Arctander, 1960).
   Bergamot oil (terpeneless) is a colourless essential oil with a sweeter but similar odour.

Aromatherapy uses

Uses include: anxiety, depression; headaches; sinus congestion, asthma, bronchitis, emphysema and influenza; digestive disorders, nausea, flatulence, dyspepsia; acne, boils, cold sores, eczema, psoriasis, wounds; insect repellent; halitosis and sore throat (Ryman, 1991; Lawless, 1992; Rose, 1992a; Price, 1993; Sheppard-Hanger, 1995).

Scientific comment
The use of the FCF essential oil (without the phototoxic furanocoumarins) is almost obligatory if the patient is to go out in the open or on a sunbed following massage. There is also the problem of potential sensitisation, which is not relieved by using the FCF essential oil; it is therefore inadvisable to massage the essential oil onto the skin. However, bergamot essential oil used as a fragrance has potentially beneficial relaxant effects, as found in brain experiments in humans (A14).

Herbal use

No traditional uses have been documented in most parts of the world bar Italy, where it is used for fever (especially in malaria) and also worms. It has become used more recently for respiratory and renal infections (Lawless, 1992).

Food and perfumery uses

Food   Bergamot oil (FEMA 2153) is used in various baked goods, frozen diary, meats, candies, beverages, chewing gum and Earl Grey tea (Fenaroli, 1997). The coumarin in bergamot is permitted in most goods at 2 mg/kg, but chewing gum can contain 50 mg/kg, alcoholic drinks 10 mg/kg and caramel confectionary 10 mg/kg.

Perfumery Bergamot oil (terpeneless) is produced mainly for perfumery especially florals (Arctander, 1960).

Chemistry

Major components

	% (Lawrence, 1976–2001)	EU sensitisers
Linalyl acetate	23–35	
Limonene	19–38	42
Linalool	4–29	15
γ-Terpinene	4–13	
β-Pinene	3–13	
Citral	trace–1	0.5
	Total =	57.5

Minor components

Furocoumarins make up approximately 0.44% of the expressed oil and this accounts for the phototoxicity. Removal of these furanocoumarins makes the oil non-phototoxic. Trace components which contribute to the odour include: (−)-guaienol, (+)-spathulenol, nerolidol, farnesol and b-sinensal (Ohloff, 1994).

Adulteration

The oily-herbaceous dry-out is characteristic of a good bergamot oil and a lack of this suggests adulteration. Synthetic, cheap linalool, limonene and linalyl acetate are used, as well as bitter orange, lime, lemon oil; synthetic or natural citral and terpinyl acetate is also added and diethylphthalate is used as diluent.

Toxicity

Acute toxicity (A22)

Oral LD_{50} Bergamot expressed >10 g/kg body weight (rat).

Dermal LD_{50} >20 g/kg body weight root oil (rabbit).

Irritation and sensitisation

No irritation reported at 30% (human), but 3/20 dermatitis patients were affected (Rudzki *et al.*, 1976). Note: contains potential sensitisers.

Phototoxicity

Exposure to sunlight or UV light as on sunbeds following skin application of the expressed oil causes pigmentation of the skin known as berloque dermatitis, and can even cause burns. The degree of phototoxicity is directly correlated to the furanocoumarin content (see also citrus oils). There is a natural progression of severity from bergamot > lime > bitter orange > lemon > grapefruit > sweet orange > tangerine > mandarin > tangelo. When the level of furanocoumarins is reduced below 0.0075%, phototoxicity is avoided (Lawrence, 2004). However, this does not take into account idiosyncratic responses in more sensitive individuals. FCF oils only should be used.

New IFRA regulations state that natural extracts containing furocoumarin-like substances may be used in cosmetic products, provided that the total concentration of furocoumarin-like substances in the finished cosmetic product does not exceed 1 ppm. These extracts include bergamot oil and all citrus expressed oils.

Bioactivities

Pharmacological activities *in vitro* and *in vivo*

Smooth muscle Bergamot oil (commercial) had an initial spasmogenic action followed by a spasmolytic effect on electrically stimulated smooth muscle of the guinea-pig *in vitro* (A2; Lis-Balchin *et al.*, 1996a). Adulteration of the oil cannot be ruled out.

Uterus Bergamot oil (commercial) caused decreased and subsequent cessation of spontaneous contractions of the rat uterus *in vitro*; this effect was also shown by its major components (A3; A4; Lis-Balchin and Hart, 1997b).

Other activities Bergamot oil had a sedative effect as shown by contingent negative variation studies (A14). Linalool has a glutamatergic and anticonvulsant action (Elisabetsky *et al.*, 1999; see lavender for full details). Experiments on the motility of mice showed that certain oils containing linalool, like bergamot, had a sedative effect (A14). Contingent negative variation studies also showed a sedative effect (A14) but this contrasted with the smooth muscle results above, which showed both a stimulant and sedative effect *in vitro*.

Antimicrobial activities

Antibacterial activity

Relative data: 22–23/25 different bacteria and 20/20 *Listeria monocytogenes* varieties affected

(A1; Lis-Balchin and Deans, 1997; Lis-Balchin *et al.*, 1998a). Other studies showed that 11/25 bacteria were affected (Deans and Ritchie, 1987); 1/5 bacteria were affected by the vapour (Maruzella and Sicurella, 1960).

Antifungal activity

Relative data (% inhibition): *Aspergillus niger* 13–70%, *A. ochraceus* 30–31%, *Fusarium culmorum* − 34–89% (A1). Poor antifungal activity was shown against 15 fungal species and the terpeneless oil was even less effective (Maruzella and Liguori, 1958).

Antioxidant action

One of two samples studied showed antioxidant action (Lis-Balchin *et al.*, 1998a). This suggests that an antioxidant had probably been added to the positively affected sample. The use of antioxidants is widespread, as the essential oil has a short lifespan otherwise.

Clinical studies

Two patients with localised and disseminated bullous phototoxic skin reactions developing within 48–72 hours after exposure to bergamot aromatherapy oil and subsequent UV exposure were described. One patient had no history of direct contact with aromatherapy oil but developed bullous skin lesions after exposure to aerosolised aromatherapy oil in a sauna and subsequent UVA radiation in a tanning salon. This report highlights the potential health hazard related to the increasing use of psoralen-containing aromatherapy oils (Kaddu *et al.*, 2001).

Use in pregnancy and lactation: contraindications

FCF bergamot oil should be used on the skin and not the pure extracted oil due to the furanocoumarin-induced burning effect. There is also the potential danger of sensitisation due to the limonene and linalool content. The lack of studies on the effects of the essential oil in pregnancy and parturition and the cessation of contractions shown in animal studies *in vitro*, suggest that caution should be observed. The essential oil should not be used in aromatherapy massage during these times and during lactation. The fragrance could be used sparingly.

Pharmaceutical guidance

There is scant pharmacological information available for bergamot oil, expressed or distilled. Oil of bergamot possesses photosensitive and melanogenic properties because of the presence of furocoumarins, primarily bergapten (5-methoxypsoralen [5-MOP]). Bergamot oil, even if FCF, contains a high percentage of sensitisers (limonene and linalool 57.5%). The distilled essential oil contains an even higher percentage (80.4%). The presence of furanocoumarins and/or sensitisers poses potential dangers from both the sensitization aspect and phototoxicity. However, due to its pleasant odour and relaxation potential in brain studies in humans (A14), the aroma could be beneficial for stress relief when used as a fragrance.

Use in babies and young children

Due to the immaturity and the delicate nature of the skin of babies and young children, it is inadvisable for any essential oils to be used in massage, however much the essential oil has been diluted in the carrier oils. This is also a necessary precaution due to the possibilities of sensitisation of the children at this young age through skin or air-borne odorant effects (see Chapters 5 and 7).

Instillation or administration of essential oils near the baby or young child's nose is not only not recommended, but distinctly inadvisable, as there have been numerous cases reported of severe toxicity and even death from such applications (see Chapter 7).

Buchu Leaf Oil

CAS numbers

USA: 68650-46-4; EINECS: 84649-93-4

Species/Botanical name

Agathosma betulina (Berg.) Pillans (Rutaceae)

Synonyms

Barosma betulina Bart. & Wendl., round buchu, short buchu, mountain buchu, bookoo, buku and bucco

Other species

Agathosma crenulata (L.) Pillans, syn. *Barosma crenulata* (L.) Hook. (oval buchu); *Agathosma serratifolia* (Curt.) Spreeth, syn. *Barosma serratifolia* (Curt.) Willd. (long buchu)

Safety

CHIP details
Xn; R10, 22 (A26)

EU sensitiser total
21.5 (based on limonene and linalool) (A27)

GRAS status
Granted (Fenaroli, 1997).

Extraction, source, appearance and odour

Extraction
A volatile oil is obtained by steam distillation of the leaves. Yield: 1.0–3.5% (Arctander, 1960).

Source
Southern Africa.

Appearance and odour
The oil from *A. betulina* is a yellow to brownish-yellow liquid, which goes viscous on ageing. It has a peculiar strong, bitter-sweet, minty-camphoraceous, penetrating, medicinal smell which most people find distasteful. The oil from *Agathosma crenulata* has a more minty and citrusy odour. Buchu is used in folk medicines in Southern Africa (Nijssen and Maarse, 1986; Simpson, 1998).

Aromatherapy uses

Buchu is not to be used in aromatherapy (Lawless, 1992) and is ignored in most aromatherapy books, but the essential oil appears in many aromatherapy oil lists on the Internet.

Scientific comment
Although used extensively in herbal medicine for centuries, the presence of pulegone (*A. crenulata*) and ρ-diosphenol and diosphenol (*A. betulina*) in the essential oils (Posthumus *et al.*, 1996), which have toxicant properties, including irritation and sensitisation, makes the use of buchu essential oils in aromatherapy massage very dangerous. Their use as fragrances, too, is rather doubtful as they have an unpleasant catty odour and no apparent function when used by inhalation.

Herbal uses

The two species of buchu (*Agathosma betulina*, *A. crenulata*) originate from the Cape area of South Africa; the indigenous people introduced the herbs to the European settlers and the plants were taken to Europe and used medicinally, especially as a diuretic (British Pharmacopoeia, 1821, quoted by Grieve, 1937/1992). Buchu species leaves, used as buchu brandy, tincture, vinegar or a tea, were used as antiseptics, for gravel, inflammation, stomach complaints and 'catarrh' of the bladder and are currently used for stimulating perspiration in rheumatism and gout, treating cholera, kidney disease, haematuria, calculus, infections of bladder, urethra, prostate and as a digestive tonic and externally the embrocation or buchu vinegar for local application to treat rheumatism, bruises, contusions, sprains and fractures and cleaning wounds (Grieve, 1937/1992; Watt and Breyer-Brandwijk, 1962; Simpson, 1998). Buchu is considered to be a urinary antiseptic and has diuretic properties and is used for cystitis, urethritis, prostatitis and specifically for acute catarrhal cystitis (BHP, 1960; Wren, 1988; Chevallier, 1996).

Food and perfumery uses

Food Buchu leaf oil (FEMA 2169) is used in foods such as gooseberry, cassis, peach, blueberry and other tart-type fruit products, with tropical fruits and as a replacement for blackcurrant bud flavour in food (Kaiser *et al.*, 1975; Nijssen, Maarse, 1986), which has made it more popular in recent years (Fenaroli, 1997).

Perfumery It is sometimes used in perfumes like chypres and as a 'catty' odour in various perfumes (Arctander, 1960).

Chemistry

Major components

	% (Posthumus et al., 1996)	
	A. crenulata	A. betulina
Limonene	24.1	26.8
Menthone	3.6	10.8
Isomenthone	11.8	26.6
Isopulegone	6.6	0.8
Pulegone	46.7	3.3
cis-Acetylthiol-p-menthan-3-one	4.9	trace
trans-Acetylthiol-p-menthan-3-one	0.4	trace
Diosphenol	0.3	15.4
p-Diosphenol	0.2	12.5
cis-3-Mercapto-p-menthan-3-one	1.2	0.6
trans-3-Mercapto-p-menthan-3-one	1.5	2.8

Adulteration

Dilution with solvents and admixing of different species accounts for most of the adulteration.

Toxicity

Acute toxicity

Oral and dermal LD_{50} values have not been determined for either essential oil.

Other toxicities

The essential oil of *A. crenulata* especially contains a high concentration of pulegone, a known hepatotoxin (De Smet *et al.*, 1993). The oil may cause gastrointestinal and renal irritation and *A. betulina* should be avoided in kidney infections (Mabey, 1988).

Bioactivities

Pharmacological activities *in vitro* and *in vivo*

Smooth muscle *A. betulina* and *A. crenulata* had somewhat different effects on the electrically stimulated guinea-pig ileum *in vitro*: at high concentration, the two oils had an initial spasmogenic activity followed by spasmolysis (Lis-Balchin *et al.*, 2001); at lower concentrations, *A. betulina* had only a spasmolytic action. The spasmolytic action was post-synaptic, not atropine-like and did not involve adrenoceptor or guanylyl cyclase activation. In the presence of the phosphodiesterase inhibitor Rolimpar the spasmolytic action of *A. betulina* was significantly increased whilst that due to *A. crenulata* was also increased but not to a significant level, suggesting a mode of action for the oils involving cyclic adenosine monophosphate. In addition, *A. betulina* appeared to block calcium channels but this was not seen with *A. crenulata*, possibly because the initial spasmogenic activity complicates the study of its spasmolytic action, but more likely because it behaved like the essential oils of lavender and geranium (Lis-Balchin *et al.*, 2001). Diosmin has shown anti-inflammatory activity against carrageenan-induced rat paw oedema (Farnsworth and Cordell, 1976).

No scientific evidence has been found to justify the herbal uses, although reputed diuretic and anti-inflammatory activities are probably attributable to the irritant nature of the essential oil.

Antimicrobial activities

Antibacterial activity

Neither *A. betulina* nor *A. crenulata* essential oil demonstrated antimicrobial action against *Enterococcus hirae* and *Pseudomonas aeruginosa* and very low activity was observed against *Escherichia coli*, *Saccharomyces cerevisiae* and *Staphyloccocus aureus*, suggesting little potential for these oils as antimicrobial agents/preservatives (Lis-Balchin *et al.*, 2001).

Antifungal activity

None found.

Use in pregnancy and lactation: contraindications

The safety of buchu oils has not been established even for their acute toxicity, and the potential toxicity and irritant action of the essential oils together with the pulegone content which has been linked to abortion, contraindicate their usage during pregnancy and lactation.

Pharmaceutical guidance

In view of the lack of documented toxicity data, together with the presence of pulegone (*A. crenulata*) and ρ-diosphenol and diosphenol (*A. betulina*) (Posthumus *et al.*, 1996), which have toxicant properties, including irritation and sensitisation, the use of buchu essential oils should be avoided in aromatherapy massage. Their use as fragrances is rather doubtful as they have catty and unpleasant odours, but on dilution they can prove reasonably odorific to some people, though unlikely to be relaxing.

Use in babies and young children

Due to the immaturity and the delicate nature of the skin of babies and young children, it is inadvisable for any essential oils to be used in massage, however much the essential oil has been diluted in the carrier oils. This is also a necessary precaution due to the possibilities of sensitisation of the children at this young age through skin or air-borne odorant effects (see Chapters 5 and 7).

Instillation or administration of essential oils near the baby or young child's nose is not only not recommended, but distinctly inadvisable, as there have been numerous cases reported of severe toxicity and even death from such applications (see Chapter 7).

Cajuput Oil

CAS numbers

USA: 8008-98-8; EINECS: 84580-37-1

Species/Botanical name

Melaleuca leucadendron L. (Myrtaceae)

Synonyms

M. cajeputi, *M. quinquenervia* (S.T. Blake), white tea-tree, broad-leaved tea-tree, paper-barked tea-tree, swamp tea-tree, punk tree and white-wood. Also known locally as tea-tree. Cajeput oil, cajuput essence, oleum cajuputi

Other species

Eucalyptus globulus, naiouli

Safety

CHIP details

Xn; R, 65; 40%; S62 (A26)

RIFM recommended safety of use limits

4% (A23)

EU sensitiser total

14 (based on limonene and linalool) (A27)

GRAS status

Granted (Fenaroli, 1997).

Extraction, source, appearance and odour

Extraction

This essential oil is steam distilled from the leaves of *Melaleuca leucadendron*, a tree growing in the Moluccas and adjacent islands (Arctander, 1960).

Source

Moluccas, Malaya, Indonesian archipelago and the Philippines.

Appearance and odour

Colourless, pale yellow or green liquid. The green colour is not essential, and may be removed by distillation; it is due chiefly to the presence of copper, and partly to the presence of some altered chlorophyll. The odour of the oil has been stated to resemble the combined fragrance of camphor, rosemary and cardamom; it is fresh, eucalyptic and camphoraceous with fruity-sweet body notes (Arctander, 1960).

Aromatherapy uses

Uses include: Insect bites, oily skin, spots; arthritis, rheumatism, muscular aches and pains; asthma, bronchitis, colds, sinusitis, sore throat; cystitis, urethritis, urinary infection; viral infections, flu, abscess, acne, dermatitis, eczema, toothache, neuralgia, sciatica (Ryman, 1991; Lawless, 1992; Rose, 1992a; Price, 1993; Sheppard-Hanger, 1995).

Scientific comment

Cajuput essential oil has strong antimicrobial and spasmolytic properties on smooth muscle *in vitro*, but it is doubtful whether the dilution used in aromatherapy massage could alleviate all the maladies and muscular conditions listed.

Herbal uses

No traditional essential oil uses have been documented and most of the data are for whole herbal extracts (Wren, 1988; Blumenthal *et al.*, 2000; Barnes *et al.*, 2002) except for Felter and Lloyd (1898): cajuput oil was used as a carminative; powerful diffusive stimulant, diaphoretic and antispasmodic; internally, used in chronic rheumatism, hysteria, colic, spasms or cramps of the stomach or bowels, Asiatic cholera, congestive dysmenorrhoea, hiccough, nervous dysphagia, in the typhoid stage of fevers, nervous vomiting; removing worms; chronic laryngitis, chronic bronchitis, catarrh of the bladder. Externally: application to rheumatic, neuralgic and other pains, i.e. a mild rubefacient; nervous headache. Applied to the cavity of a carious tooth, it apparently alleviates toothache (Felter and Lloyd, 1898).

Food and perfumery uses

Food   Cajuput (FEMA 2225) is used in various baked goods, frozen diary, meats, candies and beverages (Fenaroli, 1997).

Perfumery   Cajuput is not used to any great extent in perfumes (Arctander, 1960).

Chemistry

Major components

	% (Lawrence, 1976–2001)
1,8-Cineole	14–69
α-Pinene	8
β-Pinene	1
Limonene	trace–10
Linalool	3–4
Geraniol	trace–0.4

Adulteration

Because of its high price, oil of cajuput is subject to adulteration. It is very similar to *Eucalyptus globulus*, and the latter is thus often sold as cajuput. Eucalyptus (pharmaceutical oil) is often admixed with small amounts of terpinyl acetate, terpinyl propionate and higher esters of terpineol. Oils of rosemary or turpentine, combined with camphor and bruised cardamom seeds, and appropriately tinted with milfoil resin, have been sold as genuine cajuput oil. Oil of camphor has been used as an adulterant. Oils of lavender, origanum, and rosemary are frequently used for adulteration (A8).

Toxicity

Acute toxicity (A22)

Oral LD$_{50}$ >4 g/kg body weight (rat).

Dermal LD$_{50}$ >5 g/kg (rabbit).

Irritation and sensitisation (A22)

None recorded at 4% in humans; undiluted oil may irritate mucous membranes.

Phototoxicity

None reported.

Other toxicities

Cajuput oil is reported to be oestrogen-like and therefore caution is advised in pregnancy, but no references were supplied to support this statement (Sheppard-Hanger, 1995).

Bioactivity

Pharmacological activities *in vitro* and *in vivo*

Smooth muscle   Cajuput oil had an initial spasmogenic action followed by a weak spasmolytic effect on electrically stimulated guinea-pig ileum *in vitro* (A2; Lis-Balchin *et al.*, 1996a).

Uterus   There was a decrease in the spontaneous contractions in the rat uterus when cajuput oil was applied (A3; A4; Lis-Balchin and Hart, 1997b).

Antimicrobial activities

Antibacterial activity

Relative data: Activity was shown against 21/25 different bacterial species and 19/20 *Listeria monocytogenes* varieties (A1; Lis-Balchin and Deans, 1997; Lis-Balchin *et al.*, 1998a). Cajuput oil had a good antibacterial effect against 3/5 bacteria (Maruzella and Henry, 1958), four bacterial species (Friedman *et al.*, 2002) and the vapour against 1/5 bacteria (Maruzella and Sicurella, 1960).

Antifungal activity

Relative data (% inhibition): Activity was very poor, even showing enhancement of fungal growth (A1): *Aspergillus niger* −12%, *A. ochraceus* −30%, *Fusarium culmorum* −1%. Some activity was reported against five fungi (Maruzella, 1960) and low activity against 15 fungi (Maruzella and Liguori, 1958).

Use in pregnancy and lactation: contraindications

There is insufficient evidence to show that cajuput oil is safe to use and, due to a possible cessation of spontaneous contractions as shown in animal studies *in vitro*, which would pose a possible risk during any phase of pregnancy and parturition, caution is advised. *Eucalyptus globulus*, which has a similar chemical composition, is to be preferred for both massage and use as a fragrance.

Pharmaceutical guidance

Due to the high cineole and terpene content the essential oil should be used with caution and internal usage avoided. A loss of contractions in the uterus when the essential oil was used in the uterus of the rat *in vitro* has been reported, but no other pharmacological data (other than the spasmogenic action on the ileum followed by spasmolysis *in vitro*) and very few antimicrobial studies are available. This essential oil is very similar to *Eucalyptus globulus* essential oil and has no added benefit, especially as it is frequently adulterated or substituted by the former.

Use in babies and young children

Due to the immaturity and the delicate nature of the skin of babies and young children, it is inadvisable for any essential oils to be used in massage, however much the essential oil has been diluted in the carrier oils. This is also a necessary precaution due to the possibilities of sensitisation of the children at this young age through skin or air-borne odorant effects (see Chapters 5 and 7).

Instillation or administration of essential oils near the baby or young child's nose is not only not recommended, but distinctly inadvisable, as there have been numerous cases reported of severe toxicity and even death from such applications (see Chapter 7).

Camphor Oil

CAS numbers

USA: 8008-51-3; EINECS: 92201-50-8

Species/Botanical name

Cinnamomum camphora (L.) Nees & Ebermeier (Lauraceae)

Synonyms

C. camphora Siebs.

Safety

CHIP details
None; R10 (A26)

RIFM recommended safety of use limits
White camphor: 20 (A23)

EU sensitiser total
White camphor: 25.5 (based on limonene and linalool) (A27)

GRAS status
Yellow and white camphor (Fenaroli, 1997).

Extraction, source, appearance and odour

Extraction
A volatile oil is obtained by steam distillation of trees in Japan (hon-sho), Formosa (hon-sho and yu-sho) and China (yu-sho and apopiu oil). The crude oil contains considerable amonts of crystalline camphor, which is removed by filter-pressing and then the essential oil is vacuum-rectified to yield extra camphor and three fractions (Arctander, 1960):

1. White camphor oil – the light fraction or 860–880 oil, containing cineole and monoterpenes; 6% of the crude oil. Serves as a starting point in the synthesis of monoterpenes and oxygenated derivatives.
2a. Brown camphor oil – the medium-heavy oil or 1070 oil, containing up to 80% safrole and some terpineol; 6–7% of the total essential oil. The safrole content is a starting product for the synthesis of heliotropin, vanillin, etc. and terpineol is separated off as a by-product. The safrole is now considered a carcinogen and therefore this fraction is not used.
2b. Yellow camphor oil – the residual essential oil after removing safrole from the brown oil, known also as 960–980 oil; it still has a sassafras odour.
3. Blue camphor oil – the heaviest fraction, which contains sesquiterpenes; this is rarely used.

Source
Japan, Taiwan, China and France.

Appearance and odour
White camphor oil has a cineolic odour (Arctander, 1960).

Aromatherapy uses

Camphor is not greatly acknowledged in the aromatherapy literature but a few sources give several uses including: acne, inflammation, spots, insect prevention, arthritis, muscular aches and pains, rheumatism, sprains, bronchitis, chills, coughs, colds, fever, infectious disease; bruises, cuts, debility, neuralgia and sciatica (Lawless, 1992; Price, 1993).

Scientific comment

It is surprising that camphor is not widely acclaimed by aromatherapists as it is included in the components of so many useful medicinal mentholated products, such as Vicks VapoRub, tiger balm, etc. which are effective respiratory and muscular ointments and liniments.

Herbal uses

Camphor has many uses in cough medicines, muscular ointments and liniments (Wren, 1988; Blumenthal *et al.*, 2000; Barnes *et al.*, 2002). It is well-known as camphorated oil (see Chapter 7, page 84). In the past, camphor was said to protect against infection and a lump of camphor was sometimes worn around the neck; it was also used for respiratory and nervous diseases (Lawless, 1992).

Food and perfumery uses

Food   Yellow and white camphor is used in foods (FEMA 2231) (Fenaroli, 1997).

Perfumery   Camphor is used for perfuming detergents and cheap household products (Arctander, 1960).

Chemistry

Major components

White camphor oil

	% (Lawrence, 1976–2001)
1,8-Cineole	30
α-Pinene	7
Camphor	51
Terpineol	2
Sesquiterpenes	variable
Limonene	trace–25
Linalool	trace–0.5

Adulteration

This is a cheap product so the oil is not generally adulterated, but there is a great variability in the composition. Camphor is used in paints as a solvent, and in adulteration of different essential oils or used as the main base for rosemary, Spanish sage, thyme, lavandin, etc. Camphor fractions are also used as adulterants in many essential oils (A8; see also Chapter 4).

Toxicity

Acute toxicity (A22)

Oral LD_{50} White >5 ml/kg (rat); yellow >5 g/kg (rat); brown 4 ml/kg (rat).

Dermal LD_{50} White >5 ml/kg (rabbit); yellow >4 g/kg (rabbit); brown 2.5 g/kg (rabbit).

Irritation and sensitisation (A22)

White: None reported at 20% in humans; yellow 4%; brown 4%.

Phototoxicity

None reported.

Other toxicities

The white camphor normally used in aromatherapy is relatively non-toxic but has a considerable sensitisation potential. Safrole imparts a carcinogenic action (see nutmeg oil monograph) and therefore the darker, more crude extracts of camphor are potentially toxic. In large doses camphor is a narcotic and irritant; in small doses it is sedative, anodyne, antispasmodic, diaphoretic and anthelmintic. Very small doses of camphor stimulate and large doses depress. Large doses cause oesophageal and gastric pain, vomiting, slow and enfeebled and subsequently intermittent pulse, dizziness, drowsiness, dimness of sight, pallid, cold skin, muscular weakness, cyanosis, spasms, muscular rigidity and convulsions. Several deaths have resulted from its use. Mental confusion may follow its excessive use. Its effects in small doses are transient, and are not followed by depression or exhaustion. It exerts an influence on the brain and nervous system, exhilarating and relieving pain, is an excitant to the vascular system, and irritates mucous tissues, which are in proximity with it. When given in the solid form, it is capable of producing ulceration of the gastric mucous membrane (Felter and Lloyd, 1898).

Many cautions are found in the aromatherapy literature without scientific backing, including avoidance during pregnancy and in people with seizure disorders, high blood pressure or asthma. It is said to antidote homeopathic remedies. It should not be used on children under 5 years or animals. Most of the above are references to the pure crystalline camphor.

Bioactivities

Pharmacological activities *in vitro* and *in vivo*

Smooth muscle   White camphor oil had a strong spasmogenic effect on electrically stimulated guinea-pig ileum *in vitro* (A2; Lis-Balchin et al., 1996a).

Uterus   There was a decrease in the spontaneous contractions in the rat for oil *in vitro* (A3; A4; Lis-Balchin and Hart, 1997b).

Other activities   It is used to allay nervous excitement, subdue pain, arrest spasm, and sometimes to induce sleep. Occipital headache, from mental overwork, is relieved by small oral doses and external application. It acts beneficially as a diaphoretic and sedative, and is also valuable in gout, neuralgia, dysmenorrhoea, painful diseases of the urinary organs – acting as a sedative, anodyne and antispasmodic. It is said to act as an aphrodisiac (small doses), exciting the reproductive organs, causing considerable heat in the urethra and nocturnal emissions, but it can also act as an anti-aphrodisiac (large doses) and to reduce urino-genital irritation. It is used in many embrocations and liniments for rheumatic, neuralgic and deep-seated pains, sprains, chilblains and chronic cutaneous diseases. It has been found to be beneficial in asthma and spasmodic cough. The administration of opium will (surprisingly) best neutralize the evil effects of an overdose of camphor and small and repeated doses of alcohol may also be given (Felter and Lloyd, 1898). Vincent Van Gogh is known to have drunk camphor and absinthe, together with turpentine. These gave him severe medical problems but probably helped him to paint fantastic pictures (Bonkovsky *et al.*, 1992).

Antimicrobial activities

Antibacterial activity
Relative data (white camphor): There was a strong antibacterial effect against 25/25 different bacterial species and 16/20 *Listeria monocytogenes* varieties *in vitro* (A1; Lis-Balchin and Deans, 1997; Lis-Balchin *et al.*, 1998a). There was a very low activity against five respiratory pathogens *in vitro* (Inouye *et al.*, 2001).

Antifungal activity (A1)
Relative data (% inhibition): *Aspergillus niger* 95%, *A. ochraceus* 96%, *Fusarium culmorum* 0%.

Use in pregnancy and lactation: contraindications

There seems no problem with the use of camphor oil, used at very dilute concentrations in a carrier oil in aromatherapy massage, but there is a potential sensitisation risk, and a possible effect of a decrease in the spontaneous contractions of the uterus as shown in the rat *in vitro*.

Pharmaceutical guidance

The use of camphor in medicinal products obtained over the counter includes a vast number of very effective respiratory and muscular ointments, liniments and embrocations which have been used for over 50 years, posing no great problems (e.g. Vick VapoRub, tiger balm). However, VapoRub, an ointment used to relieve decongestion, is commonly used recreationally in conjunction with 'club drugs' such as MDMA (ecstacy). The use of camphor in aromatherapeutic dilutions in massage does not pose a problem except for its possible sensitisation and narcotic effect; however there is no scientific evidence for its effectiveness in the numerous conditions mentioned in aromatherapy books.

Use in babies and young children

Due to the immaturity and the delicate nature of the skin of babies and young children, it is inadvisable for any essential oils, especially this essential oil, to be used in massage, however much the essential oil has been diluted in the carrier oils. This is also a necessary precaution due to the possibilities of sensitisation of the children at this young age through skin or air-borne odorant effects (see Chapters 5 and 7).

Instillation or administration of essential oils near the baby or young child's nose is not only not recommended, but distinctly inadvisable, as there have been numerous cases reported of severe toxicity and even death from such applications (see Chapter 7).

Carrot Seed Oil

CAS numbers

USA: 8015-88-1; EINECS: 84929-61-3

Species/Botanical name

Daucus carota L. subsp. *carota* (Umbelliferae)

Synonyms

Daucus, Queen Anne's lace

Safety

CHIP details

Xn; R10, 65; 50%; S62 (A26)

RIFM recommended safety of use limits

4% (A23)

EU sensitiser total

3.3 (based on geraniol, limonene and linalool) (A27)

GRAS status

Granted (Fenaroli, 1997).

Extraction, source, appearance and odour

Extraction

A volatile oil is obtained by steam distillation of the seeds. Yield is 0.66–1.65% (Arctander, 1960).

Source

France and Hungary.

Appearance and odour

A yellow or amber to pale orange-brown liquid with dry, woody, root-like, earthy odour following the initial sweet and fresh notes; the tenacious undertone and dry-out is very heavy (Arctander, 1960).

Aromatherapy uses

Uses include: scanty periods, glandular problems, premenstrual tension; muscular pain, toxin accumulation, gout, arthritis, rheumatism; acne, dermatitis, eczema, psoriasis, wrinkles; anaemia, anorexia, colic, indigestion, liver congestion (Ryman, 1991; Lawless, 1992; Rose, 1992a; Price, 1993; Sheppard-Hanger, 1995).

Scientific comment

Carrot seed essential oil differs in action from the whole herb and has potent CNS-depressant, spasmodic and antispasmodic, hypotensive and cardiac-depressant activities as well as potential photosensitising properties when applied to the skin. Its use in aromatherapy may therefore be detrimental rather than beneficial.

Herbal uses

Wild carrot is stated to possess diuretic, antilithic and carminative properties. Traditionally, it has been used for urinary calculus, lithuria, cystitis, gout and specifically for urinary gravel or calculus. Carrot seeds are said to be abortifacient (Chevallier, 1996; Barnes *et al.*, 2002).

Food and perfumery uses

Food Carrot seed oil (FEMA 2244) is used in spicy foods and sauces (Fenaroli, 1997).

Perfumery It is used in perfumery for its herbaceous, fatty-woody notes in chypres, oriental and aldehydic perfumes (Arctander, 1960).

Chemistry

Major components

	% (Lawrence, 1976–2001)
α-Pinene	1–14
Camphene	0.3–0.7
β-Pinene	0.4–4.5
Sabinene	2–32
Limonene	trace–2.5
Linalool	trace–7
β-Caryophyllene	0.3–4
Geranyl acetate	1–34
Carotol	5–67
Daucol	trace–10

Minor components

Furanocoumarins: 8-Methoxypsoralen and 5-methoxypsoralen (0.01–0.02 µg/g fresh weight). Coumarin, β-bisabolene, geraniol, caryophyllene oxide, *trans*-β-farnesene, *trans*-β-bergamotene, thujopsene, *p*-cymene, terpinolene also occur from trace to several per cent.

Adulteration

D-Limonene is added (although it should be the L-form); other synthetic components e.g. α-pinene and other monoterpenes are also used (A8; see also Chapter 4).

Note: The seed essential oil differs entirely from carrot root expressed oil, which is rich in the vitamin A precursor carotene and does not have any essential oil. This is often misquoted in aromatherapy books.

Toxicity

Acute toxicity (A22)

Oral LD$_{50}$ >5 g/kg (rat).

Dermal LD$_{50}$ >5 g/kg (rabbit).

The oil is considered to be non-toxic (Leung, 1980; Tisserand and Balacs, 1995).

Irritation and sensitisation (A22)

The oil is reported to be generally non-irritating and non-sensitising (A22). However, hypersensitivity reactions, occupational dermatitis and positive patch tests have been reported for wild carrot (Mitchell and Rook, 1979; Ceska *et al.*, 1986). The essential oil contains very small amounts of terpinen-4-ol, which is associated with the renal irritancy of juniper oil.

Phototoxicity

Wild carrot has a slight photosensitising effect due to the furanocoumarins, which are known photosensitisers (Ceska *et al.*, 1986).

Bioactivities

Pharmacological activities *in vitro* and *in vivo*

Smooth muscle Carrot seed oil had a slight spasmolytic effect on guinea-pig ileum *in vitro* (A2; Lis-Balchin *et al.*, 1996a). Smooth muscle relaxant activity shown by reducing acetylcholine-induced contractions in the ileum in the rabbit, antagonism of acetylcholine in isolated frog skeletal muscle and a direct depressant effect on cardiac muscle in the dog was shown in the related

D. carota var. *sativa* seed essential oil (Gambhir *et al.*, 1966; Bhargava *et al.*, 1967).

Uterus There was a decrease in the spontaneous contractions in the rat uterus for carrot seed oil (A3; A4; Lis-Balchin and Hart, 1997b). Relaxant action on the rat uterus was shown by *D. carota* var. *sativa* seed essential oil. Oestrogenic activity, shown by the inhibition of ovarian hypertrophy in hemicastrated rats, was probably due to the small amounts of coumarin (a weak phytooestrogen) present (Kaliwal and Rao, 1981). Significant antifertility activity of 60% in rats was found for wild carrot (Prakash, 1984) but disputed by results in pregnant rats fed oral doses of aqueous, alcoholic and petrol extracts (Lal *et al.*, 1986). Weak oestrogenic activity (Prakash, 1984; Kant *et al.*, 1986) and inhibition of implantation (Prakash, 1984) has been documented for seed extracts (Kant *et al.*, 1986) but no data have been found for the pure essential oil.

Other activities *In vitro* cardiotonic activity (Gambhir *et al.*, 1966) and vasodilation of coronary vessels of the isolated cat heart have been shown for carrot seed essential oil (A22). *D. carota* var. *sativa* seed oil showed central nervous system effects similar to those of barbiturates (Bhargava *et al.*, 1967), including CNS hypnotic effects in the rat, hypotension in the dog (Gambhir *et al.*, 1966) and anticonvulsant activity in the frog.

Antimicrobial activities

Antibacterial activity

Relative data: The activity was very slight against 3/25 different bacterial species and 0/20 *Listeria monocytogenes* varieties (A1; Lis-Balchin and Deans, 1997; Lis-Balchin *et al.*, 1998a).

Antifungal activity

Activity was very low (% inhibition): *Aspergillus niger* 7%, *A. ochraceus* 0%, *Fusarium culmorum* 24% (A1). Limited antifungal activity has been documented, with activity exhibited against only one (*Botrytis cinerea*) out of nine fungi tested (Guérin and Réveillère, 1985).

Use in pregnancy and lactation: contraindications

Both spasmogenic and spasmolytic actions on smooth muscle *in vitro* have been reported and a decrease in the spontaneous contractions in the uterus *in vitro*. In view of this, and the documented mild oestrogenic activity and potentially irritant nature of the essential oil, excessive doses of carrot essential oil massaged into the skin during pregnancy and lactation should be avoided.

Pharmaceutical guidance

Animal studies have yielded data on a variety of pharmacological actions including CNS-depressant, spasmodic and antispasmodic, hypotensive and cardiac-depressant activities. The seed oil of wild carrot contains terpinen-4-ol, the diuretic component in juniper essential oil. Excessive doses may affect existing hypo- and hypertensive, cardiac and hormone therapies and slight irritation of kidneys may be experienced due to the minimal amounts of terpinen-4-ol; this is based on oral intake. In the absence of any data for dermal effects other than the presence of furanocoumarins, which are known photosensitisers, and some irritation effects carrot seed essential oil should be used with caution on the skin. The odour of the essential oil does not endear it as a fragrance for most people.

Use in babies and young children

Due to the immaturity and the delicate nature of the skin of babies and young children, it is inadvisable for any essential oils, especially this essential oil with photosensitiser potential, to be used in massage, however much the essential oil has been diluted in the carrier oils. This is also a necessary precaution due to the possibilities of sensitisation of the children at this young age through skin or air-borne odorant effects (see Chapters 5 and 7).

Instillation or administration of essential oils near the baby or young child's nose is not only not recommended, but distinctly inadvisable, as there have been numerous cases reported of severe toxicity and even death from such applications (see Chapter 7).

Cassia Oil

CAS numbers

USA: 8007-80-5; EINACS: 84961-46-6

Species/Botanical name

Cinnamomum cassia Bl. (Lauraceae)

Synonyms

Cassia bark, cassia lignea, Chinese cinnamon, *Cinnamomum aromaticum* Nees, false cinnamon, cinnamomi cassiae aetheroleum, oleum cassiae, oleum cinnamomi, oleum cinnamomi cassiae

Note: Not to be mistaken with cassie oil (*Acacia farnesiana* (Leguminosae)) used as an absolute or concrete in perfumery, which contains methyl salicylate, farnesol, geraniol, *o*-cresol and β-ionone.

Pharmacopoeias

In Chinese, European and Japanese Pharmacopoeias. Chinese and Japanese Phamacopoeias also include cassia bark, which may be known as cinnamon bark. In some countries cassia oil is known as cinnamon oil.

Safety

CHIP details
Xn; R21, 43; 0%; S24, 36/37 (A26)

EU sensitiser total
100 (due to cinnamaldehyde, 90%; cinnamyl alcohol, 0.2%; coumarin, 4%; eugenol, 7%) (A27)

GRAS status
Granted (Fenaroli, 1997).

Extraction, source, appearance and odour

Extraction
A volatile oil is obtained by steam or water distillation of the dried bark, leaves and twigs of the tree (Arctander, 1960). Cassia oil BPC is distilled from the leaves and twigs (Wren, 1988).

Source
China and USA (where most of the essential oil is distilled).

Appearance and odour
A dark brown liquid with a strong, spicy, warm and woody-resinous odour and a sweet, balsamic undertone. The tannins in the bark cause the dark colour if copper stills are used. The rectified essential oil is yellowish (Arctander, 1960).

Aromatherapy uses

No aromatherapy uses are given for cassia essential oil application on the skin and it is not often mentioned in books. Cassia oil apparently stimulates the pancreas (Rose, 1992a), but the mode of application is not given. In one manual (Sheppard-Hanger, 1995) many uses are given for cassia essential oil: skin, circulation, cardiovascular and immune system, digestive and genito-urinary, but cautions are given as to its dermal irritation and sensitisation. If inhaled it apparently has effects on the brain and mind, e.g. stimulating, insomnia, debility and depression (Sheppard-Hanger, 1995).

Scientific comment

Due to the toxicity of the essential oil and its adulteration with many sensitisers, the essential oil should not be used. Cinnamon essential oil can be substituted instead.

Herbal uses

Traditionally only the bark has been used medicinally; it is widely used in Chinese herbal medicine mainly for vascular disorders, otherwise in the same way as cinnamon and is a yang tonic (Wren, 1988; Chevallier, 1996; see also cinnamon oil monograph). The activity is strongly based on cinnamaldehyde, which has been shown to be a CNS stimulant at low doses and depressant at high doses; it is spasmolytic; hypotensive, hypoglycaemic, reduces platelet aggregation; aqueous extracts are anti-allergenic (Wren, 1988).

It has been used for flatulent dyspepsia, flatulent colic, diarrhoea, the common cold, and specifically for colic or dyspepsia with flatulent distension and nausea (British Herbal Medicine Association, 1983).

Food and perfumery uses

Food Similar to cinnamon. Cassia (FEMA 2258) is used more in foods than perfumery, e.g. liqueur flavours, cherry flavours (Fenaroli, 1997).

Perfumery The essential oil is not widely used due to the dark colour (Arctander, 1960).

Chemistry

Cassia oil (ISO 3216: 1994).

Major components

	%
Benzyldehyde	1–5
Salicylic aldehyde	trace
Acetophenone	trace
Phenylethylalcohol	trace–0.2
trans-Cinnamaldehyde	75–90%
Cinnamylacetate	trace–4
Eugenol	trace–1
Coumarin	trace
Cinnamic alcohol	trace–0.2
trans-o-Methoxy-cinnamaldehyde	trace
o-Methoxy-cinnamaldehyde	trace

Adulteration

Cassia is a grossly adulterated essential oil. Synthetic cinnamaldehyde is often added which has phenylpentadienal as a by-product at 400–500 ppm, but one can detect it at 2% adulteration. The essential oil is usually made synthetically using the components and Sumatran benzoin, etc. (A8; Arctander, 1960; see also Chapter 4).

Toxicity

Acute toxicity (A22)

Oral LD$_{50}$ 2.8 g/kg (rat).

Dermal LD$_{50}$ 0.32 g/kg (rabbit).

Irritation and sensitisation (A22)

Reports of allergic reactions, mainly to cassia oil, are numerous (Mitchell and Rook, 1979; Tisserand and Balacs, 1995). Cinnamaldehyde in toothpastes and perfumes has also caused contact sensitivity (Mitchell and Rook, 1979). Cassia oil has caused dermal and mucous membrane irritation, which has been ascribed to cinnamaldehyde (Tisserand and Balacs, 1995; see also cinnamon oil monograph; A22). A temporary estimated acceptable daily intake of cinnamaldehyde is 700 μg/kg body weight.

Phototoxicity

None reported.

Bioactivities

Pharmacological activities *in vitro* and *in vivo*

Smooth muscle Cassia oil had a spasmolytic effect on guinea-pig ileum *in vitro* (A2; Lis-Balchin *et al.*, 1996a).

Uterus There was a decrease in the spontaneous contractions in the rat uterus *in vitro* for cassia oil; mixing several other essential oils with the essential oil also had a relaxant effect (A3; A4; Lis-Balchin and Hart, 1997b).

Other activities Both the essential oil and cinnamaldehyde, the major component, are active in CNS stimulation, sedation, hypothermic and antipyretic actions (Leung, 1980; Hikino, 1985); also catecholamine release from the adrenal glands, weak papaverine-like action, increase in peripheral blood flow, hypotension, bradycardia and hyperglycaemia (Hikino, 1985). The contribution of cinnamaldehyde to the overall therapeutic efficacy of cassia as a herb has, however, been doubted (Hikino, 1985). The essential oil-free herbal preparations have shown anti-ulcerogenic properties; anti-inflammatory activity; antiplatelet aggregation and antithrombotic and antitumour actions (Wren, 1988; Chevallier, 1996; Barnes *et al.*, 2002).

Antimicrobial activities

Antibacterial activity

Relative data: Cassia oil had a strong antibacterial effect against 23/25 different bacteria and 20/20 *Listeria monocytogenes* varieties (A1; Lis-Balchin and Deans, 1997; Lis-Balchin *et al.*, 1998a).

Antifungal activity

The essential oil was very active (% inhibition): *Aspergillus niger* 87%, *A. ochraceus* 89%, *Fusarium culmorum* 54% (A1).

Use in pregnancy and lactation: contraindications

Due to the allergic dermatitic reactions possible with this highly sensitising essential oil and the possible effect of decreasing spontaneous contractions as seen in the uterus *in vitro*, the essential oil should not be applied to the skin during pregnancy, parturition and lactation. It could be used infrequently, in very small volumes, as a fragrance.

Pharmaceutical guidance

Cassia essential oil is widely used as a flavouring agents in foods, and in pharmaceutical and cosmetic preparations. However, skin contact with cassia bark oil is likely to cause an allergic reaction, especially in sensitive people, as the sensitisation value is 100%. Cassia oil is therefore one of the most hazardous oils (A29), especially as it is often adulterated, and should not be used on the skin. It could be used as a fragrance in low concentrations.

Use in babies and young children

Due to the immaturity and the delicate nature of the skin of babies and young children, it is inadvisable for any essential oils, especially this essential oil with very high sensitisation potential, to be used in massage, however much the essential oil has been diluted in the carrier oils. This is also a necessary precaution due to the possibilities of sensitisation of the children at this young age through skin or air-borne odorant effects (see Chapters 5 and 7).

Instillation or administration of essential oils near the baby or young child's nose is not only not recommended, but distinctly inadvisable, as there have been numerous cases reported of severe toxicity and even death from such applications (see Chapter 7).

Cedarwood Oil

CAS numbers

USA: 68608-32-2; EINECS: 91722-61-1

Species/Botanical name

Juniperus virginiana L. (Cupressaceae)

Synonyms

Virginian cedarwood

Other species

Juniperus mexicana Spring. (Cupressaceae) (Texas cedarwood), *Cedrus atlantica* Manetti (Pinaceae) (Atlas cedarwood, 'Moroccan' cedarwood, Lebanon cedarwood). Other species of minor importance to the essential oil industry include *Juniperus ashei* Buch. (Texas cedarwood), *Juniperus funebris* Endl. (Chinese cedarwood), *Cedrus libani* A. Rich., *Cedrus deodora* (d. Don) G. Don. F. (deodar). Japanese cedarwoods include hiba oil, hinoki oil and sugi oil.

Note: None of the cedarwoods must be confused with *Thuja occidentalis* L., which gives cedarleaf oil, which is toxic.

Safety

CHIP details

Xn; R65; 60%; S62 (A26)

RIFM recommended safety of use limits

Virginia *Juniperus virginiana* L. 1%; Atlas *Cedrus atlantica* Manetti 8% (A23)

EU sensitiser total

0 (A27)

GRAS status

Granted (Fenaroli, 1997).

Extraction, source, appearance and odour

Extraction

A volatile oil is obtained by steam distillation of comminuted barks of the trees (Arctander, 1960).

Source

USA, Morocco, East Africa and China.

Appearance and odour

Virginian oil is colourless to pale yellow to orange-yellow; oily-woody, sweet, resinous, pleasant; very persistent. It dries out to a more woody, less balsamic odour. It is rectified to a colourless liquid. Cedrene, the main component is converted to cedrenol on ageing. Light sesquiterpene fractions containing mainly cedrene are produced and converted into interesting perfume compounds. The essential oil is used extensively in perfumes, especially for soaps, as a fixative and cost-reducer for vetiver, sandalwood, patchouli and guaiacwood oils. It is often used in air-fresheners (Arctander, 1960).

Texas oil is brown to reddish-brown or can be redistilled to colourless.

Texas oil may become solid in cold weather (crude). It has a pleasant, sweet-woody, somewhat tar-like or cade-like and smoky odour. Later, on drying, it becomes balsamic-like and shows great tenacity with a sweet-woody dry-out. The rectified oil is less tar-like in odour as well as less cade-like and smoky. It has a pencil-sharpener-like odour on dry-out. A heavy fraction consisting of cedrol and cedrenol is often isolated. The light sesquiterpenoid fraction can be converted into very interesting perfumery compounds.

All the Texas oils, crude and rectified and the fractions are used in perfumery. The colourless rectified oil is preferred and blends with ionones, cinnamic alcohol, patchouli, amber bases, etc. (Arctander, 1960).

Atlas oil is similar to Virginian. Atlas oil is yellowish to orange or deep amber coloured viscous liquid; odour is peculiar and not that pleasant when undiluted: slightly camphoraceous-cresylic with a sweet and tenacious woody undertone, reminiscent of cassie and mimosa, but not as delicate as the floral oils (Arctander, 1960).

Aromatherapy uses

Cedarwood oil uses include: acne, scabs with pus, dermatitis, psoriasis, seborrhoea of the scalp, dandruff and alpaca, alopecia, falling hair, dandruff;

arthritis, rheumatism, bronchitis, coughs, sinusitis, cystitis, nervous tension, stress-related disorders; calming and soothing to nervous tension and anxious states; a tonic to the glandular and nervous systems, genito-urinary tract inflammation or burning pain; acts as sexual stimulant (Ryman, 1991; Lawless, 1992; Rose, 1992a; Price, 1993; Sheppard-Hanger, 1995).

Scientific comment

Cedarwood essential oils are relatively non-toxic and pleasantly scented, but there is no scientific evidence that they could alleviate all the conditions mentioned above. Massage itself can benefit both stress-related conditions and muscular aches. Cedarwood could be of use as a relaxant used as a fragrance, possibly replacing pine essential oil in the bath.

Herbal uses

No traditional uses for cedarwood essential oil have been documented; most of the data is for whole herbal extracts. The cedarwoods are said to be: antiseborrhoeic, pulmonary and genito-urinary antiseptic; antispasmodic; astringent; balsamic; decongestant (venous); diuretic; emmenagogue; emollient; expectorant; fungicidal and insecticidal (Wren, 1988; Blumenthal *et al.*, 2000; Barnes *et al.*, 2002).

Food and perfumery uses

Food Not used except for temporary usage for Virginian cedarwood essential oil.

Perfumery Atlas cedarwood is used in many perfumes as a fixative and for its unique odour which blends well with labdanum products and any woody and woody-floral materials (Arctander, 1960).

Chemistry

Major components

	% (Lawrence, 1976–2001)
Cedrol	1–32
α-Cedrene	15–31
β-Cedrene	1–8
Thujopsene	14–35

Minor components

There are numerous other sesquiterpenes, including: α- and β-acoradiene, α-himachalene, α- and β-chamigrene, α- and γ-himachalene, γ-curcumene, α-selinene, cuparene, α- and β-alaskene, widdrol, *trans*-3-thujopsanone, α-bisabolol and 8-cedren-13-ol. All the cedarwood oils of commerce contain a group of chemically related compounds, the relative proportions of these depending on the plant species from which the oil is obtained. These compounds include cedrol and cedrene, and while they contribute something to the odour of the whole oil they are also valuable to the chemical industry for conversion to other derivatives with fragrance applications.

The three types of commercial cedarwood oils are often admixed and are often of very similar composition; however, different ISOs exist:

Virginian (ISO 4724: 1984) *Juniperus virginiana* L. Cupressaceae: Cedrol max 14%
Texas (ISO 4725: 1986) *Juniperus mexicana* Schiede Cupressaceae: Cedrol min 35% to max 48% as alcohols and by gas chromatography 20% min.

Adulteration

All commercial cedarwood oils seem to be blended together and have similar compositions; they are also substituted for each other. They are relatively cheap so there is no real problem of adulteration with synthetic components (A8; see also Chapter 4).

Toxicity

Acute toxicity (A22)

Oral LD₅₀ Texas, Virginian and Atlas >5 g/kg (rat).

Dermal LD₅₀ Texas, Virginian and Atlas >5 g/kg (rabbit).

Irritation and sensitisation (A22)

None reported at 8%.

Phototoxicity

None found.

Bioactivities

Pharmacological activities *in vitro* and *in vivo*

Smooth muscle There was a spasmolytic action on smooth muscle of the electrically stimulated guinea-pig *in vitro* for all cedarwoods studied (commercial Atlas, Chinese, Texas and Virginian).

The sesquiterpenes, unlike monoterpenes, have a spasmolytic action (A2; Lis-Balchin *et al.*, 1996a).

Uterus There was a decrease in the spontaneous contractions in the rat uterus. Mixing several other essential oils with the cedarwood oils (commercial Atlas, Chinese, Texas and Virginian) also had a relaxant effect (A3; A4; Lis-Balchin and Hart, 1997b).

Other activities Cedarwood had a weak therapeutic effect on experimentally induced tuberculosis in the guinea-pig, but it was combined with sub-effective doses of dihydrostreptomycin (A22). There was some influence of cedar essence (red cedarwood Virginian) on spontaneous activity and sleep of rats and human daytime nap (Sano *et al.*, 1998).

Antimicrobial activities

This was very low due to the high proportion of inactive sesquiterpenes.

Antibacterial activity

Relative data: Cedarwood essential oils (commercial Atlas, Chinese, Texas and Virginian): 2–4/25 different bacteria were affected; 0/20 *Listeria monocytogenes* varieties (A1; Lis-Balchin and Deans, 1997; Lis-Balchin *et al.*, 1998a). No activity was reported against five bacteria (Yousef and Tawil, 1980); the vapour of Texas cedarwood slightly inhibited 2/5 bacteria (Maruzella and Sicurella, 1960).

Antifungal activity

Relative data (% inhibition): Cedarwood essential oils (commercial Atlas, Chinese, Texas and Virginian) had very low activity: *Aspergillus niger* 0–8%, *A. ochraceus* 0–17%, *Fusarium culmorum* 0–14% (A1). 1/15 fungi were affected by cedarwood essential oil (Maruzella and Liguori, 1958).

No antioxidant activity found (Lis-Balchin *et al.*, 1996a).

Use in pregnancy and lactation: contraindications

There was a loss of spontaneous contractions in the uterus when the essential oil was used *in vitro*, and no clinical studies have been undertaken to test their safety during pregnancy. The essential oils should therefore be used sparingly on the body during pregnancy, parturition and lactation. The essential oils could be used as a fragrance throughout.

Pharmaceutical guidance

The cedarwood essential oils seem to have no adverse effects and scant information is available on their bioactivities. They seem to be inactive apart from a relaxant action on smooth and uterine muscle *in vitro*. There is no reason to suggest that they are toxic and the sensitiser value is nil, making them acceptable as aromatherapy oils for massage. Their depth lies in their pleasant odour and they should therefore also be used as fragrances.

Use in babies and young children

Due to the immaturity and the delicate nature of the skin of babies and young children, it is inadvisable for any essential oils to be used in massage, however much the essential oil has been diluted in the carrier oils. This is also a necessary precaution due to the possibilities of sensitisation of the children at this young age through skin or air-borne odorant effects (see Chapters 5 and 7).

Instillation or administration of essential oils near the baby or young child's nose is not only not recommended, but distinctly inadvisable, as there have been numerous cases reported of severe toxicity and even death from such applications (see Chapter 7).

Celery Seed Oil

CAS numbers

USA: 8015-90-5; EINECS: 89997-35-3

Species/Botanical name

Apium graveolens (Apiaceae/Umbelliferae)

Synonyms

Apii fructus, celery fruit, celery seed, smallage

Safety

CHIP details
Xn; R10, 65; 80%, S62 (A26)

RIFM recommended safety of use limits
4% (A23)

EU sensitiser total
79.1% (based largely on its limonene content) (A27)

GRAS status
Granted (Fenaroli, 1997).

Extraction, source, appearance and odour

Extraction
The essential oil is obtained by steam distillation of the seeds. Yield: 2–3% (Arctander, 1960).

Source
India, Holland, Hungary, USA and China.

Appearance and odour
A pale yellow to orangey liquid. The odour is spicy-warm, sweet and rich and 'soup-like', long-lasting and powerful, slightly fatty and resembles the actual seed rather than the herb itself. It has the most diffusive odour and a penetrating flavour (Arctander, 1960).

Aromatherapy uses

Very few references in aromatherapy books exist and most are concerned with the herb. Apparently the essential oil is used for: arthritis, toxins in blood, gout, rheumatism; dyspepsia, flatulence, liver congestion, jaundice; amenorrhoea, increasing milk flow, cystitis; neuralgia, sciatica (Ryman, 1991; Lawless, 1992; Rose, 1992a; Sheppard-Hanger, 1995).

Scientific comment
The uses mentioned by aromatherapists are taken directly from herbal uses and no scientific evidence has been provided for the aromatherapeutic benefits. Massage itself benefits many stress conditions as well as muscular and arthritic pain.

Herbal uses

Celery is an ancient herb, used in Pharaonic Egypt and China. It apparently has antirheumatic, sedative, mild diuretic and urinary antiseptic properties. It has been used for arthritis, rheumatism, gout, urinary tract inflammation, cystitis, and specifically for rheumatoid arthritis with mental depression and also as an aphrodisiac (Wren, 1988; Chevallier, 1996; Blumenthal *et al.*, 2000; Barnes *et al.*, 2002).

Food and perfumery uses

Food Celery seed oil (FEMA 2271) is used in numerous foods: dairy, condiments, soups, puddings, beverages (both alcoholic and non-alcoholic), etc. (Fenaroli, 1997).

Perfumery Used frequently but in small amounts for imparting warm notes in floral and oriental perfumes and lavender bouquets, aldehydic and fantasy perfumes (Arctander, 1960).

Chemistry

Major components

	% (*Lawrence, 1976–2001*)
Limonene	8–68
β-Selinene	10–60
Caryophyllene	1–4
β-Elemene	1–4
n-Butyl phthalide	trace–23
n-Butyl-4*n*,5-dihydrophthalide	6–9

There are also numerous other monoterpenes and sesquiterpenes in variable concentrations. The most important ingredients for the characteristic odour are sedanenolide (*n*-butyl-4*n*, 5-dihydrophthalide) and sedanolic acid anhydride. Furanocoumarins include: apigravin, apiumetin, apiumoside, bergapten, celerin, celereoside, isoimperatorin, isopimpinellin, osthenol, rutaretin, seselin, umbelliferone; 8-hydroxy-5-methoxypsoralen also occurs in trace amounts (Innocenti *et al.*, 1976; Bos *et al.*, 1986).

Adulteration

The essential oil is frequently adulterated with synthetic limonene, which is then counteracted for its harshness by the addition of several other synthetic components present in the original essential oil (A8; see also Chapter 4).

Toxicity

Acute toxicity (A22)

Oral LD$_{50}$ >5.0 g/kg (rat).

Dermal LD$_{50}$ >5 g/kg (rabbit).

Irritation and sensitisation

In humans 4% seed oil caused no effects (A22). However, celery is a frequent food allergen, not only raw but also cooked and as a spice, and it can produce various reactions of immediate type, from oral contact urticaria to anaphylactic shock. Most celery-allergic patients suffer from hay fever and show a skin sensitisation to mugwort. The modified prick test with native celery root has proved to be the best method for detecting celery sensitisation, showing a positive result in 88.6% of people. The scratch test with celery salt is positive in 70.5%, intracutaneous testing with commercial extract in 63.5% and the RAST (radioallergosorbent) test with celery sticks in 66% of the patients. Cross-reactivity amongst the Apiaceae is the cause of the many positive results obtained with carrot, parsley, anise, fennel and caraway, the carrot allergy being of clinical importance in 50% of cases, including one with a history of anaphylactic shock after ingestion of raw carrots (Wuthrich and Dietschi, 1985).

Phototoxicity

Contact with the herb in sunlight has been reported to cause phototoxicity in men harvesting celery (Martindale, 1999). Photosensitivity reactions have also occurred due to external contact with celery stems (Mitchell and Rook, 1979; Austad and Kavli, 1983; Berkley *et al.*, 1986) and were probably associated with the furanocoumarins (Ashwood-Smith *et al.*, 1985; Chaudhary *et al.*, 1985; Barnes *et al.*, 2002). Celery soup caused severe phototoxicity during PUVA therapy (Boffa *et al.*, 1996). Allergic and anaphylactic reactions to celery have occurred after oral ingestion of the stems (Forsbeck and Ros, 1979; Déchamp *et al.*, 1984), probably mediated by IgE antibodies (Pauli *et al.*, 1985).

Bioactivities

Pharmacological activities *in vitro* and *in vivo*

Smooth muscle   Celery oil had a strong spasmogenic effect on electrically stimulated smooth muscle of the guinea-pig ileum *in vitro*. Limonene had a similar effect (A2; Lis-Balchin *et al.*, 1996a).

Uterus   There was a decrease in the spontaneous contractions in the rat when celery oil, limonene and the other components were introduced to rat uterus *in vitro*. Mixing several other essential oils with celery oil also had a relaxant effect (A3; A4; Lis-Balchin and Hart, 1997b).

Other activities   Celery plant extracts had anti-inflammatory activity in the mouse ear test and against carrageenan-induced rat paw oedema (Lewis *et al.*, 1985), also a hypotensive effect in rabbits and dogs after intravenous administration (Leung, 1980) and hypoglycaemic activity (Duke, 1985). Apigenin showed potent antiplatelet activity *in vitro* (Teng *et al.*, 1988).

Celery juice has been shown to exhibit choleretic activity and the phthalide constituents possess diuretic activity (Stahl, 1973). In mice, sedative and antispasmodic activities were shown for phthalide constituents (Duke, 1985).

Antimicrobial activities

Antibacterial activity

Relative data: There was strong activity against 17/25 different bacterial species and 19/20 *Listeria monocytogenes* varieties (A1; Lis-Balchin and Deans, 1997; Lis-Balchin *et al.*, 1998a). Celery seed oil has been reported to have bacteriostatic activity against several bacteria (Kar and Jain, 1971).

Antifungal activity

Relative data (% inhibition): *Aspergillus niger* 13–25%, *A. ochraceus* 35–48%, *Fusarium culmorum* 31–36% (A1).

Clinical studies

Hypotensive activity was shown in 88% of hypertensive patients given a celery plant extract (Leung, 1980).

Use in pregnancy and lactation: contraindications

Due to the decrease in the spontaneous contractions of the uterus in animal studies *in vitro*, the possible effect on the menstrual cycle, its uterine stimulant activity (Farnsworth, 1975; Duke, 1985) and its supposed abortifacient effect (Farnsworth, 1975), together with the possible phototoxic and/or sensitisation reaction, celery oil should not be massaged in pregnancy, parturition nor lactation. The use of the essential oil as a fragrance is not considered dangerous, but it is not a pleasant odour for most people and is over-effusive.

Pharmaceutical guidance

Celery oil contains phototoxic compounds (furanocoumarins), which may cause photosensitive reactions and the essential oil may also precipitate allergic reactions in susceptible people. The extremely high sensitisation value suggests great caution in its usage. In view of all its possible deleterious effects and in the absence of any beneficial effects, celery seed oil should not be recommended in aromatherapy.

Use in babies and young children

Due to the immaturity and the delicate nature of the skin of babies and young children, it is inadvisable for any essential oils to be used in massage, however much the essential oil has been diluted in the carrier oils. This is also a necessary precaution due to the possibilities of sensitisation of the children at this young age through skin or air-borne odorant effects (see Chapters 5 and 7).

Instillation or administration of essential oils near the baby or young child's nose is not only not recommended, but distinctly inadvisable, as there have been numerous cases reported of severe toxicity and even death from such applications (see Chapter 7).

Chamomile German Oil

CAS numbers

USA: 8002-66-2; EINECS: 84082-60-0

Species/Botanical name

Matricaria recutita L. (Asteraceae/Compositae)

Synonyms

Chamomilla recutita (L.) Rauschert, Hungarian chamomile, *Matricaria chamomilla* L., matricaria flowers, sweet false chamomile, wild chamomile

Safety

CHIP details
None

RIFM recommended safety of use limits
4% (A23)

EU sensitiser total
0.4 (based on linalool) (A27)

GRAS status
Granted (Fenaroli, 1997).

Extraction, source, appearance and odour

Extraction
Steam distillation of the flowers is the normal procedure (Arctander, 1960), but extraction of the volatile oil of chamomile flowerheads using supercritical carbon dioxide has been shown to be more efficient at keeping the concentration of chamazulene high (Vuorela *et al.*, 1990), as is alcohol or chloroform extraction. Yield of essential oil: 0.24–1.9%.

Source
Egypt and Eastern Europe.

Appearance and odour
When fresh, it is a dark blue, somewhat viscous liquid which lightens with ageing. It has a sweet, herbaceous-coumarin-like odour with a fruity undertone. In its concentrated form it is almost nauseating and many people find it unpleasant, especially its dry-out note which in fresh oils is animalistic (Arctander, 1960).

Aromatherapy uses

Uses include: acne, cuts, insect bites, hair-care; earache, inflammations; toothache, teething pains, wounds; arthritis, muscular pains, neuralgia, sprains; dyspepsia, colic, indigestion, nausea; dysmenorrhoea, menopausal problems, vaginitis, menorrhagia; headache, insomnia, migraine, stress-related complaints; tonic for the old and children; allergies, hay fever; premenstrual tension, cystitis; diarrhoea in children, gastric ulcers, bruises, burns. Added to bath: removes tension and weariness (Ryman, 1991; Lawless, 1992; Rose, 1992a; Price, 1993; Sheppard-Hanger, 1995).

Scientific comment

Although the herb has many acceptable uses in herbal medicine and the essential oil is also used for a variety of conditions as stated below, the essential oil has not been studied in aromatherapy. German chamomile essential oil is regarded as anti-inflammatory and useful for various skin, respiratory and ano-genital conditions based on its herbal usage, which is either at a high concentration given topically or orally, neither of which can equate to very low concentrations massaged into the skin. The fragrance may be useful for respiratory conditions in higher concentrations than those used in aromatherapy massage, but also for relaxation, as was noted in experiments on the human brain (A14) and the massage itself can contribute significantly to alleviating many symptoms of stress and also muscular pain. It is most unlikely that the other chamomile essential oils, with entirely different chemical compositions, could have the same desired effect, although frequently substituted for the German essential oil.

Herbal uses

German chamomile oil is a carminative, antispasmodic, mild sedative, anti-inflammatory, antiseptic and has anticatarrhal properties. It has been used topically for haemorrhoids, mastitis and leg ulcers and the herb was approved for use for: gastro-intestinal spasms and inflammatory diseases of the gastrointestinal tract and externally for skin and mucous membrane inflammation and bacterial skin diseases including oral cavity and gums. It is also approved for inflammations and irritations of the respiratory tract (by inhalation) and ano-genital inflammation (baths and irrigation) (Blumenthal et al., 2000).

Food and perfumery uses

Food German chamomile (FEMA 2273) is used in many foods (Fenaroli, 1997).

Perfumery It is used in high-class perfumes to introduce a warm, rich undertone during all stages of evaporation (Arctander, 1960).

Chemistry

Major components

	% (Lawrence, 1976–2001)
(–)-α-Bisabolol	4–77
Chamazulene	1–18
(–)-α-Bisabolol oxide A	0–66
(–)-α-Bisabolol oxide B	3–59
(–)-α-Bisabolone oxide A	2–9
cis-Spiroethers	2–20
trans-Spiroethers	1–5
-en-yn-dicycloether	1–19
Farnesene	15–28

Minor components

Other sesquiterpenes: cadinene, furfural, spanthu-lenol and proazulenes (matricarin and matricin). Chamazulene, which gives the blue colour to the essential oil, is formed from matricin during steam distillation and is destroyed on storage, especially under light. This results in a lighter colour of blue which can turn pale green, yellow or brown.

Adulteration

Fresh German chamomile essential oil or a chamazulene extract is frequently mixed into the essential oil in small amounts when the essential oil ages to intensify or change the yellow colour to the blue. Solvent extracts of *M. recutita* with a more intense blue colour are often mixed in with the essential oil. Chamazulenes, extracted from

various plants such as the balsam apple (*Populus balsamifera*) or blue oil-producing angelica root, are also used but apparently do not give the same medicinal strength (Schilcher, 1984).

Note: Moroccan chamomile (*Ormenis mixta*; *Anthemis mixta*) is available on the market as a cheaper chamomile. It has a totally different chemical composition (and odour). Main components (Toulemonde and Beauverd, 1984) are: α-pinene (15%), limonene (8%), santolina alcohol (32%), artemisia alcohol (2.5%), β-caryophyllene (1.5%) and bisabolene (2.5%). To use such a chamomile and expect similar results to German or Roman chamomile is naïve, as nothing is known about its bioactivity and it remains untested for toxicity. Chamazulene is often added and the resultant essential oil sold as German chamomile.

Toxicity

Acute toxicity (A22)

Oral LD$_{50}$ Essential oil <5 g/kg (rabbit), 2.5 mL/kg (mouse) (Ikram, 1980); (–)-α-bisabolol 15 mL/kg (Habersang et al., 1979).

Dermal LD$_{50}$ Essential oil <5 g/kg (rabbit) (A22). The subacute oral toxicity of (–)-α-bisabolol is 1.0–2.0 mL/kg (rats and dogs) (Habersang et al., 1979).

LD$_{50}$ (intraperitoneal injection) cis-Spiroether 670 mg/kg (mouse) (Breinlich and Scharnagel, 1968).

Irritation and sensitisation

No effects were noted in either animals or humans even when used undiluted on the skin (A22). Allergic reactions to 'chamomile' are common, but most reports do not state the species: many cases are due to the family Compositae and cross-sensitisation to both German chamomile and Umbelliferae exist (Hausen, 1979; Mitchell and Rook, 1979; Hausen et al., 1984). Most of the reports are not dealing with the essential oil but with the whole herb (Barnes et al., 2002). Symptoms include abdominal cramps, a tight sensation in the throat, upper airway obstruction and pharyngeal oedema (Benner and Lee, 1973), diffuse pruritus and urticaria (Casterline, 1980). Chamomile tea (which would have essential oils present in small concentrations) has exacerbated existing allergic conditions and a chamomile enema caused asthma and urticaria (Mitchell and Rook, 1979). There was a positive patch test with Kamillosan (chamomile-containing ointment) in a patient with hypersensitivity to chamomile (Rudzki and Rebandel, 1998). The allergenic properties due to chamomile have been attributed to sesquiterpene lactones, found in many Compositae (Hausen et al., 1984) and to matricarin (Mitchell and Rook, 1979).

Azulene, which is found in tobacco smoke, in cosmetic formulations including hair dyes (as a skin-conditioning agent) was included in several animal studies of anti-inflammatory actions. Azulene effects at the cellular level included inhibition of respiration and growth; relatively low oral toxicity was seen in acute animal studies; azulene was not mutagenic in an Ames test, with and without metabolic activation. These data were clearly found to be insufficient to support the safety of azulene in cosmetics and additional data were needed to make a safety assessment including: skin penetration (then both a 28-day dermal toxicity study to assess general skin and systemic toxicity and a reproductive and developmental toxicity study); one genotoxicity study in a mammalian system, then a 2-year dermal carcinogenesis study using National Toxicology Program methods; also skin irritation and sensitisation in animals or humans; and ocular toxicity (Final Report, 1999a).

Bisabolol is used in a wide range of cosmetic formulations as a skin conditioning agent at low concentrations ranging from 0.001% in lipstick to 1% in underarm deodorants. Tests indicated that: bisabolol can enhance the penetration of 5-fluorouracils; no evidence of sensitisation or photosensitisation was found; short-term oral exposure using rats produced inflammatory changes in several organs. Bisabolol was negative in bacterial and mammalian genotoxicity tests, and it did not produce reproductive or developmental toxicity in rats and is considered safe to use in cosmetics (Final Report, 1999b).

Bioactivities

Pharmacological activities in vitro and in vivo

Smooth muscle There was a strong spasmolytic action on smooth muscle of guinea-pig *in vitro* (A2; Lis-Balchin et al., 1996a). Antispasmodic activity on the isolated guinea-pig ileum has also been shown for bisabolol (Achterrath-Tuckermann et al., 1980; Mann and Staba, 1986). (−)-α-Bisabolol activity was found to be comparable to that of papaverine, while the total volatile oil was considerably less active (Mann and Staba, 1986). Smooth muscle relaxant properties for a *cis*-spiroether were

also shown (Breinlich and Scharnagel, 1968; Holzl et al., 1986).

Uterus There was a reduction in intensity of the spontaneous contractions of rat uterus *in vitro* to their complete cessation with higher dosage (A3; A4; Lis-Balchin and Hart, 1997b).

Skeletal muscle Phrenic nerve diaphragm and diaphragm direct of rat *in vitro* gave 100% decrease in twitch (Lis-Balchin and Hart, 1997c).

Other activities These are mainly after oral intake. German chamomile oil (oral) increased bile secretion and concentration of cholesterol in the bile in cats and dogs (Ikram, 1980). A higher dose (0.2 mL/kg) caused hypotension and acted as a cardiac and respiratory depressant (Ikram, 1980). Regeneration of liver tissue in partially hepatectomised rats was attributed to the azulene constituents (Mann and Staba, 1986). The essential oil has reduced the serum concentration of urea in rabbits with experimentally induced uraemic conditions (Grochulski and Borkowski, 1972).

German chamomile has anti-allergic and anti-inflammatory activities (Tubaro et al., 1984; Mann and Staba, 1986), which are partly due to azulene and probably act by inhibiting histamine release. Oxidation of arachidonic acid was shown by extracts of the plant, the active compounds included chamazulene, *cis*-en-yn spiroether and (−)-α-bisabolol (Jacovlev et al., 1979). Matricin was a more effective anti-inflammatory agent than chamazulene (Jakovlev et al., 1983; Mann and Staba, 1986). Chamazulene inhibited the formation of leukotriene B4 in intact cells (by blocking the chemical peroxidation of arachidonic acid) but matricine showed no effect at low concentration, therefore chamazulene may contribute to the anti-inflammatory activity of chamomile extracts by inhibiting the leukotriene synthesis (Safayhi et al., 1994). Anti-ulcerogenic activity (ulcers induced by indometacin, stress or ethanol) in rats was shown for (−)-α-bisabolol, where the development was inhibited (Szelenyi et al., 1979; Mann and Staba, 1986). (−)-α-Bisabolol had a significant protective effect on the gastrotoxicity of acetyl salicylic acid (Torrado et al., 1995).

Evaluation of massage with essential oils including German chamomile on childhood atopic eczema showed initial positive effects, though not significantly different to massage alone. However, after a break of a few weeks the eczema got worse, suggesting a possible sensitisation reaction (Anderson et al., 2000).

Inhalation of chamomile oil vapour decreased stress-induced increases of plasma adrenocorticotrophic hormone (ACTH) level in ovariectomised rat. The plasma ACTH level decreased further when diazepam was administered along with inhaling chamomile oil vapour (Yamada *et al.*, 1996). Activities on the CNS of the mouse of seven plant extracts given orally, including *Matricaria chamomilla*, were studied and showed a sedative effect at high dosage (Della Loggia *et al.*, 1981).

Teratogenicity studies gave contradictory results: in rats, rabbits and dogs, (–)-α-bisabolol was found to increase the number of fetuses reabsorbed and reduced the body weight of live offspring (Habersang *et al.*, 1979). However, (–)-α-bisabolol given orally to pregnant rats had no effect on the fetus (Isaac, 1979).

Antimicrobial activities

It is often impossible to determine which chamomile essential oil was used in a particular study, so only essential oil results from well-identified oils are shown.

Antibacterial activity
Relative data: Very low activity is found: 2–5/25 different bacteria (A1; Lis-Balchin and Deans, 1997; Lis-Balchin *et al.*, 1998a) and 1/25 (Deans and Ritchie, 1987). 0–1/20 *Listeria monocytogenes* varieties were affected (A1) and in another study, 1/5 (Aureli *et al.*, 1992). Samples of so-called Moroccan oil showed higher activities, but this is from a different species or an adulterated essential oil (A1; Lis-Balchin and Deans, 1997; Lis-Balchin *et al.*, 1998a).

Antifungal activity
Relative data (% inhibition): There was moderate activity against: *Aspergillus niger* 62–63%, *A. ochraceus* 40–56%, *Fusarium culmorum* 25–75% (A1).

Antioxidant activity
A strong antioxidant activity was found (Lis-Balchin *et al.*, 1998a). An ethanolic extract of the entire plant has been reported to inhibit the growth of poliovirus and herpes virus (Suganda *et al.*, 1983) but the essential oil may not be involved at all.

Clinical studies

Several studies were conducted on German chamomile extracts, but not the essential oil, which

showed anti-inflammatory, antipeptic and antispasmodic activities on the human stomach and duodenum (Mann and Staba, 1986), also anti-inflammatory effects and wound-healing properties (Blumenthal *et al.*, 2000). In a double-blind trial, 50 mg α-bisabolol and 3 mg chamazulene/100 g in an extract was tested on 14 patients with weeping wound areas after dermabrasion of tattoos and the time taken for healing and the drying process was statistically significantly decreased as judged by the doctor (Glowania *et al.*, 1987).

Positive psychological effects, including mood swings, were obtained using the essential oil (Roberts and Williams, 1992). Oral dosage of an extract caused deep sleep in 10/12 patients during cardiac catherisation (Mann and Staba, 1986).

Use in pregnancy and lactation: contraindications

German chamomile herbal preparations are said to affect the menstrual cycle (Farnsworth, 1975) and extracts are reported to be uterotonic; however, this was not proven as yet for the essential oil (Shipochliev, 1981; Mann and Staba, 1986). There was a decrease of spontaneously induced contractions in the rat uterus *in vitro* with increasing doses of German chamomile essential oil. These results suggest that the excessive use of chamomile essential oil during pregnancy, parturition and lactation should be avoided, but the usual concentrations of the essential oil used in aromatherapy massage should not prove a safety hazard. The fragrance could be used throughout.

Pharmaceutical guidance

Although the German chamomile herb should be avoided by individuals with a known hypersensitivity to any members of the Asteraceae/Compositae family, due to allergic reactions and cross-sensitivities, it is unclear whether the essential oil could have the same effect. It is also not known whether it precipitates an allergic reaction or exacerbates existing symptoms (e.g. in asthmatics). Excessive doses orally may interfere with existing anticoagulant therapy, because of the coumarin constituents, but this has not been demonstrated for dermal application.

German chamomile oil is different from Roman chamomile oil and aromatherapy uses should not be judged by using data from the latter and the other species (Moroccan) as the three essential oil compositions are entirely different. The toxicity of German chamomile essential oil is low and there should be no safety hazard associated with normal aromatherapy massage use nor its use as a fragrance. The odour was found to have a relaxant effect on the human brain (A14), therefore could be used either alone, or in conjunction with massage for a more profound relaxant effect.

Use in babies and young children

Due to the immaturity and the delicate nature of the skin of babies and young children, it is inadvisable for any essential oils to be used in massage, however much the essential oil has been diluted in the carrier oils. This is also a necessary precaution due to the possibilities of sensitisation of the children at this young age through skin or air-borne odorant effects (see Chapters 5 and 7).

Instillation or administration of essential oils near the baby or young child's nose is not only not recommended, but distinctly inadvisable, as there have been numerous cases reported of severe toxicity and even death from such applications (see Chapter 7).

Chamomile Roman Oil

CAS numbers

USA: 8015-92-7; EINECS: 84082-60-0

Species/Botanical name

Chamaemelum nobile (L.) All. (Asteraceae/Compositae)

Synonyms

Anthemis nobilis L.

Safety

CHIP details

Xn; R10, 65; 15%; S62 (A26)

RIFM recommended safety of use limits

4% (A23)

EU sensitiser total

7 (based on geraniol, citronellol, limonene and linalool) (A27)

GRAS status

Granted (Fenaroli, 1997).

Extraction, source, appearance and odour

Extraction

Steam distillation of flowers and herbal tops. Yield: 0.4–1.75% (Arctander, 1960).

Source

Egypt, Morocco, UK and most of Europe.

Appearance and odour

A colourless to faintly blue essential oil, the colour fading within a few weeks. Chamazulene is formed from a natural precursor during steam distillation of the oil, and varies in yield depending on the origin and age of the oil (Williams, 1996). It has a sweet, herbaceous, somewhat fruity-warm and tea-like odour, which is diffusive but has little tenacity (Arctander, 1960).

Aromatherapy uses

Aromatherapists give many uses for Roman chamomile essential oil, often based on those of German chamomile essential oil, which include: calming the mind, insomnia, easing anxiety, tension, anger, worries, fear; pain such as neuralgia, headaches, toothache, earache; menstrual problems; gastrointestinal problems, gastritis, diarrhoea, colitis, peptic ulcers, flatulence, inflammation of the bowels; genito-urinary tract problems; liver problems such as jaundice; skin problems, burns, blisters, inflamed wounds, ulcers, boils, dermatitis, hypersensitive skin, dry, itchy skin, puffiness; broken capillaries, low elasticity and tissue strength (Ryman, 1991; Lawless, 1992; Rose, 1992a; Price, 1993; Sheppard-Hanger, 1995).

Scientific comment

Due to the confusion over which of the chamomile essential oils (German or Roman) has been used in a number of recent studies, little is actually proven regarding Roman chamomile oil activity. There is very little anti-inflammatory potential as this essential oil has a different chemical composition to that of German essential oil, and it has virtually no antimicrobial activity. There is evidence that the Roman essential oil has an antispasmodic action on smooth muscle *in vitro* and that it has some relaxing properties shown in human brain studies, although it is unclear in some of the studies whether this species was used (A14). Massage itself could alleviate a number of stress symptoms and the fragrance alone could be useful for relaxation due to its pleasant relaxant odour or combined with massage for a stronger relaxant effect.

Herbal uses

Chamomile oil is a stomachic, antiemetic and mild sedative when taken orally. It has been used for dyspepsia, nausea, vomiting of pregnancy, anorexia, dysmenorrhoea and especially for flatulent dyspepsia due to mental stress. It is used as a lotion for toothache, earache and neuralgia and a cream or ointment for wounds, sore nipples and nappy rash. It is also used as a shampoo for blonde hair

(Wren, 1988; Chevallier, 1996; Blumenthal *et al.*, 2000; Barnes *et al.*, 2002).

Moroccan chamomile essential oil was originally produced solely for the perfumery and fragrance trades, but is still used as a substitute for Roman and German chamomile oils.

Food and perfumery uses

Food Roman chamomile (FEMA 2272, 2274) is used in many foods (Fenaroli, 1997).

Perfumery It is used in perfumes to a small extent (Arctander, 1960).

Chemistry
Major components

	Average % (Lawrence 1976–2001)
α-Pinene	0.5
β-Pinene	0.3
Isobutyl angelate	3.4
Methyl angelate	16
3-Methyl pentenyl isobutyrate	12
2-Methyl butyl angelate	4–25
3-Methyl butyl angelate	4–6
3-Methyl pentyl isovalerate	21

Another example of chemical composition of an essential oil from a different source showed:

α-Pinene	18.0
β-Pinene	2.9
Amyl butyrate + methyl angelate	1.9 + 4 (5.9)
Butyl angelates	1.0, 12.1, 9.5 (21.6)
Linalool	0.4
Amyl angelates	3, 7.2, 7.3, 1.0 (18.5)
Isopropyl tiglate	11.2

Minor components
Chamazulene 0–trace; sesquiterpene lactones 0.6% (A22), including nobilin, 3-epinobilin, 1,10-epoxynobilin, 3-dehydronobilin and anthemol (Hausen, 1979; Casterline, 1980; Hausen *et al.*, 1984; Mann and Staba, 1986; A22). This essential oil has one of the largest percentage of esters of all essential oils. These are very different to the usual esters of, for example, geranium, lavender, palmarosa, etc. Angelic and tiglic acid esters (85%) predominate; there are also esters of methyl butyric acid, methacrylic acid, isobutyric acid and

acetic acid. There is always difficulty in identifying many of these esters as they come in batches of dozens of peaks, which often consist of many different esters. The many peaks of, for example, angelates, are therefore often grouped together to give an overall percentage and the actual identification varies from one analytical chemist to another: the actual gas chromatographic pattern gives the best guide, but only to those with experience.

Adulteration
As the odour of this essential oil is very distinctive, it is difficult to sell it as German chamomile, even if it contains considerable amounts of blue chamazulene. However, the lower price of Moroccan chamomile, which is chemically different from both, encourages substitution (see also German chamomile monograph).

Toxicity
Acute toxicity (A22)
Oral LD$_{50}$ >5 g/kg (rats).

Dermal LD$_{50}$ >5 g/kg (rabbit).

Irritation and sensitisation
Roman chamomile oil is non-irritant and non-sensitising to human skin and mildly or non-irritant in animal models.

Allergic reactions
Cases of allergic and anaphylactic reactions to various chamomile plants and Asteraceae in general have been reported (see German chamomile oil monograph). The allergenic principles are thought to be the sesquiterpene lactones (e.g. nobilin) (Mann and Staba, 1986). Allergic contact dermatitis of the nipple from Roman chamomile ointment has been reported in lactating women (McGeorge and Steele, 1991).

Phototoxicity
None reported.

Drug interaction
Excessive doses may interfere with anticoagulant therapy due to the coumarin constituents.

Bioactivities

German and Roman chamomile are said to possess similar pharmacological activities; however, the results of various assays *in vitro*, given below, prove otherwise. Moroccan chamomile has a totally different composition (see German chamomile oil monograph).

Pharmacological activities *in vitro* and *in vivo*

Smooth muscle   There was an initial strong contractile action followed by a spasmolytic action on electrically stimulated smooth muscle of guinea-pig *in vitro* (A2; Lis-Balchin *et al.*, 1996a).

Uterus   There was a reduction in intensity to complete cessation of spontaneous contractions with higher dosage in the rat uterus *in vitro* (A3; A4; Lis-Balchin and Hart, 1997b).

Other activities   Although the essential oil has apparent anti-allergic and anti-inflammatory properties, these are mainly due to azulene and bisabolol – which are not found to any great extent in the essential oil (see German chamomile oil monograph).

The essential oil has shown anti-inflammatory activity (carrageenan rat paw oedema test), and antidiuretic and sedative effects following intraperitoneal administration of doses up to 350 mg/kg body weight to rats (Melegari *et al.*, 1988). The essential oil has sedative properties as shown by contingent negative variation studies, but the exact species was not given so it could have been the German essential oil (A5). A comfortable feeling was engendered by the odours of lavender, eugenol, chamomile and sandalwood in that order from highest to lowest effect. Significant changes in alpha 1 waves were observed after inhalation of eugenol or chamomile. These results showed that alpha 1 activity significantly decreased under odour conditions in which subjects felt comfortable (Masago *et al.*, 2000).

Antimicrobial activities

It is often impossible to determine which chamomile was used in any particular study, so only essential oil results from well-identified oils are shown.

Note: Samples of so-called Moroccan oil showed higher activities, but it is a different species, if not an adulterated essential oil.

Antibacterial activity

Relative data: Only 3–5/25 different bacteria were affected (A1; Lis-Balchin, Deans, 1997; Lis-Balchin *et al.*, 1998a, also 1/25 (Deans and Ritchie, 1987) and 0/20 *Listeria monocytogenes* varieties were affected (A1; Lis-Balchin and Deans, 1997;

Lis-Balchin *et al.*, 1998a) and in another report: 1/5 (Aureli *et al.*, 1992).

Antifungal activity

Relative data (% inhibition): Activity was very low against: *Aspergillus niger* −1–39%, *A. ochraceus* 5–26%, *Fusarium culmorum* −18–62% (A1). Note that there were two negative values, indicating fungal growth promotion!

Antioxidant activity

No antioxidant activity found (Lis-Balchin *et al.*, 1996a).

Miscellaneous activity

This is apparently the same as for German chamomile, although their chemical compositions are totally different. Roman chamomile is said to have sedative properties; however, the spasmogenic action found initially for the commercial Roman chamomile oils suggests both activities. Sedative, anti-inflammatory and antidiuretic effects were induced in rats by essential oils of two varieties of *Anthemis nobilis* (Rossi *et al.*, 1988) named 'white-headed' or double flowered and 'yellow-headed', which had considerable morphological differences and yielded essential oils with different composition: the white-flowered one was more anti-inflammatory.

Use in pregnancy and lactation: contraindications

Roman chamomile extracts may have abortifacient properties and may possibly affect the menstrual cycle (Farnsworth, 1975). In view of this, as well as the decrease and even cessation of uterine contractions *in vitro* in rats, and the potential for allergic reactions, the excessive use of chamomile on the skin during pregnancy and lactation should be avoided.

Pharmaceutical guidance

The bioactivity of Roman chamomile oil is rather confused in the literature with that of German chamomile. Due to the total differences in chemical composition, similar bioactivity is not expected. Limited pharmacological data are available for Roman chamomile, although many actions have been reported for German chamomile. Roman chamomile is of low toxicity and antimicrobial activity, although allergic reactions (mainly contact dermatitis) have been reported (Mitchell and Rook, 1979). In view of possible allergic reactions and cross-sensitivities (see German chamomile oil monograph), Roman chamomile is best avoided where hypersensitivity to any member of the Asteraceae/Compositae family has been shown, as it may also may precipitate an allergic reaction or exacerbate existing symptoms (e.g. asthma). There is no reason other than its possible allergic action to ban the use of this essential oil in aromatherapy massage and the use of the fragrance alone has been shown to be relaxant in studies on the human brain (A14). Combining massage with the fragrance could increase the relaxant effect, which may benefit many stress-related and muscular conditions.

Use in babies and young children

Due to the immaturity and the delicate nature of the skin of babies and young children, it is inadvisable for any essential oils to be used in massage, however much the essential oil has been diluted in the carrier oils. This is also a necessary precaution due to the possibilities of sensitisation of the children at this young age through skin or air-borne odorant effects (see Chapters 5 and 7).

Instillation or administration of essential oils near the baby or young child's nose is not only not recommended, but distinctly inadvisable, as there have been numerous cases reported of severe toxicity and even death from such applications (see Chapter 7).

Cinnamon Oil

CAS numbers

Bark: USA: 8015-91-6; EINECS: 283-479-0
Leaf: USA: 8007-80-5; EINACS: 283-479-0

Species/Botanical name

Cinnamomum zeylanicum Garc. ex Blume Nees (Lauraceae)

Synonyms

Cinnamomum verum J.S. Presl., true cinnamon, Ceylon cinnamon, aetheroleum cinnamomi zeylanici, ceylon cinnamon bark oil, cinnam. oil, cinnamoni zeylanicii corticus aetheroleum, esencia de canela, essence de cannelle de Ceylan, oleum cinnamomi, zimtöl

Other species

Cinnamomum burmanii (Nees) Bl., *Cinnamomum loureirii* Nees, Saigon cinnamon, *Laurus cinnamomum* (see also cassia oil monograph)

Pharmacopoeias

European Pharmacopoeia includes oil from both the bark and the leaf. Japanese Pharmacopoeia specifies oil from either *Cinnamomum cassia* or *Cinnamomum zeylanicum*.

Safety

CHIP details
Bark: Xn; R21, 43; 0%; S24, 36/37; leaf: none (A26)

RIFM recommended safety of use limits
Bark: 1%; leaf: 10% (A23)

EU sensitiser total
Bark: 89.5 (based on cinnamaldehyde); leaf: 95.5 (eugenol) plus cinnamyl alcohol, benzyl benzoate, limonene and linalool) (A27)

GRAS status
Both (Fenaroli, 1997).

Extraction, source, appearance and odour

Extraction
The essential oil is obtained by steam/water distillation of the bark or leaf of the tree. The different parts of the plant give an essential oil of totally different composition. Yield of the bark essential oil is up to 4% (Arctander, 1960).

Source
Sri Lanka, India, Burma, Indo-China and the Indonesian archipelago. Distillation is carried out in the USA and Europe to give a better quality oil.

Appearance and odour
Bark oil is a yellowish or brownish liquid, becoming darker and thicker by age and exposure to the air, with the characteristic odour of cinnamon – an extremely powerful, diffusive, warm, spicy and tenacious odour with a dry-out which is dry, powdery, dusty and warm and a sweetish, spicy, and burning taste (Arctander, 1960).

Leaf oil is yellow to brownish-yellow oil of spicy, warm, rather harsh odour, lacking the body of the bark oil. It is somewhat similar to both the clove bud and stem essential oil (Arctander, 1960).

Aromatherapy uses

Uses include: insect bites, oily skin, spots, abscess, acne, dermatitis, eczema; arthritis, rheumatism, muscular aches and pains; asthma, bronchitis, colds, sinusitis, sore throat; cystitis, urethritis, urinary infection; viral infections, flu; toothache, neuralgia, sciatica (Ryman, 1991; Lawless, 1992; Rose, 1992a,b; Price, 1993; Sheppard-Hanger, 1995).

Scientific comment

Cinnamon has been used for many thousands of years both as a vapour and in drinks and foods as preservative and for preventing infection (e.g. in mincemeat and the ingredient of 'beaks' worn by doctors in the sixteenth century as described in Chapter 2). Cinnamon essential oil has a high sensitisation index for both bark and clove, due to cinnamaldehyde and eugenol respectively (which are also irritant), which suggests that massage with the essential oils is ill-advised and the vapour alone should be used in moderation. The many uses stated by aromatherapists have not been credited with scientific evidence, however, massage alone can alleviate many stress and muscular conditions.

Herbal uses

Cinnamon is said to be antispasmodic, carminative, orexigenic, antidiarrhoeal, antimicrobial, refrigerant and anthelmintic. It has been used for anorexia, intestinal colic, infantile diarrhoea, common cold, influenza, and specifically for flatulent colic and dyspepsia with nausea (Wren, 1988; Chevallier, 1996; Blumenthal et al., 2000; Barnes et al., 2002).

Conventional uses

Pharmacopoeial: Cinnamon bark oil has properties and uses similar to those of cinnamon. It is also included in preparations for musculoskeletal and joint disorders and for respiratory tract disorders (Martindale, 2004), such as aromatic cardamom tincture, compound cardamom tincture, concentrated cinnamon water and tolu-flavour solution (BP 2003).

Food and perfumery uses

Food   Cinnamon bark oil (FEMA 2291) and leaf oil (FEMA 2292) are used in numerous processed foods and drinks (Fenaroli, 1997).

Perfumery   Leaf oil is used in perfumery in preference to bark oil, where its spicy notes blend in to produce woody-oriental perfumes (Arctander, 1960).

Chemistry

Major components

| | % (Lawrence, 1976–2001) | |
	Bark	Leaf
Cinnamaldehyde	60–75	1.3–2.0
p-Cymene	0.6–1.2	0.4–1.2
α-Pinene	0.2–0.6	0.2–1.0
Eugenol	0.8	70–96
Cinnamyl acetate	5.0	0.8–1.7
Caryophyllene	1.4–3.3	1.9–5.8
Benzyl benzoate	0.7–1.0	2.7–3.5

Minor components

Benzaldehyde, cuminaldehyde, phenols (4–10%) including, methyl eugenol and safrole, also phellandrene, eugenol acetate (the amount dependent on distillation conditions), methyl n-amyl ketone (giving characteristic notes) and linalool.

The bark and leaf oils differ in their main component: bark has cinnamaldehyde, the leaf oil has eugenol (the latter is commonly used in dentistry).

Apart from its use in food, cinnamon bark is used in dental preparations, gargles, dentifrices and perfumery, especially oriental perfumes where the warmth and spiciness of even 1% cinnamon bark oil gives great potential.

A cinnamon leaf oil of Chinese origin, *Cinnamomum japonicum* Sieb., contains a high concentration of safrole (60%) and only about 3% eugenol.

Cinnamon bark oil, Ceylon (Ph. Eur. 4.8) is obtained by steam distillation of the bark of the shoots of *Cinnamomum zeylanicum* (*C. verum*). It contains 55–75% cinnamaldehyde and less than 7.5% eugenol.

Cinnamon leaf oil, Ceylon (Ph. Eur. 4.8) is obtained by steam distillation of the leaves of *C. zeylanicum* (*C. verum*). It contains less than 3% cinnamaldehyde and 70–85% eugenol.

Adulteration

Cinnamon bark oil is often cut with cinnamon leaf oil and vice versa. Other adulterants used include canella bark oil (bark oil), clove and bay leaf oil (for the leaf oil). Synthetic eugenol and cinnamaldehyde are also used. Diluents can include fuel oil, kerosene and petroleum. Artificial cassia oil is often provided under the cinnamon bark oil label.

Clove leaf oil is often used to cut cinnamon leaf oil, being cheaper. Other diluents and components used are similar to those above (A8; see also Chapter 4).

Toxicity

Acute toxicity (A22)

Oral LD$_{50}$ Cinnamon bark 3.4 g/kg (rat); cinnamon leaf 2.7 g/kg (rat).

Dermal LD$_{50}$ Cinnamon bark 690 mg/kg body weight (rabbit); cinnamon leaf >5 g/kg (rabbit).

Irritation and sensitisation (A22)

Cinnamon bark oil contains cinnamaldehyde, which is an irritant and sensitising agent. An 8%

cinnamon bark oil produced sensitisation reactions in 18/25 and 20/25 subjects, but even a 0.01% dilution produced a reaction. Cinnamon oil burns were found in a child, where the oil had been in contact with the skin for 48 hours (Sparks, 1985). Many workers in a Swedish spice factory showed pruritus and skin irritation, particularly from cinnamon powder; patch test reactions to cinnamaldehyde were found in 11/25 factory workers and on prick testing 6/25 workers reacted to cinnamaldehyde (Meding, 1993).

Guinea-pig maximization tests (GPMT) performed with cinnamon compounds showed a certain degree of cross-reactivity between cinnamaldehyde, cinnamyl alcohol and cinnamic acid as animals sensitised to cinnamaldehyde reacted to the challenge with the three substances. Animals sensitised to cinnamyl alcohol reacted to cinnamyl alcohol and cinnamaldehyde, but not to cinnamic acid. Cinnamic acid did not sensitize. The study suggests that cinnamaldehyde is the 'true' allergen, while cinnamyl alcohol and cinnamic acid are transformed in the skin to cinnamaldehyde, before contact allergic reactions can occur (Weibel et al., 1989).

Sixteen patients developed a variety of oral lesions following a change in the toothpaste they used; mucosal biopsy demonstrated features consistent with the application of a topical medicament; patch testing towards the components of the toothpastes indicated that the flavouring agent cinnamaldehyde was the most likely responsible agent. Avoidance of the implicated toothpastes resulted in a considerable improvement in clinical signs and symptoms, whereas rechallenge in ten patients resulted in recurrence of symptoms in eight patients (Lamey et al., 1990).

The cinnamon component of chewing gum was discovered to be the aetiologic agent in an oral leukoplakic lesion that was clinically thought to be a squamous cell carcinoma; the case was unusual because of the leukoplakia noted as all other previously reported cases described erythematous patches only (Mihail, 1992).

Food or flavouring intolerance has been demonstrated in 14 out of 80 patients with oro-facial granulomatosis. Provoking molecules included cinnamaldehyde, carvone and piperitone, although a wide range of food or flavourings may be implicated; the reaction does not seem to involve an IgE-mediated response (Patton et al., 1985).

Fifty-six patients with chronic urticaria were patch tested with particular reference to the immediate weal response to a range of materials and this was followed by challenge tests to most of the same components. Positive immediate patch tests were commonly seen with balsam of Peru and cinnamon and this appears to be a reaction in many normal subjects. Positive challenge tests in patients who also had positive immediate patch tests to the same substance occurred in two patients with cinnamon and two patients with cloves (Warin and Smith, 1982).

Cinnamon and citronellol oil mixture is used for the detection of allergy to perfumes (Rudzki et al., 1976).

Leaf essential oil, with its highly sensitising and irritating eugenol content, is also very dangerous (see clove oil monograph).

New EU and IFRA guidance (European Union cosmetics) states that the concentration of cinnamic aldehyde in the finished cosmetic product should not exceed 0.1%. These extracts are: cassia oil and cinnamon bark oil; also cinnamyl alcohol-containing products should not be used such that the level in finished cosmetic products exceeds 0.8% (based on test results showing sensitising potential).

Drug interaction
Cinnamon leaf oil containing high eugenol concentrations is not recommended for people on anticoagulant therapy. The possible impairment of liver function by eugenol suggests caution in people with liver impairment, alcoholics and those on paracetamol.

Other toxicities
Cinnamon oil is easily obtained from pharmacies in 5–10 mL amounts for use as a flavouring agent and in craft items. Over a five-month period the Pittsburgh Poison Center (PPC) documented 32 cases of cinnamon oil abuse; all cases involved males aged 11–16 years and were reported to the PPC by school nurses. Sucking on toothpicks or fingers which had been dipped in cinnamon oil was the primary method of abuse. A rush or sensation of warmth, facial flushing and oral burning were the experiences reported by the users. Some children complained of nausea or abdominal pain but no systemic effects were reported. Eight patients with dermal exposure had irritation ranging from erythema to welts, which resolved after thorough soap and water decontamination. Two ocular exposures resulted in mild irritation and were successfully treated with irrigation or dilution (Perry et al., 1990).

Cinnamon aldehydes found in cinnamon-flavoured gums can incite mucosal alterations at points of contact with the oral mucosa. These alterations may include inflammation and epithelial proliferation, but as a rule the changes are reversible and promptly resolve when gum-chewing activity is discontinued. A 24-year-old woman developed a squamous cell carcinoma of the tongue following persistent and prolonged exposure to cinnamon-flavoured gum. Prompt withdrawal of cinnamon products is encouraged in heavy gum chewers who develop cinnamon-related oral lesions. For those lesions that do not promptly resolve upon cinnamon withdrawal diagnostic biopsy should be considered (Westra et al., 1998). Raw cinnamon (*Cinnamon zeylanicum*) is tumorigenic, inducing squamous papillomas in some and poorly differentiated carcinomas in others (Balachandran and Sivaramkrishnan, 1995).

Bioactivities

Pharmacological activities *in vitro* and *in vivo*

Smooth muscle Cinnamon leaf oil had a spasmolytic effect on electrically stimulated guinea-pig ileum *in vitro* (A2; Lis-Balchin et al., 1996a).

Uterus Cinnamon leaf decreased the spontaneous contractions in the rat uterus *in vitro* to zero (A3; A4; Lis-Balchin and Hart, 1997b).

Other activities Cinnamaldehyde increased plasma catecholamine concentration in anesthetised dogs given through intradermal (i.d.) or intravenous (i.v.) routes. Almost all the increased plasma catecholamine induced by i.v. or i.d. cinnamaldehyde was epinephrine. It was concluded that cinnamaldehyde entering the circulatory system reaches the adrenals and releases catecholamines through a mechanism(s) independent of the cholinergic system (Harada et al., 1976; Barnes et al., 2002).

Weak tumour-promoting activity on mouse skin and weak cytotoxic activity against HeLa cells was shown for eugenol (Leung, 1980).

Antimicrobial activities

Antibacterial activity

Relative data: Cinnamon leaf had a very strong antibacterial effect against 24/25 different bacteria 20/20 *Listeria monocytogenes* varieties (A1; Lis-Balchin and Deans, 1997; Lis-Balchin et al., 1998a). Cinnamon oil showed the highest bacteriostatic and fungistatic activities out of 22 essential oils tested (Yousef and Tawil, 1980). Cinnamon bark oil showed strong activity against several

respiratory tract bacteria (Inouye et al., 2001). Both cinnamon bark and leaf essential oil showed strong activity against four bacterial species (Friedman et al., 2002). A carbon dioxide extract of cinnamon bark (0.1%) suppressed completely the growth of numerous microorganisms including *Escherichia coli*, *Staphylococcus aureus* and *Candida albicans* (Leung, 1980).

There was strong antimicrobial action of cinnamon bark oil and clove bud oil *in vitro* against oral bacteria (Saeki et al., 1989). Oils of cinnamon, clove, bay and thyme were the most potent antimicrobials against *Campylobacter*, *Salmonella*, *E. coli*, *Staphylococcus aureus* and *Listeria* (Smith-Palmer et al., 1998). Cinnamon (alcoholic extract) was the most effective for inhibitory activity against *Helicobacter pylori* (Tabak et al., 1996).

Antifungal activity

Relative data (% inhibition): Strong activity was shown against *Aspergillus niger* 95%, *A. ochraceus* 94%, *Fusarium culmorum* 74% (A1). Mycelial growth of aflatoxin-producing *Aspergillus parasiticus* was halted by 0.1% cinnamon, thyme, oregano or cumin essential oils compared with 0.2–1% coriander, black pepper, mugwort, bay or rosemary essential oils (Tantaoui-Elaraki and Beraoud, 1994).

Anti-lice activity

Essential oils of cinnamon leaf, aniseed, red thyme, tea tree, peppermint and nutmeg were effective (*in vitro*) against lice (*Pediculus humanus*) in a single study (Veal, 1996).

Clinical studies

These were using extracts not essential oils and also *trans*-cinnamaldehyde and O-methoxycinnamaldehyde against resistant *Candida* and candidiasis in HIV patients (Barnes et al., 2002).

Use in pregnancy and lactation: contraindications

Neither cinnamon leaf or bark oil is recommended for massage during pregnancy due to the possible cessation of spontaneous contractions in the uterine muscle and the irritant nature of the essential oils. Either essential oil can be used as a fragrance.

Pharmaceutical guidance

Both the bark and leaf oils of cinnamon have many adverse effects and great caution must be shown in their usage. Contact with cinnamon bark or oil on the skin is not advised as they are dermal and mucous membrane irritants and sensitisers and may cause an allergic reaction (Weibel *et al.*, 1989). The essential oils should not be taken internally. The International Fragrance Association (IFRA) recommends that the bark oil should not be used above 0.2% and is best avoided. Cinnamon leaf oil containing high eugenol concentrations is not recommended for people on anticoagulant therapy. Also, because of possible adulteration with the bark essential oil it should be avoided. The possible impairment of liver function by eugenol suggests caution in people with liver impairment, alcoholics and those on paracetamol. There is also the problem of adulteration with a high safrol-containing cinnamon species, which is carcinogenic.

The recent reports of cinnamon oil abuse and the fact that cinnamaldehyde provokes an increase in adrenaline levels in the blood suggests that the essential oil is liable to be used as a drug of abuse. Inhalation of concentrated vapours should be avoided, but both essential oils can be used occasionally as fragrances in moderate concentrations.

Use in babies and young children

Due to the immaturity and the delicate nature of the skin of babies and young children, it is inadvisable for any essential oils, especially these essential oils with strong irritant and sensitisation potential, to be used in massage, however much the essential oil has been diluted in the carrier oils. This is also a necessary precaution due to the possibilities of sensitisation of the children at this young age through skin or air-borne odorant effects (see Chapters 5 and 7).

Instillation or administration of essential oils near the baby or young child's nose is not only not recommended, but distinctly inadvisable, as there have been numerous cases reported of severe toxicity and even death from such applications (see Chapter 7).

Citronella Oil

CAS numbers

Ceylon: USA: 8000-29-1; EINECS: 289-753-6;
Java: USA: 8000-29-1; EINECS: 289-753-6

Species/Botanical name

Cymbopogon nardus L.(Rendle) (Poaceae, formerly Gramineae)

Synonyms

Andropogon nardus L., *Andropogon nardus* Ceylon de Jong. Essential oil from *Cympobogon nardus* is commercially known as Ceylon-type citronella oil and the oil from *Cymbopogon winterianus* is called Java citronella oil. Citronellae aetheroleum, oleum citronellae.

Other species

Cymbopogon winterianus Jowitt

Pharmacopoeias

In European Pharmacopoeia.

Safety

CHIP details

Ceylon: Xn; R10, 65; 15%; S62; Java: none (A26)

RIFM recommended safety of use limits

1% (A23)

EU sensitiser total

Ceylon citronella and Java citronella essential oils have a value of 45.1 and 46.1% respectively (based on citral, eugenol, geraniol, citronellol, limonene and linalool) (A27).

GRAS status

Granted (Fenaroli, 1997).

Extraction, source, appearance and odour

Extraction

The essential oil is obtained by steam distillation of the dried grass (Arctander, 1960).

Source

Sri Lanka, Java, Formosa, Taiwan, Indonesia, India, China and Argentina.

Appearance

A pale to dark yellow liquid. The Ceylon oil has a warm floral, lemony, woody odour with a rose nuance and a fresh top-note of citronellal, more pleasant than the Java type. The Java essential oil is darker with a more pronounced aldehyde note. Java-type oil has a fresh, citrusy, somewhat lemon-like odour; it has the image of a cheap perfumery product for household soap (Arctander, 1960).

Aromatherapy uses

Citronella essential oil uses include: fatigue, headache, migraine, neuralgia, rheumatism, arthritis pain, depression; speeding up heart-beat; stomach ache, colitis, intestinal parasites; excessive perspiration, oily skin and hair; insect repellant (Ryman, 1991; Lawless, 1992; Rose, 1992a; Price, 1993; Sheppard-Hanger, 1995).

Scientific comment

Citronella essential oil has a relaxant effect on smooth muscle and a moderate antimicrobial effect, but due to its potential irritation and sensitisation potential due to citral, which should be avoided (Geldof *et al.*, 1992), it cannot be recommended for massaging into the skin. Massage alone can relieve many stress-related and muscular problems and citronella could be used with massage just as a fragrance.

Herbal uses

It was apparently used as a herbal remedy for colds, fatigue, headache, neuralgia (Lawless, 1992) but citronella, like Moroccan chamomile, clary sage, geranium, rosewood, vetiver and ylang ylang were originally produced solely for the perfumery and fragrance trades, so have no traditional uses.

Food and perfumery uses

Food Citronella oil (FEMA 2308) is used in numerous foods and beverages (Fenaroli, 1997).

Perfumery It is used in many perfumes. Ceylon-type oil is useful in fresh floral compounds for all purposes. Java essential oil, in low dosage, can impart freshness even in high-class perfume compounds. The oil is useful in herbal compounds for cosmetic purposes, such as shampoos (Arctander, 1960).

Chemistry

Major components
Citronella (Sri Lanka): ISO 3849:2003.

	%
α-Pinene	2.2
Camphene	7.6
Myrcene	0.8
Limonene	11.3*
cis-Ocimene	2.1
Citronellal	14.7
Borneol	4.8
Citronellol	6.2*
Geraniol	17.0*
Bornyl acetate	0.5
Citronellyl acetate	1.1
Geranyl acetate	2.1
trans-Methyl isoeugenol	10.1

*Sensitisers.

Ceylon citronella oil consists of ±60% monoterpene alcohols (calculated as geraniol) and ±10% aldehydes. Java citronella oil contains not less than 35% monoterpene alcohols and a minimum of 35% aldehydes, mainly citronellal. The odour of freshly cut grass is due to *cis*- or (*Z*)-3-hexenol and *trans*- or (*E*)-2-hexenal, also called leaf alcohol and leaf aldehyde respectively; the scent of hay is due to coumarin and dihydrocoumarin. These compounds are formed from coumarinic acid derivatives during drying of the grass. Citronella grasses belong to one of the most extensive plant families in the world, consisting of more than 500 genera with over 5000 species. The group of aromatic tropical grasses includes the genus *Cymbopogon*, which comprises about 40 species. Others are lemongrass oil from *Cymbopogon citratus* (DC) Stapf. or *Cymbopogon flexuosus* Stapf. and palmarosa oil from *Cymbopogon martinii* (Roxb.) Stapf. var. *motia*, also known as *Cymbopogon martinii* (Roxb.) Wats var. *martinii*. There is also gingergrass oil from *Cymbopogon martinii* Stapf., var. *sofia*, which has a harsher, terpeny,

somewhat fatty, herbal and cumin-like odour with a rose nuance and a woody undertone. Gingergrass oil contains ±35% monoterpene hydrocarbons, mainly limonene, and ±50% menthadienols. It has a harsh odour (BACIS). The oil does not contain the camphene-borneol notes characteristic of the Ceylon citronella oil.

One type of labelling for citronella oil Java type is expressed in total geraniol and citronellal, e.g. 85/35, which means that this oil contains a maximum of 85% geraniol and citronellal and various alcohols, and a minimum of 35% aldehydes, calculated as citronellal. A good oil should contain at least 40% citronellal and it may contain up to 95% total geraniol.

Citronella (Ph. Eur. 4.8) contains 30.0–45.0% citronellal, 9.0–15.0% citronellol, 2.0–4.0% citronellyl acetate, less than 2.0% geranial, 20.0–25.0% geraniol, 3.0–8.0% geranyl acetate, 1.0–5.0% limonene, and less than 2.0% neral.

Adulteration
Citronella is a cheap essential oil, produced from a grass, which is easily grown, therefore adulteration is unlikely. However, citronella itself is used to adulterate geranium and rose oils. The two types of citronella essential oil are often mixed (A8; see also Chapter 4).

Toxicity

Acute toxicity (A22)
Oral LD$_{50}$ >5 g/kg (rat).

Dermal LD$_{50}$ 3.4–6.7 g/kg (rabbit).

Irritation and sensitisation (A22)
Applied neat to rabbit skin citronella oil caused irritation. None at 8% (human); 5/22 patients with dermatitis were sensitive to citronella oil (A22). Several cases of eczematous, contact-type hypersensitivity have been reported; also folliculitis, papulovesicular eczema of hands (A22). It is noted as a primary irritant in perfumery.

Bioactivities

Pharmacological activities *in vitro* and *in vivo*
Smooth muscle Citronella oil had a strong spasmolytic effect on electrically-stimulated guinea-pig ileum *in vitro* (A2; Lis-Balchin *et al.*, 1996a).

Uterus There was a decrease in the spontaneous contractions in the rat uterus when citronella oil and its main components were applied *in vitro* (A3; A4; Lis-Balchin and Hart, 1997b).

Antimicrobial activities

Antibacterial activity
There was moderate activity against 14/25 different bacterial species (Deans and Ritchie, 1987) and the vapour was effective against 2/5 bacteria (Maruzella and Sicurella, 1960). Citronella essential oil had moderate activity against five bacteria (Friedman *et al.*, 2002).

Antifungal effect
Low activity was found against 14/15 fungi, which was mainly fungistatic (Maruzella and Liguori, 1958) and against 5/5 fungi (Maruzella, 1960). Mixed with cedarwood and other essential oils it was used against mosquitoes before DDT, etc. was available.

Use in pregnancy and lactation: contraindications

There is a loss of spontaneous contractions in the uterus when the essential oil was applied *in vitro*, which suggests caution of usage during pregnancy and parturition. There is also the problem of irritation and sensitisation when applied on the skin, especially if sensitive, which is more likely during pregnancy. It could possibly be used sparingly as a fragrance.

Pharmaceutical guidance

There is scant pharmacological information available regarding citronella and, due to its irritation and sensitisation potential, it should not be used in massage, especially on sensitive or damaged skin. It may be used as a fragrance in low concentrations.

Use in babies and young children

Due to the immaturity and the delicate nature of the skin of babies and young children, it is inadvisable for any essential oils to be used in massage, however much the essential oil has been diluted in the carrier oils. This is also a necessary precaution due to the possibilities of sensitisation of the children at this young age through skin or air-borne odorant effects (see Chapters 5 and 7).

Instillation or administration of essential oils near the baby or young child's nose is not only not recommended, but distinctly inadvisable, as there have been numerous cases reported of severe toxicity and even death from such applications (see Chapter 7).

Clary Sage Oil

CAS numbers

USA: 8016-63-5; EINECS: 84775-83-7

Species/Botanical name

Salvia sclarea L (Labiatae)

Synonyms

Clary wort, clear eye, common clary, eye-bright

Safety

CHIP details
None

RIFM recommended safety of use limits
8% (A23)

EU sensitiser total
22.7 (based on geraniol 2%, limonene 0.7% and linalool 20%) (A27)

GRAS status
Granted (Fenaroli, 1997).

Extraction, source, appearance and odour

Extraction
The essential oil is obtained from steam distilled tops of the herb (Arctander, 1960). Different plant species of *Salvia* give an essential oil of totally different composition (see sage oil monograph).

Source
Southern Europe, Russia, USA and Morocco.

Appearance and odour
Salvia sclarea is a colourless to pale yellow or olive liquid. The strong, pungent and penetrating (disliked) odour of fresh plant material of *Salvia sclarea* largely disappears during steam distillation and the oil has a fresh, floral, dry, sweet-herbaceous, weedy odour with a bitter-sweet undertone and an amber-like or tobacco- and tea-like note and a balsamic nuance dry-out, which is not pleasant for everybody (Arctander, 1960).

Clary sage should be distilled fresh, otherwise a considerable amount of volatile oil is lost by evaporation. The essential oil yield is approximately 0.1–0.15%.

Concrete: Appearance: green, wax-like mass (Arctander, 1960).

Aromatherapy uses

Uses include: depression, nervous tension, fatigue, stress; strengthening the nervous system (nervine); skin conditions, gastric complaints; controlling menstrual spasms and labour pains; haemorrhoids, varicose veins, diabetes, menopause, premenstrual syndrome, vaginitis, epilepsy, inflammation and wrinkles. It is apparently mildly intoxicating and euphoric and enhances dreaming (Ryman, 1991; Lawless, 1992; Rose, 1992a; Price, 1993; Sheppard-Hanger, 1995).

Scientific comment

Clary sage has an immense reputation in aromatherapy, but no real scientific proof exists for its usage. Its high linalool content makes it liable to cause sensitisation and the odour is also very unpleasant to most people. The essential oil is said to be very sedative and large doses can induce narcotic effect; however, this is unlikely to alleviate most of the conditions listed above and massage itself has a beneficial effect on stress-related symptoms and muscular problems.

Herbal uses

Clary sage essential oil was originally produced solely for the perfumery and fragrance trades but the herb was used in the Middle Ages for digestion, kidney, uterine and menstrual complaints, menopause, cleansing ulcers and nerve tonic. It cools inflammation and is useful for throat and respiratory infection. Nowadays it is used for digestive conditions and kidney disease. The seeds were used to treat eye infection, hence the name 'clear eye'. It was also used in a decoction for drawing out splinters (Wren, 1988; Lawless, 1992; Chevallier, 1996).

Food and perfumery uses

Food Clary sage oil (FEMA 2321) is used in major food products: frozen dairy desserts, candy, baked goods, gelatins and puddings, condiments, relishes and non-alcoholic beverages, also alcoholic beverages (vermouths, etc.) and especially in liqueurs (to flavour wines and liqueurs with a muscatel flavour), other wine essences and grape flavours. Highest average maximum use level reported is about 0.016% (155 ppm) for the oil in alcoholic beverages (Fenaroli, 1997).

Perfumery It is used in perfumery in chypres bases, fougeres, orientals and modern creations, especially with aldehydic notes; it is also used as a modifier for bergamot and lavender oils (Arctander, 1960) and has a somewhat wine-like odour and is reminiscent of ambergris (Guenther, 1948–52). It lends tenacity to colognes. The dry-out is tobacco- and tea-like with a balsamic nuance (Arctander, 1960). It blends well with most oils, especially bergamot, jasmine, juniper, lavender, neroli, petitgrain, pine, frankincense, vetiver, geranium, sandalwood, cedarwood and citrus. Clary sage oil is used as a fragrance component in soaps, detergents, creams, lotions and perfumes. Maximum use level reported for the oil in perfumes is 0.8% (Arctander, 1960).

Chemistry

Major components

	% (Lawrence, 1976–2001)
Linalyl acetate	63–80 (5% in concrete)
Linalool	8–28
β-Caryophyllene	1–2
Sclareol	0.8–2 (70% in concrete)
Germacrene D	0.4–4

Minor components
Over 250 components and the trace ones give the characteristic odour: main olfactively characteristic is salvial-4(14)-en-1-one, also dihydropyran, some cyclic ethers, gamma-lactones, (+)-spathulenol, (+)-isospathulenol and sclareol. After the essential oil is removed by distillation, the crude material is used as a source of sclareol, which can be solvent extracted from the plant and converted to sclareolide; both of which are used in the flavouring of tobaccos.

Adulteration
Synthetic linalool and linalyl acetate may be added or lavender/lavandin oils or *Mentha citrata* oil, etc.

Toxicity

Acute toxicity
Oral LD$_{50}$ >5 g/kg (rat).

Dermal LD$_{50}$ 2 g/kg body weight (rabbit).

Irritation and sensitisation
Clary sage oil from this species was irritant to abraded rabbit skin when applied under occlusion. No irritation or sensitisation was observed for humans at 8% (Opdyke, 1974; A22). In several cases of dermatitis attributed to sage, positive patch test reactions were obtained from the mucous membranes but not from the skin (A22).

Clary sage oil produced positive reactions in 2/60 perfumery workers who had dermatitis (Gutman and Somov, 1968). In another study 1/200 dermatitis patients were affected (Rudzki *et al.*, 1976).

Phototoxicity
None reported.

Bioactivities

Pharmacological activities *in vitro* and *in vivo*

Smooth muscle There was an initial spasmogenic effect followed by a spasmolytic effect on guinea-pig ileum *in vitro* (A2; Lis-Balchin *et al.*, 1996a).

Uterus The essential oil and some of its components caused a decrease in the spontaneous contractions of rat uterus *in vitro* (A3; A4; Lis-Balchin and Hart, 1997b).

Other activities *Salvia sclarea* oil and its main components have some anti-inflammatory and peripheral analgesic action (Moretti *et al.*, 1997). *Salvia sclarea* had a spasmolytic effect on smooth muscle. A 5% emulsion of the essential oil in physiological solution given intravenously to cats (5–10 mg/kg) increased respiratory volume and depressed blood pressure. Guinea-pigs given the essential oil in doses of 35 mg/kg intraperitoneally after preliminary sensitisation with egg albumen went into anaphylactic shock. The spasmolytic effect is considered to be chiefly myotropic (Shipochliev, 1968).

Antimicrobial activities

Antibacterial activity
Relative data: Moderate action was shown against 11–18/25 different bacteria and 9–15/20 *Listeria monocytogenes* species, in different commercial

samples (A1; Lis-Balchin and Deans, 1997; Lis-Balchin *et al.*, 1998a); 1/5 bacteria were affected by the vapour (Maruzella and Sicurella, 1960).

Antifungal activity

Relative data (% inhibition): *Aspergillus niger* 72–92%; *A. ochraceus* 91–96%; *Fusarium culmorum* 67–69% (A1). Other work showed slight action against 3/5 fungi (Maruzella, 1960).

Use in pregnancy and lactation: contraindications

This essential oil is quoted widely in the aromatherapy literature as being oestrogenic, but clear scientific evidence has not been forthcoming. However, due to the spasmolytic effect on the uterus *in vitro*, caution should be used in pregnancy and parturition. Sensitisation due to the linalool present may also occur.

Pharmaceutical guidance

Clary sage has an immense reputation in aromatherapy, but no real scientific proof exists for its use. The presence of linalool in large quantities makes it liable to cause sensitisation. The odour is also very unpleasant to most people. The essential oil is said to be very sedative and large doses can induce narcotic effect and cause headaches. It is reputed to slow one down, and brings on a feeling of euphoria, making concentration difficult. The effect of clary sage can be comparable to that of cannabis in some people, who feel drugged after using the essential oil in aromatherapy massage (Tisserand and Balacs, 1995). Caution should therefore be used with this essential oil.

Use in babies and young children

Due to the immaturity and the delicate nature of the skin of babies and young children, it is inadvisable for any essential oils to be used in massage, however much the essential oil has been diluted in the carrier oils. This is also a necessary precaution due to the possibilities of sensitisation of the children at this young age through skin or air-borne odorant effects (see Chapters 5 and 7).

Instillation or administration of essential oils near the baby or young child's nose is not only not recommended, but distinctly inadvisable, as there have been numerous cases reported of severe toxicity and even death from such applications (see Chapter 7).

Clove Oil

CAS numbers

Bud/leaf/stem: USA: 8000-34-8; EINECS: 84961-50-2

Species/Botanical name

Syzygium aromaticum (L.) Merr. & Perry (Myrtaceae)

Synonyms

Caryophyllus aromaticus L., *Eugenia aromatica* (L.) Baill., *Eugenia caryophyllata* Thunb., *Eugenia caryophyllus* (Spreng.) Bull. & Harr., Ol. caryoph., caryophylli floris aetheroleum, esencia de clavo, essence de girofle, nelkenöl, oleum caryophylli

Pharmacopoeias

In European and Japanese Pharmacopoeias. Also in United States National Formulary.

Safety

CHIP details
Bud: Xn; R65; 15%; S62; leaf: Xn; R21/22; 15%; S36/37, 62; stem: Xn; R65; 15%; S62 (A26)

RIFM recommended safety of use limits
Bud: 4%; leaf: 2%; stem: 4% (A23)

EU sensitiser total
92.3 (based on eugenol, 92% and isoeugenol, 0.3%) (A27)

GRAS status
Granted (Fenaroli, 1997).

Extraction, source, appearance and odour

Extraction

A volatile oil is obtained by steam/water distillation of the buds or stems. To extract the whole of the oil from cloves, there must be repeated cohobations. Yields: clove bud oil: 15–18% essential oil; stem oil: 4–6%; leaf oil: 2% (Arctander, 1960).

Source
Madagascar, Indonesia, Comoro and Zanzibar. Distillation is mainly done in Europe or the USA.

Appearance and odour
Bud oil is colourless to yellow-brown, darkening on ageing, with a strong clove aroma. Leaf oil is yellow (rectified) to dark brown (crude) when fresh, but turns dark violet on ageing in iron vessels. It has a eugenol odour with a harsh, phenolic, slightly sweet, with burnt notes; overall it has woody and dry notes. The rectified oil is yellow and smells sweeter, less harsh and burnt and more like eugenol than the crude. Stem oil is somewhat similar to the leaf oil – pale yellow to straw yellow with a strong spicy, woody odour (Arctander, 1960).

Clove bud absolute is also produced from clove bud concrete. Also clove bud oleoresin (Arctander, 1960).

Aromatherapy uses

Uses include: insect bites; oily skin, spots; arthritis, rheumatism, muscular aches and pains; asthma, bronchitis, colds, sinusitis, sore throat; cystitis, urethritis, urinary infection; viral infections, flu; abscess, acne, dermatitis, eczema, toothache, neuralgia, sciatica (Ryman, 1991; Lawless, 1992; Rose, 1992a; Price, 1993; Sheppard-Hanger, 1995).

Scientific comment

Clove essential oil is both a stimulant and a relaxant as shown by different parameters of study (A14), but of more relevance is its stimulant action on the human brain. It is also an extremely potent antimicrobial. However, its sensitisation potential is exceedingly high and its use on the skin should be limited. The fragrance can, however, be used to combat microbial infection and as a stimulant, although the use of the massage combined with the fragrance could be contradictory.

Herbal uses

Clove is used as a carminative, antiemetic, toothache remedy and counter-irritant. Cloves are considered to be a stimulant and to improve the memory; they are used as an aphrodisiac in India. They also apparently stimulate and strengthen the uterine muscle contractions in labour (Wren, 1988; Chevallier, 1996; Blumenthal *et al.*, 2000; Barnes *et al.*, 2002).

Conventional uses

Pharmacopoeial: Clove oil itself is a carminative, used in the treatment of flatulent colic and for toothache (applied directly). Mixed with zinc oxide, it is used as a temporary anodyne dental filling, although eugenol is often preferred. Clove oil is included as a counter-irritant in preparations for musculoskeletal and joint disorders (Martindale, 2004), such as aromatic cardamom tincture (BP 2003).

Food and perfumery uses

Food   Clove oil (FEMA 2323 (bud), FEMA 2325 (leaf) and FEMA 2328 (stem)) are used in a wide variety of foods and beverages. Bud oil is also used in pharmaceutical and dental products (Fenaroli, 1997). In humans, the accepted daily intake of eugenol is up to 2.5 mg/kg body weight (Martindale, 1989).

Perfumery   Bud oil is used in perfumery in orientals and to form the basis of carnation, rose and honeysuckle perfumes. Rectified leaf oil is used in spicy perfumes and low-grade cosmetics and soaps. Stem oil again is used in oriental type perfumes (Arctander, 1960).

Chemistry

Major components

	% (Lawrence, 1976–2001)		
	Clove bud	Leaf	Stem
Eugenol	36–90*	75–90	85–95
Eugenyl acetate	11–27	trace–10	trace–5
β-Caryophyllene	trace–16	15–19	2.5–3.5
α-Humulene	trace–2	1.5–2.5	0.3–0.4

* Should contain 82–88% eugenol.
Oil of clove leaf (ISO 3141: 1997).
ISO for clove stem: 3143: 1997 and clove bud: 3142: 1997

Minor components

Methyl salicylate, methyl eugenol, benzaldehyde, methyl amyl ketone and α-ylangene.

All the essential oils are used in the production of eugenol especially the stem and leaf oils, which are cheaper.

Clove oil (Ph. Eur. 4.8) is a clear yellow liquid obtained by steam distillation from clove containing 75.0–88.0% of eugenol.

Clove oil (USNF 22) is a volatile oil distilled with steam from clove. It contains not less than 85.0% of phenolic substances, chiefly eugenol.

Adulteration

Clove bud oil is the most expensive of these essential oils and is commonly adulterated by the other two essential oils, or substituted by them. The price of the synthetic eugenol and isoeugenol is higher than that of the essential oils, therefore unlikely to be used (A8; see also Chapter 4).

Toxicity

Acute toxicity (A22)

Oral LD_{50}   Clove bud >2.7–3.7 g/kg; clove leaf 1.4 g/kg; clove stem 2–3.7 g/kg (rat).

Dermal LD_{50}   Clove bud >5 g/kg; clove leaf 1.2 g/kg; clove stem >5 g/kg (rabbit).

Irritation and sensitisation (A22)

Clove bud oil: None at 5% (human) and at 0.2% in dermatoses patients. At 20% in an ointment 2/25 subjects showed dermal irritation – erythema.
Clove leaf oil: None at 5%.
Clove stem oil: None at 10% and at 0.2% in dermatoses patients; at 20% in an ointment, 2/25 subjects showed dermal irritation – erythema.

Note: Clove oil is now considered a very hazardous sensitiser. Clove oil is a dermal and mucous membrane irritant; it has caused contact dermatitis, cheilitis and stomatitis, mainly due to eugenol, which also has sensitising properties (Mitchell and Rook, 1979). A woman had right infra-orbital anaesthesia after trying to apply clove oil directly to the neck of an upper premolar to relieve toothache a year before and the oil had spilt onto her face. She had a dry, erythematous region extending from the inferior eyelid to the upper lip and within it sensation was reduced to that of deep pressure and she had anhidrosis. The clove spillage caused minor transient irritation followed by permanent local anaesthesia, presumably due to a direct neurotoxic effect (Isaacs, 1983).

Phototoxicity

None reported in the literature, however, personal experience of putting undiluted clove oil on a cold sore in bright sunlight led to severe burns and spread of the viral sores down the chin with a concomitant phototoxic reaction.

Drug interactions

Eugenol is a powerful inhibitor of platelet activity and caution must be exercised for patients on anticoagulant therapy, even aspirin (Tisserand and Balacs, 1995; see also cinnamon oil monograph).

Bioactivities

Pharmacological activities *in vitro* and *in vivo*

Smooth muscle Relative data: Clove oils had a spasmolytic effect on electrically stimulated guinea-pig ileum *in vitro* (A2; Lis-Balchin et al., 1996a).

Uterus Clove oil and eugenol caused a dramatic decrease in the spontaneous contractions of rat uterus *in vitro* (A3; A4; Lis-Balchin and Hart, 1997b).

Other activities Eugenol is probably responsible for the anodyne and mild antiseptic properties of clove oil (Leung, 1980). Eugenol is applied directly to the tooth in the case of toothache but repeated applications may result in damage to the gingival tissue (Martindale, 1989). Eugenol, eugenol acetate and methyl acetate exhibited trypsin-potentiating activity and clove oil has both antihistaminic and antispasmodic properties (Leung, 1980). Clove essential oil is both a stimulant (contingent negative variation studies) and a relaxant (smooth muscle studies) (A14).

Antimicrobial activities

The strong antimicrobial action of clove oils is universally accepted.

Antibacterial activity

Relative data: Clove oil (commercial) was effective against 24/25 different bacterial species and 20/20 *Listeria monocytogenes* varieties (A1; Lis-Balchin and Deans, 1997; Lis-Balchin et al., 1998a). Oils of bay, cinnamon, clove and thyme were the most effective against *Campylobacter, Salmonella, E. coli, Staphylococcus aureus* and *Listeria* (Smith-Palmer et al., 1998). Strong antibacterial action was shown against four different bacterial species (Friedman et al., 2002) and against 24/25 different species (Deans and Ritchie, 1987); 5/5 *Listeria* varieties were affected (Aureli et al., 1992); clove oil vapour affected 2/5 bacteria (Maruzella and Sicurella, 1960).

Antifungal activity

Clove bud and leaf oils: Relative data (% inhibition): *Aspergillus niger* 95%; *A. ochraceus* 94%; *Fusarium culmorum* 74% (A1).

Variable results were obtained for the clove bud, leaf and stem oils, giving from poor to good results against 5/5 fungal species (Maruzella, 1960); clove oil was active against 15/15 fungi (Maruzella and Liguori, 1958). Clove and cinnamon oils were very effective on the growth of aflatoxin production by *A. flavus* (Sinha et al., 1993).

Antioxidant action

Clove bud and leaf oils had strong antioxidant activity (Lis-Balchin et al., 1996a).

Clinical studies

A tincture of cloves (15% in 70% alcohol) was effective in treating athlete's foot (Leung, 1980).

Use in pregnancy and lactation: contraindications

The clove oils are very irritant and also potential sensitisers; they are also capable of dramatically decreasing the spontaneous contractions of rat uterus *in vitro* and may therefore prove hazardous in pregnancy and parturition. Neither clove oils nor eugenol are recommended in aromatherapy massage, but can be used as a fragrance in small doses.

Pharmaceutical guidance

The pharmacological properties of clove oils are mainly linked to the main component eugenol, which has both irritant and sensitisation potentials. It is therefore advisable not to massage clove oils on the skin in aromatherapy. Their pleasant, possibly stimulant aroma, as shown by studies on the human brain (A14), can however prove beneficial.

Warnings: Do not use in the bath. Do not use as a local rub for any rheumatic or painful conditions. Do not store the oil in a plastic container as it dissolves it rapidly.

Caution must be observed with patients on anticoagulant therapy, even aspirin (see also cinnamon oil monograph), as eugenol is a powerful inhibitor of platelet activity. People with kidney, liver disease, prostatic cancer or alcoholism should apparently avoid clove oils, although this warning was for oral intake. Avoid massage with this essential oil where there is damaged skin (Tisserand and Balacs, 1995). As aromatherapy often includes medicinal application of essential oils, the use of clove essential oil must be carefully controlled as a remedy in toothache (where it can cause damage to the gingival tissue) and in athlete's foot (where it can be painful and severely damage the skin).

Use in babies and young children

Due to the immaturity and the delicate nature of the skin of babies and young children, it is inadvisable for any essential oils, especially these irritant and sensitising essential oils, to be used in massage, however much the essential oil has been diluted in the carrier oils. This is also a necessary precaution due to the possibilities of sensitisation of the children at this young age through skin or air-borne odorant effects (see Chapters 5 and 7).

Instillation or administration of essential oils near the baby or young child's nose is not only not recommended, but distinctly inadvisable, as there have been numerous cases reported of severe toxicity and even death from such applications (see Chapter 7).

Cornmint Oil

CAS numbers

USA: 68917-18-0; EINECS: 90063-97-1

Species/Botanical name

Mentha arvensis var. *piperascens* Holmes

Synonyms

Field mint, Japanese mint

Other species

Mentha spicata L. (spearmint), *Mentha viridis*, L., *Mentha × piperita* L. (Lamiaceae), hybrid of *M. spicata × M. aquatica* L. (peppermint)

Safety

CHIP details

Xn; R22 (A26)

RIFM recommended safety of use limits

8% (A23)

EU sensitiser total

7% (based on limonene) (A27)

GRAS status

Granted (Fenaroli, 1997).

Extraction, source, appearance and odour

Extraction

A volatile oil is obtained by steam distillation of freshly harvested, flowering sprigs. Cornmint is dementholised by freezing the essential oil and retrieving 40% of the menthol by precipitation. The now dementholised essential oil still contains 55% menthol which can be converted, together with the bitter menthone, by chemical means, to isomers of menthol; the menthol is then removed again (Arctander, 1960).

Source

USA, China, India, South America, Italy and Japan.

Appearance and odour

Cornmint is a pale yellow or almost colourless essential oil, similar to peppermint, but stronger due to extra menthol and has a bitter-sweet odour with a harsh-woody undertone and a bitter-herbaceous dry-out (Arctander, 1960).

Aromatherapy uses

See peppermint oil monograph.

Scientific comment

See peppermint oil monograph.

Herbal uses

Known in China as Bo He, cornmint has been used for thousands of years for colds, sore throats, sore mouth and tongue, toothache, lowering temperature, dysentery and diarrhoea (Chevallier, 1996). See also peppermint oil monograph.

Other uses

Mint oil (usually dementholised cornmint) is used in a cream (Uddermint) to prevent and treat mastitis in cows (from Teisen Products Ltd, Redditch, UK).

Food and perfumery uses

Cornmint is not listed for food usage but is often used as peppermint essential oil after dementholisation. Spearmint (FEMA 3032) is used in similar products (Fenaroli, 1997).

All mints have a cool feeling on the mucous membranes in the nose and mouth and on the skin. They are used in toothpastes.

Perfumery   Limited usage (Arctander, 1960).

Chemistry

| | % (Lawrence, 1976–2001) | | |
	Peppermint	Spearmint	Cornmint*
Menthol	27–50	0.1–0.3	65–80 (38)
Menthone	13–32	0.7–2	3–15 (31)
Isomenthone	2–10	trace	1.9–4.8 (12)
1,8-Cineole	5–14	1–2	0.1–0.3 (0.2–0.8)
Limonene	1–3	8–12	0.7–6.2 (10)
Carvone	0	58–70	0

*Brackets indicate values for dementholised cornmint oil.

Adulteration

Cornmint is cheaper than peppermint as it grows wild and is frequently used to dilute or even be a substitute for the peppermint oil. Adulteration is difficult to detect even when it is added at 85% to pure peppermint oil, as the colour test for menthofuran remains constant, even when it is diluted. Dementholised cornmint, mainly from Brazil and China, has a cineole:limonene ratio >1 and a different range of esters and alcohols. Cornmint has *trans*-sabinene hydrate (just before L-menthone) (A8; see also Chapter 4).

Toxicity

Acute toxicity (A22)

Oral LD$_{50}$ >1.2–2.9 g/kg (rat); 3.1 g/kg (mouse).

Dermal LD$_{50}$ >5 g/kg (rabbit).

Irritation and sensitisation (A22)

Menthol may irritate the eyes. May be harmful if ingested in quantity.

Phototoxicity
None reported.

Other toxicities
See peppermint oil monograph for numerous toxicities associated with menthol alone or in peppermint.

Bioactivities

Pharmacological activities *in vitro* and *in vivo*

Smooth muscle None found.

Other uses

Anti-inflammatory effects of L-menthol were greater than those of mint oil using human monocytes *in vitro* (Juergens *et al.*, 1998). The authors suggest that these data support the use of clinical trials to investigate L-menthol for treatment of chronic inflammatory problems such as bronchial asthma, colitis and allergic rhinitis. Calcium antagonist activity of menthol was shown on gastrointestinal smooth muscle (Taylor *et al.*, 1985). When inhaled by rabbits, eucalyptol improved lung compliance values (Zanker *et al.*, 1980). Nasal inhalation of L-menthol reduces respiratory discomfort associated with breathing (Nishino *et al.*, 1997).

See peppermint oil monograph for further bioactivities associated with menthol.

Antimicrobial activities

The effects of the essential oil of Japanese mint (*Mentha arvensis* L.) were assessed on the proliferation of *Helicobacter pylori*, *Salmonella enteritidis*, *Escherichia coli* O157:H7, methicillin-resistant *Staphylococcus aureus* (MRSA) and methicillin-sensitive *Staphylococcus aureus* (MSSA) and showed that the essential oil inhibited the proliferation of each strain and the effects were almost the same against antibiotic-resistant and anti-biotic-sensitive strains of *Helicobacter pylori* and *S. aureus* (Imai *et al.*, 2001).

See peppermint oil monograph for further antimicrobial data.

Clinical studies

In a randomised, controlled clinical trial, 20 healthy subjects inhaled 75% menthol in eucalyptus oil or one of two placebos prior to having a cough induced. Results showed that menthol inhalation caused a significant reduction in induced cough, and can be considered an effective antitussive agent for induced cough (Morice *et al.*, 1994).

See also peppermint oil monograph for further data.

Use in pregnancy and lactation: contraindications

Cornmint is a major adulterant or substitute for peppermint essential oil, therefore most of the dangers of peppermint must be considered, especially as the level of menthol can often be higher than that in peppermint, which can be more hazardous. There is a loss of spontaneous contractions in the rat uterus when menthol and peppermint essential oil is administered *in vitro*. Cornmint oil should therefore only be used with caution as a fragrance, but not massaged into the skin during pregnancy, parturition or lactation.

Pharmaceutical guidance

Cornmint essential oil can be equated with peppermint essential oil due to the adulteration and frequent substitution of cornmint for peppermint essential oil. In both cases, the most active component is menthol and can be the cause of severe problems, especially in young children. Peppermint oil is useful for many illnesses when taken internally, and for respiratory conditions when used with other volatiles. Cornmint essential oil, like peppermint oil, is an irritant and can cause hypersensitivity reactions, mainly due to menthol (Martindale, 1992). Reactions include erythematous skin rash, headache, bradycardia, muscle tremor and ataxia. Idiopathic atrial fibrillation and exacerbation of asthma have also occurred. Cornmint oil should be avoided in cases of obstruction of bile ducts, gallbladder inflammation, gallstones and severe liver damage (Blumenthal *et al.*, 2000). Preparations containing peppermint oil should not be used on the face, particularly the nose, of infants and small children (Blumenthal *et al.*, 2000).

Its usefulness in aromatherapy has to be judged against its possible sensitisation when applied on the skin and possible fibrillation or asthmatic symptoms when used as a volatile.

Use in babies and young children

Due to the immaturity and the delicate nature of the skin of babies and young children, it is inadvisable for any essential oils, especially cornmint or menthol-containing products, to be used in massage, however much the essential oil has been diluted in the carrier oils. This is also a necessary precaution due to the possibilities of sensitisation of the children at this young age through skin or air-borne odorant effects (see Chapters 5 and 7).

Instillation or administration of essential oils near the baby or young child's nose is not only not recommended, but distinctly inadvisable, as there have been numerous cases reported of severe toxicity and even death from such applications (Blumenthal *et al.*, 2000; see Chapter 7). Even mint water, wrongly prepared by a pharmacist, caused a baby's death recently (Bunyan, 1998; *Evening Standard*, 1998).

Cubeb Oil

CAS numbers

USA: 8007-87-2; EINECS: 90082-59-0

Species/Botanical name

Piper cubeba L. f. (Piperaceae)

Synonyms

Cubeba officinalis, tailed pepper, cubeb berry, false pepper

Safety

CHIP details
Xn; R65; 70%; S62 (A26)

RIFM recommended safety of use limits
8% (A23)

EU sensitiser total
1.8 (based on limonene and linalool) (A27)

GRAS status
Granted (Fenaroli, 1997).

Extraction, source, appearance and odour

Extraction
A volatile oil is obtained by steam distillation of the unripe seeds of the berries growing on the vine (Arctander, 1960).

Source
Indonesia, Sri Lanka and the Malayan peninsula.

Appearance and odour
A pale yellow to greenish-yellow to bluish-green (also sometimes colourless) slightly viscous essential oil with a dry, spicy, woody, camphoric, peppery odour. During the distillation there is an ammoniacal odour (also witnessed with black pepper, allspice and ginger) (Arctander, 1960).

Aromatherapy uses

Uses include: bronchitis, catarrh, congestion, coughs, sinusitis; flatulence, indigestion, piles; cystitis, leucorrhoea, urethritis; skin rashes and inflammations (Ryman, 1991; Lawless, 1992; Rose, 1992a; Price, 1993; Sheppard-Hanger, 1995).

Scientific comment
Cubeb essential oil is used very seldom, but can be the base-note in a triple essential oil mixture, so is used by the more adventurous aromatherapists. The essential oil has no particular components to make it interesting and there are no recent data on its bioactivity apart from some antimicrobial work, where it shows virtually no antifungal activity. It is unlikely to remedy any of the maladies indicated above, but massage alone can alleviate many stress and muscular conditions.

Herbal uses

Formerly considered by the Abbess St. Hildegarde of Bingen (1098–1179) to be a great tonic for the nervous system, an antiseptic and vulnerary (Brunn and Epiney-Burgard, 1989), cubeb is nowadays used as a urinary antiseptic, also to treat gonorrhoea, gleet, leucorrhoea, catarrh of the urinary bladder, chronic inflammation of the bladder, abscess of the prostate, chronic laryngitis and bronchitis, and dyspepsia due to an atonic condition of the stomach. The essential oil is said to be mildly stimulant, expectorant, stomachic and carminative. It acts more particularly upon mucous tissues, arresting excessive discharges, especially from the urethra (Felter and Lloyd, 1898; Wren, 1988; Chevallier, 1996).

Food and perfumery uses

Food Cubeb oil (FEMA 2339) is used in a wide range of foods and beverages (Fenaroli, 1997).

Perfumery It is used in cosmetic products such as soap where peppery undertones are needed, carnation base and in artificial essential oil construction (Arctander, 1960).

Chemistry

Major components

	% (Lawrence, 1976–2001)
α-Thujene	trace–2
α-Pinene	2
Sabinene	5
α-Cubebene	7
β-Cubebene	11
Copaene	10
β-Elemene	1
β-Caryophyllene	4
allo-Aromadendrene	4
γ-Humulene	5
β-Bisabolene	2
ε-Cadinene	9
Calamene	4
Cubebol	10
Nerolidol	4
Cubenol	4
Cesarone	4

Adulteration

Addition of clove leaf oil sesquiterpenes, cedrela oil, copaiba oil, *Schinus molle* oil, fractions of essential oils like false cubebs, etc. Cubeb oleoresin is also produced, containing at least 50% of cubeb oil (A8; see also Chapter 4).

Toxicity

Acute toxicity (A22)

Oral LD$_{50}$ <5 g/kg (rat).

Dermal LD$_{50}$ >5 g/kg (rabbit).

Irritation and sensitisation (A22)

At full strength it was irritating to intact and abraded skin of rabbit, but at 8% was non-irritating in humans.

Phototoxicity

No reaction reported in mice.

Bioactivities

Pharmacological activities *in vitro* and *in vivo*

No data found.

Antimicrobial activities

Antibacterial activity

Antibacterial activity was shown against 14/15 different bacterial species (A22). There was a weak action against 1/5 bacteria and other oils tested with cubeb showed decreased activity (Maruzella and Henry, 1958). The vapour inhibited 1/6 bacteria (Maruzella and Sicurella, 1960).

Antifungal activity

No activity was found against 12 pathogenic fungi (A22) and only weak activity against 4/15 fungi (Maruzella and Liguori, 1958).

Other activity

The essential oil is apparently antiviral in rats as well as antibacterial *in vitro* (A22).

Use in pregnancy and lactation: contraindications

As there are no data on the pharmacological effects and absolutely no information on effects during pregnancy, etc. the use of cubeb essential oil is not recommended during pregnancy, parturition or lactation.

Pharmaceutical guidance

There is scant information on the bioactivity, especially on the pharmacological effects, and there is no justification according to the chemical composition to consider this essential oil active, though there is some antibacterial effect, but not antifungal. The use of cubeb essential oil is therefore not recommended in aromatherapy.

Use in babies and young children

Due to the immaturity and the delicate nature of the skin of babies and young children, it is inadvisable for any essential oils to be used in massage, however much the essential oil has been diluted in the carrier oils. This is also a necessary precaution due to the possibilities of sensitisation of the children at this young age through skin or air-borne odorant effects (see Chapters 5 and 7).

Instillation or administration of essential oils near the baby or young child's nose is not only not recommended, but distinctly inadvisable, as there have been numerous cases reported of severe toxicity and even death from such applications (see Chapter 7).

Cypress Oil

CAS numbers
USA: 8013-86-3; EINECS: 84696-07-1

Species/Botanical name
Cupressus sempervirens (Cupressaceae)

Synonyms
Italian or Mediterranean cypress

Other species
Cypress spp. from Brazil, Japan and Kenya

Safety
CHIP details
Xn; R10, 65; 70%; S62 (A26)

RIFM recommended safety of use limits
4% (A23)

EU sensitiser total
7.4 (based on limonene 6.6% and linalool 0.8%) (A27)

Extraction, source, appearance and odour
Extraction
A volatile oil is obtained by steam distillation of the leaves (needles) and twigs of the evergreen tree (Arctander, 1960).

Source
Cyprus, southern European coasts, North Africa and Spain.

Appearance and odour
A pale yellow, pale olive-green or almost colourless essential oil of sweet-balsamic yet refreshing odour, reminiscent of pine needle, juniper berry and cardamom essential oils and a unique dry-out which is delicate, sweet and tenacious rather like labdanum-ambre. Partially deterpenised essential oil is often made by fractional distillation and used in perfumery (Arctander, 1960).

Aromatherapy uses
Cypress oil uses include: circulatory problems; coughs, flu, rheumatism, excess fluids; broken veins on the face. It is said to be: a styptic, expectorant, diuretic, sudorific, vasoconstrictor, vermifuge, vulnerary and 'the healer for blood, sweat, and tears' (Ryman, 1991; Lawless, 1992; Rose, 1992a; Price, 1993; Sheppard-Hanger, 1995).

Scientific comment
There are virtually no bioactivity data available for this essential oil, so the aromatherapy uses are based entirely on herbal usage, which is mainly using the water-soluble components and at best an alcoholic extract containing very little essential oil. There is therefore little justification for suggesting that cypress oil alleviates any of the conditions listed above. However, massage itself can alleviate many stress and muscular conditions and cypress essential oil can be used as a fragrance in conjunction with this therapy to provide a pleasant odour.

Herbal uses
In Ancient Egypt, cypress was burnt with juniper and pine for clearing the atmosphere in temples and Aristotle said it was conducive to health (Manniche, 1999). It was also one of the ingredients in myrtle unguent (Manniche, 1999) and other medicinal preparations for haemorrhoids and other vasoconstrictive uses (Dioscorides). The Ancient Greeks mashed the cones and steeped them in wine to treat dysentery, coughing up of blood and coughs; it is still used as such. It was used as an inhalant in whooping cough (Webster's, 1938). Hippocrates recommended cypress for haemorrhoids with bleeding. It is applied externally as an astringent for varicose veins and taken internally for coughs, colds, flu and rheumatic aches (Ryman, 1991; Chevallier, 1996).

Food and perfumery uses

Food   Not used.

Perfumery   It is used in perfumes as a modifier for pine, citrus colognes, fougeres and chypres and modern aldehydic fragrances. Partially deterpenised essential oil is also used in perfumery (Arctander, 1960).

Chemistry
Major components

	% (Lawrence, 1976–2001)
α-Pinene	39–53
β-Pinene	1–1.5
Sabinene	trace–1
δ-3-carene	19–21
Myrcene	3
Limonene	2–3
α-Terpinyl acetate	4–6
Cedrol	2–4

Minor components
Numerous other mono- and sesquiterpenes.

Adulteration
Other evergreens are often added for distillation. Many cypress species essential oils are used as adulterants together with synthetic pinenes, camphene and other components, such as juniper berry oil, pine needle oil, etc. (A8).

Toxicity
Note: Chinese medicine does not always distinguish between cypress and thuya, which is highly poisonous (Tisserand and Balacs, 1995).

Acute toxicity (A22)
Oral LD$_{50}$ >5 g/kg (rat).

Dermal LD$_{50}$ >5 g/kg (rabbit).

Irritation and sensitisation (A22)
Not irritating when applied to backs of hairless mice and pigs; moderately irritating when applied under 24 hours occlusion to both intact and abraded rabbit skin. Five per cent in petrolatum was not irritating or sensitising (human).

Phototoxicity
None reported.

Bioactivities
Pharmacological activities *in vitro* and *in vivo*
Smooth muscle   No data found.

Uterus   No data found.

Other activities
One study has shown that inhalation of an essential oil causes a different subjective perception of fragrance depending on the type of work. For example, inhalation of cypress after physical work produced a much more favourable impression than before work, in contrast to orange, which produced an unfavourable impression after physical work when compared with that before work (Sugawara *et al.*, 1999).

Antimicrobial activities
Antibacterial activity
Low to moderate activity was shown against five different bacterial species (Friedman *et al.*, 2002).

Antifungal activity
No data found.

Use in pregnancy and lactation: contraindications

There are no pharmacological data on this essential oil and no studies on its effect in pregnancy, parturition or lactation, therefore cypress essential oil cannot be recommended at these times.

Pharmaceutical guidance

There are virtually no bioactivity data available for this essential oil, and herbal usage, which is mainly using the water-soluble component and at best an alcoholic extract containing very little essential oil, cannot be taken as an indication of essential oil effects. There is therefore little justification for the use of cypress essential oil in aromatherapy. However, massage itself can alleviate many stress and muscular conditions and the cypress fragrance could be a pleasant addition.

Use in babies and young children

Due to the immaturity and the delicate nature of the skin of babies and young children, it is inadvisable for any essential oils to be used in massage, however much the essential oil has been diluted in the carrier oils. This is also a necessary precaution due to the possibilities of sensitisation of the children at this young age through skin or air-borne odorant effects (see Chapters 5 and 7).

Instillation or administration of essential oils near the baby or young child's nose is not only not recommended, but distinctly inadvisable, as there have been numerous cases reported of severe toxicity and even death from such applications (see Chapter 7).

Elecampane Oil

Species/Botanical name

Inula helenium L. (Asteraceae/Compositae)

Synonyms

Alant, *Aster helenium* (L.) Scop., *Aster officinalis* All., *Helenium grandiflorum* Gilib., *Aster grandiflorum*; horseheal, inula, scabwort, yellow starwort; wild sunflower

Safety

CHIP details
No data

RIFM recommended safety of use limits
0.1 (A22)

EU sensitiser total
No data (A27)

Extraction, source, appearance and odour

Extraction
A volatile oil is obtained by steam distillation of the herb; Yield is 1–4% (Arctander, 1960).

Source
France, Germany, Belgium, China and India.

Appearance and odour
Elecampane oil is a viscous dark yellow or brownish liquid, often containing whitish crystals, with a dryish, woody, honey-like odour. It blends well with cananga, cinnamon, labdanum, lavender, mimosa, frankincense, patchouli, sandalwood and bergamot (Arctander, 1960).

Aromatherapy uses

Elecampane is not used to any great extent and most aromatherapy books advise no aromatherapy use. However, uses include: scabies, itch mite, acne; acute and chronic bronchitis, sinus infections; palpitations and erythema, although there is a stipulation that it is a hazardous essential oil with irritant and sensitiser properties on the skin (Sheppard-Hanger, 1995).

Scientific comment

Elecampane essential oil may cause an allergic reaction, particularly in individuals with an existing allergy or sensitivity to other plants in the Asteraceae family. There is also a lack of acute toxicity data, so the use of elecampane essential oil is not recommended in aromatherapy massage. It is possible that limited inhalation of the essential oil could alleviate sinus problems, but this could be accomplished by numerous other essential oils, which are not so potentially hazardous.

Herbal uses

Specific indications and uses in the past include: cough, of a teasing, persistent character, accompanied with substernal pain, and profuse secretion; atony of abdominal viscera, with engorgement and relaxation; catarrhal discharges (Felter and Lloyd, 1898). Elecampane has expectorant, antitussive, diaphoretic and bactericidal properties and is used for bronchial/tracheal catarrh, cough associated with pulmonary tuberculosis and dry irritating cough in children; nausea, diarrhoea. Alantolactone has been used as an anthelmintic in the treatment of roundworm, threadworm, hookworm and whipworm infection (Wren, 1988; Chevallier, 1996; Barnes *et al.*, 2002).

Food and perfumery uses

Food Food flavouring category N2: elecampane can be added to foodstuffs in small quantities (Council of Europe, 1981). In the USA, elecampane is only approved for use in alcoholic beverages (Leung, 1980).

Perfumery Not used.

Chemistry (Lawrence, 1976–2001)
Major and minor components
Mainly contains sesquiterpene lactones including alantolactone, isoalantolactone and dihydroalantolactone (eudesmanolides), alantic acid and azulene;

β- and γ-sitosterols, stigmasterol and damara-dienol (sterols), friedelin. Alant camphor (helenin) was observed in the root of elecampane as early as 1760, as it sometimes crystallizes on old roots (Felter and Lloyd, 1898).

Adulteration

The usual solvent adulterations are used (A8; see also Chapter 4).

Toxicity (A22)

Acute toxicity

Oral LD$_{50}$ Not studied.

Dermal LD$_{50}$ Not studied.

Irritation and sensitisation

The essential oil and both its components, alanto-lactone and isoalantolactone (Stampf *et al.*, 1982), have sensitising properties and elecampane has caused allergic contact dermatitis (Mitchell and Rook, 1979).

Phototoxicity

None reported.

Bioactivities

Pharmacological activities *in vitro* and *in vivo*

Smooth muscle   The essential oil showed a potent relaxant effect on guinea-pig ileal and tracheal muscle. Phasic contractions of the ileal myenteric plexus–longitudinal muscle preparation were inhibited by elecampane root, as well as by clove, thyme and angelica root oil (Reiter and Brandt, 1985).

Other activities   Elecampane infusion has showed a pronounced sedative effect in mice (Leung, 1980). Alantolactone showed hypotensive, hyperglycaemic (large doses) and hypoglycaemic (smaller doses) actions in animals. Other species showed varying pharmacological actions (Barnes *et al.*, 2002). Alantolactone has been used as an anthelmintic in the treatment of roundworm, threadworm, hookworm and whipworm infection (Martindale, 1989).

It showed anti-inflammatory effects in animals and stimulated the immune system (Wagner, 1985).

Antimicrobial activities

Antibacterial activity

Alantolactone and isoalantolactone have shown considerable bactericidal and fungicidal properties *in vitro* (Leung, 1980).

Use in pregnancy and lactation: contraindications

In view of the lack of toxicity data for this essential oil and the possible allergic reaction, the use of elecampane during pregnancy, parturition and lactation should be avoided.

Pharmaceutical guidance

The pharmacological actions of elecampane are apparently due to the sesquiterpene lactone constituents, in particular alantolactone and isoalantolactone. Elecampane essential oil may cause an allergic reaction, particularly in individuals with an existing allergy or sensitivity to other plants in the Asteraceae family. It may also interfere with existing hypoglycaemic and antihypertensive treatment. In view of the lack of acute toxicity data, the use of elecampane essential oil is not recommended in aromatherapy massage.

Use in babies and young children

Due to the immaturity and the delicate nature of the skin of babies and young children, it is inadvisable for any essential oils to be used in massage, however much the essential oil has been diluted in the carrier oils. This is also a necessary precaution due to the possibilities of sensitisation of the children at this young age through skin or air-borne odorant effects (see Chapters 5 and 7).

Instillation or administration of essential oils near the baby or young child's nose is not only not recommended, but distinctly inadvisable, as there have been numerous cases reported of severe toxicity and even death from such applications (see Chapter 7).

Eucalyptus Oils

CAS numbers

E. globulus/*E. citriodora*: USA: 8000-48-4
E. globulus: EINECS: 84625-32-1
E. citriodora: EINECS: 85203-56-1

Species/Botanical name

Eucalyptus globulus Labill. (Myrtaceae)

Synonyms

Fevertree, gum tree, tasmanian blue gum (*E. globulus*), ésencia de eucalipto, essence d'eucalyptus rectifiée, eucalypti aetheroleum, oleum eucalypti

Other species

Other species with a similar odour include *E. radiata* R.T. Baker, *E. polybractea* and *E. smithii*. Other species with different odours include *E. citriodora* Hooker syn., lemon-scented gum. Also *E. macurthurii*, which is rich in geranyl acetate; *E. stagierana*, which is rich in citral and limonene; *E. australiana* var., which is rich in phellandrene; and *E. dives* var. rich in piperitone. Over 700 other species occur, but not many are used as essential oils in aromatherapy. The most commonly used are *E. globulus* and *E. citriodora*.

Pharmacopoeias

In Chinese, European, Japanese and Polish Pharmacopoeias.

Safety

CHIP details
E. globulus: Xn; R10, 15; 70%; S62
E. citriodora: None; R10 (A26)

RIFM recommended safety of use limits
10% for all (A23)

EU sensitiser total
E. globulus 5; *E. radiata* 5; *E. citriodora* 20.3 (A27)

GRAS status
E. globulus granted (Fenaroli, 1997).

Extraction, source, appearance and odour

Extraction
Extraction is by steam distillation of the leaves of the tree (Arctander, 1960). The different species can give an essential oil of totally different composition.

Source
China, Australia, Portugal, Brazil, South Africa, Indonesia and former Soviet Union.

Appearance and odour
E. globulus and *E. radiata* oils are colourless to pale yellow with a camphoraceous aroma (Arctander, 1960). *E. citriodora* is colourless to pale yellow with a strong and very fresh rosy-citronella-like, citrusy odour with a sweet, balsamic-floral dry-out note. It is a source of citronellal and hydroxy-citronellal. *E. citriodora* flourished when supplies of citronella oil from East Asia were limited in the 1950s (Arctander, 1960).

Aromatherapy uses

The uses are largely based on the conventional uses of eucalyptus essential oils in products such as Vicks ointment, inhalants and liniments used for respiratory and muscular problems. Uses of the cineole-rich essential oils (e.g. *E. globulus*) include: acne, athlete's foot, blisters, burns, cold sores, dandruff, herpes, insect bites, nappy rash, spots, wound healing, warts; effects on the immune system; debility, neuralgia, headaches, chicken-pox, flu, measles; poor circulation; decongestion; asthma, bronchitis, emphysema (with infection), catarrh coughs, tuberculosis, sinusitis, whooping cough, tonsillitis, plus ear, nose and throat infections; genito-urinary tract infections (e.g. thrush, vaginitis, cystitis). Similar uses are given for *E. citriodora*, which has a completely different chemical composition (Ryman, 1991; Lawless, 1992; Rose, 1992a; Price, 1993; Sheppard-Hanger, 1995).

Scientific comment

Eucalyptus globulus essential oil and other essential oils from species rich in eucalyptol have antiseptic and expectorant properties, especially if inhaled. However, the benefits of eucalyptol can outweigh the dangers in susceptible individuals and children. The essential oil is not recommended for skin application at high concentrations and therefore there is a likelihood that low aromatherapeutic dilutions will not have any effect on the majority of the maladies listed above. Massage alone can alleviate many muscular and circulatory conditions and the odour of the essential oil may have beneficial results on respiratory function.

Herbal uses

Eucalyptus oil, *Eucalyptus globulus*, is an Approved Herb and used for catarrhs of the respiratory tract (internal and external application) and externally for rheumatic complaints. The actions are listed as: secretomotory, expectorant, mildly antispasmodic and mild local hyperaemic. It is used in cough medicines, sweets, pastilles; in inhalation mixtures; in liniments, ointments (e.g. Vicks VapoRub); as rubefacient, decongestant and antiseptic. It is used in many pharmaceutical preparations as a flavouring (e.g. dentifrices). It is applied topically as an insect repellent (diluted in water) or used over the temporal areas of the forehead for tension headaches (Wren, 1988; Chevallier, 1996; Blumenthal *et al.*, 2000; Barnes *et al.*, 2002; for other uses see A19, A20, A21).

Food and perfumery uses

Food E. *globulus* (FEMA 2466) is used in many foods and beverages (Fenaroli, 1997). In the USA, eucalyptus is approved for food use and eucalyptol is listed as a synthetic flavouring agent (Leung, 1980).

Perfumery E. *globulus* has limited use in perfumery, as does E. *citriodora*. E. *globulus* has considerable usage in medicinal products like vapour rubs and inhalants (Arctander, 1960).

Chemistry

Major components

	% (typical commercial oil) (Lawrence, 1976–2001)		
	E. globulus	E. radiata	E. citriodora
1,8-Cineole	80–91*	84	0.6
α-Pinene	6.1	1.6	0.8
Citronellal	0	0	85.0
Menthone	0	0	3.7
Citronellol	0	0	4.7 up to 15
Limonene	5	5	15
Linalool	0	0	0.3

*Often as low as 60% in some studies (e.g. in Portuguese essential oil).

Minor components

In all three species there are numerous monoterpenes and sesquiterpenes (aromadendrene, alloaromadendrene, globulol, epiglobulol, ledol, viridiflorol); citronellyl acetate is found from trace to 13% in E. *citriodora*. E. *polybractea* and E. *smithii* contain about 90% 1,8-cineole. E. *macurthurii* is rich in geranyl acetate; E. *stagierana* is rich in citral and limonene; E. *australiana* var. rich in phellandrene; E. *dives* var. is rich in piperitone.

Oleum eucalypti is the rectified essential oil, containing no less than 70% eucalyptol (Martindale, 1992). It is the Pharmacopoeia grade eucalyptus oil (BAN, USAN) and is rectified from the essential oils of many high 1,8-cineole-containing *Eucalyptus* species.

Eucalyptus oil (Ph. Eur. 4.8) from E. *globulus*, E. *polybractea* and E. *smithii* contains not less than 70% w/w cineole. Soluble 1 in 5 of alcohol (70%).

Standards for eucalyptus oils are as follows: British Standard Specifications for E. *citriodora* (BS 2999/23, 1972) and for E. *globulus* (BS 2999/ 53, 1975). Eucalyptus oil (BPC 1973), internal usage: 0.05–0.2 mL. Oil for local application: 30 mL oil to 500 mL lukewarm water.

Adulteration

The two main species sold, E. *globulus* and E. *radiata*, are very cheap, therefore adulteration is unlikely. These oils are often redistilled or rectified to give the Pharmacopoeia grade oil, which has less cough-producing aldehydes and terpenes and can therefore be used in cough medicines. E. *citriodora* is not usually adulterated with synthetic citronellal, as this is more expensive than the whole essential oil. It could however be used in place of citronella, when the price of the latter rises (A8; see also Chapter 4).

Toxicity

Acute toxicity (A22)

Dermal LD_{50} E. *globulus* $>$ 5 g/kg (rabbit); E. *radiata* untested; E. *citriodora* 2.5 g/kg (rabbit)

Oral LD$_{50}$ *E. globulus* 4.4 g/kg (rat); *E. radiata* untested; *E. citriodora* >5 g/kg (rat).

Irritation and sensitisation (A22)

Only *E. globulus* and *E. radiata* have been tested and showed nil effect at 10% (human), though hypersensitivity for *E. globulus* has been reported. There is also the sensitisation potential of *E. citriodora*.

Phototoxicity

None reported.

Other toxicities

Eucalyptus globulus was found to be non-teratogenic in mice (A22).

In humans, applied externally, eucalyptus oil is considered generally non-toxic, non-sensitising and non-phototoxic (Tisserand and Balacs, 1995). However, a 6-year-old girl who had a eucalyptus oil preparation rubbed on much of her body for an itchy rash developed slurred speech and muscle weakness, and became unconscious; the ointment was removed and she recovered with no long-term problems (Burkhard *et al.*, 1998). Undiluted eucalyptus oil is toxic and should not be taken internally. An evaluation of 109 paediatric poisoning accidents involving eucalyptus oil in Victoria, Australia revealed that 74% gained access via a home vapouriser unit, often placed at ground level, and in most instances between 5 and 10 mL was consumed (Day *et al.*, 1997). In fact, eucalyptus oil is much more toxic by the oral route than by any other: oral (child) TD$_{Lo}$ = 218 mg/kg; oral (man) TD$_{Lo}$ = 375 mg/kg NIOSH 1975. Eucalyptus oil poisoning symptoms include: epigastric burning, nausea, vomiting, dizziness, muscular weakness, miosis and feeling of suffocation; cyanosis, delirium and convulsions may occur. Deaths have been recorded from as little as 3.5 mL (Martindale, 1982). Death is usual after ingestion of 30 mL, following severe cardiovascular, respiratory and central nervous effects (Tisserand and Balacs, 1995). A 3-year-old boy has survived the ingestion of about 10 mL of eucalyptus oil and an adult has survived ingestion of 60 mL; under 5 mL has apparently been fatal in an adult, although this is atypical; a 10-year-old boy died within 15 hours of ingesting about 30 mL of eucalyptus oil. Signs included shortness of breath and vomiting coming on in minutes (Tisserand and Balacs, 1995).

A survey of the literature found that essential oils of 11 plants potentially induced seizures, including: eucalyptus, fennel, hyssop, pennyroyal, rosemary, sage, savin, tansy, thuja, turpentine and wormwood. The cases of two healthy adults and one child with seizures related to absorption of oils were described (Burkhard *et al.*, 1999). In a survey of 109 cases of ingestion by children of eucalyptus oil, three became unconscious after taking between 5 mL and 10 mL of pure eucalyptus oil, but all patients recovered. The author concluded that ingestion of eucalyptus oil may cause significant problems in infants and young children (Tibballs, 1995). Forty-two cases of eucalyptus oil poisoning over 7 years were reviewed in children under the age of 14. Of 41 cases investigated, 80% of children were asymptomatic, including four who drank over 1 ounce (30 mL) of eucalyptus oil. No long-term effects were noted. The author concludes that eucalyptus oil may be less toxic than currently believed (Webb and Pitt, 1993).

A 53-year-old woman had chronic eczema, resistant to standard therapy, which was traced to allergic air-borne dermatitis from a year-long use of aroma lamps in her home. She had inhaled lavender, jasmine and rosewood, but also tested as allergic to laurel (bay), eucalyptus and pomerance. Her dermatitis eventually resolved with steroid treatment (Schaller and Korting, 1995).

Oily solutions of eucalyptus oil were formerly used in nasal preparations, but this use is now considered unsuitable as the vehicle inhibits ciliary movements and may cause lipoid pneumonia (Martindale, 2004).

Drug interaction

Eucalyptus oil induces the detoxification enzyme system of the liver, thus the effects of other drugs can be weakened and/or shortened (Blumenthal *et al.*, 2000).

Bioactivities

Pharmacological activities *in vitro* and *in vivo*

Smooth muscle *Eucalyptus globulus*, *E. radiata* and *E. citriodora* had a spasmolytic effect on electrically stimulated smooth muscle of the guinea-pig *in vitro* (A2; Lis-Balchin *et al.*, 1996a). The action of *E. citriodora* was very strong, whilst there was very little effect with *E. radiata* at the same concentration; 1,8-cineole showed a rise in tone (A2; Lis-Balchin *et al.*, 1996a).

Uterus *Eucalyptus globulus*, *E. radiata* and *E. citriodora* all caused a decrease in the spontaneous contractions of rat uterus; as did 1,8-cineole, limonene and other components in the eucalyptus essential oils (A3; A4; Lis-Balchin and Hart, 1997b).

Other activities Hypoglycaemic activity was noted in eucalyptus extracts not containing the essential oil (Barnes *et al.*, 2002). Expectorant activities have been shown for eucalyptus oil and for eucalyptol; the latter probably being responsible for the effect (Leung, 1980). *E. globulus* (alcoholic and hexane extracts) inhibited IgE-dependent histamine release from RBL-2H3 cells (Ikawati *et al.*, 2001). Lung compliance values in rabbits improved with inhalation of eucalyptol and eucalyptus oil (Zanker *et al.*, 1980).

Eucalyptus oils reduced inflammation by acting as antioxidants and interfering with leukocyte (white blood cell) activation: the authors suggest that this may buffer biochemical damage triggered by infections (Grassmann *et al.*, 2000). Eucalyptus extract was found to have significant dose-dependent anti-inflammatory effects when used against induced, localized acute and chronic inflammation in rodents. The authors concluded that the study affirmed the traditional use of eucalyptus for these conditions of pain and inflammation (Atta and Alkofahi, 1998). However, 1,8-cineole, a main component of eucalyptus oil, was found to produce inflammatory swelling when injected into the paws of rats. The mechanism appears to involve mast cell degranulation (involved in allergic reactions), and was inhibited by antihistamines (Santos and Rao, 2000).

1,8-Cineole, an active component in eucalyptus oil, was used as a model substance in order to study skin absorption of volatile oils. Absorption into the skeletal muscle following application to the skin was studied and large differences in absorption were found depending on the method of application. Applying the 1,8-cineole on the skin with an applicator improved bioavailability in the skeletal muscle by 320% over laying the oil on the skin with an occlusive dressing (Weyers *et al.*, 2000).

Using human epidermis, the abilities of 26 different terpenes to enhance the permeability of 5-fluorouracil (a chemotherapy agent) through skin were tested. Cineole was shown to enhance the effect of 5-fluorouracil much more than limonene (Moghimi *et al.*, 1988).

A eucalyptus-based insect repellent was compared with DEET (*N,N*-diethyl-meta-toluamide) for protection against biting from mosquitoes. Both repellents provided over 98% protection for over 8 hours (Trigg, 1996). *E. globulus* essential oil was found to kill the larvae of two mosquito species;

maximum effectiveness was seen after 48 hours of exposure to the oil (Monzon *et al.*, 1994).

Quwenling, a mosquito repellent derived from lemon eucalyptus extract (*E. citriodora*), was compared with DEET when tested against five mosquito species. The duration of protection of Quwenling was generally shorter than that of DEET (Schreck and Leonhardt, 1991).

Antimicrobial activities

Antibacterial activity

Relative data: Against 25 different bacteria: *E. globulus* 14/25; *E. radiata* 20/25; *E. citriodora* 10/25; and 1,8-cineole 16/25 (A1; Lis-Balchin and Deans, 1997; Lis-Balchin *et al.*, 1998a). These were commercial samples and their purity and authenticity could not be guaranteed although gas chromatography was carried out. Rectified eucalyptus oil vapour was active against 2/5 bacteria (Maruzella and Sicurella, 1960). There are also several reports of the activity of unnamed eucalyptus oils (probably *E. globulus*): 5/5 bacteria were affected (Yousef and Tawil, 1980); 11/25 bacteria (Deans and Ritchie, 1987). Activity against 20 *Listeria monocytogenes* species was also shown to vary in the commercial samples (A1; Lis-Balchin and Deans, 1997; Lis-Balchin *et al.*, 1998a): *E. globulus* 6/20; *E. radiata* 20/20; *E. citriodora* 20/20 and 1,8-cineole 0/20. *Eucalyptus alba*, *E. citriodora*, *E. deglupta*, *E. globulus*, *E. saligna* and *E. robusta* essential oils showed good antibacterial activity, particularly against *Pseudomonas aeruginosa* (Cimanga *et al.*, 2002).

The antibacterial activity of the Australian tea tree oil and other oils from the family Myrtaceae were tested against 12 common strains of bacteria, including *Escherichia coli*, *Staphylococcus aureus* and *Salmonella choleraesuis*. Tea tree had the highest antibacterial activity, and was effective against all bacteria except *P. aeruginosa*. Both tea tree and manuka oil had significant antibacterial effects on various strains of antibiotic-resistant *Staphylococcus* species (Harkenthal *et al.*, 1999). Essential oils from eucalyptus, lemongrass, peppermint and palmarosa were tested against a strain of *E. coli*. All four oils killed the strain at very low dilutions (Pattnaik *et al.*, 1995a). A strain of *P. aeruginosa* harbouring a plasmid was not inhibited by large concentrations of essential oils of eucalyptus (or lemongrass, palmarosa or peppermint), showing resistance to the oils (Pattnaik *et al.*, 1995b). An extract of *E. globulus* had strong *in vitro* antimicrobial activity against *Staph. aureus*, *E. coli*, *P. aeruginosa* and *Candida albicans* (Navarro *et al.*, 1996).

Antifungal activity

Relative data (% inhibition) against three filamentous fungi was very low (A1):

	E. globulus	E. radiata	E. citriodora
Aspergillus niger	24	35	61
A. ochraceus	−18*	36	78
Fusarium culmorum	0	0	0

*Promoted fungal growth!

Five types of eucalyptus oils were moderately active against 5/5 fungi; an unspecified eucalyptus oil was active against 4/5 fungi (Maruzella and Sicurella, 1960) and against 15/15 fungi, while the 1,8-cineole was only active against 11/15 (Maruzella and Liguori, 1958). E. citriodora was effective against Candida spp. (Asre, 1994). Good activity was found against 5/5 fungi (Yousef and Tawil, 1980). The ability of essential oils to inhibit five species of fungi was evaluated and compared with the effects of miconazole, a common OTC (over the counter) treatment for vaginal yeast infection. The six eucalyptus species used all markedly inhibited fungal growth (Rai et al., 1999). The essential oils were also tested against 22 bacterial strains and 12 fungi strains by the disc diffusion method. Essential oil of eucalyptus was effective against all 22 bacterial strains and 11 of the fungi strains (Pattnaik et al., 1996).

From the relative data it appears that some Eucalyptus species (E. globulus and E. radiata) have strong antibacterial activity, but E. citriodora is almost inactive in comparison. However the activity against fungi is opposite to the antibacterial effect and is negatively correlated to the concentration of eucalyptol (1,8-cineole), i.e. the greater the content, the lower the antifungal activity: E. globulus and E. radiata are poorly antifungal, if not promoting growth, and E. citriodora is relatively good as an antifungal agent (see A1 and A6). However, there is wide variation in results from different studies, indicating differences in the essential oils used and their possible degree of adulteration.

Other activities

In vitro antiviral activity against influenza type A has been documented only for water-soluble fractions (Wren, 1988; Barnes et al., 2002).

Clinical studies

In a clinical trial, nasal respiratory cells from 45 healthy people were exposed to varying concentrations of a mixture of menthol, eucalyptus oil and pine needle oil, eucalyptus oil alone, and pine needle oil alone. High concentrations of essential oils reduced the ciliary beat frequency (Riechelmann et al., 1997). Individuals were exposed to 5 minutes of camphor, eucalyptus or menthol vapour. No effect on nasal resistance to airflow was reported, but a majority of subjects reported a cold sensation in the nose and a feeling of improved airflow (Burrow et al., 1983).

In a controlled clinical trial, the effect of Eucalyptamint, a topically applied counterirritant, was studied on ten healthy people. Significant increases in skin temperature, muscle temperature and blood flow occurred and lasted approximately 45 minutes. The researchers concluded that Eucalyptamint may be useful for pain relief or as a passive warm-up for athletes (Hong and Shellock, 1991).

Using extracts rather than the essential oil, a clinical trial involving 15 people compared eucalyptus extract-containing chewing gum, funoran-containing chewing gum, and a control gum on plaque formation. Plaque formation was significantly reduced with both the eucalyptus and the funoran gum compared with the control (Sato et al., 1998). A plant preparation containing tinctures of various herbs including eucalyptus has been used successfully in the treatment of chronic suppurative otitis (Shaparenko et al., 1979).

Effects on headache were studied in 32 healthy people in a double-blind, placebo-controlled, randomised crossover study. The test chemicals were applied to large areas of the forehead and temples. The eucalyptus oil had little influence on pain, but did have a muscle-relaxing effect, whilst headache pain was relieved with a combination of peppermint oil and ethanol (Gobel et al., 1994).

Use in pregnancy and lactation: contraindications

The safety of eucalyptus oil has not been established in pregnant or nursing women. Eucalyptus oil should definitely not be taken internally during pregnancy, but massage with the essential oil (greatly diluted) and use of the fragrance should not pose a threat, as there is such a long-standing usage of eucalyptus products. See below for cautions.

Pharmaceutical guidance

Antiseptic and expectorant properties have been shown for eucalyptus essential oils containing eucalyptol (1,8-cineole), which is considered to be the main component responsible for the action. The undiluted oil is toxic if taken internally and should not be applied to the skin undiluted. Moreover, the oil may aggravate bronchial spasms in asthmatics and should not be taken internally by those with severe liver diseases and inflammatory disorders of the gastrointestinal tract and kidney (Blumenthal et al., 2000). It also should not be used in large doses by individuals with low blood pressure (Brinker, 1997). These effects could be initiated by the use of eucalyptus essential oils externally, due to respiratory system absorption. As eucalyptus oil activates certain enzyme systems in the liver, it can weaken or shorten the action of other types of medications, including pentobarbital, aminopyrine and amphetamine (Blumenthal et al., 2000).

In rare cases, after taking eucalyptus preparations nausea, vomiting and diarrhoea may occur. This may also happen after external application.

Species other than *E. globulus* and *E. citriodora* should not be used as these have not been tested toxicologically. *Ravensara aromatica*, which has a similar odour, should not be used as it is also untested.

Use in babies and young children

Due to the immaturity and the delicate nature of the skin of babies and young children, it is inadvisable for any essential oils to be used in massage, however much the essential oil has been diluted in the carrier oils. This is also a necessary precaution due to the possibilities of sensitisation of the children at this young age through skin or air-borne odorant effects (see Chapters 5 and 7).

Instillation or administration of essential oils near the baby or young child's nose is not only not recommended, but distinctly inadvisable, as there have been numerous cases reported of severe toxicity due to the risk of laryngeal spasm and subsequent respiratory arrest (Schultz et al., 1998; see Chapter 7).

Fennel Oil

CAS numbers

USA: 8006-84-6; EINECS: 84455-29-8

Species/Botanical name

Foeniculum vulgare Miller var. *dulce* (Umbellifeae)

Synonyms

Foeniculum vulgare Miller subsp. *capillaceum* (Galib.) Holmboe (sweet fennel), aetheroleum foeniculi, esencia de hinojo, essência de funcho, oleum foeniculi

Other species

Foeniculum vulgare Miller subsp. *vulgare* Miller (bitter fennel), foeniculi amari, fructus aetheroleum

Pharmacopoeias

In European, Japanese and Polish Pharmacopoeias. Also in United States National Formulary.

Safety

CHIP details
Xn; R10, 65; 20%; S62 (A26)

RIFM recommended safety of use limits
4% (A23)

EU sensitiser total
0.8 (based on low limonene content) (A27)

GRAS status
Granted (Fenaroli, 1997).

Extraction, source, appearance and odour

Extraction
A volatile oil is obtained by steam distillation of the dried ripe fennel seed (Arctander, 1960).

Source
Spain, Eastern Europe and Java.

Appearance and odour
Sweet fennel oil is colourless or pale yellow to greenish with a characteristic smell of anise, fresh and spicy (Arctander, 1960). Bitter fennel oil is colourless to pale yellow with a sharp, warm-camphoraceous, herbaceous odour, initially earthy, later sweet, anisic and spicy (Arctander, 1960).

Aromatherapy uses

Sweet fennel essential oil uses include: bruises, pyorrhoea, cellulites, obesity, oedema, rheumatism; asthma, bronchitis; anorexia, colic, constipation, dyspepsia, flatulence, hiccup, nausea; amenorrhoea, menopausal problems; labour pains, period pains and insufficient milk production in lactation (Lawless, 1992; Rose, 1992a; Price, 1993; Sheppard-Hanger, 1995).

Scientific comment
The aromatherapy uses are based on herbal uses of fennel essential oil and the whole herb and have not been scientifically proven to be effective at low concentrations when applied to the skin. Massage alone can alleviate various stress and muscular problems.

Herbal uses

Fennel essential oil has a folk reputation to increase milk secretion, promote menstruation, facilitate birth, alleviate the symptoms of the male climacteric, and increase libido. These effects are attributed to polymers of anethole, such as dianethole and photoanethole (Albert-Puleo, 1980). Also said to be affected are peptic discomforts, such as mild, spastic disorders of the gastrointestinal tract, catarrhs of the upper respiratory tract, especially in children, feeling of fullness, flatulence; stimulation of gastrointestinal motility and, in higher concentrations, antispasmodic. Fennel herb itself is indicated for digestive debility, anorexia, belching, hiccupping or reflux, persistent epigastric pain relieved by warmth or pressure, with slippery coating on the tongue and slow pulse rate, intestinal cramps, colic. It helps to dilute urinary salts and dissolve stones; open obstructions of the liver, spleen and gall (Grieve, 1937/1992; Wren, 1988; Chevallier, 1996; Blumenthal *et al.*, 2000; Barnes *et al.*, 2002; Dr Phyto, 2005).

Food and perfumery uses

Food   Sweet fennel oil (FEMA 2483) is used in a wide range of foods and beverages. Bitter fennel oil (FEMA 2481) is used in bitter drinks (Fenaroli, 1997).

Perfumery   Both are used in a limited number of perfumes (Arctander, 1960).

Chemistry

Major components
Sweet fennel:

	% (Lawrence, 1976–2001)
trans-Anethole	30–75
Fenchone	1–25
Methyl chavicol	1–7
Limonene	1–55
α-Pinene	1–15

Bitter-fennel fruit oil (Ph. Eur. 4.8) contains 12.0–25.0% fenchone and 55.0–75.0% anethole.

Fennel oil (USNF 22) has a congealing temperature not lower than 3°C. It is soluble 1 in 1 of alcohol (90%).

Adulteration
Sweet fennel, the more prized fennel in the perfumery industry, is often adulterated with the bitter fennel. Various synthetic components can be added, such as *trans*-anethole, *cis*-anethole (more toxic), fenchone, methyl chavicol and limonene. Various other essential oil fractions are also used. A type of fennel, finocchio, is often marketed under the misnomer of anise, another culinary herb (*Pimpinella anisum* L.), which has led to market and consumer confusion. Both plants contain high levels of anethole in the essential oil, imparting the licorice-like aroma and taste (A8; Simon, 1990; see also Chapter 4).

Toxicity

Acute toxicity (A22)

Oral LD$_{50}$ Bitter fennel seed oil >4.5 g/kg; sweet fennel seed oil >3.8 g/kg (rat).

Dermal LD$_{50}$ Bitter fennel seed oil >5 g/kg; sweet fennel seed oil >5 g/kg (rabbit).

Irritation and sensitisation (A22)
Both bitter and sweet fennel oils had nil effect at 4% (human). Undiluted sweet fennel proved severely irritating to mice and moderately to rabbit. Anethole has allergenic properties (see anise).

Phototoxicity
None reported.

Other toxicities
Soreness, dryness and cracking of lips and perioral skin occurred in an individual using a herbal (fennel) toothpaste; anethole was reported to be the sensitising agent (A22).

Bioactivities

Pharmacological activities *in vitro* and *in vivo*

Smooth muscle   Sweet fennel oil had a strong spasmogenic effect on electrically stimulated smooth muscle of the guinea-pig *in vitro* (A2; Lis-Balchin *et al.*, 1996a). Limonene and pinenes had a similar effect, whilst fenchone was spasmolytic. Fennel oil increased phasic contractions of muscle cells at high concentrations and had a relaxant effect at low concentrations; fennel contracted tracheal muscle (Reiter and Brandt, 1985). Contractions were also shown with anethole both in the smooth intestinal muscle and trachea (Reiter and Brandt, 1985; Saleh *et al.*, 1996).

Uterus   There was a decrease in the spontaneous contractions in the rat uterus when sweet fennel oil, limonene and other components were applied *in vitro*. Mixing several other essential oils with fennel oil also had a relaxant effect (A3; A4; Lis-Balchin and Hart, 1997b).

Fennel oil is mildly oestrogenic, similarly to aniseed oil, due to the anethole content (Albert-Puleo, 1980) (see aniseed oil monograph). Pharmacological effects on the isolated rat uterus were studied using oxytocin (0.1, 1 and 10 mg/mL) and prostaglandin E$_2$ (PGE$_2$) (5×10^{-5} mol/L) to induce muscle contraction. Administration of different doses of essential oil reduced the intensity of oxytocin and PGE$_2$-induced contractions significantly (25 and 50 g/mL for oxytocin and 10 and 20 g/mL PGE$_2$, respectively). Fennel essential oil also reduced the frequency of contractions induced by PGE$_2$ but not with oxytocin (Ostad *et al.*, 2001).

Skeletal muscle Fennel essential oil showed a contracture and inhibition of the twitch response to nerve stimulation in the phrenic nerve–diaphragm muscle *in vitro*. The same effect was shown by dill, frankincense and nutmeg (Lis-Balchin and Hart, 1997c).

Other activities Fennel oil has increased liver regeneration in partially hepatectomised rats and has shown anti-inflammatory action (Wren, 1988). Following the oral administration of an acetone extract of *Foeniculum vulgare* seeds for 15 days in male rats, total protein concentration was found to be significantly decreased in testes and vas deferens and increased in seminal vesicles and prostate gland. There was a decrease in activities of acid and alkaline phosphatase in all these regions, except that alkaline phosphatase was unchanged in vasa. In female rats, oral administration of the extract for 10 days led to vaginal cornification and changes to the oestrus cycle. While moderate doses caused increase in weight of mammary glands, higher doses increased the weight of oviduct, endometrium, myometrium, cervix and vagina also. The results seem to confirm the oestrogenic activity of the seed extract (Malini *et al.*, 1985).

Antimicrobial activities

Antibacterial effects were low, but antifungal effects were moderate to good.

Antibacterial activity
Relative data: Activity was shown against 6/25 different bacterial species (A1; Lis-Balchin, Deans, 1997; Lis-Balchin *et al.*, 1998a); and using the same bacteria in another study 6/25 were again affected (Deans and Ritchie, 1987); 0/20 *Listeria monocytogenes* varieties were affected (A1; Lis-Balchin and Deans, 1997; Lis-Balchin *et al.*, 1998a); sweet fennel vapour affected only 1/5 bacteria (Maruzella and Sicurella, 1960); but *Listeria monocytogenes* and *Salmonella enteritidis* inhibition was shown by a synergistic mixture of essential oils of anise, fennel and/or basil with methyl paraben (Fyfe *et al.*, 1997). Fennel seed oil showed a moderate effect against four different bacteria (Friedman *et al.*, 2002).

Antifungal activity
Relative data (% inhibition): *Aspergillus niger* 95%, *A. ochraceus* 78%, *Fusarium culmorum* 66% (A1). Fennel showed poor activity against 4/5 fungi

and a good reaction against one of them (Maruzella, 1960); it affected 11/15 fungi to some extent (Maruzella and Liguori, 1958).

Use in pregnancy and lactation: contraindications

Due to the oestrogenic potential of fennel oil, including a decrease in the spontaneous contractions in the rat uterus when sweet fennel oil, limonene and other components were applied *in vitro*, it should not be used during pregnancy, parturition and lactation.

Pharmaceutical guidance

Fennel is used extensively as a spice and is widely used in conventional pharmaceuticals for its carminative, expectorant and flavouring properties. It contains anethole and estragole, which are structurally related to safrole, a known hepatotoxin and carcinogen. Anethole was reaffirmed as GRAS in 1997 on the basis of the recognised metabolic detoxication of *trans*-anethole in humans at low levels of exposure (1 mg/kg body weight). Fennel oil should not be taken orally for an extended period of several weeks (Blumenthal *et al.*, 2000) and should be avoided by persons with known sensitivity to anethole and by people with cancer (Tisserand and Balacs, 1995): these cautions should also apply in aromatherapy. Anethole-high oils in general should be avoided (Zondek and Bergman, 1938; Albert-Puleo, 1980) as in rare cases allergic reactions may occur, affecting the skin and respiratory system in humans.

Use in babies and young children

Due to the immaturity and the delicate nature of the skin of babies and young children, it is inadvisable for any essential oils, especially this essential oil containing a known toxicant and carcinogen, to be used in massage, however much the essential oil has been diluted in the carrier oils. This is also a necessary precaution due to the possibilities of sensitisation of the children at this young age through skin or airborne odorant effects (see Chapters 5 and 7).

Instillation or administration of essential oils near the baby or young child's nose is not only not recommended, but distinctly inadvisable, as there have been numerous cases reported of severe toxicity and even death from such applications (see Chapter 7).

Frankincense Oil

CAS numbers

USA: 8016-36-2; EINECS: 8050-07-5

Species/Botanical name

Boswellia carterii Birdw. (Burseraceae)

Synonyms

Olibanum; Arabic: mogar (tree); sheehaz (resin). Somali: mohor (tree); beyo (resin)

Other species

Boswellia serrata Roxburgh or *Boswellia thurifera* Colebrooke, syn. *Indian olibanum*, salai guggul; *B. frereana*, syn. Somali: yagar (tree); maidi (resin)

Safety

CHIP details
Xn; R10, 65; 90%; S62 (A26)

RIFM recommended safety of use limits
Absolute: 3%; essential oil: 8% (tentative) (A23)

EU sensitiser total
17.9 (based on limonene) (A27)

GRAS status
Granted (Fenaroli, 1997).

Extraction, source, appearance and odour

Extraction
An oleo-gum resin obtained from cuts in trees and falling to the ground as tears is steam distilled to give the essential oil or solvent-extracted to give an absolute. Distillation is carried out in Europe under precise conditions, as is solvent extraction. Olibanum resinoid is extracted with solvents, usually benzene and usually diluted with diethylphthalate 15–25% (Arctander, 1960).

Source
Eritrea, Yemen, India, Ethiopia, Kenya and Somalia.

Appearance and odour
The essential oil of *B. carterii* is colourless to yellowish/green or amber-green with a diffusive, fresh-terpeney, almost green-lemon-like odour but not terebinthinate. It has a certain pepperiness mellowed with a rich, sweet-woody, balsamic undertone. It can be tenacious (depending on distillation procedure) with a cistus-like, amber-type, balsamic dry-out note.

The absolute is a solid but plastic mass of pale amber colour with the characteristic odour of olibanum. It is free from the terebinthinate (paint-can) odour. It has a fresh, balsamic, yet dry and resinous, slightly green odour with a characteristic fruity-green top-note (rather like unripe apples) and great tenacity (Arctander, 1960).

Olibanum resinoid is a dark amber to orange or reddish-brown, almost solid, plastic-like mass of non-pourable consistency. This contains 7–10% essential oil.

Boswellia frereana Birdw., the yagar of the Somalis, yields a fragrant resin of a lemon odour. It contains no gum, and is employed in the East as a masticatory (Arctander, 1960).

Aromatherapy uses

Uses include: blemishes on skin, scars, wounds, dry and mature complexions, wrinkles; asthma, bronchitis, catarrh, coughs, laryngitis; cystitis, dysmenorrhoea, leucorrhoea; anxiety, nervous tension and stress-related conditions (Ryman, 1991; Lawless, 1992; Rose, 1992a; Price, 1993; Sheppard-Hanger, 1995).

Scientific comment

Although none of the aromatherapy uses have been scientifically proven, the fact that frankincense has been burnt in offerings to the gods for thousands of years must be of significance in at least imparting a fragrance for relaxation, meditation and perhaps more profound CNS stimuli. Burnt resin, however, has a completely different chemical composition to the essential oil and therefore a different bioactivity. The use of massage alone can alleviate many symptoms of stress and the use of the very stimulating essential oil as a fragrance alone could prove beneficial.

Herbal uses

The gum resin was used as an incense from early Egyptian times and was also highly prized enough as a medicine to warrant being given to the Baby Jesus as one of three pricely treasures. Dioscorides mentioned the use of the gum in treating skin disorders, ophthalmology, haemorrhages and pneumonia. Olibanum has received some interest more recently in traditional medicine: China is the largest market for all the resins, mainly for use in traditional Chinese medicine. In Europe and Latin America, substantial amounts of Eritrean-type olibanum are used as incense by the Orthodox and Roman Catholic Churches (approaching 500 tonnes in 1987). Similar quantities are imported into North African and the Middle Eastern countries where it is used for chewing (the higher quality 'maidi' type from Somalia is used. Smaller quantities of lower grade maidi are employed in the Middle East for burning in the home (see Chapter 2).

Research into the use of frankincense as an anti-inflammatory, anti-athritic, anti-ulcerogenic, anti-asthmatic and cure for ulcerative colitis are being instigated (see bioactivity).

Food and perfumery uses

Food   Olibanum oil (FEMA 2816) is used in a variety of foods and beverages (Fenaroli, 1997).

Perfumery   The essential oil is used in fine perfumery in citrus colognes and also many incense-like perfumes, oriental, floral, masculine perfumes, etc. (Arctander, 1960).

The absolute is used as a fixative in many perfumes and provides the exotic/oriental effect with its fresh-balsamic notes (Arctander, 1960).

Chemistry

Major components
Olibanum (frankincense) (1993) sample *Boswellia carterii* Birdw.:

	% (Lawrence, 1976–2001)	
	% range	High levels (country)
α-Thujene	0–6	61 (India)
α-Pinene	0–43	43 (Aden/Yemeni)
Camphene	trace–2	2 (Yemeni)
p-Cymene	trace–1	8 (Aden)
Limonene	trace–11	
Verbenone	trace–6.5	6.5 (Yemeni)
Octanol	trace–13	12.7 (Somali)
Octyl acetate	0–52	52 (Eritrea)
Incensol	0–2.4	2.4 (Eritrea)
Incensyl acetate	0–3.4	3.4 (Eritrea)

There is a wide variation in the composition of different olibanum oils from different sources, different species and also time of distillation. The Chemical Manufacturers Association International grading system is based on the pinene content, where grade 1 is 37–42%, but other olibanum oils, such as those from India, have a pleasant odour despite a lower pinene content.

Adulteration
Many of the components are added as synthetics, especially α-pinene.

The residue after distillation consists of resins and water-soluble gum and is odourless; a true olibanum resin can be extracted from this and is used as a diluent, imparting no quality or odour to the olibanum resinoid (A8; see also Chapter 4).

Toxicity

Acute toxicity (A22)
Oral LD$_{50}$ >5 g/kg (rat).
Dermal LD$_{50}$ >5 g/kg (rabbit).

Irritation and sensitisation (A22)
Nil at 8%.

Phototoxicity
Untested.

Bioactivities

Pharmacological activities *in vitro* and *in vivo*

Smooth muscle   Olibanum oil had a strong spasmogenic effect on electrically stimulated smooth muscle of the guinea-pig *in vitro* (A2; Lis-Balchin *et al.*, 1996a).

Uterus   There was a decrease in spontaneous contractions of the uterus in the rat when olibanum oil was added *in vitro*; mixing several other essential oils with olibanum oil also had a relaxant effect (A3; A4; Lis-Balchin and Hart, 1997b).

Skeletal muscle   Contracture of skeletal muscle and inhibition of the twitch response to nerve stimulation was seen with essential oils of clary sage, dill, fennel, frankincense and nutmeg (Lis-Balchin and Hart, 1997c).

Other activities Salai guggal (*Boswellia serrata*) was described as a non-redox inhibitor of leukotriene biosynthesis (Ammon, 1996).

Carrageenan- or dextran-induced oedema and formaldehyde-induced arthritis were reduced by *Boswellia* alcoholic extract salai guggal (AESG). It was equally effective in adrenalectomised rats. In formaldehyde and adjuvant arthritis, AESG produced prominent anti-arthritic activity. It inhibited inflammation-induced increase in serum transaminase levels and leukocyte counts, but it lacked any analgesic or antipyretic effects and no significant effect was seen on cardiovascular, respiratory and central nervous systems. The gestation period or parturition time in pregnant rats or onset time of castor oil-induced diarrhoea was unaffected by AESG (Singh and Attal, 1986). Preliminary effective studies of *B. serrata* gum resin in patients with ulcerative colitis have been conducted (Gupta *et al.*, 1997).

Anti-inflammatory, anti-arthritic and anti-ulcerogenic use of boswellic acid compositions has been patented as US Patent 5,629,351 and a bone/joint inflammation treatment with a mixture including 470 mg *Boswellia* extract as US Patent 5,888,514.

Clinical studies

The gum resin of *B. serrata*, known in the Indian Ayurvedic system of medicine as salai guggal, contains boswellic acids, which have been shown to inhibit leukotriene biosynthesis. In a double-blind, placebo-controlled study, bronchial asthma was reduced in 70% of 40 patients treated with gum resin at 300 mg three times daily for 6 weeks (Gupta *et al.*, 1998). Two cases of therapy with frankincense and myrrh in children have been described (Michie and Cooper, 1991).

Antimicrobial activities

Antibacterial effects were very strong, but antifungal effects were very poor.

Antibacterial activity

Relative data: Strong effect was shown against 23/25 different bacterial species and 18/20

Listeria monocytogenes varieties (A1; Lis-Balchin and Deans, 1997; Lis-Balchin *et al.*, 1998a). Strong effects against four different species were also reported (Friedman *et al.*, 2002).

Antifungal activity

Relative data (% inhibition): *Aspergillus niger* 7%; *A. ochraceus* 65%; *Fusarium culmorum* 28% (A1). Generally poor action was obtained against 5/5 fungi (Maruzella, 1960).

Use in pregnancy and lactation: contraindications

Frankincense essential oil has not been studied for use in massage, but the fact that there is a spasmolytic effect on the uterus *in vitro* suggests caution in its usage. The burnt incense and fragrance poses no apparent threat.

Pharmaceutical guidance

Frankincense essential oil differs in its chemical composition depending on source and mode of production. It is therefore difficult to generalise as to its bioactivity. There does not seem to be any apparent danger in its use, though the high limonene content in some commercial essential oils may add to its possible sensitisation potential, especially when used in massage. The use of the essential oil fragrance alone, and also burning the resin, poses no danger. The fragrance may act as a stimulant due to its limonene content and that of other monoterpenes, whilst the burnt resin may be more relaxing.

Use in babies and young children

Due to the immaturity and the delicate nature of the skin of babies and young children, it is inadvisable for any essential oils to be used in massage, however much the essential oil has been diluted in the carrier oils. This is also a necessary precaution due to the possibilities of sensitisation of the children at this young age through skin or air-borne odorant effects (see Chapters 5 and 7).

Instillation or administration of essential oils near the baby or young child's nose is not only not recommended, but distinctly inadvisable, as there have been numerous cases reported of severe toxicity and even death from such applications (see Chapter 7).

Geranium Oil

CAS numbers

USA: 8000-46-2; EINECS: 90082-51-2

Species/Botanical name

Pelargonium species and cultivars are obtained from *Pelargonium capitatum* × *P. radens* and *P. capitatum* × *P. graveolens*, etc., originating in southern Africa, and not from the genus *Geranium* (Lis-Balchin, 2002a). Geranium oil does not originate from *P. odoratisssimum*, which is apple-scented, nor from *Geranium maculatum* (which is not only the wrong species but also has no odour) nor from any other *Geranium* species, such as *G. robertianum* (herb robert) and *G. macrorrhizum* (yielding zdravetz oil in Bulgaria; see also Chapter 4).

Synonyms

Rose geranium, poor-man's rose, aetheroleum pelargonii, oleum geranii, pelargonium oil, rose geranium oil

Safety

CHIP details
Xn; R65; 15%; S62 (A26)

EU sensitiser total
69.5 (based on citral 1.5%, geraniol 18%, citronellol 40% and linalool 10%) (A27)

GRAS status
Granted (Fenaroli, 1997).

Extraction, source, appearance and odour

Extraction
The essential oil is produced by steam distillation of the leaves and flowers of the flowering herb (Arctander, 1960). The term rose geranium implies either a particular cultivar or sometimes the fact that rose petals were distributed on top of the geranium leaves during the distillation.

Source
Egypt, China and the Comores, with some recent production from plants grown in India and South Africa. Plants had previously been grown in southern France, Morocco, Algeria and Tunisia.

Appearance and odour
Various shades of amber-yellow to greenish-yellow colour are found. The odour is characteristic of the origin, but mainly rose-like with a varying minty note (Arctander, 1960).

Aromatherapy uses

The uses include: premenstrual tension and menopausal problems, inflammation and congestion of the breasts; stimulating and cleansing the lymphatic system and hence the immune system; circulatory problems, haemorrhoids and phlebitis; sore throats, tonsillitis, asthma, and excess mucus. Geranium essential oil is apparently known for its beneficial use on all skin types; ringworm, general infections, acne, burns, bruises, shingles, herpes, eczema, dermatitis; normalising sebaceous gland activity and sebum secretion (Ryman, 1991; Lawless, 1992; Rose, 1992a; Price, 1993; Sheppard-Hanger, 1995).

Scientific comment

Geranium essential oil was originally produced solely for the perfumery and fragrance trades, however geranium oil is commonly used in aromatherapy, based on the misinterpretation by original aromatherapists of old English herbals (Culpeper, 1653), which referred to the real *Geranium* genus (e.g. *G. robertianum*) and not *Pelargonium*. The usages of the geranium extracts mentioned in old herbals (antidiarrhoeal) are mainly associated with their tannin content and other water-soluble chemicals (e.g. flavonoids) in the leaves. Essential oils are steam-distilled volatiles and do not contain these components. 'Geranium oil's' major attributes were given as its vulnerary powers and its power to mend fractures and eliminate cancers (Valnet, 1982) taken straight out of the old herbals; the directions for oral use are given as for herb Robert. Geranium oil is both a sedative and a stimulant, based on human brain contingent negative variation studies (A14). The use of massage can be beneficial for stress-related and muscular conditions and combining this with the odour used as a fragrance could magnify the relaxant effect in some people or may cause a contradictory effect.

Herbal uses

Many *Pelargonium* species have been used in the past as traditional medicines in southern Africa with mainly antidysenteric properties (Watt and Breyer-Brandwijk, 1962) (e.g. root of *P. transvaalense* and *P. triste* and the leaves of *P. bowkeri* and *P. sidaefolium*). Some *Pelargonium* species were also used to treat specific maladies (e.g. *P. cucullatum* for nephritis, *P. tragacanthoides* for neuralgia, *P. luridum* and *P. transvaalense* root for fever, *P. grossularioides* for menstrual flow) (Pappe, 1868; Watt and Breyer-Brandwijk, 1962). The latter was also used as an emmanogogue and abortifacient by both Zulus and Boers and has recently been studied further (Lis-Balchin and Hart, 1994) and shown to have spasmogenic properties on the uterus and smooth muscle preparations *in vitro*. *P. reniforme* and *P. sidoides* extracts (not containing the essential oil) are currently used in the herbal remedy Umckaloabo (produced in Germany) for respiratory ailments due to its strong antimicrobial properties. It also has immunomodulatory properties, leishmanicidal activity and interferon-like properties (Lis-Balchin, 2002a, ch.24). One aromatherapist has realised that there was no traditional, esoteric or medicinal use of the essential oil before 1900, as geranium oil was created for the fragrance trade (Sheppard-Hanger, 1995).

Food and perfumery uses

Food   Geranium rose oil (FEMA 2508) is used in: baked goods, frozen diary, gelatin and pudding, non-alcoholic and alcoholic beverages, hard candy and chewing gum. Concentrations of 30–300 ppm are used (Fenaroli, 1997).

Perfumery   Geranium oil and concoctions using geranium oil components have long been used in making artificial rose oil or 'rose extenders' (Curtis and Williams, 1996). Rhodinol ex geranium is used in numerous modern perfumery and cosmetic products (Arctander, 1960).

Chemistry

Major components

	% (Lawrence, 1976–2001)
Citronellol	28–58
Geraniol	7–19
Linalool	3–10
Isomenthone	4–7
Citronellyl formate	5–12
Geranyl formate	1–4

Quality specification of the essential oil: the ISO defines geranium oil as 'The oil obtained by steam distillation of the fresh or slightly withered herbaceous parts of *Pelargonium graveolens* L'Heritier ex Aiton, *Pelargonium roseum* Willdenow and other undefined hybrids which have given rise to differing ecotypes in the various geographical areas' (ISO 4731: 1972). The specification does not include the Bulgarian geranium oil distilled from *Geranium macrorrhizum*, known as zdravetz oil.

ISO 4731 has set the concentration for citronellol content at a minimum 42%/maximum 55% for Bourbon geranium oil; 35/58% for Moroccan; 40/58% for Egyptian and 40/58% for Chinese oils. Other physicochemical values are also given, but these may now be academic as the greatest production is apparently from China (Quinhua, 1993), the oil resembling Bourbon, and considerable variation is found in the chemical composition (Lawrence, 1992, 1994) with notable incidence of apparent adulteration (Lis-Balchin, 2002a, ch.1).

The apparent geographical source had on the whole no correlation with the chemical composition of commercial geranium oils (Lis-Balchin et al., 1996b) except for the presence or absence of the relevant sesquiterpene: i.e. 10-epi-γ-eudesmol in Egyptian oils (3–7%) and guaia-6.9-diene (1–7%) in the Bourbon and China oils. A Moroccan oil contained both these sesquiterpenes. The proportions of the main components (i.e. citronellol, geraniol, linalool, isomenthone, citronellyl formate and geranyl formate) were not consistent for any geographical source. See Table 1.

Note: The essential oil composition of geranium oil differs completely from that of a true *Geranium robertianum* oil (Pedro et al., 1992) or that of *G. macrorrhizum* (Ognyanov, 1985).

Adulteration

Geranium oil contains mainly citronellol and geraniol and their esters, therefore can be easily

Table 1   Physicochemical characteristics of geranium oils from different sources

	Bourbon	*Morocco*	*Egypt*
Relative density at 20°C	0.884–0.892	0.883–0.900	0.887–0.892
Refractive index at 20°C	1.462–1.468	1.464–1.472	1.466–1.470
Optical rotation at 20°C	−8 to −14	−8 to −13	−8 to 212
Acid value maximum	10	10	6
Ester value	52–78	35–80	42–58
Ester value after acetylation	205–230	192–230	210–235
Carbonyl value expressed as isomenthone	58	58	Not given
Apparent citronellol (rhodinol) content	42–55	35–58	40–58

concocted from cheaper essential oils and adjusted to the recommended ISO standards with low-priced synthetics. The most expensive geranium oil was always Bourbon (Guenther, 1948–1952), and it increased in tonnage as well as value over some years, surprisingly, on the small volcanic island of Réunion. This was partly due to the increase in geranium oil production in China, which being very similar to that of Bourbon would often get accepted as such (Verlet, 1992).

Toxicity

Acute toxicity (A22)
Oral LD$_{50}$ >5 g/kg (rats).
Dermal LD$_{50}$ 2.5 g/kg (rabbit).

Irritation and sensitisation
Geranium oil applied undiluted to abraded or intact rabbit skin for 24 hours under occlusion was found to be moderately irritant, but applied to backs of hairless mice it was not irritating (Urbach and Forbes, 1972). Human patch test (closed) to 10% geranium oil in petrolatum produced no irritation after 48 hours (Kligman, 1973). A maximisation test on 25 volunteers using 10% in petrolatum produced no sensitisation (Kligman, 1973).

Phototoxicity
Not found for geranium oil (Urbach and Forbes, 1972).

Other toxicities
There are very few, scattered references to toxicity, and all references are due to contact dermatitis and sensitisation. Most of the references are to the geranium oil and the main components geraniol (Lovell, 1993). Pelargonium plants themselves have caused hand dermatitis (Anderson, 1923) and sensitisation (Rook, 1961; Hjorth, 1969) and dermatitis to perfumes containing geranium oil has been shown in a few cases (Klarmann, 1958). Ointments containing geraniol (e.g. 'Blastoestimulina') were reported to cause sensitisation when used in the treatment of chronic leg ulcers (Romaguera et al., 1986; Guerra et al., 1987), although the patients were also sensitive to other ointments which contained no essential oils. Geraniol was found to give a positive patch test in over 1.2% cases when used at 1% in white petrolatum with 5% sorbitan sesquioleate (Frosch et al., 1998). Although the sensitisation to geraniol using a maximization test proved negative (A22), the allergen may be geraniol as cross-reactions often occurred with citronella (Keil, 1947), however, the main sensitiser in citronella is citronellal, with citronellol less reactive; geraniol was even weaker, as was citral. In two cases, strong reactions were obtained with 1% solutions of citronellal and weaker ones with citronellol, geraniol and geranyl acetate. In 23/23 cases no response was found using lemon oil, suggesting specificity of the response. In a lemon oil sensitisation case, α-pinene gave a greater response than β-pinene: this is due to the close similarity between limonene and α-pinene (due to an exposed methylene radical). Recent Japanese studies on patients with ordinary cosmetic dermatitis and pigmented cosmetic dermatitis, who showed a positive allergic responses to a wide range of fragrances (Nakayama, 1998), gave rise to a list of common cosmetic sensitisers and primary sensitisers, which included geranium oil and geraniol. D-Limonene, although present in small quantities in geranium oil, has shown many sensitisation reactions (see Chapter 7).

Bioactivities

Pharmacological activities *in vitro* and *in vivo*

Smooth muscle Geranium oil had a spasmolytic effect on electrically stimulated smooth muscle of the guinea-pig ileum *in vitro* (A2; Lis-Balchin *et al.*, 1996a). However, *P. grossularioides* essential oil had a spasmogenic effect (Lis-Balchin and Hart, 1994). Antispasmodic action of citronellol, geraniol and linalool on mouse small intestine was reported (Imaseki and Kitabatake, 1962). The majority of pelargonium oils and their components produce a relaxation of smooth muscle through a mechanism involving adenylate cyclase and a rise in the concentration of the secondary messenger cyclic AMP (Lis-Balchin and Hart, 1997a, 1998a; Lis-Balchin, 2002a, ch.11). There is some evidence of calcium channel blockade, but only at high concentrations. Preliminary results using more hydrophilic (methanolic) extracts of *Pelargonium* species and cultivars and their teas indicate that most have a contractile effect initially, which is followed by a relaxation (Lis-Balchin, 2002a, ch.11). There is also some evidence that a few methanolic extracts use calcium channels at normal concentrations.

Uterus The essential oils of *P. grossularioides*, as well as its water-soluble and methanolic extracts, were all spasmogenic on the rat uterus (Lis-Balchin and Hart, 1994). This is in contrast to all other 'geranium oils' (*Pelargonium* species) and their components, such as geraniol and linalool, and all other commercial oils studied, which had a spasmolytic action on the uterus (A3; A4; Lis-Balchin and Hart, 1997b).

Skeletal muscle Geranium oil caused an increase in tone and reduction of contraction in skeletal muscle (chick biventer and rat phrenic nerve–diaphragm) (Lis-Balchin and Hart, 1997c).

Physiological actions There is little direct scientific evidence for the physiological effectiveness of geranium oil apart from some studies on animal movement (A5). There are miscellaneous physiological reactions attributed to a geranium component, linalool: a hypoglycaemic effect in normal and streptozotocin-diabetic rats (Afifi *et al.*, 1997); a hepatic peroxysomal and microsomal enzyme induction in rats (Roffey *et al.*, 1990), also shown by geraniol (Chadba *et al.*, 1984); and choleretic and cholagogic activity of a mixture of linalool and α-terpineol (Gruncharov, 1973; Peana *et al.*, 1994). Linalool has a dose-dependent sedative

effect on the CNS of rats, which could be caused by its inhibitory activity on glutamate binding in the cortex (Elisabetsky *et al.*, 1995).

Psychological actions The main action of essential oils is probably on the primitive, unconscious, limbic system of the brain, which is not under the control of the cerebrum or higher centres (Lis-Balchin, 1997; Lis-Balchin, 2002b, ch.13). Many fragrances have been shown to have an effect on mood and, in general, pleasant odours generate happy memories, more positive feelings and a general sense of well-being (Warren and Warrenburg, 1993). Geranium oil has both a sedative and stimulant effect on the contingent negative variation brain waves in human volunteers (A14).

Antimicrobial activities

Antibacterial action

Relative values: 8 to 19/25 bacteria were inhibited by different commercial oil samples (A1; G7, G10; Ger paper); the variation between samples could not be correlated with the chemical composition of the samples; 3 to 16/20 strains of *Listeria monocytogenes* were affected by the same 16 different geranium oil samples (Lis-Balchin, 2004a). Geranium oil was most effective against the dairy products organism *Brevibacterium linens* and the toxin-producing *Yersinia enterocolitica*, but, in contrast, with *Klebsiella pneumoniae* and *Escherichia coli* its presence resulted in enhancement of growth (Deans and Ritchie, 1987). In other studies 12/22 bacteria and 12/12 fungi (three yeast-like, nine filamentous) were inhibited (Pattnaik *et al.*, 1996). The antimicrobial activity of commercial geranium essential oils, which are often adulterated with synthetics, was much greater than that of an authentic oil, but this had a similar pharmacological effect on smooth muscle (spasmolytic). The odour can be even more appreciated by perfumers than the real essential oil (Lis-Balchin, 2002a, ch.1).

Synergistic activity: In a study into the potential usage of mixtures of plant volatile oils as synergistic antibacterial agents in foods, 'geranium oil' was used in a mixture with nutmeg and bergamot oils, but no synergistic effect was found (Lis-Balchin and Deans, 1997b).

The antimicrobial activity of pelargonium oil components (Dorman and Deans, 2000) showed the following ranking order of activity: linalool > geranyl acetate > nerol > geraniol > menthone > β-pinene > limonene > α-pinene. Compared with more phenolic compounds, these activities are relatively modest. The bacteria showing the greatest levels of inhibition were *Clostridium sporogenes* > *Lactobacillus plantarum* > *Citrobacter freundii* > *Escherichia coli* > *Flavobacterium suaveolens*.

Antifungal activity

Relative values: Different commercial geranium oil samples showed inhibition against *Aspergillus niger* 0–94%; *A. ochraceus* 12–95%; *Fusarium culmorum* 40–86% (A1).

Antioxidant activity

Pelargonium species, including the commercial geranium oil, have been shown to have antioxidative properties (Fukaya *et al.*, 1988; Youdim *et al.*, 1999; Dorman and Deans, 2000), although these properties had very variable activities in different commercial samples of 'geranium oil' (Lis-Balchin *et al.*, 1996a).

Clinical studies

No evidence has been provided by clinical studies for the uses to which geranium oil is put, for example in childbirth (Burns and Blaney, 1994). However, there is pharmacological evidence for the decrease and even cessation of uterine contractions in animal experiments, which could prove harmful (Lis-Balchin, 2002a, ch.11). Furthermore, although 'geranium' oils are very active on many different animal tissues *in vitro* (Lis-Balchin *et al.*, 1997b), there is no proof as yet as to whether minute amounts (as used in aromatherapy massage) can have direct action on target organs or tissues rather than through the odour pathway (Vickers, 1996), despite some evidence that certain essential oil components can be absorbed either through the skin or lungs (Jager *et al.*, 1992; Buchbauer *et al.*, 1993b).

Unconfirmed and unpublished reports of the efficacy of geranium essential oil for treatment of pain have appeared in advertisements for certain topical 'medicines' over several years. It is known that certain essential oils and their components have a nociceptive effect in animal experiments (Hart *et al.*, 1994; Santos and Rao, 2000; Hajhashemi *et al.*, 2002; Barocelli *et al.*, 2004).

The results of a clinical trial using Neuragen (containing geranium essential oil) for relief of pain associated with diabetic peripheral neuropathy (DPN) showed that of 29 patients completing the feedback survey, at least 20 patients (69%) noted improvement in pain, usually within minutes of applying Neuragen topically. The trial of Neuragen (Origin BioMedicinals Inc.) was conducted by health practitioners in Sacramento, California between May and September 2004 in collaboration with DiabetesinControl.com and the Yolo County Peripheral Neuropathy Support Groups.

DPN is characterized by numbness, tingling or burning pain in the feet and hands, and can affect 40% of diabetics. Other positive effects of Neuragen have been reported across North America for post-shingles pain, fibromyalgia, causalgias radiculopathies, phantom limb pain, Bell's palsy, trigeminal neuralgias, mysofascial pain, HIV and other chronic nerve pain. Treatment with topical application of Neuragen and also undiluted geranium essential oil has led to severe side-effects, which are not reported by the manufacturer. A report from a user of geranium oil who applied it topically to scalp, cheek, and wrist, in spots where he suffered allodynia led to more and more local stinging; a bout of tremor of the hands just when the geranium oil regime was instigated; growing sensitisation to the geranium oil (personal correspondence). As much as 40–50 drops of geranium oil were used per day, usually applied to the same places. It is possible that some of the alleviation of pain was due to the inhalation of the geranium essential oil.

Use in pregnancy and lactation: contraindications

Due to the lack of experimental evidence as to the effect of geranium oil on the uterus and the cessation of contractions in animal experiments *in vitro*, caution should be exercised during pregnancy and especially during parturition. The incidence of any other adverse effects is very low, however. Use as a fragrance should be without adverse effects.

Pharmaceutical guidance

Geranium oil is relatively safe but has recently acquired a very high sensitiser value from the EU, which warrants restriction of the usage on the skin, especially by susceptible people or those with dermatitis. It can be used safely as a fragrance and the odour has proved to be both relaxant and stimulant on the human brain (A14). The use of the fragrance together with massage could therefore be complementary and relaxant, or contradictory if the odour is disliked.

Use in babies and young children

Due to the immaturity and the delicate nature of the skin of babies and young children, it is inadvisable for any essential oils to be used in massage, however much the essential oil has been diluted in the carrier oils. This is also a necessary precaution due to the possibilities of sensitisation of the children at this young age through skin or air-borne odorant effects (see also Chapters 5 and 7).

Instillation or administration of essential oils near the baby or young child's nose is not only not recommended, but distinctly inadvisable, as there have been numerous cases reported of severe toxicity and even death from such applications (see Chapter 7).

Ginger Oil

CAS numbers
USA: 8007-08-7; EINECS: 84696-15-1

Species/Botanical name
Zingiber officinale Roscoe (Zingiberaceae)

Safety
CHIP details
Xn; R65; 90%; S62

EU sensitiser total
2.3 (based on 0.7% citral, 1% limonene and 0.6% linalool)

GRAS status
Granted.

Extraction, source, appearance and odour
Extraction
A volatile oil is obtained from the dried pulverised ginger rhizome by steam distillation, then the ginger residue is dried and solvent extracted to get the oleoresin (Arctander, 1960; Lawrence and Reynolds, 1984).

Source
India, China, Africa and Australia.

Appearance and odour
A pale yellow to yellow essential oil with a warm, spicy, fresh-woody, aromatic odour, said to be reminiscent of citrus, lemongrass, coriander, etc. The sweet and heavy undertone is tenacious, sweet and rich and almost balsamic-floral. Ginger oil differs according to origin: the African oil is heavier and darker in colour. It tends to thicken and darken on exposure to air (resinification) (Arctander, 1960).

Aromatherapy uses
Uses include: sharpening the senses, aiding memory, tiredness and nervous exhaustion; colds, influenza, sore throats; cooling the body if feverish through perspiration evaporation; phlegmatic bronchial conditions; digestive conditions of nausea and vomiting, travel sickness; circulatory stimulant, poor circulation to the extremities; rheumatism, muscular aches, sprains; reinstating menstrual flow and dysmenorrhoea; aphrodisiac and useful for cases of impotence (Ryman, 1991; Lawless, 1992; Rose, 1992a; Price, 1993; Sheppard-Hanger, 1995).

Scientific comment
It is unlikely that most of the uses given above could be accomplished by massaging the ginger essential oil, as many of the herbally active components are absent. Massage itself can alleviate many stress-related problems and the ginger fragrance may relieve nausea in some people.

Herbal uses
Ginger is carminative, diaphoretic and antispasmodic. It has been used for colic, flatulent dyspepsia and flatulent intestinal colic. Nowadays, its use in the prevention of nausea and vomiting, particularly motion (travel) sickness, is of interest and also its use as a digestive aid and in the treatment of inflammatory conditions, such as osteoarthritis and rheumatoid arthritis (Wren, 1988; Chevallier, 1996; Blumenthal *et al.*, 2000; Barnes *et al.*, 2002).

Food and perfumery uses
Food Ginger oil (FEMA 2522) is used in a large number of foods and beverages (Fenaroli, 1997).

Perfumery It is used in perfumery in oriental and floral fragrances (Arctander, 1960).

Chemistry

Ginger (Nigeria) *Zingiber officinale* Roscoe:

Major components

	%
α-Pinene	3
Camphene	8.3
β-Phellandrene	9.6
Linalool	0.8
Borneol	0.8
Neral	1.4
Geranyl acetate	0.9
α-Zingiberene	29
β-Bisabolene + α-farnesene	14
β-Sesquiphellandrene	9.9

Minor components

Other sesquiterpenes include zingiberol, zingiberenol, ar-curcumene, β-sesquiphellandrol (*cis* and *trans*). There is wide variation in the composition of ginger oils from different origins (Lawrence, 1976–2001).

Adulteration

Ginger is produced in large quantities and is relatively cheap, therefore adulteration is not common. Galanga oil can be used as an adulterant. Ginger oleoresin may be added to give a more ginger-like odour (A8; see also Chapter 4).

Toxicity

Acute toxicity (A22)

Oral LD$_{50}$ >5 g/kg (rat).
Dermal LD$_{50}$ >5 g/kg (rabbit).

Irritation and sensitisation (A22)

None at 4% (human), but ginger oil products can cause dermatitis in hypersensitive people.

Phototoxicity (A22)

A minor effect was noted.

Bioactivities

Pharmacological activities *in vitro* and *in vivo*

Smooth muscle Ginger oil had a slight spasmolytic effect on the electrically stimulated smooth muscle of the guinea-pig ileum *in vitro* (A2; Lis-Balchin *et al.*, 1996a).

Uterus There was a decrease in the spontaneous contractions in the rat when ginger oil was introduced *in vitro* (A3; A4; Lis-Balchin and Hart, 1997b).

Other activities Ginger oil showed anti-inflammatory activity in rats with induced severe chronic adjuvant arthritis (Sharma *et al.*, 1994) and at 33 mg/kg administered orally for 26 days caused a significant suppression of paw and joint swelling, compared with controls. Extracts of ginger (not essential oils) administered by oral or intraperitoneal routes have shown antiemetic, antithrombotic, antimicrobial, anticancer, antioxidant and anti-inflammatory properties (Barnes *et al.*, 2002). Also, ginger has been reported to have hypoglycaemic, hypo- and hypertensive, cardiac, prostaglandin and platelet aggregation inhibition, antihypercholesterolaemic, cholagogic and stomachic properties.

Ginger was also found to reduce platelet synthesis of prostaglandin endoperoxides, thromboxane and prostaglandins. In rats, cholesterol absorption was impaired by ginger oleoresin containing small proportions of essential oil given intragastrically (Gujral *et al.*, 1974). Antihypercholesterolaemic activity was also shown by dried ginger rhizome given to rats fed a cholesterol-rich diet and to those with existing hypercholesterolaemia (Giri *et al.*, 1984).

A hypoglycaemic effect in both non-diabetic and alloxan-induced diabetic rabbits and rats (where it was significant) was shown by fresh ginger juice given orally (Sharma and Shukla, 1977).

An acetone extract of ginger, possibly containing some essential oil, administered intraduodenally showed a cholagogic action in rats (Yamahara *et al.*, 1985). Extracts of ginger or constituents of ginger (usually water-soluble) have been shown to have cancer chemopreventive and cytotoxic or cytostatic activity *in vitro* and *in vivo* (animals) and mutagenic activity was shown by an ethanolic ginger extract in some *Salmonella typhimurium* strains, although ginger juice showed antimutagenic activity (Barnes *et al.*, 2002). The combination of standardised extracts of ginger (water-soluble) and *Ginkgo biloba* administered intragastrically, assessed in the elevated plus-maze test, was found to have an anxiolytic effect at lower doses, but appeared to have an anxiogenic effect at higher doses in rats (Hasenohri *et al.*, 1996).

Clinical studies

The powdered root of ginger, not the essential oil, was shown to be effective in preventing seasickness and vomiting, although in another study ginger was ineffective in the prevention of motion sickness induced by a rotating chair (Barnes *et al.*, 2002). A systematic review of six randomised controlled trials of ginger preparations involving patients with nausea and vomiting following operations, morning sickness, seasickness and cancer chemotherapy-induced nausea showed that the difference between the ginger and placebo groups was statistically non-significant when the data were pooled (Barnes *et al.*, 2002). Oral raw ginger reduced thromboxane B2 concentrations in serum collected after clotting in seven women, indicating a reduction in eicosanoid synthesis associated with platelet aggregation (Srivastava, 1989).

Antimicrobial activities

Antibacterial activity

There was a very low effect on 7/25 different bacterial species (Deans and Ritchie, 1987); ginger oil vapour affected 1/5 bacteria (Maruzella and Sicurella, 1960). There was no effect on five *Listeria monocytogenes* varieties (Aureli *et al.*, 1992).

Sesquiterpenes from ginger rhizomes showed *in vitro* activity against rhinovirus IB (Denyer *et al.*, 1994).

Antifungal activity

Antifungal activity was virtually absent: no action was found against five fungi (Maruzella, 1960) and only slight fungistatic action against 8/15 fungi (Maruzella and Liguori, 1958).

Antioxidant activity

Antioxidant activity was reported in ginger constituents *in vitro* (Surh *et al.*, 1998).

Use in pregnancy and lactation: contraindications

Ginger is said to be an abortifacient (Taroeno *et al.*, 1989) and uteroactivity has been documented for a related species. This may not involve the essential oil; however, a decrease in the spontaneous contractions in the rat when ginger oil was introduced *in vitro* suggests caution during pregnancy and parturition.

Pharmaceutical guidance

Ginger essential oil is relatively safe and should not contain oleoresin components, which are thought to be the main active principles in ginger in the pharmacological actions (e.g. the hypoglycaemic, antihypercholesterolaemic, anti-ulcer and inhibition of prostaglandin synthesis). The use of ginger as a prophylactic remedy against motion sickness is contentious. It seems likely that ginger may act by a local action on the gastrointestinal tract, rather than by a centrally mediated mechanism. The effect of ginger vapour has been shown to be very remedial.

Excessive doses of the root may interfere with existing cardiac, antidiabetic or anticoagulant therapy. An oleoresin component, (6)-shogaol, has been reported to affect blood pressure (initially decrease then increase) *in vivo*. However, ginger oil may not be involved in these activities.

Ginger essential oil can therefore be used in aromatherapy massage or used as a fragrance.

Use in babies and young children

Due to the immaturity and the delicate nature of the skin of babies and young children, it is inadvisable for any essential oils to be used in massage, however much the essential oil has been diluted in the carrier oils. This is also a necessary precaution due to the possibilities of sensitisation of the children at this young age through skin or air-borne odorant effects (see Chapters 5 and 7).

Instillation or administration of essential oils near the baby or young child's nose is not only not recommended, but distinctly inadvisable, as there have been numerous cases reported of severe toxicity and even death from such applications (see Chapter 7).

Ho Leaf Oil

CAS numbers

USA: 8022-91-1; EINECS: 91745-89-0

Species/Botanical name

Cinnamomum camphora L. Nees & Eberneier (Lauraceae)

Synonyms

Cinnamomum camphora Sieb.

Safety

RIFM recommended safety of use limits
10% (A23)

CHIP details
None

EU sensitiser total
90.6 (90% linalool, 0.4 geraniol, 0.2 limonene) (A27)

Extraction, source, appearance and odour

Extraction
A volatile oil is obtained by steam distillation of the leaves of the tree (Arctander, 1960).

Source
Taiwan, Japan, Brazil and China.

Appearance and odour
Ho leaf oil is a colourless oil with a clean, sweet, delicately floral, somewhat woody odour reminiscent of linalool (Arctander, 1960).

Aromatherapy uses

This should be the same as for rosewood oil, due to the similarity in chemical composition. Most aromatherapy books do not list ho leaf oil, but aromatherapists are being made aware of the potential of using ho leaf (which is replenishable yearly) rather than rosewood (produced by destruction of the trees, which are now under threat of extinction).

Scientific comment

See above and rosewood monograph.

Herbal uses

None recorded, but see rosewood monograph.

Food and perfumery uses

Food No FEMA number has been given to ho leaf oil, but it is included temporarily in the list for food use. Its uses in many foods and drinks are similar to those of rosewood (Fenaroli, 1997).

Perfumery It is used in numerous perfumes due to its odour and low cost, also for the isolation of linalool and production of linalyl esters. Acetylated ho leaf oil is a good substitute for linalyl acetate in cosmetic products such as soaps (Arctander, 1960).

Chemistry

Major components

	% (Lawrence, 1976–2001)
Linalool	85–95
Linalyl acetate	2–5
Geraniol	trace–0.4
Limonene	trace–0.2
Terpenes, various types	trace–0.5

Adulteration

Synthetic linalool and linalyl acetate is frequently used as the basis of the essential oil. Rosewood oil is similar and preferred by perfumers (A8; see also Chapter 4).

Toxicity

Acute toxicity (A22)

Oral LD$_{50}$ >3.8 g/kg (rat).

Dermal LD$_{50}$ >5 g/kg (rabbit).

Irritation and sensitisation (A22)

None at 10% (human).

Note: High sensitisation potential. The chemotype normally used is linalool-rich and does not contain camphor and safrole; this chemotype is therefore non-toxic, in contrast to the latter (Tisserand and Balacs, 1995), and its only possible effect is sensitisation.

Phototoxicity
None reported.

Bioactivities

Pharmacological activities *in vitro* and *in vivo*

Smooth muscle Ho leaf oil had a spasmolytic effect on the electrically stimulated smooth muscle of the guinea-pig ileum *in vitro*. Linalool had a similar effect (A2; Lis-Balchin *et al.*, 1996a). Similar results were obtained by another group (Reiter and Brandt, 1985).

Uterus There was a decrease in the spontaneous contractions in the rat for ho leaf oil, linalool, limonene and other components. Mixing several other essential oils with ho leaf oil also had a relaxant effect (A3; A4; Lis-Balchin and Hart, 1997b).

Skeletal muscle Linalyl acetate showed a decrease in the twitch and a delayed increase in resting tone in the rat phrenic nerve–diaphragm. Linalool showed a decrease in the twitch only (Lis-Balchin and Hart, 1997c).

Other activities Linalool is relaxant (see lavender oil monograph). Evidence for the sedative properties of linalool after inhalation in animals was provided as it significantly decreased the motility of 'normal' test mice as well as that of animals rendered hyperactive or 'stressed' by an intraperitoneal dose of caffeine (Buchbauer *et al.*, 1991, 1993a,b). The dose-dependent sedative effect of linalool on the CNS of rats (Elisabetsky *et al.*, 1995) may be caused by its inhibitory activity on glutamate binding in the cortex (Elisabetsky *et al.*, 1995). There are many psychological, physiological and biochemical effects of linalool and lavender, with linalool as its main component (see lavender oil monograph). The effect of linalool and lavender on guinea-pig ileum correlated with its chemical profile and the relaxant effect shown in aromatherapy (A11, A12).

Antimicrobial activities

Antibacterial effect
Relative data: Ho leaf oil was active against 23/25 different bacterial species and 15/20 *Listeria*

monocytogenes varieties (A1; Lis-Balchin and Deans, 1997; Lis-Balchin *et al.*, 1998a). Linalool showed good effects against four bacteria (Friedman *et al.*, 2002).

Antifungal activity
Relative data (% inhibition): *Aspergillus niger* 73%; *A. ochraceus* 93%; *Fusarium culmorum* 81% (A1).

Antioxidant activity
A slight antioxidant effect was noted (Lis-Balchin *et al.*, 1996a).

Use in pregnancy and lactation: contraindications

Like the similar rosewood oil, ho leaf oil has sensitisation potential and caused a decrease in the spontaneous contractions in the uterus *in vitro*, therefore it should not be used in massage during pregnancy, parturition or lactation. It can be used as a fragrance in low concentrations, as the odour of rosewood has been shown to be relaxant on the human brain (A14).

Pharmaceutical guidance

Due to its high content of linalool, this is a relaxant essential oil, as shown by brain wave effects, and should be regarded as a good substitute for rosewood oil, which is in limited supply because the tree from which it is produced is now an endangered species. Only the potential sensitisation effect presents a risk, but mainly in sensitive people.

Use in babies and young children

Due to the immaturity and the delicate nature of the skin of babies and young children, it is inadvisable for any essential oils to be used in massage, however much the essential oil has been diluted in the carrier oils. This is also a necessary precaution due to the possibilities of sensitisation of the children at this young age through skin or air-borne odorant effects (see Chapters 5 and 7).

Instillation or administration of essential oils near the baby or young child's nose is not only not recommended, but distinctly inadvisable, as there have been numerous cases reported of severe toxicity and even death from such applications (see Chapter 7).

Hyssop Oil

low BP

CAS numbers
USA: 8006-83-5; EINECS: 84603-66-7

Species/Botanical name
Hyssopus officinalis (Lamiaceae syn. Labiatae)

Synonyms
Azob

Safety
CHIP details
Xn; R10, 22, 65; 20%; S62 (A26)

RIFM recommended safety of use limits
4% (A23)

EU sensitiser total
1 (A27)

GRAS status
? (Fenaroli, 1997).

Extraction, source, appearance and odour
Extraction
A volatile oil is obtained by steam distillation of the herb (Arctander, 1960).

Source
Hungary, Italy and Bulgaria.

Appearance and odour
Hyssop oil is colourless to pale yellow-green, sweet, aromatic, herbaceous and camphoraceous, with a warm-aromatic, spicy undertone (Arctander, 1960).

Aromatherapy uses
Uses include: raising low blood pressure; tonic for weakness; respiratory problems, especially where thick mucus is present; stimulating effect on the heart; gargle for sore throats and loss of voice; inhalations for coughs and sore throats; influenza, bronchitis, cystitis, urinary stones, wounds, emphysema, hay fever, multiple sclerosis, pneumonia, asthma; digestion; stomach cramp, appetite; menstrual problems; clearing effect on the mind, feeling of alertness and clarity; bruises (applied in a cold compress as soon as possible); hot compresses for rheumatism; scars; dermatitis, eczema (Ryman, 1991; Lawless, 1992; Rose, 1992a; Price, 1993; Sheppard-Hanger, 1995).

Scientific comment
Most of the uses of hyssop essential oil are based entirely on its herbal usage, where there are many active principles that are, however, absent from the essential oil. There is no scientific evidence that any of the conditions can benefit muscular problems. The use of a potentially dangerous essential oil in the massage mixture could prove damaging rather than alleviating.

Herbal uses
Hyssop originated in the Mediterranean area and has long been considered a sacred and healing herb. In the tenth century the Benedictine monks used it in the making of liqueurs. It was also used in food preparation, to ward off lice, to heal wounds, to reduce swelling and to fight cancer. It is used as a carminative, pectoral, stimulant and sedative; for bronchitis, coughs, colds and for asthma. It contains an anti-inflammatory (ursolic acid) and an expectorant (marrubiin). There is some danger of causing epileptic fits (Wren, 1988; Chevallier, 1996).

Food and perfumery uses
Food Hyssop oil (FEMA 2591) is used in a variety of foods and beverages, for example in Chartreuse and other liqueurs (Fenaroli, 1997).

Perfumery It is used in spicy, cologne-type perfumes; soaps and cosmetics (Arctander, 1960).

Chemistry

Major components
Hyssopus officinalis Linn., hyssop (ISO 9841: 1991):

	%	
	Min	Max
α-Pinene	1.0	1.5
β-Pinene	13.5	23
Sabinene	2	3
Myrcene	1	2
Limonene	1	4
Myrtenylmethylether	1	3
Pinocamphone	5.5	17.5
β-Bourbonene	1.5	2
Isopinocamphone	34.5	50
β-Caryophyllene	1	3
Alloaromadendrene	1.5	2
Germacrene D	2	3
γ-Cardinene	2	2.5
Apathulenol	0.5	2

Minor components
Phellandrene (0.7–1%), camphene (0.1–0.4%), cis-ocimene (0.1–3.6%), trans-ocimene (0.3–0.5%), p-cymene (0.1–0.9%), calamenene (trace), nerolidol (0.1–1%), spathulenol (0.7–2.2%), terpinen-4-ol (0.1%), α-terpineol (1–1.8%), myrtenol (0.4–2.2%), elemol (0.4–1.7%); bornyl acetate, methyl myrtenate (2%); α-thujone (trace–0.08%), β-thujone (0.1–0.3%), carvacrol (trace); methyl chavicol (0.1–1.3%), methyl eugenol (0.1–0.5%), 1,8-cineole (0.6%), caryophyllene oxide (0.2%).

Adulteration
Cedarleaf oil, camphor oil or its fractions, lavandin, myrtle and sage oils are used as adulterants (A8; Arctander, 1960; see also Chapter 4).

Toxicity

Acute toxicity
Oral LD_{50} >5 g/kg (rat).

Dermal LD_{50} >5 g/kg (rabbit).

Irritation and sensitisation
No irritation or sensitisation at 4% dilution on humans (A22).

Phototoxicity
No phototoxic effects reported (A22).

Other toxicities
Neurotoxicity was investigated in 65 male and female rats given hyssop intraperitoneally at progressively increasing doses; the components thujone and pinocamphone were also tested (Millet et al., 1981). The animals were equipped with four skull electrodes for EEG and convulsions were elicited by all the oils, but varied according to the plant. For hyssop, the dose for no effect was 0.08 g/kg; convulsions were at 0.13 g/kg and it was lethal at 1.25 g/kg. A daily repeated subclinical dose of hyssop oil (0.02 g/kg) for 15 days precipitated convulsions after just 5 days, but the rats returned to normal after cessation of injections. Convulsions were shown for pinocamphone at a lower dose of 0.05 g/kg. This suggests that small doses every day for a short time could produce convulsions (Millet et al., 1981).

In humans, neurotoxicity studies have shown a period of latency of a few minutes to 2 hours following poisoning by hyssop: the patients vomited and had convulsions, resembling epileptic fits, sometimes with cyanosis (Millet et al., 1981; Tisserand and Balacs, 1995). The cases included: 30 drops of hyssop oil taken for a common cold; repetitive intake in an asthmatic 6-year-old girl who had 2–3 drops of hyssop oil per day, but during a dyspnoeic crisis, she received half a teaspoonful of hyssop; 10 drops of hyssop oil taken 'for flu' during two consecutive days and on the second day the convulsions appeared (see also Chapter 7).

Bioactivities

Pharmacological activities in vitro and in vivo
Smooth muscle   No data found.

Antimicrobial activities

Antibacterial activity
Hyssop showed a good antibacterial effect against 5/5 different species of bacteria (Friedman et al., 2002); in another study only one of four bacteria were affected (Morris et al., 1979).

Antifungal activity
No data found.

Use in pregnancy and lactation: contraindications

It is contraindicated for children under 2 years of age and the use of this essential oil during breastfeeding may also endanger the infant. The oil is a neurotoxin and the recommendation is to avoid the oil during pregnancy (Tisserand and Balacs, 1995).

Pharmaceutical guidance

Hyssop is a dangerous essential oil showing the ability to initiate convulsions even when taken in small repeated doses. The two toxic ketones pinocamphone and isopinocamphone have caused epilepsy and this essential oil remains on the danger list (see also sage oil monograph). Hyssop essential oil is not to be used, even in very small doses, in epilepsy, fever and in young children under 5, nor in patients with high blood pressure. The essential oil should not be taken orally (Tisserand and Balacs, 1995). It is generally recommended that hyssop essential oil should not be used in any way.

Use in babies and young children

Due to the immaturity and the delicate nature of the skin of babies and young children, it is inadvisable for any essential oils to be used in massage, however much the essential oil has been diluted in the carrier oils. This is also a necessary precaution due to the possibilities of sensitisation of the children at this young age through skin or air-borne odorant effects (see Chapters 5 and 7).

Instillation or administration of essential oils near the baby or young child's nose is not only not recommended, but distinctly inadvisable, as there have been numerous cases reported of severe toxicity and even death from such applications (see Chapter 7).

Jasmine Absolute

CAS numbers

USA: 8022-96-6; EINECS: 90045-94-6

Species/Botanical name

Jasminum grandiflorum L. (Oleaceae)

Synonyms

Royal jasmine, Catalonian and Spanish jasmine

Other species

Jasminum officinale L. (Poet's jasmine, white jasmine), *J. sambac* (L.) Aiton (Arabian jasmine)

Safety

CHIP details
None

RIFM recommended safety of use limits
4% (A23)

GRAS status
Granted (Fenaroli, 1997).

Extraction, source, appearance and odour

Extraction

An absolute is obtained by volatile solvent extraction of the flowers to give a concrete and then this is reprocessed in absolute alcohol (Arctander, 1960). The flowers are picked at dawn, since they are the most fragrant at daybreak; this is done delicately by young girls. Flowers from higher altitudes are of a finer quality than those of lower altitudes. Jasmine flower oil is extracted immediately after the flowers are collected by solvents or by enfleurage (Arctander, 1960). Poet's jasmine is native to the Himalayas of western China. Royal jasmine is usually grafted onto Poet's jasmine rootstocks as this is much more cold tolerant. *J. sambac* has been used to flavour teas and is reported to have antimicrobial activity (Simon *et al.*, 1990).

Source

Egypt, India, China and Morocco.

Appearance and odour

Dark orange to brown absolute (darkening on ageing) with an intense exotic, highly diffusive odour, with a waxy-herbaeous, oily-fruity and tea-like undertone (Arctander, 1960).

Aromatherapy uses

Jasmine absolute is used in aromatherapy as a holistic treatment for apathy, fear, hysteria, hypochondria, uterine disorders, childbirth, muscle relaxation and coughs; depression; calming, purifying, cleansing, aphrodisiac, balancing; general skin care on all skin types, muscular spasms, stress; headaches; uplifting; inspirational and mood lifting; inspiring confidence, creativity and imagination (Tisserand, 1977; Ryman, 1991; Lawless, 1992).

Scientific comment

Studies *in vivo* have shown that jasmine absolute stimulates, probably due to psychological impact. *In vitro*, however, it sedates muscle, which is a physiological action. Massage alone alleviates various stress conditions and muscle spasms and there is little evidence that the jasmine absolute has any further benefits. The concentration of the jasmine and the particular idiosyncrasies of each individual patient would govern the bioactivity achieved and could be completely different in different individuals and, indeed, in the same patient on different occasions (see Chapter 6).

Herbal uses

As a medicinal plant, jasmine has traditionally been considered an aphrodisiac and calmative. The roots and leaves of some jasmine species have been used in folk medicine for headaches, insomnia, pain due to rheumatism and bone dislocations and as an anthelmintic, active against ringworm and tapeworm. In China, the flowers were used for hepatitis, liver cirrhosis and dysentery and the related *J. sambac* flowers for conjunctivitis, dysentery, skin ulcers and tumours (Lawless, 1992).

The plant has been employed against some forms of cancer (Simon, 1984).

Food and perfumery uses

Food Jasmine absolute (FEMA 2598), concrete (FEMA 2599) and oil (FEMA 2600) are used in various foods and beverages (Fenaroli, 1997).

Perfumery It is used in most perfumes in very small proportions to impart a floral note; especially in high-class floral and oriental perfumes (Arctander, 1960). It blends well with most oils, especially clary sage, rose, sandalwood and citrus oils.

Chemistry

Major components

	% (Lawrence, 1976–2001)
Benzyl acetate	24–27
Benzyl benzoate	11–15
Linalool	4–6
Indole	3–5
Eugenol	2.5–3.4
Isojasmone	2.4–3.3
Farnesene	2–3.5
Phytols	9–28

Sensitisation is likely on the skin of sensitive individuals as this is not only an absolute (therefore contains components other than volatiles) it also has sensitisers like benzyl benzoate, farnesene, eugenol and linalool present.

Minor components

Methyl jasmonate occurs up to 0.5% in jasmine absolute and is the most characteristic compound for the jasmine odour. *cis*-Jasmone, up to 3%, also has the odour character of jasmine. Jasminlactone is present in jasmine absolute and in a wide range of other essential oils: it has a lactonic, coconut-like, fruity odour with characteristics of jasmone. Dihydro- and isojasmone also add to the odour.

Adulteration

Because of its high price, due to the delicate nature of production and low yield, adulteration of this absolute is very common, using synthetic components like indole, cinnamic aldehyde, *cis*-jasmone, farnesene, benzyl benzoate, benzyl acetate and fractions or whole oils, such as ylang ylang (A8; see also Chapter 4).

Toxicity

Acute toxicity (A22)

Oral LD$_{50}$ >5 g/kg (rat).

Dermal LD$_{50}$ >5 g/kg (rabbit).

Irritation and sensitisation
None at 3% (human), but sensitive people may be affected.

Phototoxicity
None reported.

Bioactivities

Pharmacological activities *in vitro* and *in vivo*

Smooth muscle Jasmine absolute had a spasmolytic effect on guinea-pig ileum *in vitro* (Lis-Balchin *et al.*, 2002). The mechanism of action was post-synaptic and probably mediated via cAMP but not cGMP. The mode of action *in vitro* resembled that of geranium, lavender and peppermint oils. Some calcium channel blockade may also be involved at higher concentrations.

Skeletal muscle Jasmine absolute decreased the tone of phrenic nerve–diaphragm preparations in the rat (Lis-Balchin and Hart, 1997c).

Uterus There was a decrease in the spontaneous contractions in the rat uterus with jasmine absolute, limonene and the other components (A3; A4; Lis-Balchin and Hart, 1997b). Mixing several other essential oils with jasmine absolute also had a relaxant effect.

Other activities There was a stimulant action on mice activity (Buchbauer, 1993) and contingent negative variation brain waves (A14). The contradictory effects *in vitro* and *in vivo* are probably due to the solely physiological effects of jasmine absolute *in vitro* (producing a relaxation) compared with those *in vivo*, where it has a strong psychological input, producing a stimulant effect in humans and enhanced movement in animals.
  Jasmine absolute is apparently a galactagogue and so promotes the flow of breast milk (BACIS archives). In contrast, in India, jasmine flowers are traditionally applied as a poultice to the breasts to suppress milk flow after a stillbirth. The galactogogue theory perhaps evolved from a misinterpretation of information given in *A Modern Herbal* (Grieve, 1937/1992), which said: 'and an oil

obtained from the roots [of *Jasminum sambac*] is used medicinally to arrest the secretion of milk'. Since jasmine absolute is produced from the flowers, it seems unreasonable to assume that it has a similar lactation-inhibiting effect. One study involved 60 women and compared the efficacy of bromocriptine (a lactation-inhibiting drug) with the application of jasmine flowers (*J. sambac*) to the breasts; both treatments produced a significant reduction in milk production (Abraham *et al.*, 1979). It was postulated that both tactile and olfactory stimuli of the flowers were responsible for the suppression of lactation. In another study (Shrivastav *et al.*, 1988), the mechanism of jasmine (botanical source unspecified) was discussed, including the possibility that when the fragrance is inhaled, aromatic molecules may travel via an olfactory pathway to the hypothalamus, which then conveys an inhibitory effect on the pituitary gland.

Antimicrobial activities

None reported.

Use in pregnancy and lactation: contraindications

Jasmine absolute should be restricted during pregnancy and lactation for two main reasons: first, it is an absolute and therefore contains other non-volatile components, which can have a sensitisation effect (together with its volatile components); second, there may be a decrease in the spontaneous contractions of the uterus, as shown in rat studies *in vitro*.

Pharmaceutical guidance

Sensitisation could occur as there are considerable numbers of sensitisers present (e.g. benzyl benzoate, farnesene, eugenol and linalool) and it is an absolute, therefore not entirely composed of volatile components. It is advisable not to use jasmine absolute in aromatherapy massage.

The jasmine odour has been shown to have a stimulating effect on human brain waves (A14). It also has an idiosyncratic effect on people, which may be influenced by the concentration: low concentrations may be relaxing whilst high concentrations are stimulating.

Use in babies and young children

Due to the immaturity and the delicate nature of the skin of babies and young children, it is inadvisable for any essential oils and especially absolutes to be used in massage, however much the essential oil/absolute has been diluted in the carrier oils. This is also a necessary precaution due to the possibilities of sensitisation of the children at this young age through skin or air-borne odorant effects (see Chapters 5 and 7).

Instillation or administration of essential oils near the baby or young child's nose is not only not recommended, but distinctly inadvisable, as there have been numerous cases reported of severe toxicity and even death from such applications (see Chapter 7).

Juniper Oil

CAS numbers

USA: 8002-68-4; EINECS: 84603-69-0

Species/Botanical name

Juniperus communis L. (Pinaceae, Cupressaceae)

Synonyms

Essence de Genièvre, juniper berry oil, juniperi aetheroleum, oleum juniperi, wacholderöl

Other species

Juniperus oxycedrus, Juniperus phoenicea, Juniperus virginiana

Pharmacopoeias

In European Pharmacopoeia.

Safety

CHIP details
Xn; R10, 65; 90%; S62

EU sensitiser total
4.5 (due to limonene)

GRAS status
Granted.

Extraction, source, appearance and odour

Extraction
A volatile oil is obtained by steam distillation of the unfermented berries or the fermented berries, as a by-product of gin distillation. The fermented juniper fruits are distilled and the terpenic oil fraction is separated from the gin distillate, yielding the cheaper commercial juniper oil. Juniper oil (Ph. Eur. 4.8) is obtained by steam distillation from the ripe, non-fermented berry cones of *Juniperus communis*; a suitable antioxidant may be added.

Source
Eastern Europe and India.

Appearance and odour
A colourless to pale yellowish essential oil with a fresh, yet warm, rich-balsamic, woody-sweet, and pine-like odour, which is characteristic (Arctander, 1960).

Aromatherapy uses

Juniper berry essential oil uses include: anxiety, nervous tension, stress-related problems, poor memory; strengthening, uplifting and clearing of negative influences; leucorrhoea, cystitis, cellulites, dropsy, fluid retention, menstrual pains, genital warts, stimulation of the kidneys and bladder (aids passing urine and kidney stones, and relieves urine retention when the prostate gland is enlarged); eliminating uric acid, arthritis, rheumatism, gout, sciatica, stiffness; haemorrhoids, stimulating circulation, and cleansing the blood of toxins; acne, dermatitis, oily skin, blocked pores, varicose veins, cellulite, eczema, ulcers, abscesses, oedema, dermatosis and wounds (Lawless, 1992; Sheppard-Hanger, 1995).

Scientific comment

Although there are many positive benefits of the herb given orally, there is no scientific evidence to show that there would be any benefit in massaging the dilute essential oil in aromatherapy. The doubts over its use in cosmetics (Final Report, 2001b) suggest caution in its use in massage and it is unlikely that the odour alone could alleviate any of the complaints, although massage itself can benefit many stress-related and muscular symptoms.

Herbal uses

Culpeper (1826) stated that juniper oil 'expelleth all wind out of the body, and also the stone and gravel, terms and urine; it removes all fevers, jaundice, dropsy, gout and colic; it cures gonnorhoea; it opens all obstructions of the liver, spleen, gall and lungs and cures ulcers and tumours in those places. It helps all disease of the head, as vertigo, megrim, convulsions, etc., it provokes sweat and expels both plague and poison.'

Traditionally, it has been used for cystitis, flatulence, colic and applied topically for rheumatic pains in joints or muscles (Barnes *et al.*, 2002). Juniper apparently possesses diuretic, antiseptic, carminative, stomachic and antirheumatic properties (Grieve, 1937/1992). More recently, juniper oil has been used as a carminative and in herbal remedies for urinary tract infections and muscle and joint pain (Martindale, 1973). Juniper berries are approved for dyspepsia (Blumenthal *et al.*, 2000).

Food and perfumery uses

Food   Juniper berry oil (FEMA 2604) is used in a wide range of food and beverages. Juniper berries are widely used as a flavouring component in gin.

Perfumery   The essential oil is used in perfumery for its fresh, balsamic notes and to modify pine notes and in fougeres, chypres, colognes, aftershaves.

Chemistry

Major components
Juniper berry, *Juniperus communis* L. Cupressaceae (ISO 8897: 1991):

	% (Analyst *109*, 1343–1351 (1984))	
α-Thujene	2.8	
α-Pinene	35	(33–71)
Camphene	0.3	
Sabinene	5	(trace–27)
Myrcene	9.3	(5–18)
α-Phellandrene	0.4	
p-Cymene	2.1	
Limonene	1.2	(2–9)
α-Terpinene	3.7	
Terpinolene	1.8	
Linalool	0	
Terpinen-4-ol	9.6	(4–10)
α-Terpineol	0.9	
Bornyl acetate	0.3	
α-Cubebene	0.4	
α-Copaene	0.5	
β-Elemene	1.9	
β-Caryophyllene	1.9	
α-Humulene	1.5	
Germacrene D	0	
δ-Cadinene	2.8	

Adulteration
True juniper berry oil is rare as the fermented berries are more economical and abundant, and berries take 2 years to ripen. Many synthetic components like pinenes, camphene, myrcene or fractions of turpentine oil can be added. Different juniper oils (e.g. wood or twig oils) are added as well as essential oils from different species.

Toxicity (A22)

Acute toxicity
Oral LD$_{50}$ >5–8 g/kg (rat).

Dermal LD$_{50}$ >5 g/kg (rabbit).

LD$_{50}$ (intraperitoneal injection)   3 g/kg (mice) (A22).

Irritation and sensitisation
None at 8% (human). When tested at full strength, it produced irritation in 2/20 people after a 24-hour exposure. Dermatitic reactions have occurred with juniper extracts with positive patch tests (Mitchell and Rook, 1979).

Phototoxicity
None found.

Other toxicities
No harm to kidneys was seen after 100, 300 or 900 mg juniper oil/kg or terpinen-4-ol (10 mg% of oil) at 400 mg/kg for 28 days with rats (Schilcher and Leuschner, 1997). However, excessive doses of terpinen-4-ol may cause kidney irritation (Duke, 1985). Symptoms from oral overdose include: pain in or near the kidneys, strong diuresis, albuminuria, haematuria, purplish urine, tachycardia, hypertension and, rarely, convulsions, metrorrhagia and abortion. Following external application of the essential oil burning, erythema, inflammation with blisters and oedema occurred (Duke, 1985).

Essential oils derived from other juniper species are used solely as fragrance ingredients. The chemical compositions of *J. communis* oil and *J. communis* extract are similar, both containing a wide variety of terpenoids and aromatic compounds, with the occasional aliphatic alcohols and aldehydes, and, more rarely, alkanes (Final Report, 2001b). The principal component of *J. oxycedrus* tar is cadinene, a sesquiterpene, but cresol and guaiacol are also found. Acute studies using animals show little toxicity of the oil or tar. The oils derived from *J. communis* and *J. virginiana* and *J. oxycedrus* tar were not skin irritants in animals. The oil from *J. virginiana* was not a sensitiser, and the oil from *J. communis* was not phototoxic in animal tests. *J. oxycedrus* tar had some sensitisation and was genotoxic in several assays but no genotoxicity data were available for any of the extracts. Clinical tests showed no evidence of irritation or sensitisation with any of the tested oils. The study concluded that the available data are insufficient to support the safety of these ingredients in cosmetic formulations until further studies have been carried out. This therefore suggests caution with skin application of juniper essential oil.

Bioactivities

Pharmacological activities *in vitro* and *in vivo*

Smooth muscle A slight spasmolytic effect was noted in guinea-pig ileum (A2; Lis-Balchin *et al.*, 1996a).

Uterus Uterine stimulant activity was found for the essential oil (Farnsworth, 1975). An antifertility effect has been described for a juniper extract, though not the essential oil itself, when given orally to rats on days 1–7 of pregnancy: this was dose-dependent (Agrawal OP *et al.*, 1980). An abortifacient effect was also found when the extract was given on days 14–16 (Agrawal OP *et al.*, 1980; Final Report, 2001b). The data on antifertility was both confirmed (Prakash, 1984) and later disputed (Prakash *et al.*, 1985). Anti-implantation was reduced to 60–70% (Prakash, 1984).

Other activities The essential oil components have diuretic, gastrointestinal, antiseptic and irritant properties (Leung, 1980). The diuretic activity is due to terpinen-4-ol, which increases the glomerular filtration rate (Tyler, 1993). This could be irritant to the kidneys. No evidence of teratogenicity was reported. Anti-inflammatory, hypertensive and astringent activities were shown for the extract given orally to rats (Barnes *et al.*, 2002).

When perceptional changes due to the odour of juniper (as well as ylang ylang, orange, geranium, cypress, bergamot and spearmint essential oils) in relation to type of work were studied, for mental work inhalation of juniper seemed to create a favourable impression after work, whereas geranium and orange both produced an unfavourable impression (Sugawara *et al.*, 1999).

Antimicrobial activities

Antibacterial activity

There was a moderate effect against four different bacterial species (Friedman *et al.*, 2002).

Antifungal activity

Activity was weak on 6/15 fungi (Maruzella and Liguori, 1958) and twice-rectified essential oil had no effect on five fungi (Maruzella, 1960).

Other activities

Antiviral activities have only been shown with non-essential oil extracts, which were water-soluble (Barnes *et al.*, 2002).

Uses in pregnancy and lactation: contraindications

Taken orally as a herb, juniper is contraindicated in pregnancy due to its abortifacient, antifertility and anti-implantation properties and effect on the menstrual cycle and other data (Final Report, 2001b). There seems to be insufficient data for its safe use in cosmetics, and therefore its use in aromatherapy massage cannot be advised during pregnancy, parturition and lactation.

Pharmaceutical guidance

External application of the oil may cause an irritant reaction, but some later studies showed no hazards (Tisserand and Balacs, 1995). Juniper has been confused with savin (*Juniperus sabina*) in the literature and this may be the reason for believing that the oil is toxic. Prolonged oral use may cause gastrointestinal irritation and there is a risk of renal damage with high doses (Martindale, 1993). Because of the doubts raised about its use in cosmetics, juniper oil should not be used in aromatherapy massage, but its use as a fragrance should not cause concern.

Use in babies and young children

Due to the immaturity and the delicate nature of the skin of babies and young children, it is inadvisable for any essential oils to be used in massage, however much the essential oil has been diluted in the carrier oils. This is also a necessary precaution due to the possibilities of sensitisation of the children at this young age through skin or air-borne odorant effects (see Chapters 5 and 7).

Instillation or administration of essential oils near the baby or young child's nose is not only not recommended, but distinctly inadvisable, as there have been numerous cases reported of severe toxicity and even death from such applications (see Chapter 7).

Kanuka Oil

CAS numbers

USA:8015-64-3; EINECS: 84775-71-7

Species/Botanical name

Kunzea ericoides (Myrtaceae)

Synonyms

White tea tree

Safety

CHIP details

Xn; R10, 65; 95%; S62 (A26)

RIFM recommended safety of use limits

Not stated

EU sensitiser total

Not given

Extraction, source, appearance and odour

Extraction

Essential oils are obtained by steam distillation of the leaves and branchlets (Arctander, 1960).

Source

Australia.

Appearance and odour

A pale yellow liquid.

Aromatherapy uses

Few books mention kanuka, although it appears on many Internet sites. Uses include: muscular pain and swelling relief, sprains, strains, sports injuries, relaxing skin.

Scientific comment

The variability in the manuka and kanuka essential oils suggests caution in their usage, as does the fact that the oils have not been scientifically tested for toxicity (see also Chapters 5 and 8). Tea tree oil (*Melaleuca* species) would be more acceptable for use in aromatherapy, though with caution (see tea tree oil monograph).

Herbal uses

The folk-medicinal uses of the New Zealand 'tea-tree' oils are related to both manuka and kanuka. For example the leaves of both species were used as vapour baths for colds; an infusion was very astringent and various uses were found for concoctions, including urinary complaints and as a febrifuge (Brooker *et al.*, 1987). Kanuka was applied to scalds and burns, used to stop coughing and as a sedative; it was also used against dysentery. The decoction of boiled leaves and bark was used to treat stiff backs, etc. Seed capsules were boiled to give a decoction for external application to treat inflammation or to be drunk for diarrhoea; the capsules or leaves were also chewed for dysentery. The water from boiled bark was used for treating inflamed breasts and also to treat mouth, throat and eye problems (Cook, 1777; Polack, 1840; Neill, 1884; Poverty Bay, 1930; Adams, 1945; McDonald, 1975).

The antibacterial activity of honeys derived from kanuka and manuka blossom against *Staphylococcus aureus* was shown by Allen *et al.* (1991) and more recently manuka honey was shown to be active against *Helicobacter pylori* (Somal *et al.*, 1994).

Food and perfumery uses

Food None found.

Perfumery None found.

Chemistry

Major components

	% (Perry et al., 1997a,b; Porter, 1998)
α-Pinene	66.5–68
α-Terpinene	4.4–5
Limonene	1–1.2
γ-Terpinene	0.8–1

Adulteration

Admixing of different species and even the same species from a different location can give very different results, both in chemical composition and activity (Perry *et al.*, 1997a,b; Porter, 1998; Porter and Wilkins, 1999) (see also tea tree oil monograph).

Toxicity

Acute toxicity
Not determined.

Irritation and sensitisation
Not determined.

Phototoxicity
None reported.

Bioactivities

See also tea tree oil monograph.

Pharmacological activities *in vitro* and *in vivo*

Smooth muscle Kanuka had an initial spasmogenic action on the electrically stimulated guinea-pig ileum *in vitro* (Lis-Balchin and Hart, 2000; Lis-Balchin *et al.*, 2000). α-Terpineol and terpinen-4-ol produced a substantial spasmolytic action, while α-terpinene, β-pinene and (−)α-pinene produced an initial contraction followed by spasmolysis at the same concentration; the (+)α-pinene enantiomer produced only a spasmogenic response. 1,8-Cineole produced a rise in tone of the electrically induced contractions. The activity of *Melaleuca* oils resembles kanuka to some extent as the oil has an initial spasmogenic action followed by a potent spasmolytic action. The mechanism of the latter action was apparently neither via cAMP nor cGMP nor acting as potassium channel openers at low concentrations, but some evidence was obtained for action as calcium channel blockers at higher concentrations (Lis-Balchin and Hart, 2000; see tea tree essential oil monograph).

Uterus A decrease in the force of the spontaneous contractions in the rat was obtained (Lis-Balchin and Hart, 2000; Lis-Balchin *et al.*, 2000; see also tea tree oil monograph).

Skeletal muscle Using the rat phrenic nerve–diaphragm, kanuka had no activity at the same concentration as that of manuka, which decreased the tension and caused a delayed contracture. The action on chick biventer muscle was similar for all three oils (tea tree oil monograph).

Antimicrobial activities

See also tea tree oil monograph.

Antibacterial activity
Relative data: 12/25 different bacteria and 19/20 *Listeria monocytogenes* varieties were affected (Lis-Balchin and Hart, 2000; Lis-Balchin *et al.*, 2000). In comparative studies, the antimicrobial activities showed greater differences between different samples of kanuka (and manuka) than between them and *Melaleuca* samples. Tests at a commercial laboratory also provided positive unpublished data on the antimicrobial effects of kanuka (Cooke and Cooke, 1991).

Antifungal activity
Relative data (% inhibition): *Aspergillus niger* 0–1%, *A. ochraceus* 10–27%, *Fusarium culmorum* 0–16% (Lis-Balchin and Hart, 2000; Lis-Balchin *et al.*, 2000). The antifungal activity of kanuka was inversely proportional to its strong antibacterial activity. There was a very strong negative correlation between the pure kanuka samples and the antifungal activity, compared with the more effective antifungal activity of manuka; the mixture of kanuka/manuka showed an intermediate antifungal activity (see also tea tree oil monograph).

The antibacterial and antifungal activity was stronger for *Melaleuca* oils than for manuka and kanuka oils (see tea tree oil monograph). Different samples of the New Zealand manuka and kanuka oils showed considerable variation, whilst *Melaleuca* oils remained more constant. However, the production of more potent *Melaleuca* oils (labelled as therapeutic) by some Australian companies, which contain a higher percentage of terpinen-4-ol and lower 1,8-cineole indicates that there is an expected difference in antimicrobial activity.

Antioxidant activity
The antioxidant activity of kanuka samples was less consistent than that of manuka, while *Melaleuca* showed no activity (tea tree oil monograph, Table 6). The antioxidant activity of the 'tea-tree' oils was very variable, the manuka samples showing more effectiveness than one of the kanuka samples and the kanuka/manuka mixture. Only γ-terpinene and terpinen-4-ol showed antioxidant potential. The latter are also the most potent antibacterial agents

and possibly exert some of this activity through their antioxidant action.

Clinical studies

No clinical studies have been documented.

Use in pregnancy and lactation: contraindications

There are no studies on the effect of the *Melaleuca* essential oil on the uterus other than the *in vitro* studies in rat, which showed a decrease in the spontaneous contractions (there is therefore a possible caution for the use of essential oils during childbirth, as they could stop contractions and thereby put the baby, as well as the mother at risk). As this essential oil has also not been properly assessed toxicologically, it cannot be recommended for use in pregnancy, parturition or during lactation.

Pharmaceutical guidance

There is scant pharmacological information available for kanuka essential oil and the variability in both the kanuka and its closely related species, manuka essential oils, with which it can be distilled, suggests caution in their usage, as does the fact that the oils have not been tested for toxicity.

There is also little evidence that either kanuka (*Kunzea ericoides*) or manuka (*Leptospermum scoparium*) have great potential (Lis-Balchin *et al.*, 1996a, 1998b), although, based on folk medicinal usage, they are said to have remarkable powers of healing (Brooker *et al.*, 1987). Kanuka cannot at present be recommended for aromatherapy massage and its use as a fragrance is limited due to its unpleasant odour.

Note: See also pharmaceutical guidance in the tea tree oil monograph.

Use in babies and young children

Due to the immaturity and the delicate nature of the skin of babies and young children, it is inadvisable for any essential oils to be used in massage, however much the essential oil has been diluted in the carrier oils. This is also a necessary precaution due to the possibilities of sensitisation of the children at this young age through skin or air-borne odorant effects (see Chapters 5 and 7).

Instillation or administration of essential oils near the baby or young child's nose is not only not recommended, but distinctly inadvisable, as there have been numerous cases reported of severe toxicity and even death from such applications (see Chapter 7).

Lavender Oil

CAS numbers

Lavender: USA: 8000-28-0; EINECS: 90063-37-9
Lavandin: USA: 8022-15-9; EINECS: 91722-69-9

Species/Botanical name

Lavandula angustifolia P. Miller, *L. vera*

Synonyms

Lavandula officinalis (Chaiz.), true lavender, English lavender oil, esencia de alhucema, esencia de espliego, essência de alfazema, huile essentielle de lavande, lavandulae aetheroleum, lavendelöl, lavender flower oil, oleum lavandulae

Pharmacopoeias

In European Pharmacopoeia.

Other species

Lavandula latifolia (L.), *L. viridis*, *L. stoechas*
Lavandins: Lavandin abrialis (*Lavandula angustifolia* P. Miller × *Lavandula latifolia* (L.) Medikus), lavandin grosso (*Lavandula angustifolia* P. Miller × *Lavandula latifolia* (L.) Medikus)

Safety

CHIP details

Lavender: Xn; R65; 15%; S62
Lavandin: None (A26)

EU sensitiser total

Lavender oil: coumarin: below 0.1%; geraniol, 1.1; limonene, 0.6; linalool, 38; total: 39.7 (A23)

Lavender and lavandin absolute: coumarin: 6; geraniol, 0.3; limonene, 0.7; linalool, 28; total: 35

Lavandin oil: coumarin: below 0.1%; geraniol, 0.4; limonene, 1; linalool, 37; total: 38.4

GRAS status

Granted (Fenaroli, 1997).

Extraction, source, appearance and odour

Extraction

Steam-distilled tops and flowers give the essential oil. The different parts of the plant give an essential oil of totally different composition (Wiesenfeld, 1999).

Lavender oil (Ph. Eur. 4.8) is obtained by steam distillation from the fresh flowering tops of *Lavandula angustifolia* (*L. officinalis*). It is miscible with alcohol (90%), with ether, and with fatty oils.

Source

France, Spain and Bulgaria.

Appearance and odour

The true oil (*Lavandula angustifolia*) is almost colourless and has a sweet, floral, herbaceous, refreshing odour with a pleasant, balsamic-wood undertone and a fruity-sweet top-note (Arctander, 1960).

Lavandins are like true lavender with some camphor tones. The oil is colourless to pale yellow in all cases. Lavandin oil was first produced in the late 1920s, but production has since escalated well above that of true lavender. The yield is higher and the price is therefore lower (Arctander, 1960).

Lavender absolute and concrete (*L. angustifolia* P. Miller or *L. officinalis*) is produced from direct extraction of the herb with solvents (concrete) and thence extraction with absolute alcohol to give the lavandin absolute. Both are a viscous dark green liquid of herbaceous odour, resembling the flowering plant; the concrete is more solid (Arctander, 1960; Lis-Balchin, 2002b, ch.16).

Aromatherapy uses

Lavender is the most used essential oil of all in aromatherapy. Its greatest attribute is said to be as a relaxant. Aromatherapists' uses include: headache, nervous tension, exhaustion, emotional extremes, spiritual balance, passive/aggressive personalities or manic–depressive states; cardiac tonic; hypertension, atherosclerosis, palpitations, arteritis, peripheral circulatory deficiencies; stroke prophylaxis; respiratory system problems: bronchitis, asthma, catarrh, colds, laryngitis, infection in general; muscular spasm and pain, strains, cramps plus rheumatic pain; it is said to clear the spleen and liver, increase gastric secretion; to aid digestion of fats; nausea, vomiting; scanty or painful periods, cystitis, thrush, leucorrhoea; it reportedly aids childbirth pain and speeds delivery; skin conditions, growth of new cells; it has a balancing action on sebum; burns including sunburn, acne, eczema, psoriasis, abscesses, boils, carbuncles, fungal growth, swellings, scarring and infective wounds, soothing skin pain, irritations and parasitic infections.

Scientific comment

The relaxant effect of lavender and linalool on guinea-pig ileum smooth muscle showed a positive correlation with its chemical profile and the relaxant effect shown in aromatherapy (A11; A12), adding weight to the holistic relaxant theory. Lavender essential oil has shown a relaxant effect on animal motion, contingent negative variation and various other physiological and psychological parameters in humans (A14).

Many of the attributes of lavender oil were mistakenly taken from herbals, e.g. Culpeper (1653), who used alcoholic extracts or teas, not distilled essential oils. There was also an interest in astrology: every plant had an assigned planet, hence *L. angustifolia* is associated with Mercury and now also has a 'yang' quality (Tisserand, 1977). The species referred to was also misinterpreted (see below). René-Maurice Gattefossé (1937/1993), the so-called pioneer of modern aromatherapy, actually used perfumes, or at most deterpenated essential oils, and not pure natural plant essential oils. The fact that some extracts of *L. angustifolia* have a strong spasmogenic action (dried flowers and fresh leaves) is somewhat disturbing as so many modern herbal and aromatherapy books state that the teas are sedative; they are often prescribed for upset stomachs. It has been concluded (Lis-Balchin, 2002b, chs 1, 3, 23) that the information on lavender has been mistakenly transcribed from early herbals, like those of Culpeper (1653), where *L. spica*, a more camphoric lavender was used medicinally and not the very floral *L. angustifolia*. The spasmolytic results shown for the water-soluble extracts of the more camphoraceous *L. stoechas* support the well-quoted action of the camphoraceous spike lavender over the centuries and emphasise the confusion.

Herbal uses

Lavender drops were used for fainting and red lavender (lavender mixed with rosemary and cinnamon bark, nutmeg and sandalwood and macerated in spirit of wine for several days) was used for indigestion (Grieve, 1937/1992). Paramedical uses appear in many modern books (Wren, 1988), where *L. angustifolia* is stated to be a carminative, spasmolytic, tonic and antidepressant. Numerous uses have been suggested for *L. angustifolia* (Bertram, 1995), but many of these are identical to those quoted in the old herbals (Gerard, 1597; Culpeper, 1653), which were referring to a different species! These include: nervous headache, neuralgia, rheumatism, depression, insomnia, windy colic, fainting, toothache, sprains, sinusitis, stress and migraine.

Conventional uses

The British Pharmacopoeia officially recognised red lavender for 200 years. In the eighteenth century it was known as palsy drops and red hartshorn. British Pharmaceutical Codex (BPC) products included: compound lavender tincture (BPC 1949) (dose: 2–4 mL) and lavender spirit (BPC 1934) (dose: 0.3–1.2 mL).

Food and perfumery uses

Food Lavandin oil (FEMA 2618), lavender oil (FEMA 2622), spike lavender oil (FEMA 3033) and lavender absolute (FEMA 2620) and even concrete (FEMA 2621) are used as natural food flavours in baked goods, frozen dairy, soft candy, gelatin, pudding, non-alcoholic and alcoholic beverages at levels from 4 to 44 ppm (Fenaroli, 1997).

Perfumery The lavender and lavandin oils have widespread usage in perfumery and cosmetic products: in colognes, lavender waters, fougeres, chypres, florals, non-florals, etc. (Arctander, 1960).

Chemistry

Major components

Lavender oil, *Lavandula angustifolia* P. Miller, oil of french lavender (ISO 3515: 1987):

	Min	Max	
trans-β-Ocimene	2	6	
cis-β-Ocimene	4	10	
Octanone-3	–	2	
1,8-Cineole	–	1.5	lavandins 6–20; spike 25–37
Limonene	–	0.5	
Camphor	–	0.5	lavandins 0.4–12; spike 9–60
Linalool	25	38	lavandins 24–41; spike 11–54
Linalyl acetate	25	45	lavandins 2–34; spike 0.8–15
Terpinen-4-ol	2	6	
Lavandulol	0.3		
Lavandulyl acetate	2		lavandins 3.5; spike 0
α-terpineol	–	1	

Specification of the essential oil: 'The oil obtained by steam distillation of recently picked lavender flowers (*Lavandula angustifolia* P. Miller) either growing wild or cultivated in France'. The established chromatographic profile includes the main identifying components (as above). The main components of *L. angustifolia* of commerce (Naef and Morris, 1992) are linalool (25–38%) and linalyl acetate (25–45%).

Oil of lavandin abrialis (*L. angustifolia* P. Miller × *L. latifolia* (L.) Medikus), France has a requirement for a minimum linalyl acetate content of 27%/37% maximum and linalool 28%/38% with camphor at 7/11% maximum. Oil of lavandin grosso (*L. angustifolia* P. Miller × *L. latifolia* (L.) Medikus), France also has an ISO. The commercial hybrids, lavandins, have variable concentrations of 1,8-cineole and camphor, absent from the *L. angustifolia* P. Miller, which provide the harsher notes. The 'rhodinol content', consisting of citronellol, geraniol, nerol, neryl acetate and geranyl acetate, together amounting to a very small percentage of the total composition, gives a sweet, rose-like odour to the lavandin oils, with small differences between the cultivars (Lis-Balchin, 2004b). The chemical composition of L. 'Grosso' varies with the method of extraction: steam-distilled and CO_2-extracted samples showed differences in linalool and linalyl acetate compared with an absolute (Pellerin, 1991) (see also spike lavender monograph). Other oils from different species are not usually on the commercial market (for descriptions see Lis-Balchin, 2002a, ch.24).

Terpeneless lavender oil is produced by careful vacuum distillation and a 'topping off' of about 10% of the oil is sufficient to make it mellower and softer and more soluble in dilute alcohol and of course it has increased stability and is more useful in foods and perfumes. This terpeneless lavender essential oil was used by Gattefossé for healing his burnt hand!

Adulteration

Adulteration of lavender oils is primarily with lavandin oil and its fractions (as it is so much cheaper, being produced in at least a ten-fold excess). Other synthetic and natural fractions include: acetylated lavandin, synthetic linalool and linalyl acetate, fractions of ho leaf oil and rosewood oil, terpinyl propionate, isobornyl acetate, terpineol, fractions of rosemary, aspic oil, lavandin, etc. The lavender essential oil may be totally synthetic (G1; Lis-Balchin, 1995, 2002b, ch.16).

Toxicity

Acute toxicity (A22)

Oral LD$_{50}$ Lavender and lavandin oils: >5 g/kg (rat).

Dermal LD$_{50}$ >5 g/kg body weight (rabbit).

Irritation and sensitisation

Lavender: nil at 10%; Lavandin: nil at 5%. Little or no irritation to human and animal skin was shown (BIBRA Working Group, 1994), but it has caused sensitisation. Patch tests have shown a few allergies due to photosensitisation and also pigmentation (Nakayama *et al.*, 1976; Brandao, 1986). Dermatitis occurred in sensitive people (Rudzki *et al.*, 1976) and an occupational allergy to a lavender shampoo used by a hairdresser was reported (Menard, 1961; Brandao, 1986). Facial 'pillow' dermatitis due to lavender oil allergy was described (Coulson, 1999), also facial psoriasis caused by contact allergy to linalool and hydroxycitronellal in an aftershave (De Groot and Liem, 1983). Patch testing using lavender oil at 20% in petrolatum on patients suspected of suffering from cosmetic contact dermatitis over a 9-year period in Japan (Sugiura *et al.*, 2000) showed a dramatic increase in 1997, which coincided with the importation of the aromatherapy trend for using lavender oil and dried flowers. There is also the danger of airborne contact allergic dermatitis through overuse of essential oils and their storage (Schaller and Korting, 1995), which produced a severe response in a woman who had been active with essential oils in aromatherapy.

Phototoxicity

Some cases of photosensitisation and pigmentation have been reported (BIBRA Working Group, 1994).

Other toxicities

Toxicities of lavender essential oils have been reported for centuries: Culpeper (1653) said that lavender (*L. vera*) 'provokes menses of women, and expels both a stillborn child and afterbirth' (the only reference to lavender as an abortifacient). Its principal effect following administration by oral, injection or inhalation routes to rodents, was sedation.

Bioactivities

Pharmacological activities *in vitro* and *in vivo*

Smooth muscle Relative data: Different commercial samples of lavender showed either a relaxation or an initial contraction followed by relaxation in the electrically stimulated guinea-pig ileum (A2; Lis-Balchin *et al.*, 1996a) (Table 1). When 'waters' of lavender were applied to the intestine of dogs *in vivo* they were reported to increase activity, which was sometimes followed by relaxation and decreased peristaltic activity (Plant, 1920). Linalool relaxed the small intestine of the mouse (Imaseki and Kitabatake, 1962); a spasmolytic action on rabbit and guinea-pig gut by the essential oil of a different lavender species (*L. spica* L.) was reported (Shipochliev, 1968); *L. angustifolia* P. Miller essential oil relaxed both longitudinal and circular muscles of the guinea-pig ileum (Izzo *et al.*, 1996); linalool relaxed the longitudinal muscle of guinea-pig ileum (Reiter and Brandt, 1985). Spasmolytic activity of *L. dentata* L. oil and its components 1,8-cineole and α- and β-pinene was reported on rat duodenum (Gamez *et al.*, 1990). There appears therefore to be good agreement that the oils of lavender are spasmolytic on intestinal muscle, although another group reported that with some commercial samples the spasmolytic action is preceded by a contraction on guinea-pig ileum (Lis-Balchin *et al.*, 1996a,b; Lis-Balchin and Hart, 1999a).

Recent experiments using three different extracts of several *Lavandula* species, including a cold methanolic extract, a tea made with boiling water and a hydrosol (the water remaining after steam/water distillation), showed that methanolic extracts of *L. angustifolia* dried flowers, *L. angustifolia* fresh flowers and fresh leaves, assessed separately, *L. stoechas* leaves and *L. viridis* leaves have a spasmolytic action on the guinea-pig ileum. All the teas and hydrosols, except for *L. angustifolia* dried flowers and *L. angustifolia* fresh leaves were also spasmolytic, while the water-soluble tea extract of *L. angustifolia* dried flowers and the leaves of *L. angustifolia* showed an initial spasmogenic action (Lis-Balchin, 2002b, ch.12). There was a spasmolytic action of linalool on tracheal muscle (Brandt, 1988).

Smooth muscle Mode of action: All essential oils of different lavenders showed a post-synaptic effect on the guinea-pig ileum and none possessed atropine-like activity (Lis-Balchin and Hart, 1999a) nor appeared to stimulate adrenoceptors. Lavender oil and linalool appeared to mediate a spasmolytic action on intestinal smooth muscle via a rise in

Table 1 Contraction (C) and or relaxation (R) for extracts and essential oils in electrically stimulated guinea-pig ileum (smooth muscle) *in vitro*

Plant	Extract	Tea	Hydrosol	Essential oil
L. angustifolia (dried flowers)	R (+ baseline C)*	C/R	C/R	R
L. angustifolia (fresh flowers)	R	R	R	R
L. angustifolia (leaves)	R	R (low) C/R (high)	C/R	R
L. stoechas (leaves)	R	R	R	R
L. stoechas 'pedunculata' (leaves)	R	R	R	R
L. viridis (leaves)	R	N/A	R	R

*(+ baseline C) indicates that there is a distinct contraction rather than an increase in tone as shown by the other samples where C is shown.
From Lis-Balchin *et al.* (2001).

cAMP (Lis-Balchin and Hart, 1999a). There is no evidence of the use of calcium channels except at very high concentrations; this is in contrast to other essential oils (Vuorela *et al.*, 1997). There is no evidence for potassium channel opening. In a study on the rat duodenum, the essential oil from *L. dentata* L. and its component 1,8-cineole inhibited calcium-induced contractions (Gamez *et al.*, 1988). There is recent evidence to show that the methanolic extracts of *L. angustifolia* (dry flowers, fresh flowers and fresh leaves) are calcium channel blockers as are the leaves of *L. viridis* and *L. stoechas* (Lis-Balchin, 2002b, ch.13).

Uterus Lavender oil, linalool, linalyl acetate, α- and β-pinene and 1,8-cineole reduced spontaneous uterine contractions in the rat at concentrations that were spasmolytic on intestinal muscle (A3; A4; Lis-Balchin and Hart, 1997b).

Skeletal muscle Action of the essential oil of *L. angustifolia* P. Miller on skeletal muscle and also linalool and linalyl acetate produced a reduction in the size of the contraction in response to stimulation of the phrenic nerve and also when the muscle was stimulated directly (Lis-Balchin and Hart, 1997a). Thus the action would appear to be myogenic, however similar results were interpreted as showing a local anaesthetic action (Ghelardini *et al.*, 1999) and similar conclusions were obtained from experiments on mouse neuromuscular junction (Re *et al.*, 2000), i.e. that linalool has a local anaesthetic action. Linalyl acetate also caused an increase in baseline or resting tone (Lis-Balchin and Hart, 1997a), while limonene caused a rise in tone, with a decrease in the size of the contractions.

Other activities Percutaneous absorption: Lavender oil was not absorbed within 2 hours of application to the intact shaved abdominal skin of the mouse (Meyer and Meyer, 1959).

Physiological actions Evidence for the sedative properties of the essential oil of lavender after inhalation in animals was shown as it significantly decreased the motility of 'normal' test mice as well as that of animals rendered hyperactive or 'stressed' by an intraperitoneal dose of caffeine (Buchbauer *et al.*, 1991, 1993b). The main constituents of this oil, linalool and linalyl acetate, elicited a similar effect, which was dose related. (−)-Linalool, when applied to 14 healthy subjects by percutaneous administration (inhalation of the fragrance was prevented by means of breathing masks), induced a decrease of systolic blood pressure and a smaller decrease of skin temperature, compared with a corresponding control group receiving a placebo, but had no effects on subjective evaluation of well-being (Heuberger *et al.*, 2004). Other parameters were also unaffected (blood oxygen saturation, breathing rate, eye-blink rate, pulse rate, skin conductance, surface electromyogram and diastolic blood pressure). The absorption of linalool from percutaneous application of lavender oil (Jager *et al.*, 1992) provided some evidence for the aromatherapeutic use of lavender.

Stress and travel sickness of pigs was reduced by lavender straw, measured by concentrations of cortisol in the pigs' saliva (Bradshaw *et al.*, 1998). The dose-dependent sedative effect of linalool on the CNS of rats (Elisabetsky *et al.*, 1995) may be caused by its inhibitory activity on glutamate binding in the cortex (Elisabetsky *et al.*, 1995). Potentiation of GABA$_A$ receptors expressed in *Xenopus* oocytes by perfumes and phytoncides, including lavender oils and lavender perfumes (shown by benzodiazepine, barbiturates, steroids and anesthetics, which induce an anxiolytic, anticonvulsant and sedative effect), was investigated (Aoshima *et al.*, 1999). Swiss mice showed sedation after lavender oil (1/60 in olive oil) was administered orally (Guillemain *et al.*, 1989). Lavender inhalation showed a similar effect (Komori and Hamamoto, 1997). The positive effect of lavender oil as treatment for insomnia was indicated in a limited study of four geriatrics (Hardy *et al.*, 1995).

A Japanese patent application for the usage of several monoterpenes (which can be incorporated into food such as chewing gums) as brain stimulants and/or enhancers of brain activity has been filed (Nakamatsu, 1995). Certain central neurotropic effects of lavender essential oil and were shown (Atanassova-Shopova and Roussinov, 1970a). A more detailed account of physiological and other effects has been published recently (Lis-Balchin, 2002b, ch.12).

Other properties of lavender oil or its components A study on mast cell-mediated immediate type allergic reactions induced by an irritant in test animals showed a dose-dependent beneficial effect of lavender oil administered either topically or intradermally (Kim *et al.*, 1999). Lavender flowers had a protective effect against enzyme-dependent lipid peroxidation (Hohmann *et al.*, 1999). Lipid peroxidation and lipid metabolism studies in patients with chronic bronchitis showed normalisation of the level of total lipids by lavender oil (Siurin, 1997). Inhalation of lavender oil had no effect on the content of cholesterol in the blood, but reduced its content in the aorta and atherosclerotic plaques (Nikolaevskii et al., 1990). Linalool showed only marginal effects on lipid peroxidation of polyunsaturated fatty acids (Reddy and Lokesch, 1992). Anticonvulsive effects of inhaling lavender oil vapour were shown (Yamada et al., 1994) and similar effects occurred with linalool in glutamate-related seizure models (Elisabetsky et al., 1999).

A hypoglycaemic effect of various species of lavender was shown (Gamez et al., 1987a,b). Linalool leads to a hepatic peroxysomal and microsomal enzyme induction in rats (Chadba and Madyastha, 1984; Roffey et al., 1990) and choleretic and cholagogic activity of Bulgarian lavender oil and a mixture of linalool and α-terpineol was found (Gruncharov, 1973; Peana et al., 1994).

The antinociceptive and gastroprotective effects of orally administered or inhaled *Lavandula hybrida* Reverchon 'Grosso' essential oil, and its principal constituents linalool and linalyl acetate, were evaluated in rodents (Barocelli et al., 2004). Either when orally administered (100 mg/kg) or inhaled for 60 minutes, lavender essential oil significantly reduced the acetic acid-writhing response in a naloxone-sensitive manner. In the hot plate test, analgesic activity observed after oil inhalation was inhibited by naloxone, atropine, mecamylamine pretreatment, suggesting the involvement of opioidergic as well as cholinergic pathways. Linalool and linalyl acetate did not produce significant analgesic response. Oral or inhalatory treatment with analgesic doses of the essential oil did not affect mice spontaneous locomotor activity (in contrast to studies by Buchbauer, 1993). Lavender oil, linalool and linalyl acetate oral administration protected against acute ethanol-induced gastric ulcers but did not prevent indometacin-induced lesions, indicating no interference with arachidonic acid metabolic cascade (Buchbauer, 1993).

Carcinogenicity prevention Perillyl alcohol, a very minor component of lavender and the most important metabolite of D-limonene, is a chemopreventative and chemotherapeutic agent (Reddy et al., 1997; Bellanger, 1998), e.g. against rat liver cancer and rodent mammary and pancreatic tumours (Crowell, 1999). Pancreatic tumours were inhibited completely by geraniol at 20 g/kg diet and 50% by perillyl alcohol at 40 g/kg diet in hamsters. Patents

have been taken out for various uses of perillyl alcohol including: antibiotic and antifungal action (US Patent 5 110 832) and carcinoma regression (US Patent 5 414 019).

Contemporary patents for lavender include: wound treatment (US Patent 4 318 906); treating skin and scalp conditions (US Patent 4 855 131); minor skin irritations, promoting healing, resisting insects (US Patent 5 620 695); fly and mosquito attractant (US Patent 5 635 174) and control of dermatomycoses and dermatophytoses of skin ailments (US Patent 5 641 481).

Psychological actions Most clinical studies initiated by aromatherapists used lavender oil and showed little, if any, benefit (Vickers, 1996; Cooke and Ernst, 2000; Lis-Balchin, 2002b, ch.1). There was no significant difference shown between the use of aromatherapy (with lavender), massage and periods of rest in an intensive care unit (Dunn et al., 1995). Aromatherapy massage on four patients with severe dementia and disturbed behaviour proved detrimental for most (Brooker et al., 1997). Scientific research into the psychological (often referred to as psychopharmacological) effects of lavender is limited, but there is a long history of it being regarded and used as a sedative or calming agent (Lis-Balchin, 2002b, ch.14). The effects on cells and brain tissues also suggests both reduction in electrical activity and an anticonvulsant effect.

Both laboratory and clinically based studies reveal that responses to lavender may be determined not only by these pharmacological sedative effects but by individual, situational and expectational factors independent of the lavender odour itself (Lis-Balchin, 2002b, ch.13). Many fragrances have been shown to have an effect on mood, and in general, pleasant odours generate happy memories, more positive feelings and a general sense of well-being (Warren and Warrenburg, 1993). Inhalation of lavender was found to have a sedative effect on humans (judging by contingent negative variation studies) (Torii et al., 1988; Kubota et al., 1992; Manley, 1993; A14). This was in agreement with the reduced motility in mice (Kovar et al., 1987; Ammon, 1989; Buchbauer, 1992; Jager et al., 1992; A14).

Lavender oil administered in an aroma stream showed modest efficacy in the treatment of agitated behaviour in patients with severe dementia. Nine patients (60%) showed an improvement, five (33%) showed no change and one patient (7%) showed a worsening of agitated behaviour during aromatherapy compared with placebo. A comparison of the group median Psychogeriatric Assessment Scales (PAS) scores during aromatherapy showed a significant improvement in agitated behaviour during aromatherapy compared with placebo (Holmes *et al.*, 2002).

Many other studies on humans have been published. Inhalation studies using rosemary oil versus lavender oil using EEG and simple maths computations showed that lavender increased α-power, suggesting drowsiness, whilst rosemary instigated decreased frontal alpha and beta power, suggesting increased alertness with faster and more accurate results in the maths (Diego *et al.*, 1998). These results seem to show that odour has an effect on performance *per se*, but when the investigators lied to their subjects that odour would be given (Knasko *et al.*, 1990) an improvement was again shown in carrying out tasks, i.e. mind over matter! However, it was also shown that lavender had a stimulant effect on decision times in human experiments (Karamat *et al.*, 1992). Subjects in a group given ambient odour of dimethyl sulphide were less happy than those in the lavender group on both odour and non-odour days (Knasko, 1992). The effect of ambient odours of lavender and cloves on cognition, memory, affect and mood of 72 volunteers showed that lavender adversely influenced arithmetic reasoning (Ludvigson and Rottman, 1989). Lavender (at imperceptible levels) reduced the number of errors made in arithmetical and concentration tasks compared with the number made when jasmine was used (Degel and Koster, 1999) and reduced stress in flight controllers (Leshchinskaia *et al.*, 1983).

Some periodontal diseases can be treated with a mixture of essential oils including lavender (Sysoev *et al.*, 1990; Yamahara *et al.*, 1994). Lavender oil was said to be suitable for prevention and treatment of decubitus ulcers, insect bites, athlete's foot and skin rash and can also be used for the topical treatment of acne, prevention of facial scarring and blemishes of the face and body (Hartwig, 1996; Karita, 1996). The essential oil of lavender was used in a mixture as a hair growth stimulant and for the treatment of alopecia areata (Hay *et al.*, 1998) and in a pilot study to determine possible novel, safe pediculicides in children (Weston *et al.*, 1997). Skin penetration enhancers, especially for the transdermal absorption of various drugs and medicaments have included lavender oil with nifedipine (Thacharodi *et al.*, 1994). Lavender oil is used as a component in topical formulations to relieve the pain associated with rheumatic and musculoskeletal disorders, acting as a potent radical scavenger (Billany *et al.*, 1995).

Antimicrobial activities

Antibacterial activity

Relative data: Using seven different commercial essential oils, 13–23/25 different bacteria were affected and 0–18/20 strains of *Listeria monocytogenes* (A1; Lis-Balchin and Deans, 1997; Lis-Balchin *et al.*, 1998a). The antimicrobial activity of lavender oil against different bacterial species of lavender is moderate, in contrast to the considerable antimicrobial status awarded to lavender by aromatherapists (Lis-Balchin, 2002b, ch.15). Lavender was most effective against *Enterococcus faecalis* out of 25 bacteria, but *Klebsiella pneumoniae* had enhanced growth (Deans and Ritchie, 1987)! The genus *Bacillus* has been shown to be susceptible to lavender oil (Deans and Ritchie, 1987; Jean *et al.*, 1991; Lis-Balchin *et al.*, 1998a). Other reports for lavender showed action against 3/5 bacteria (Yousef and Tawil, 1980); vapour showed 1/5 (Maruzella and Sicurela, 1960); lavandin vapour 1/5; spike vapour 2/5. Spike lavender showed lower activity against 18/25 different bacterial species (Deans and Ritchie, 1987).

Antifungal activity

Relative data: Seven different lavenders showed variable antifungal activities against three fungi: *Aspergillus niger* 57–93% inhibition; *A. ochraceus* 29–90%; *Fusarium culmorum* 8–89% (A1). Lavender and lavandin had low activity against 5/5 different fungi (Maruzella, 1960); similar effects were shown against 5/5 different fungi in other tests (Yousef and Tawil, 1980).

Antioxidant activity

Some activity was shown for some commercial lavenders and lavandins, but not for spike lavender (Lis-Balchin *et al.*, 1996b).

Use in pregnancy and lactation: contraindications

Lavender oil should now be used with caution due to its sensitisation potential and also because studies on the uterus *in vitro* show decrease in the intensity of contractions. However, its use both as a fragrance and in massage could be beneficial, provided the source of the essential oil is known and it is unadulterated.

Pharmaceutical guidance

Lavender essential oil and its hybrids are relatively safe to use except for their sensitisation potential, especially in sensitive people. Lavender essential oil is grossly adulterated with lavandins and also synthetic components and there is therefore a danger of an adverse effect through adulteration rather than the essential oil itself. The incidence of sensitisation to lavender is increasing over the years so that it may be wise not to massage children and certainly not to massage babies with the essential oil in order not to sensitise them at an early stage. The aroma of lavender has great psychological as well as physiological attributes (A14) and therefore can be recommended for use as a fragrance.

Use in babies and young children

Due to the immaturity and the delicate nature of the skin of babies and young children, it is inadvisable for any essential oils, even this supposedly safe essential oil, to be used in massage, however much the essential oil has been diluted in the carrier oils. This is also a necessary precaution due to the possibilities of sensitisation of the children at this young age through skin or air-borne odorant effects (see Chapters 5 and 7).

Instillation or administration of essential oils near the baby or young child's nose is not only not recommended, but distinctly inadvisable, as there have been numerous cases reported of severe toxicity and even death from such applications (see Chapter 7).

Lemon Balm Oil/Melissa Essential Oil

CAS numbers

USA: 8014-71-9; EINECS: 90814-71-9

Species/Botanical name

Melissa officinalis L. (Labiatae)

Synonyms

Balm, honeyplant, lemon balm, sweet balm, heart's delight, melissae folium, melissenblätter

Safety

CHIP details
Xi; R38, 43; 0%; S24, 37 (A26)

EU sensitiser total
None given by the authorities as this essential oil is mostly synthetic. It would be around 25, based on some analyses (A23).

Extraction, source, appearance and odour

Extraction
Steam-distilled leaves and tops of herb. Other plant materials/essential oils are often added to the distillation, e.g. lemon oil, verbena oil, lemongrass, citronella, etc. (Arctander, 1960).

Source
Europe.

Appearance and odour
A colourless essential oil with sweet, dry, floral-herbaceous odour. As this is the most adulterated of oils, the genuine essential oil is seldom encountered, so a description of its aroma is rather academic, as most people prefer the synthetic mixture anyway (Arctander, 1960).

Aromatherapy uses

Uses of *Melissa* include: anxiety, depression, hypertension, insomnia, migraine, hysterics, nervous crisis, tension, fear, shock, grief, and anger; stress response of elevated blood pressure; palpitations; dysmenorrhoea, menstrual regulation and infertility problems; upset stomach, indigestion, nausea, flatulence, vomiting, dyspepsia, stomach cramps asthma, allergies, bronchitis, chronic coughs, colds (with headache), fevers associated with colds and flu, muscle spasm, rheumatic pain; oily skin, acne, insect bites, cold sores, herpes, fungal infections. Advice is given in some aromatherapy books not to use this rather dangerous essential oil unless one is very proficient as it can be overpowering if used in large amounts, due to its narcotic properties (Ryman, 1991; Lawless, 1992; Rose, 1992a,b; Price, 1993; Sheppard-Hanger, 1995).

Scientific comment

The lack of any toxicological evaluations and the consistent adulteration of this essential oil, and therefore its increase in toxicological potential, make it potentially dangerous for aromatherapy use. It is unlikely that most of the listed aromatherapy uses could be proven and massage alone alleviates many stress conditions, including muscular and also some internal symptoms.

Herbal uses

Lemon balm has been used for centuries – Paracelsus called it the 'elixir of life' – and it has been associated with nervous disorders, the heart and emotions. Its genus name *Melissa* is from the Greek word for 'bee', referring to the bee's attraction to its flower and the quality of the honey produced from it (Grieve, 1937). The herb has sedative, spasmolytic and antibacterial properties and is a carminative, diaphoretic and a febrifuge, used for headaches, gastrointestinal disorders, nervousness and rheumatism (Wren, 1988; Chevallier, 1996; Barnes *et al.*, 2002). The Commission E reported sedative and carminative activity and it is now indicated for nervous sleeping disorders and functional gastrointestinal complaints (Blumenthal *et al.*, 2000). Internally it has been used for tenseness, restlessness, irritability and symptomatic treatment of digestive disorders, such as minor spasms; externally, for herpes labialis (cold sores) (ESCOP,

1997). The German Standard License for lemon balm tea approves it for nervous disorders of sleep and of the gastrointestinal tract, and to stimulate the appetite (Wichtl, 1994). It is internally a sedative and externally a topical antiviral (British Herbal Medicine Association, 1996). The hydroalcoholic lemon balm extract is a CNS sedative in animal studies; its essential oil content does not appear to play a role in this activity (Bruneton, 1995). Preparations of lemon balm have sedative, spasmolytic and antibacterial actions (Wichtl, 1994). The Ayurvedic Pharmacopoeia (AP) lists *Melissa officinalis*, along with the related Indian species *M. parviflora*, for dyspepsia associated with anxiety or depressive states, in a dried herb or alcoholic fluid extract dosage form. The AP reports its actions as carminative, antispasmodic, diaphoretic and sedative (Karnick, 1994).

Food and perfumery uses

Not used.

Chemistry

Major components

	% (Lawrence, 1976–2001)
Geranial	1–48
Neral	0.6–36
Citronellal	2–38
Linalool	0.5–3
Geranyl acetate	trace–6
Geraniol	trace–23
Caryophyllene	0.3–29

Minor components

Under 1%: *trans*-ocimene, *cis*-ocimene, methyl heptanone, 3-octanol, α-humulene, δ-cadinene and γ-cadinene; also caryophyllene oxide (3%), copaene (4%) and germacrene D (4%). There are about 200 components with a very wide range of variation in the composition of this oil.

Adulteration

Yield is very small: 0.06–0.375% v/m (volume in mass) hence the price is very high and adulteration rampant. As the cost of the real *Melissa* oil is roughly equivalent to that of rose oil (very high), most commercial oils are compounded from synthetic components and other cheaper essential oils (e.g. lemon, verbena, lemongrass, citronella, or

fractions of these) (A8; see Chapter 4). Some aromatherapists admit to this adulteration and actually prefer the odour of the adulterated essential oil (Price, 1993).

Toxicity

Acute toxicity

Oral and dermal LD_{50} values for *Melissa* are not documented. However, citral, the main component, can cause a rise in ocular tension after two weeks of daily oral dosing in monkeys (Leach and Lloyd, 1956). There are also reports of topically applied citral, at a high dose of 10 mL, causing benign prostatic hyperplasia (Scolnik *et al.*, 1994), which may be testosterone-dependent (Servadio *et al.*, 1986) or have an oestrogenic effect in rats (Geldof *et al.*, 1992); sebaceous gland proliferation (Sandbank *et al.*, 1988); may be receptor-mediated (Sandbank *et al.*, 1988). This dose is 15 times higher than that normally used in aromatherapy massage using an essential oil, like *Melissa* with about 75% citral, however it approaches a possible oral dose (Tisserand and Balacs, 1995).

Irritation and sensitisation
None documented.

Bioactivities

Pharmacological activities *in vitro* and *in vivo*
All studies were conducted on commercial samples of unknown authenticity.

Smooth muscle   Melissa oil had a weak spasmolytic effect on guinea-pig ileum *in vitro* (A2; Brandt, 1988; Lis-Balchin *et al.*, 1996a) and tracheal muscle (Reiter and Brandt, 1985). A 30% alcoholic extract of *M. officinalis* demonstrated an antispasmodic effect on rat duodenum *in vitro* (Barnes *et al.*, 2002).

Other activities   *M. officinalis* essential oil did not demonstrate sedative or sleep-inducing effects, administered intraperitoneally, however, low doses of a hydroalcoholic extract induced sleep in mice given an infrahypnotic dose of pentobarbital (Barnes *et al.*, 2002). Other studies are mainly on hydroalcoholic extracts, which may have some of the components of the essential oil present in very small amounts and were administered mainly intraperitoneally. Most showed nil effects on analgesia, but effects on lipid peroxidation *in vitro* were observed (Barnes *et al.*, 2002). Studies in mice have shown that a lemon balm extract is highly effective in reducing stress-induced behaviours and potentiating pentobarbital-induced sleep. The relaxant effect of the essential oil of *M. officinalis* and its main component, citral, on rat isolated ileum showed inhibition of contractions (Sadraei *et al.*, 2003). Citral also had a concentration-dependent inhibitory effect on contraction of rat ileum.

Antimicrobial activities

Antibacterial activity
Relative values: A commercial sample was active against 22/25 different bacterial species and against 9/20 *Listeria monocytogenes* varieties (A1; Lis-Balchin and Deans, 1997; Lis-Balchin *et al.*, 1998a). Another sample was active against 9/25 bacteria of the same species as above (Deans and Ritchie, 1987); the vapour was active against 1/5 bacterial species (Maruzella and Sicurella, 1960). Antimicrobial activity has been reported against the yeasts *Candida albicans* and *Saccharomyces cerevisiae*, and against six bacteria (Larrondo *et al.*, 1995). Citronellal and geranial as well as citronellol have a strong antibacterial effect (Deans, 2002).

Antifungal activity
Relative values (% inhibition): *Aspergillus niger* 89%; *A. ochraceus* 73%; *Fusarium culmorum* 60% (A1). The alcohols and aldehydes are again responsible for the antifungal action (Deans, 2002).

Antioxidant activity
A commercial sample had a strong antioxidant action (Lis-Balchin *et al.*, 1996a). Melissa oil was found to be relaxant, based on its contingent negative variation effect and the observation that it reduced motility in mice (A14).

Other activities
Although aromatherapy books and other literature state that melissa oil is antiviral, especially against herpes simplex virus, only the aqueous extracts of *M. officinalis* have been reported to inhibit the development of this and other viruses (Barnes *et al.*, 2002; see Chapter 6). The fat-soluble fractions were all inactive, therefore the essential oil does not apparently have any antiviral properties.

However, recently, *M. officinalis* essential oil was found to be slightly toxic on *Herpes simplex virus* type 2 (HSV-2) replication in HEp-2 cells at a very high concentration of over 100 µg/ml *in vitro* (Allahverdiyev *et al.*, 2004). Some slight reduction in replication was also noted. However, no proper control was used and there was no information on how the essential oil was obtained or in what solvent it was diluted as this could have affected the viral cells.

Clinical studies
When the antiviral effects of aqueous extracts of *M. officinalis* leaves were investigated in *Herpes simplex virus* (HSV) infection, adverse effects were often shown, such as irritation or burning sensations (Barnes *et al.*, 2002). In one study on 115 patients, a proprietary preparation of lemon balm extract in a lip balm showed efficacy in treating lip sores associated with the *Herpes simplex virus* (Wölbling and Leonhardt, 1994).

Melissa extracts, given orally, were also tested for their acute sedative effects in a randomised, double-blind, placebo-controlled, crossover study involving 12 healthy volunteers and showed virtually no effect in comparison with other plant extracts and controls (Barnes *et al.*, 2002). The sedative effects of oral combination preparations containing extracts of lemon balm and valerian (*Valeriana officinalis*), for example, were more successful, showing a very slight but non-significant improvement in sleep quality (Barnes *et al.*, 2002).

Old European medical herbals report melissa's memory-improving properties, recently corroborated as cholinergic activities identified in extracts of lemon balm (Perry *et al.*, 1998). Studies in patients with Alzheimer's syndrome and other forms of dementia have shown some benefits of aromatherapy, particularly using lemon balm and lavender oil; bright light therapy also eases restlessness and sleeping and behavioural problems. Melissa supplements were found to improve the mood and memory of 20 healthy young participants (Kennedy *et al.*, 2002).

Use in pregnancy and lactation: contraindications
In view of the gross adulteration of the essential oil, its possible deleterious effect on the uterus, possible oestrogenic effect, lack of toxicity data and possible sensitisation, the use of lemon balm during pregnancy, parturition and lactation should be avoided in massage. Use as a fragrance could be considered in small quantities.

Pharmaceutical guidance
The effects of lemon balm essential oil have not been studied to any great extent, except for animal

movements and effect on the gut *in vitro*, and its effect on human brain waves (using contingent negative variation studies) (A14). There is a lack of research investigating the safety of long-term administration of lemon balm essential oil. There is no antiviral effect from using the essential oil. People with glaucoma should avoid this essential oil (Tisserand and Balacs, 1995). A possible testosterone-dependent or oestrogenic effect on hyperplasia in rat prostate suggests caution in prostatic conditions. Children under 5 years should not be massaged with melissa oil, nor people with sensitive skins, due to the common adulteration of this oil and substitution by synthetics including citral, which is a sensitiser and possibly oestrogenic. Melissa oil is not recommended in aromatherapy massage and the fragrance is not very pleasant to most people.

Use in babies and young children

Due to the immaturity and the delicate nature of the skin of babies and young children, it is inadvisable for any essential oils, especially with this essential oil containing potential sensitisers, to be used in massage, however much the essential oil has been diluted in the carrier oils. This is also a necessary precaution due to the possibilities of sensitisation of the children at this young age through skin or air-borne odorant effects (see Chapters 5 and 7).

Instillation or administration of essential oils near the baby or young child's nose is not only not recommended, but distinctly inadvisable, as there have been numerous cases reported of severe toxicity and even death from such applications (see Chapter 7).

Lemon Oil

CAS numbers

Lemon expressed: USA: 84929-31-7; EINECS: 84929-31-7
Lemon distilled: USA: 8008-56-8; EINECS: 84929-31-7

Species/Botanical name

Citrus limonum (L.) Burm.f. (Rutaceae)

Synonyms

C. limonum Risso
Ol. limon., aetheroleum citri, citronenöl, esencia de cidra, essência de limão, essence de citron, limonis aetheroleum, oleum citri, oleum limonis
Deterpenated lemon oil BP: oleum limonis deterpenatum, terpeneless lemon oil

Pharmacopoeias

In European and Polish Pharmacopoeias. Also in United States National Formulary. Deterpenated lemon oil is in British Pharmacopoeia.

Safety

CHIP details

Lemon oil expressed: Xn; R10, 65; 90%; S62
Lemon oil distilled: Xn; R10, 65; 95%; S62

EU sensitiser value

73.3 (based on citral 3%, limonene 70% and linalool 0.3%)

GRAS status

Granted (Fenaroli, 1997).

Extraction, source, appearance and odour

Extraction

A volatile oil obtained by expression from the fresh peel of lemons. The peels can also be steam distilled to give an essential oil of a different composition.

Lemon oil (USNF 22) is volatile oil obtained by expression, without the aid of heat, from the fresh peel of the fruit of *Citrus × limon* (Rutaceae), with or without the previous separation of the pulp and the peel.

Source

Sicily, California (USA), Argentina and Spain.

Appearance and odour

The oil is yellow to orangey to greenish-yellow, if cold expressed; colourless to light yellow if distilled or rectified. Expressed oil has a short-lasting, light, fresh odour reminiscent of the peel. This is retained throughout its evaporation (Arctander, 1960).

Aromatherapy uses

There are hundreds of uses given. In many books, the lemon (juice, etc.) is quoted and the essential oil is only mentioned in passing. 'Lemon' apparently acts as a stimulant to the brain, sense organs, parasympathetic nervous system, provides awareness and connectivity between our soma and soul thereby soothing conflict between thoughts and intellect. Other uses include: varicose veins, anaemic conditions, poor circulation, hypertension, phlebitis, thrombosis, arteriosclerosis and nosebleeds; sore throats, coughs, colds and influenza; kidneys, urine excretion; stimulating the glandular system and smooth muscle tissue (therefore useful to induce labour when overdue); nephritic colic; asthma, bronchitis, catarrh, sinus infections; cellulite; broken capillaries; greasy skin and hair; mouth ulcers, herpes, acne, boils, corns, warts and balancing sebum (Ryman, 1991; Lawless, 1992; Rose, 1992a; Price, 1993; Sheppard-Hanger, 1995).

Scientific comment

Lemon essential oil is extremely adulterated and the commercial product is variable in composition and activity. There was little antimicrobial activity; the spasmogenic effect on the smooth muscle *in vitro* may have a stimulating effect as a fragrance, although it has been shown to have a sedative effect on the human brain waves (A14). The use of lemon essential oil on the skin is not recommended due to its sensitisation and phototoxic potential. It is unlikely that the essential oil could alleviate most of the conditions listed above, especially as the use of the whole fruit or lemon juice was implied by some aromatherapists. Massage itself could benefit many stress ailments and the use of the fragrance with massage could help the patient further.

Herbal uses

Most of the uses listed are for lemon juice, not the essential oil. Uses include: rheumatic conditions (as it has an alkaline effect in the body); varicose veins and bruises, strengthening capillaries and veins; preventative for infections, fevers, arteriosclerosis, bleeding gums, etc. (Wren, 1988; Chevalier, 1996).

Conventional uses

Lemon oil is used in various compound spirits for embrocation or in cough medicines, such as aromatic ammonia spirit (BP 2003) and compound orange spirit (USNF 22). The deterpenated lemon oil is used in preparations such as: compound orange spirit (BP 2003), lemon spirit (BP 2003) and lemon syrup (BP 2003).

Food and perfumery uses

Food   Lemon oil (FEMA 2625) and the terpeneless oil (FEMA 2626) are used in many different foods and beverages (Fenaroli, 1997).

Perfumery   It is used in perfumes for its refreshing note, especially in colognes and masculine-type perfume (Arctander, 1960).

Chemistry

Major components
Lemon (expressed) (ISO, 1984)

	% (range)
α-Pinene	1.8 (66–80)
Sabinene	1.9
β-Pinene	12.1 (0.4–15)
Myrcene	trace (0–13)
α-Terpinene	0.5
p-Cymene	trace (0–2)

Limonene	67
γ-Terpinene	8.6 (6–14)
Neral/nerol	1.1 (0.2–1.3)
Geranial/geraniol	1.8 (1–3)
Neryl acetate	0.5
Geranyl acetate	0.5
α-Bergamotene	0.4 (0–2.5)
β-Bisabolene	0.5

Minor components
Coumarins and psoralens (bergaptenes) cause phototoxic action. These are not found in distilled oils of furocoumarin-free redistilled oils. Cold-pressed lemon oil has a limonene content of about 80% maximum, but the 10-fold oil and 25-fold oil has a drastically reduced percentage; in fact the limonene content can decrease to almost zero on total deterpenation, raising other components to extremely high levels (Lawrence, 1976–2001).

Lemon oil (Ph. Eur. 4.8) contains a maximum of 0.5% β-caryophyllene, 0.5–2.3% geranial, 0.1–0.8% geranyl acetate, 56.0–78.0% limonene, 0.3–1.5% neral, 0.2–0.9% neryl acetate, 7.0–17.0% β-pinene, 1.0–3.0% sabinene, 6.0–12.0% γ-terpinene and a maximum of 0.6% α-terpineol.

Lemon oil (USNF 22) has a total aldehyde content, calculated as citral, not less than 2.2% and not more than 3.8% for the California-type lemon oil, and not less than 3.0% and not more than 5.5% for the Italian-type lemon oil.

Adulteration
Although not true adulteration, the use of various techniques for deterpenation after cold pressing the oil can give very different essential oils. First, lemon oil, like other citrus oils is often folded, using vacuum distillation. The lemon oil can also be 'washed' by partitioning the oil into a mixture of alcohol and water, with stirring, for 24 hours. The two methods can be used sequentially. There are also other methods of deterpenation – chromatographic and countercurrent techniques. These deterpenations are used for the benefit of the food and perfumery industry and there is often no way of telling how the citrus oils have been altered if they are bought on the commercial market. Lemon oil can be adulterated with distilled lemon oil, concentrated lemon oil, terpeneless or sesquiterpeneless lemon oil, synthetic or natural limonene, citral, turpentine, etc. Lemon oil is ten times more expensive than orange oil, therefore many adulterations involve using orange oil and its components, together with lemongrass oil, or just the citral part. UV absorbers

have to be added as otherwise it is known that the oil is not pressed. Large numbers of different UV absorbers are in use, e.g. aurapene from grapefruit (A8; see Chapter 4).

Antioxidants like butylhydroxy anisole (BHA) and butylhydroxy toluene (BHT) are usually added as the citrus oils oxidise very quickly. δ-3-Carene levels above trace show adulteration; also terpinen-4-ol 0.02% maximum (cold-pressed), 0.35% (distilled) (A8; see Chapter 4).

Toxicity

Acute toxicity (A22)

Oral LD$_{50}$ >5 g/kg (rat).

Dermal LD$_{50}$ >5 g/kg (rabbit).

Irritation and sensitisation

Nil at 10% and 100% (A22); 1/200 dermatitis patients were sensitive to lemon oil (Rudzki *et al.*, 1976). Increased adulteration has shown increased sensitisations.

d-Limonene-high oils (citrus oils) in particular will quickly degrade after opening to produce weak carcinogenic chemicals (Homberger and Boger, 1968) or will increase risk of sensitisation and skin irritation. Therefore the shelf-life of opened bottles if stored correctly is recommended to be 1 year, or 2 years if stored in a fridge. Citrus oils will last six months if stored correctly (Homberger and Boger, 1968).

Phototoxicity

This can be from high to low, depending on whether cold-pressed (high) or furocoumarin-free (very low) essential oils are used. Natural extracts containing furocoumarin-like substances may be used in cosmetic products, provided that the total concentration of furocoumarin-like substances in the finished cosmetic product does not exceed 1 ppm. These extracts include: lemon oil; lemon oil (cold pressed, California type); lemon oil (cold pressed, desert type); angelica root oil (*Angelica archangelica* L.); bergamot oil; grapefruit oil (expressed) (*Citrus paradisi* Macf.); lime oil (cold pressed, Mexican); lime oil (expressed); lime oil (expressed rectified); orange peel oil (bitter) (*Citrus aurantium* L.); and rue oil (*Ruta graveolens* L.).

Pharmacological activities *in vitro* and *in vivo*

Smooth muscle Lemon oil had a spasmogenic effect on electrically stimulated smooth muscle of the

guinea-pig ileum *in vitro*. Limonene had a similar effect (A2; Lis-Balchin *et al.*, 1996a).

Uterus There was a decrease in the spontaneous contractions in the rat for lemon oil, limonene and the other components studied. Mixing several other essential oils with lemon oil also had a relaxant effect (A3; A4; Lis-Balchin and Hart, 1997b).

Antimicrobial activities

Lemon oil has generally a poor antimicrobial capability. It is also variable, due to the different compositions of essential oil supplied.

Antibacterial activity

Relative data: poor effect was shown against 8/25 different bacterial species and 3/20 *Listeria monocytogenes* varieties (A1; Lis-Balchin and Deans, 1997; Lis-Balchin *et al.*, 1998a). Other work on the same bacterial species showed 9/25 were affected, but very poorly (Deans and Ritchie, 1987); and 13/25 (Baratta *et al.*, 1998b); 4/4 bacteria were affected mildly (Friedman *et al.*, 2002); 0/5 *Listeria* were affected (Aureli *et al.*, 1992).

Antifungal activity

Relative data: There was very poor activity against *Aspergillus niger* 4% inhibition, *A. ochraceus* 22%, *Fusarium culmorum* 0 (A1); 5/5 fungi were affected in another study (Maruzella, 1960).

Antioxidant activity

Antioxidant effect was virtually zero (Lis-Balchin *et al.*, 1996a; Baratta *et al.*, 1998b).

Other activities

Lemon oil was considered to be sedative, according to contingent negative variation brain waves (A14). A preparation containing *d*-limonene and other monoterpenes is used to dissolve gallstones (Martindale, 1972).

Male and female rats allowed to inhale the aroma of lemon essential oil while experiencing a persistent nociceptive input showed a decrease in the licking of the injected paw in both sexes. Flinching and flexing were decreased in males and increased in females in the interphase (5–20 minutes) of the formalin test. In the same animals c-Fos immunohistochemistry was used to test the degree of neuronal activation of areas belonging to the limbic system: lemon essential oil also increased c-Fos expression in the arcuate nucleus of the hypothalamus. The results indicate the ability of lemon essential oil to modulate the behavioural and neuronal responses related to nociception and pain (Aloisi *et al.*, 2002).

Oils high in *d*-limonene (citrus oils such as sweet orange, lime, lemon and grapefruit) have been shown to stimulate tumorous growths in mice on the site of topical application (Roe, 1959; Roe and Peirce, 1960). A potential antidepressant effect of lemon odour was shown in rats (Komori *et al.*, 1995).

Use during pregnancy and lactation: contraindications

The lemon expressed essential oil has been widely used but recently there have been more studies on its potential sensitisation and also its photoxicity. There is also some evidence from animal experiments that it causes a decrease in spontaneous contractions of the uterus and therefore caution is advised in the use of lemon essential oil during pregnancy and parturition. There is no risk if the essential oil is used as a fragrance in small amounts.

Pharmaceutical guidance

The main problem is the potential sensitisation of the expressed essential oil, especially after prolonged storage or allowing oxidation of the limonene to occur. The essential oil, especially the pure expressed essential oil, is also phototoxic.

Use on sensitive or damaged skin should be avoided and the essential oil should not be used on skin before being exposed to quantities of sunlight or UV light on sunbeds. Deterpenated essential oils should be used to circumvent the sensitisation and photoxicity problems when using aromatherapy massage. The lemon odour has been shown to have a relaxant effect on human brain waves (A14) and it is also refreshing, therefore could be used as a fragrance with massage for more beneficial effects and less danger of toxic effects, or used as a fragrance alone.

Use in babies and young children

Due to the immaturity and the delicate nature of the skin of babies and young children, it is inadvisable for any essential oils, especially this one with sensitisation/photosensitisation potential, to be used in massage, however much the essential oil has been diluted in the carrier oils. This is also a necessary precaution due to the possibilities of sensitisation of the children at this young age through skin or air-borne odorant effects (see Chapters 5 and 7).

Instillation or administration of essential oils near the baby or young child's nose is not only not recommended, but distinctly inadvisable, as there have been numerous cases reported of severe toxicity and even death from such applications (see Chapter 7).

Lemongrass Oil

CAS numbers

USA: 8007-02-1; EINECS: 89998-14-1 (West Indian); 91844-92-7 (East Indian)

Species/Botanical name

Cymbopogon citratus (DC) Stapf. (Graminae)

Synonyms

Cymbopogon flexuosus Stapf., *Andropogon nardus* var. *flexuosus*, melissa grass, fever grass, citronella grass, geranium grass
Essência de capim-limão, Indian melissa oil, Indian verbena oil, lemongrass oil, oleum graminis citrati

Safety

CHIP details
Xn; R65; 15%; S62 (A26)

RIFM recommended safety of use limits
4% (A23)

EU sensitiser total
84.1 due to geranial, neral, limonene, linalool, geraniol, citronellol and eugenol (A27)

GRAS status
Granted (Fenaroli, 1997).

Extraction, source, appearance and odour

Extraction
A volatile oil obtained by steam distillation of the dried or partly dried grass. It can keep 2–3% water, so must be kept dry, as the citral decomposes (Arctander, 1960).

Source
Guatemala, Madagascar and India.

Appearance and odour
A yellow/brown oil with a tinge of red, if unrectified, otherwise almost colourless. Lemongrass oil has a fresh, strongly citrusy, lemon-like, and pungent odour with herbal and leafy aspects and fatty-grassy notes. Lemongrass is related to palmarosa and citronella and has an odour reminiscent of *Melissa* and *Litsea cubeba* (Arctander, 1960).

Aromatherapy uses

Uses include: nervous exhaustion, stress, headaches, fatigue, irritability; stimulates glandular secretions, liver, digestion, and appetite; colitis, indigestion, gastroenteritis, intestinal parasites; inducing menstruation and increasing milk flow in nursing mothers; activating fibrocytes, T-lymphocytes, histocytes, granulocytes so used for fevers, infections, cholera, sore throats, laryngitis; strengthening and detoxifying connective tissues of elastin and extravascular tissues in general; arteritis, increasing circulation, stimulating lymphatic circulation and detoxification; aching muscles, arthritis, bruises, and dislocation (pain); imparting tone to the skin and balancing oily conditions, acne, athlete's foot, skin parasites, excessive perspiration, enlarged pores, cellulite. Lemongrass oil is stimulating yet relaxing (Ryman, 1991; Lawless, 1992; Rose, 1992a; Price, 1993; Sheppard-Hanger, 1995).

Scientific comment
The essential oil is strongly antispasmodic to smooth muscle of the intestine *in vitro* and also to uterine muscles and is used as a herbal tea for intestinal problems, but it may not be effective when massaged into the skin and there is no scientific evidence to support any of the aromatherapy claims made. Massage itself can alleviate many stress and muscular problems and lemongrass essential oil, used as a fragrance, with its strong antimicrobial citral could help in cases of infection and also potentially stimulate the brain (A14).

Herbal uses

The lemongrass herb is used in Ayurvedic medicine for infectious diseases and fever and as a sedative, insecticide and food flavouring. Traditional uses involve its analgesic, antidepressant, anti-inflammatory, antimicrobial, antioxidant, anti-rickets, antiseptic (strong; air-borne), astringent, carminative, deodorant, febrifuge, fungicidal, parasiticide, galactogogue, insecticidal, nervine and sedative properties. It is drunk as a tea in both India and the Caribbean for relaxing intestinal cramps and flatulence, especially in children, and for reducing fever. It is applied as a poultice externally for pain relief in arthritis and for eradicating ringworm (Lawless, 1992; Sheppard-Hanger, 1995; Chevallier, 1996).

Food and perfumery uses

Food Lemongrass oil (FEMA 2624) is used in a wide range of food and beverages (Fenaroli, 1997).

Perfumery Lemongrass is used in many types of perfumery, especially in citrusy perfume compounds for household products and as an insect repellent (Arctander, 1960).

Chemistry

Major components

	% *(Lawrence, 1976–2001)*
Geranial	40–70
Neral	25–42
Limonene	trace–15
Linalool	trace–3
Geraniol	trace–16
Citronellol	trace–1
Eugenol	trace–0.5

There is a difference between lemongrass essential oils from East and West Indies but there is often admixing in the commercial essential oils.

Adulteration

This is one of the cheapest oils and therefore unlikely to be adulterated with synthetics, but can be substituted by *Litsea cubeba* of a similar composition.

Lemongrass is a useful supplier of citral, and is used in the production of vitamin A, ionones and methyl ionones. However, synthetic citral is often added. Lemongrass is used with geranium oil and citronella and some synthetic components as a cheap rose oil (A8; see Chapter 4).

Toxicity

Acute toxicity (A22)

Oral LD$_{50}$ >5 g/kg body weight (rat).
Dermal LD$_{50}$ >5 g/kg (rabbit).

Irritation and sensitisation (A22)

None at 4% (human), but now regarded as a very sensitising essential oil due to the increased reports of sensitisation to its components and the very high total sensitisation value of 84.1.

Phototoxicity

None reported.

Bioactivities

Pharmacological activities *in vitro* and *in vivo*

Smooth muscle Lemongrass oil had a strong spasmolytic effect on electrically stimulated smooth muscle of the guinea-pig *in vitro* (A2; Lis-Balchin et al., 1996a).

Uterus There was a decrease in the spontaneous contractions in the rat when lemongrass oil and its main components were applied *in vitro* (A3; A4; Lis-Balchin and Hart, 1997b).

Other activities The essential oil increased the reaction time to thermal stimuli after both oral (25 mg/kg) and intraperitoneal (25–100 mg/kg) administration. It strongly inhibited acetic acid-induced writhings in mice. The opioid antagonist naloxone blocked the central antinociceptive effect of the essential oil, suggesting that the essential oil acts both at peripheral and central levels (Viana et al., 2000). There was an impact on cholesterol levels by the essential oil (Elson et al., 1989).

There was a stimulant action on the contingent negative variation brain waves (A14) which opposed the sedative effect on smooth muscle *in vitro* as above.

Antimicrobial activities

Antibacterial activity

Relative values: There was a strong action against 18/25 different bacterial species and 20/20 *Listeria monocytogenes* varieties (A1; Lis-Balchin and Deans, 1997; Lis-Balchin et al., 1998a). Similar strong activity was reported for several bacteria (Hammer et al., 1999a). Rectified vapour was effective against 4/5 bacteria (Maruzella and Sicurella, 1960). The essential oil was mildly to moderately effective against 23/25 different bacterial species (Baratta et al., 1998b).

Antifungal activity

Relative values (A1) (% inhibition): *Aspergillus niger* 90%, *A. ochraceus* 83%, *Fusarium culmorum* 69%. Rectified lemongrass oil was effective against

5/5 fungi (Maruzella, 1960). Lemongrass oil was effective against tinea pedis and dandruff (Asre, 1994) and 11/15 fungi (Maruzella and Liguori, 1958). The essential oil was very effective against *A. niger* (Baratta *et al.*, 1998b).

Antioxidant activity

Antioxidant activity was noted (Lis-Balchin *et al.*, 1996a; Baratta *et al.*, 1998a).

Use during pregnancy and lactation: contraindications

Due to the problems of possible sensitisation, the unknown toxicological effects on the human uterus, the effect on the uterus of a mammal *in vitro* (causing reduction and eventual cessation of spasms) and the oestrogenic potential of citral, lemongrass oil is not recommended in massage during pregnancy, parturition and lactation. The use of the fragrance itself should not prove hazardous if used in moderation.

Pharmaceutical guidance

The essential oil of lemongrass is best avoided in aromatherapy for skin application as there are apparently no benefits for its use and the sensitising potential is greatly in excess of other essential oils; the avoidance of citral-high oils is generally recommended (Geldof, 1992).

Lemongrass is best used as a citrusy perfume, which has a stimulant effect on the human brain (A14) and should not be harmful if used sparingly (see also *Litsea cubeba* oil monograph).

Use in babies and young children

Due to the immaturity and the delicate nature of the skin of babies and young children, it is inadvisable for any essential oils, especially this essential oil with strong sensitisation potential, to be used in massage, however much the essential oil has been diluted in the carrier oils. This is also a necessary precaution due to the possibilities of sensitisation of the children at this young age through skin or air-borne odorant effects (see Chapters 5 and 7).

Instillation or administration of essential oils near the baby or young child's nose is not only not recommended, but distinctly inadvisable, as there have been numerous cases reported of severe toxicity and even death from such applications (see Chapter 7).

Litsea cubeba Oil

CAS numbers

USA: 68855-99-2; EINECS: 90063-59-5

Species/Botanical name

Litsea cubeba L. (Lauraceae)

Synonyms

Litsea cubeba Pers.
May chang

Safety

CHIP details
Xi; R10, 38; 0% (A26)

RIFM recommended safety of use limits
8% (A23)

EU sensitiser total
97.2 (based on: geranial, neral, limonene, linalool and geraniol) (A27)

Extraction, source, appearance and odour

Extraction
A volatile oil obtained by steam distillation of pepper-like fruit of the tree (Arctander, 1960).

Source
China and Taiwan.

Appearance and odour
A pale yellow essential oil with an intensely fresh lemon-like, sweet odour and a soft, fruity dry-out. It has no fatty-grassy notes of the similar lemongrass (Arctander, 1960).

Aromatherapy uses

Litsea cubeba is not greatly used in aromatherapy, but can be a substitute for lemongrass oil, which bears a distinct similarity to it. This substitution is commonly done by essential oil producers if the price is to their advantage. Uses include: acne, dermatitis, greasy skin, spots, insect repellent on the skin; flatulence and indigestion; epidemics; sanitation (Lawless, 1992; Rose, 1992; Sheppard-Hanger, 1995; see also lemongrass oil monograph).

Scientific comment
The essential oil is strongly antispasmodic to smooth muscle of the intestine *in vitro* and also to uterine muscles but it may not be effective when massaged into the skin and there is no scientific evidence to support any of the aromatherapy claims made. Massage itself can alleviate many stress and muscular problems and used as a fragrance the essential oil, with its strong antimicrobial component citral, could help in cases of infection.

Herbal uses

It is planted as a windbreaker in Japan: but its herbal uses in Japan have not become apparent (see lemongrass oil monograph).

Food and perfumery uses

Food   Not used in foods.

Perfumery   Limited use in perfumes when substituting for lemongrass (Arctander, 1960).

Chemistry
Major components

	% (Lawrence, 1976–2001)
Geranial	40–52
Neral	30–42
Limonene	1–15
Linalool	trace–3
Geraniol	trace–2

Adulteration
Litsea cubeba essential oil is similar to lemongrass, therefore substitution by each other is common, depending on the price prevailing. *Litsea citrata*, planted as a windbreaker in Chinese tea groves, may also be substituted, but has a lower citral

level. Litsea is a cheap oil, therefore substitution by synthetic citral etc. is uneconomical (A8; see Chapter 4).

Toxicity

Acute toxicity (A22)

Oral LD₅₀ LD_{50} >5 g/kg (rat).

Dermal LD₅₀ LD_{50} >5 g/kg (rabbit).

Irritation and sensitisation (A22)

Nil at 8% (human), but in dermatitis patients, 3/200 and 13/450 patients were affected (Rudzki *et al.*, 1976). Many more cases of sensitisation to citral and the other components have since been reported and the sensitisation potential of the oil is very high (97.2%). It should therefore be avoided in sensitive people.

Phototoxicity

Not tested.

Bioactivities

Pharmacological activities *in vitro* and *in vivo*

Smooth muscle Litsea cubeba oil had a spasmolytic effect on electrically stimulated smooth muscle of the guinea-pig *in vitro* (A2; Lis-Balchin *et al.*, 1996a). Limonene had a similar effect.

Uterus There was a decrease in the spontaneous contractions in the rat for the oil and its major components (A3; A4; Lis-Balchin and Hart, 1997b).

Other activities The essential oil is very active due to the presence of about 80% citral. When administered intraperitoneally or by inhalation to guinea-pigs, it protected them against asthma induced by inhaled bronchoconstrictors. The oil also inhibited passive cutaneous anaphylaxis in rats and anaphylactic shock in guinea-pigs sensitised to egg albumin (US Patent Application: 0030215530, 2005).

Antimicrobial activities

Antibacterial activity

Relative data: The essential oil was very active against 16/25 different bacterial species and 18/20 *Listeria monocytogenes* varieties (A1; Lis-Balchin and Deans, 1997; Lis-Balchin *et al.*, 1998a).

Antifungal activity

Relative value (A1) (% inhibition): *Aspergillus niger* 87–95%, *A. ochraceus* 80–90%, *Fusarium culmorum* 40–64%. There was an inhibition of mycelial growth in four fungal species (Gogoi *et al.*, 1997) (see also lemongrass oil monograph).

Use in pregnancy and lactation: contraindications

Due to the lack of toxicological and pharmacological data and its possible detrimental effect on spontaneous contractions in the uterus, together with the high sensitisation potential, *Litsea cubeba* oil is not recommended during pregnancy, parturition and lactation.

Pharmaceutical guidance

The essential oil of *Litsea cubeba* is best avoided as there are apparently no benefits for its use and the sensitising potential is much higher than that of other essential oils. It can easily be replaced by the chemically similar lemongrass essential oil, but because of economic considerations, it is difficult to know when either oil is the true essential oil as it could be labelled either as lemongrass or *Litsea cubeba*.

Use in babies and young children

Due to the immaturity and the delicate nature of the skin of babies and young children, it is inadvisable for any essential oils, especially one with strong sensitisation potential, to be used in massage, however much the essential oil has been diluted in the carrier oils. This is also a necessary precaution due to the possibilities of sensitisation of the children at this young age through skin or air-borne odorant effects (see Chapters 5 and 7).

Instillation or administration of essential oils near the baby or young child's nose is not only not recommended, but distinctly inadvisable, as there have been numerous cases reported of severe toxicity and even death from such applications (see Chapter 7).

Manuka Oil

CAS numbers
USA: 8015-64-3; EINECS: 84775-71-7

Species/Botanical name
Leptospermum scoparium (Myrtaceae)

Synonyms
Manex

Related species
Kanuka (*Kunzea ericoides*)

Safety
CHIP details
Xn, R10, 65, 95%, S62 (A26)

RIFM recommended safety of use limits
Not stated

EU sensitiser total
Not given

Extraction, source, appearance and odour
Extraction
The essential oil is obtained by steam distillation of the leaves and branchlets of the tree (Arctander, 1960).

Source
Australia.

Appearance and odour
Manuka oil has a honey-like aroma, sweet yet herbaceous and medicinal.

Aromatherapy uses
Most aromatherapy books do not list manuka essential oil, but numerous Internet sites associated with aromatherapy oil supply give uses by oral intake, inhalation and external application. Uses include: sunburn, fungal skin and nail infections (e.g. athlete's foot); itching scalp, dandruff, cuts, scratches, pimples, oily skin, rashes, body odour, insect bites and stings; asthma; aching muscles.

Scientific comment
Although manuka has folk medicinal uses, the essential oil has not been tested toxicologically nor for its medicinal benefit for all the conditions listed. The many external uses listed use the essential oil simply as a chemical, using mainly its antiseptic qualities based on herbal usage. Manuka essential oil cannot therefore be condoned for general aromatherapy usage (see Chapters 5 and 8; also tea tree oil and kanuka oil monographs).

Herbal uses
The folk medicinal uses of the New Zealand 'tea-tree' oils are related to both manuka and kanuka. The leaves of both species were used as vapour baths for colds; an infusion was very astringent and various uses were found for concoctions, including urinary complaints and as a febrifuge (Brooker *et al.*, 1987). Kanuka was applied to scalds and burns, used to stop coughing and as a sedative; it was also used against dysentery. The decoction of boiled leaves and bark was used to treat stiff backs, etc. Seed capsules were boiled to give a decoction for external application to treat inflammation or drunk for diarrhoea; the capsules or leaves were also chewed for dysentery. The water from boiled bark was used to treat inflamed breasts and also to treat mouth, throat and eye problems. The emollient white gum, called pai manuka, was given to nursing babies and also used to treat scalds and burns. Chewing the bark is said to have a relaxing effect and to enhance sleep.

The antibacterial activity of honeys derived from kanuka and manuka blossom against *Staphylococcus aureus* was shown by Allen *et al.* (1991) and more recently manuka honey was shown to be active against *Helicobacter pylori* (Somal *et al.*, 1994; see also Cook, 1777; Polack, 1840; Neill, 1884; Adams, 1945; McDonald, 1975; see also tea tree oil monograph).

Food and perfumery uses

Food   None found.

Perfumery   Not used, but it apparently blends well with bay leaf, bergamot, black pepper, cajuput, cedarwood atlas, cinnamon, clove bud, elemi, ginger, juniper, lavender, nutmeg, peppermint, rose, rosemary, sandalwood, thyme, vetiver and ylang ylang.

Chemistry

Major components

	%
Terpinene-4-ol	39–41
γ-Terpinene	14–16
Flavescone	5–8
Isoleptospermone	7–8
Leptospermone	15–20
Calamenene	14

Manuka essential oil (Manex) also contains monoterpene hydrocarbons, α-cubebene, β-pinene, *p*-cymene, γ-terpinene, α-copaene, β-caryophyllene, aromadendrene, selinene, cadinene, calamanene, gurjunene, farnesene, elemene, limonene and myrcene; the oxide 1,8-cineole, linalool and esters (Perry *et al.*, 1997a,b; Porter *et al.*, 1998; Porter and Wilkins, 1999).

Lowered aroma manuka essential oil is said to be ideal for most uses as it has very low levels of pinenes and myrcene (monoterpenes >1%), but high levels of flavesone (5%), isoleptospermone (7–8%) and leptospermone (18–20%). This combination gives a high level of antimicrobial activity, particularly against Gram-positive organisms such as *Staphylococcus* and *Streptococcus*. It also has a wide range of antifungal activity (ManukaOil.com).

Leptospermone has antihelmintic properties and is closely related to compounds with similar properties in male ferns; it also has insecticidal properties, and is similar in structure to the insecticide valone (Brooker *et al.*, 1987). The presence of the triketones leptospermone, isoleptospermone and flavesone within the Manex oil identified it as a specific chemotype. Moreover, antimicrobial activity was directly related to the triketone fraction and gave Manex oil superior activity over other manuka chemotypes and kanuka essential oils. Manuka and kanuka often grow together and are difficult to differentiate morphologically. This, together with the existence of manuka chemotypes has led to the availability of commercial manuka

essential oils of variable antimicrobial activity (Perry *et al.*, 1997a,b; Porter *et al.*, 1998; Porter and Wilkins, 1999) (see also tea tree oil monograph, Tables 1–5).

Adulteration

The admixing of the different trees and shrubs gives essential oils of variable chemical compositions and bioactivity qualities (as above).

Toxicity

Acute toxicity not determined.

Irritation and sensitisation

Manuka essential oil was found to be non-irritant on 30 subjects undiluted; some irritancy was reported (Porter, 2004, unpublished report). There are a number of unconfirmed reports of dermatitis occurring in bushmen clearing kanuka scrub and also reported following aromatherapy.

Photosensitisation

None reported.

Bioactivities

See also tea tree oil monograph.

Pharmacological activities *in vitro* and *in vivo*

Smooth muscle   Manuka had a spasmolytic action on the electrically stimulated guinea-pig ileum *in vitro* (Lis-Balchin and Hart, 2000; Lis-Balchin *et al.*, 2000; see tea tree oil monograph, Table 2), while kanuka and *Melaleuca* had an initial spasmogenic action. α-Terpineol and terpinen-4-ol produced a substantial spasmolytic action, while α-terpinene, β-pinene and (−)α-pinene produced an initial contraction followed by spasmolysis at the same concentration; the (+)α-pinene enantiomer produced only a spasmogenic response. 1,8-Cineole produced a rise in tone of the electrically induced contractions.

Uterus   Manuka essential oil caused a decrease in the spontaneous contractions of rat uterus (Lis-Balchin and Hart, 2000; Lis-Balchin *et al.*, 2000; see tea tree oil monograph, Table 3).

Skeletal muscle   Manuka produced a decrease in tension, in contrast to the increase in tone or contracture shown by α- and β-pinene and also *p*-cymene (see tea tree oil monograph, Table 4;

Lis-Balchin and Hart, 2000; Lis-Balchin et al., 2000). The action of manuka was almost identical to that of *Melaleuca*, showing both a decrease in tension (through an inhibition of the twitch response to nerve stimulation) and a delayed but very profound increase in resting tone which signifies contracture whether the muscle was stimulated directly or via the phrenic nerve. The same actions were shown by clary sage, dill, fennel, frankincense and nutmeg, all of which, except clary sage, are very strongly spasmogenic on smooth muscle (Lis-Balchin and Hart, 1997). There was a difference in the effects of manuka in the two muscle tissues and indicated a rather less relaxing effect on skeletal muscle than that obviously wanted through aromatherapeutic massage: the effect of manuka on muscle fatigue or muscle cramp could thus be very detrimental. See also tea tree oil monograph.

Antimicrobial activities

See also tea tree oil monograph.

Antibacterial activity

Relative data: Effects were noted on 11–15/25 different bacteria and 0–20/20 *Listeria monocytogenes* varieties (Lis-Balchin et al., 2000; see also tea tree oil monograph, Table 1). Both tea tree and manuka oil had significant antibacterial effects on various strains of antibiotic-resistant *Staphylococcus* species (Harkenthal et al., 1999). Tests at a commercial laboratory also provided positive unpublished data on the antimicrobial effects of manuka (Cooke and Cooke, 1991).

The β-triketones can be removed from manuka oil as an almost pure extract that has much less aroma than the whole oil. Repeated tests *in vitro* show that this lowered aroma extract retains the strong, selective activity, but that the remaining part of the oil – largely sesquiterpenes – has little or no measurable antibacterial activity. The majority of manuka in New Zealand does not contain significant, measurable (<2%) levels of β-triketones and gives oil with comparatively non-selective and little antimicrobial activity. While the basic oil composition is determined genetically, it may change in individual plants within and between seasons. The β-triketone-rich manuka from East Cape can be recognised as a chemotype, but there seems to be a continuum of variation of oil composition involving both monoterpenes and sesquiterpenes in the area. Such chemical variation is reflected in the antimicrobial activity and it is therefore not

possible to generalise about the chemistry or activity of manuka oils (Porter and Wilkins, 1998; Porter et al., 1999; see also tea tree oil monograph).

Note: Australian tea tree oil is effective against a wide range of microorganisms, but comparatively high concentrations are required – typically 0.25–2% in current medical laboratory tests. Manuka oils with β-triketones are effective against a smaller range of microorganisms. However, this selective activity is particularly strong against some dermatophytic fungi and against Gram-positive bacteria – typically 0.02–0.1%. β-Triketone-rich oils and concentrates of the β-triketones have been shown to be just as effective in *in vitro* tests against antibiotic-resistant strains of bacteria as against the susceptible strains (Porter and Wilkins, 1998; Porter et al., 1999; Porter, 2004, unpublished report).

Antifungal activity

Relative data (% inhibition): *Aspergillus niger* 64–68%, *A.ochraceus* 49–87%, *Fusarium culmorum* 25–57% (Lis-Balchin and Hart, 2000; Lis-Balchin et al., 2000). Manuka displayed a stronger antifungal effect than kanuka, but was not as potent as *Melaleuca* essential oil (Lis-Balchin et al., 2000; see tea tree oil monograph, Table 5).

Antioxidant activity

There was a strong antioxidant effect for the two samples assessed (Lis-Balchin et al., 2000; see tea tree oil monograph, Table 6).

Use in pregnancy and lactation: contraindications

As there are no studies on the effect of the manuka essential oil on the uterus other than the *in vitro* studies in rat, which showed a decrease in the spontaneous contractions, and this essential oil has also not been properly assessed toxicologically, it cannot be recommended for aromatherapeutic use in pregnancy, parturition or during lactation.

Pharmaceutical guidance

Although there is scant evidence that manuka (*Leptospermum scoparium*) and kanuka (*Kunzea ericoides*) have such potential (Cooke and Cooke, 1994; Lis-Balchin et al., 1996a; 1998b), the essential oils are said to have remarkable powers of healing, based on folk medicinal usage (Brooker et al., 1987), and are being used by some aromatherapists even though there have been no safety/toxicological evaluations performed on them. There are also virtually no studies on the pharmacological effects of this 'tea tree' oil, except for Lis-Balchin *et al.* (1996a) and Lis-Balchin and Hart (1998) and therefore it cannot be recommended for aromatherapy massage. The unpleasant odour of the essential oil does not recommend its usage as a fragrance.

Note: See also pharmaceutical guidance in the tea tree oil monograph.

Use in babies and young children

Due to the immaturity and the delicate nature of the skin of babies and young children, it is inadvisable for any essential oils to be used in massage, however much the essential oil has been diluted in the carrier oils. This is also a necessary precaution due to the possibilities of sensitisation of the children at this young age through skin or air-borne odorant effects (see Chapters 5 and 7).

Instillation or administration of essential oils near the baby or young child's nose is not only not recommended, but distinctly inadvisable, as there have been numerous cases reported of severe toxicity and even death from such applications (see Chapter 7).

Marjoram Oil

CAS numbers

Sweet marjoram oil: USA: 8015-01-8; EINECS: 84082-58-6
Spanish marjoram oil: USA: 8016-33-9; EINECS: 84837-14-9
Origanum: USA: 8007-11-2; EINECS: 90131-59-2

Species/Botanical name

Origanum marjorana L. (Labiatae)

Synonyms

Majorana hortensis Moench, sweet marjoram, French marjoram

Other species

Thymus capitatus L., *Origanum virens* L., *Origanum vulgare* L. (wild oregano), *Thymus mastichina* L. (Spanish marjoram)

Safety

CHIP details

Sweet marjoram oil: Xn; R10, 65; 20%; S62 (A26)
Spanish marjoram oil: Xn; R10, 65; 97%; S62 (A26)
Origanum: Xn; R10, 21/22; 25%; S36/37, 62 (A26)

RIFM recommended safety of use limits

Origanum marjorana: 4% (A23)

EU sensitiser total

French sweet: 1 (based on geraniol 0.15%, limonene 1.8% and linalool 12%)
Spanish: 4.2 (based on limonene 1.7% and linalool 2.5%) (A27)

GRAS status

Granted (Fenaroli, 1997).

Extraction, source, appearance and odour

Extraction

A volatile oil is obtained by steam distillation of the tops of the herb: sweet from *Origanum marjorana* and Spanish from *Thymus capitatus*, etc. (Arctander, 1960).

Source

France, Spain, Egypt and Turkey.

Appearance and odour

Sweet: Yellow to yellow-green essential oil with warm, spicy, aromatic-camphoraceous and woody odour, reminiscent of nutmeg and cardamom (Arctander, 1960).
Spanish: Orange to amber essential oil with a strong, fresh, sweet-spicy, aromatic, eucalyptus-like, camphoraceous odour. The quality is very variable (Arctander, 1960).

Aromatherapy uses

No aromatherapy uses are given for the French and Spanish oregano essential oils (Lawless, 1992). Sweet marjoram is used for bruises, period problems, agitation, anxiety, depression, epilepsy, migraine headache and insomnia, neuralgia, sciatica, nervous exhaustion, arthritis, cramp, high blood pressure, palpitations, constipation, flatulence, gastritis; eczema, abcesses, boils, bronchitis, colic, diarrhoea, psoriasis, mycosis, rheumatic conditions (poultice also), lumbago, sciatica, shingles, pneumonia, stings and bites (Ryman, 1991; Rose, 1992a,b; Price, 1993; Sheppard-Hanger, 1995).

Scientific comment

Although oregano essential oil is a very potent antimicrobial, its irritant qualities do not make it acceptable for use on the skin in massage. Although used as a herb, there has been no direct scientific evidence that any of the claims for oregano essential oil are proven. There is also the problem of the variation of the oregano essential oils available on the market, which makes it even more difficult to judge their effectiveness, if any.

Herbal uses

Note: Most of the data are for whole herbal extracts. Marjoram leaf and flower, *Origanum marjorana*, syn. *Majorana hortensis* is an 'Approved Herb' (Blumenthal *et al.*, 2000) but there are no applications as a result of evaluation. Claimed uses with negative evaluation include: rhinitis and cold in infants; rhinitis in toddlers. Marjoram and marjoram oil, in combination with other herbs, are used for: appetite, digestion, strengthening of the stomach, acute and chronic gastritis, as an antispasmodic, flatulence, colic-like nervous gastrointestinal disorders, intestinal activity, supportive for acute inflammatory liver diseases, regulation of diseases involving gallstones, dry irritating coughs, swellings of the nasal and pharyngeal mucosa, inflammation of the ears, headaches, lowering the blood sugar in diabetics, promotion of milk secretion, tonic for nerves, heart and circulation system; promotion of healthy sleep, mood swings, blood builder, anorexia, sprains, bruises, lumbago, astringent, dysmenorrhoea, menstrual disturbances, urogenital bleeding and as a diuretic (Wren, 1988; Chevallier, 1996; Blumenthal *et al.*, 2000; Barnes *et al.*, 2002).

Food and perfumery uses

Food   Sweet marjoram oil (FEMA 2663) is used in a large number of foods and beverages (Fenaroli, 1997).

Perfumery   Sweet marjoram is used for its fresh, medicinal-aromatic warmth in perfumery especially in fougeres, chypres, colognes and oriental bases (Arctander, 1960).

Chemistry

Major components

	% *(Lawrence, 1976–2001)*	
	French	*Spanish*
1,8-Cineole	0–58	50–62
Linalool	4–12	trace–2.5
α-Terpinene	0	1–4
γ-Terpinene	3–17	trace–0.5
Terpinolene	14–19	10–20
α-Terpineol	2–6	2–4
Terpinen-4-ol	0–30	0
β-Caryophyllene	0–2	0–2
Limonene	trace–1.8	trace–1.7
Geraniol	trace–0.15	0

There is a wide variation in marjoram essential oils, due to the different species and instability of the genera, giving rise to numerous chemotypes. Similarities exist between these oils and ajowan, savory and thyme. Oregano imported into the USA was found to be derived from 16 plant genera and more than 40 plant species; hence oregano is described as a flavour and aroma rather than an individual plant and is usually a blend of plants. The European type of oregano comes mainly from subspecies of *O. vulgare* L. including ssp. *hirtum* (Link) Ietswaart, ssp. *virens* (Hoffmanns Link) Ietswaart and ssp. *viride* (Boiss.) Hayek (Tucker, 1989).

In contrast, Mexican oregano, also called Mexican sage, is principally gathered from the small Mexican shrub *Lippia graveolens* H.B.K. (Simon *et al.*, 1984), although leaves from other species are collected.

The essential oil of European oregano is often composed mainly of carvacrol and thymol. The proportions of each can be very variable and many chemotypes are available.

Wild marjoram contains carvacrol, often in high concentrations: it resembles the thymes rather than sweet marjoram or even Spanish marjoram.

Adulteration

Many different essential oils are used to adulterate the marjoram essential oils: tea tree, ajowan, savory, origanum or thyme oils. Synthetic components are also used (A8; see Chapter 4).

Toxicity

Acute toxicity (A22)

Oral LD$_{50}$ Sweet: 2.2 g/kg (rat); Spanish: > 5 g/kg (rat).

Dermal LD$_{50}$ Sweet: >5 g/kg (rabbit); Spanish: >5 g/kg (rabbit).

Irritation and sensitisation (A22)

Nil at 6% (human) for sweet. Undiluted oregano oil was severely irritating to mouse skin and moderately on rabbit skin. However all the essential oils are likely to damage mucous membranes at concentrations higher than 1% (Tisserand and Balacs, 1995).

Phototoxicity

Nil for Spanish; sweet untested.

Bioactivities

Pharmacological activities *in vitro* and *in vivo*

Smooth muscle Both sweet and Spanish oils had a spasmolytic effect on electrically stimulated smooth muscle guinea-pig ileum *in vitro* (A2; Lis-Balchin *et al.*, 1996a).

Uterus There was a decrease in the spontaneous contractions in the rat for both oils, and some of their components; mixing several other essential oils with marjoram oils also had a relaxant effect (A3; A4; Lis-Balchin and Hart, 1997b).

Other activities The highest doses of origanum essential oils (also chamomile, cinnamon, absinthium and mace) are depressive to rats, while the lowest doses have weak or doubtful effects, suggesting that origanum might have action on the CNS (Fundaro and Cassone, 1980).

A folk remedy for diabetes, *O. onites* oil, reduced streptozotocin-induced tissue injury without affecting blood glucose levels in rats (Lermioglu *et al.*, 1997).

Antimicrobial activities

Antibacterial activity
Different types of commercial marjoram oils and samples gave different results: Relative data: Sweet showed an effect against 15–20/25 different bacterial species and 15–20/20 *Listeria monocytogenes* varieties, while Spanish was effective against 23/25 bacteria and 20/20 *Listeria monocytogenes* (A1; Lis-Balchin and Deans, 1997; Lis-Balchin *et al.*, 1998a). Oregano and bay essential oils inhibited all organisms studied at concentrations below 2% v/v (Hammer *et al.*, 1999a). Both sweet and Spanish oregano greatly inhibited 5/5 bacteria (Friedman *et al.*, 2002).

Antifungal activity
Relative data (% inhibition) (A1):

	Sweet	*Spanish*
Aspergillus niger	55–84	16–41
A. ochraceus	66–79	8–67
Fusarium culmorum	27–46	26–39

Note: These were low values, but commercial samples were used.

Good antifungal activity was reported for *Origanum* and *Ocimum* (Afifi *et al.*, 1997). Eight yeasts were more sensitive to essential oils (allspice, cinnamon, clove, garlic, onion, oregano, savory and thyme) after sublethal heat stress (Conner and Beuchat, 1984). Nine food-borne fungi were inhibited better by oregano than by salt, thymol or carvacrol (Akgul and Kivanc, 1988).

Antioxidant activity
There was considerable antioxidant effect in 3/4 commercial samples (Dorman *et al.*, 1995b; Lis-Balchin *et al.*, 1996a). Dietary oregano essential oil had a positive effect on lipid peroxidation in chicken meat (Botsoglou *et al.*, 2002).

Use in pregnancy and lactation: contraindications

There was a loss of spontaneous contractions in the rat uterus when the essential oil was applied *in vitro*, suggesting a possible adverse effect during pregnancy and parturition, and as no clinical studies are available, caution should be paramount and the essential oils should not be used on the skin during these periods. The irritant nature of the essential oils containing thymol also excludes them from dermal application. Use as a fragrance does not appear to be disallowed as the essential oils are widely used in cooking.

Pharmaceutical guidance

There are too many different commercial marjoram oils on the market to be able to judge the effectiveness or the dangers. Sweet marjoram has a sensitisation potential which is higher than that of the Spanish oil; all the marjorams have some irritancy potential on the skin, and are likely to damage mucous membranes at concentrations higher than 1%. They should not be used at all on hypersensitive, diseased or damaged skin. Since the effectiveness for the claimed applications is not sufficiently documented, therapeutic administration of marjoram oil cannot be recommended in aromatherapy massage. However, marjoram oil can be used as a fragrance, alone or in conjunction with massage.

Use in babies and young children

Due to the immaturity and the delicate nature of the skin of babies and young children, it is inadvisable for any essential oils, especially with an irritant potential, to be used in massage, however much the essential oil has been diluted in the carrier oils. This is also a necessary precaution due to the possibilities of sensitisation of the children at this young age through skin or air-borne odorant effects (see Chapters 5 and 7).

Instillation or administration of essential oils near the baby or young child's nose is not only not recommended, but distinctly inadvisable, as there have been numerous cases reported of severe toxicity and even death from such applications (see Chapter 7).

Myrrh Oil

CAS numbers

USA: 8016-37-3; EINECS: 9000-45-7

Species/Botanical name

Commiphora myrrha var. *molmol* Engl. (Burseraceae)

Synonyms

Commiphora myrrha (Nees) Engl., Somalian or African myrrh. Somali: didin (tree), molmol (resin). Gum myrrh, myrrha

Pharmacopoeias

In European Pharmacopoeia and United States Pharmacopeia. Myrrh (Ph. Eur. 4.8) is a gum-resin, hardened in air, obtained from the stem and branches of *Commiphora molmol* and/or other species of *Commiphora*. Myrrh (USP 27) is an oleo-gum-resin obtained from the stems and branches of *Commiphora molmol* and other related species of *Commiphora* (Burseraceae) other than *C. mukul* (Martindale, 2004).

Other species

Commiphora abyssinica (Berg) Engl. (Arabian myrrh, Yemen myrrh). Other *Commiphora* species include balsamodendron myrrha.

Safety

CHIP details
Xn; R22, 65; 70%; S62 (A26)

RIFM recommended safety of use limits
Absolute: 3%; essential oil: 8% (A23)

EU sensitiser total
0 (A27)

GRAS status
Granted (Fenaroli, 1997).

Extraction, source, appearance and odour

Extraction
An oleo-gum-resin, obtained from the cuts in the stems of *Commiphora molmol*, etc. (Burseraceae) is either extracted into a solvent (tincture, usually in ethanol) or an absolute, or steam distilled to give an essential oil of a different composition. The solvent extractions are often sold as myrrh oil (Arctander, 1960).

Source
Arabia, Yemen and Somalia.

Appearance and odour
The oil is a pale yellow, pale orange, light-brown to green essential oil with a peppery, warm-spicy, pungent, sharp-balsamic odour; slightly medicinal, with a delightful lift free from terebinthinate notes. The sweetness increases to deep, warm-spicy and aromatic dry-out; the oil thickens and darkens on exposure to air and light (Arctander, 1960).

Myrrh absolute is too thick to pour and a solvent like DEP is added at 25–75% volume. The real absolute is a dark reddish-brown or orangey, viscous mass (Arctander, 1960).

Aromatherapy uses

Uses include: eczema, bruises, infection, athlete's foot, difficult-to-heal wounds; swelling; increasing the production of white blood cells; varicose veins, chapped, cracked, aged skin, thrush, herpes blisters; dry hair; mouth and gum diseases (in gargles, mouthwash and toothpaste); activating the immune system: coughs, colds, flu; regulating an overactive thyroid; increasing menstrual flow; aphrodisiac (Ryman, 1991; Lawless, 1992; Rose, 1992a,b; Price, 1993; Sheppard-Hanger, 1995).

Scientific comment
The gum and resin components and more water-soluble fractions of myrrh have anti-inflammatory, antipyretic, lipid-lowering activities in both animals

and humans. But, there is a lack of scientific data to prove that the essential oil alleviates any of the conditions mentioned above; massage itself is beneficial for many stress conditions and the fragrance, both of the essential oil and the burnt resin could be relaxing and safe in small doses.

Herbal uses

Topical treatment of mild inflammations of the oral and pharyngeal mucosa is advised (Blumenthal *et al.*, 2000): Myrrh is said to have antimicrobial, astringent, carminative, expectorant, anticatarrhal, antiseptic and vulnerary properties. Traditionally, it has been used for aphthous ulcers, pharyngitis, respiratory catarrh, common cold, furunculosis, wounds and abrasions, and specifically for mouth ulcers, gingivitis and pharyngitis (Wren, 1988; Chevallier, 1996; Barnes *et al.*, 2002).

Conventional uses

Pharmacopoieas: Myrrh is astringent to mucous membranes and the tincture is used in mouthwashes and gargles for inflammatory disorders of the mouth and pharynx; also used internally as a carminative and hypocholesterolaemic (Martindale, 1992, 2004). Myrrh tincture (BPC 1973) 2.5–5.0 mL in a glass of water several times daily is used as a gargle or a mouthwash. Pharmacopoeial preparations include myrrh topical solution (USP 27).

Food and perfumery uses

Food Myrrh oil (FEMA 2766) is used in many foods and beverages (Fenaroli, 1997).

Perfumery It is used in heavy floral and oriental perfumes as well as in forest and moss-like perfumes (Arctander, 1960).

Chemistry

Major components

	% (Lawrence, 1976–2001)
Curzerene	12
Furanoeudesma-1,3-diene	13
Curzerenone	12
Lindestrene	4

Most of the components are sesquiterpenes.

Minor components

Furanodiene, 2-methoxyfuranodiene and 4,5-dihydrofuranodiene-6-one and many monoterpenoids in trace to small amounts.

Adulteration

Opoponax and different commiphora species are often used as or with myrrh oil. Extracts are sometimes decolourised and sold as the essential oil (A8; see Chapter 4).

Toxicity

Acute toxicity (A22)

Oral LD$_{50}$ 1.7 g/kg (rat).

Dermal LD$_{50}$ Untested.

Irritation and sensitisation (A22)

Nil at 8% for essential oil and absolute; cross-sensitisation reported.

Phototoxicity

Untested.

Other toxicities

No side-effects were reported for either *C. molmol* or *C. abyssinica* but hiccup, diarrhoea, restlessness and apprehension were reported for guggulipid in humans (Barnes *et al.*, 2002). Myrrh is generally non-irritating, non-sensitising and non-phototoxic to human and animal skins (Leung, 1980). Myrrh may interfere with existing antidiabetic therapy, as hypoglycaemic properties have been documented.

Bioactivities

Pharmacological activities *in vitro* and *in vivo*

Smooth muscle Myrrh oil had a spasmolytic effect on electrically stimulated smooth muscle of the guinea-pig *in vitro* (A2; Lis-Balchin *et al.*, 1996a).

Uterus There was a decrease in the spontaneous contractions in the rat when myrrh oil was introduced; mixing several other essential oils with myrrh oil also had a relaxant effect (A3; A4; Lis-Balchin and Hart, 1997b).

Other activities There have been virtually no studies of myrrh essential oil effects and the various activities are due to various myrrh fractions, often water-soluble (Barnes *et al.*, 2002). Examples include: anti-inflammatory (carrageenan-induced inflammation and cotton pellet granuloma) and antipyretic activities in mice shown by some extracts of *C. molmol*; also hypoglycaemic activity in both normal and diabetic rats for a myrrh extract. Myrrh has astringent properties on mucous membranes (Martindale, 1989). An aqueous suspension of myrrh given to rats orally gave significant and dose-dependent protection to gastric mucosa against various ulcerogenic agents and a reduction in the tumour in mice with Ehrlich solid tumours; powdered myrrh had significant analgesic activity on mice in the hot-plate test; fura-noeudesma-1,3-dione (orally) was significantly more effective than control in the mouse writhing test; thyroid stimulation and lipid lowering properties have been shown for the related species, *Commiphora mukul* (Barnes *et al.*, 2002).

Antimicrobial activities

Both antibacterial and antifungal effects were very low.

Antibacterial activity
A slight effect was noted against 6/25 different bacterial species and 6/20 *Listeria monocytogenes* varieties (A1; Lis-Balchin and Deans, 1997; Lis-Balchin *et al.*, 1998a). Myrrh gum had moderate activity against 5/5 bacteria (Friedman *et al.*, 2002).

Antifungal activity (A1)
Aspergillus niger 0% inhibition; *A. ochraceus* 21%; *Fusarium culmorum* 4%. In another study 13/15 fungi were slightly affected (Maruzella and Liguori, 1958).

Antioxidant activity
No antioxidant properties were found (Lis-Balchin *et al.*, 1996a).

Clinical studies

Well-designed clinical studies of myrrh are lacking. Guggulipid has been reported to lower the concentration of total serum lipids, serum cholesterol, serum triglycerides, serum phospholipids and β-lipoproteins in 20 patients (Malhotra and Ahuja, 1971). The effect was comparable to that of two other known lipid-lowering drugs used in the study.

Two cases of therapy with frankincense and myrrh in children were described and myrrh has found recent pharmacological application in the reduction of cholesterol and triglycerides (Michie and Cooper, 1991).

Use in pregnancy and lactation: contraindications

Myrrh is said to affect the menstrual cycle (Leung, 1980) and the safety of myrrh taken during pregnancy has not been established, but there was a decrease in the spontaneous contractions in the rat uterus *in vitro* which suggests caution during pregnancy and parturition, especially in massage. Myrrh essential oil has a different odour to that of burnt myrrh resin, but both have a relaxant effect, which could be of benefit in small doses.

Pharmaceutical guidance

The gum and resin components and more water-soluble fractions of myrrh have anti-inflammatory, antipyretic, lipid-lowering activities possibly via a stimulant action on the thyroid gland as shown for *C. mukul* in both animals and humans. But, there is a lack of sufficient toxicity data and bioactivity data for the essential oil, therefore excessive use of myrrh should be avoided in massage, though the fragrance, both of the essential oil and the burnt resin, could be relaxing and safe in small doses.

Use in babies and young children

Due to the immaturity and the delicate nature of the skin of babies and young children, it is inadvisable for any essential oils to be used in massage, however much the essential oil has been diluted in the carrier oils. This is also a necessary precaution due to the possibilities of sensitisation of the children at this young age through skin or air-borne odorant effects (see Chapters 5 and 7).

Instillation or administration of essential oils near the baby or young child's nose is not only not recommended, but distinctly inadvisable, as there have been numerous cases reported of severe toxicity and even death from such applications (see Chapter 7).

Myrtle Oil

CAS numbers

USA: 8008-46-6; EINECS: 84082-67-7 (282-012-8)

Species/Botanical name

Myrtus communis (Myrtaceae)

Synonyms

Corsican pepper

Safety

CHIP details
Xn; R10, 65; 50%; S62 (A26)

RIFM recommended safety of use limits
4% (A23)

EU sensitiser total
16 (based on coumarin 0.2%, eugenol 0.7%, geraniol 0.8%, citronellol 0.3%, limonene 12% and linalool 2%) (A27)

Extraction, source, appearance and odour

Extraction
A volatile oil obtained from steam distillation of the leaves and twigs of the tree (Arctander, 1960).

Source
Mediterranean countries, especially Morocco and Spain, also Albania.

Appearance and odour
A pale yellow to orange-yellow or amber-coloured essential oil with a strong camphoraceous-spicy, even emerald-green, sweet-herbaceous and fresh odour. It has a top-note quality useful in perfumes and foods (Arctander, 1960).

Aromatherapy uses

Uses include: acne, haemorrhoids, open pores; asthma, pharyngitis, bronchitis, catarrh, coughs, tuberculosis; flu, infectious diseases. Myrtle essential oil is helpful in meditation and mood revitalising (Ryman, 1991; Rose, 1992a,b; Lawless, 1992; Sheppard-Hanger, 1995).

Scientific comment
There is scant data for the bioactivity of myrtle essential oil, although it has been used extensively in herbal medicine. The essential oil is not used in food and there are virtually no bioactivity data other than *in vitro* work on the smooth muscle of the guinea-pig, where there was an initial spasmogenic action followed by spasmolysis, a decrease in the contractions of the uterus in the rat. Massage alone can alleviate many stress conditions and there is no scientific evidence that myrtle essential oil will aid any of the conditions listed above.

Herbal uses

Myrtle was used in the wreaths of the Grecian and Roman victors in the Olympian and other festivities. Scriptural allusions to it are abundant, and to the Jews it was a token of peace and used in bridal decorations. According to Mohammedan tradition it was among the pure things carried by Adam from the Garden of Eden. The oil and the alcoholic solution possess anodyne properties. The powder has been applied to uterine ulcerations, suppurative wounds and ulcers and eczema. Offensive discharges and threatened gangrene were treated with a wine of myrtle. An infusion of the leaves or the tincture, diluted, has given excellent results when used as an injection in uterine prolapse, lax vaginal walls and leucorrhoea, and also dysentery. An infusion was valuable as a topical agent in catarrhal conjunctivitis, pharyngitis and bronchitis and haemorrhoids. The oil stimulates the gastric, renal and pulmonic membranes, increasing their functions. It is a soothing agent, astringent, skin conditioner, muscle relaxant; used for urinary infections as a substitute for buchu (Felter and Lloyd, 1898; Wren, 1988; Chevallier, 1996).

Food and perfumery uses

Food No FEMA.

Perfumery Myrtle blends well with: bergamot, cardamon, coriander, lavender, lemon, lemongrass, rosemary, spearmint, thyme and tea tree (Arctander, 1960).

Chemistry

Major components

	% (Lawrence, 1976–2001)
α-Pinene	8–26
1,8-Cineole	15–34
Geraniol	trace–0.5
Linalool	0.5–10
Myrtenol	0.5–1.6
Myrtenyl acetate	16–36
Geranyl acetate	1.7–2.9
Methyl eugenol	0.7–2.3
Eugenol	trace–0.3

Minor components

Many monoterpenes and sesquiterpenes.

Adulteration

Essential oils of different countries are often pooled together (A8; see also Chapter 4).

Toxicity

Acute toxicity (A22)

Oral LD$_{50}$ >5 g/kg (rat).

Dermal LD$_{50}$ >10 g/kg (rabbit).

Phototoxicity

Nil found.

Bioactivities

Pharmacological activities *in vitro* and *in vivo*

Smooth muscle Myrtle essential oil had an initial strong spasmogenic action followed by a spasmolytic action on electrically stimulated smooth muscle of the guinea-pig *in vitro* (A2; Lis-Balchin et al., 1996a).

Uterus There was a decrease in the spontaneous contractions in the rat for myrtle essential oil (A3; A4; Lis-Balchin and Hart, 1997b).

Antimicrobial activities

Antibacterial activity

Relative data: Myrtle oil showed activity against 22/25 different bacterial species and 17/20 *Listeria monocytogenes* varieties (A1; Lis-Balchin and Deans, 1997; Lis-Balchin et al., 1998a).

Antifungal activity

Relative data: Very poor antifungal activity was shown (A1): *Aspergillus niger* 10% inhibition, *A. ochraceus* 3%, *Fusarium culmorum* 15%.

Use in pregnancy and lactation: contraindications

There are scant data for the bioactivity of myrtle essential oil and it is not used in food. There are no safety data for use during pregnancy other than *in vitro* work in the rat, where there was a decrease in the contractions of the uterus. The essential oil cannot therefore be recommended for use during pregnancy, parturition and lactation.

Pharmaceutical guidance

Myrtle essential oil has not been studied in any depth and there is no scientific evidence that the essential oil can alleviate any condition when massaged into the skin, although the herb has been used extensively in herbal medicine. Avoidance of myrtle essential oil in cases of cancer has been advised (Tisserand and Balacs, 1995). There are many other essential oils which could be used for many of the ailments listed, and even massage alone could be of benefit; therefore myrtle essential oil is not recommended in aromatherapy.

Use in babies and young children

Due to the immaturity and the delicate nature of the skin of babies and young children, it is inadvisable for any essential oils to be used in massage, however much the essential oil has been diluted in the carrier oils. This is also a necessary precaution due to the possibilities of sensitisation of the children at this young age through skin or air-borne odorant effects (see Chapters 5 and 7).

Instillation or administration of essential oils near the baby or young child's nose is not only not recommended, but distinctly inadvisable, as there have been numerous cases reported of severe toxicity and even death from such applications (see Chapter 7).

Neroli Oil

CAS numbers

USA: 8016-38-4; EINECS: 72968-50-4

Species/Botanical name

Citrus aurantium L. (Rutaceae), *C. bigaradia* L.

Synonyms

Oleum aurantii florum (USP), *Citrus aurantium* L. subsp. *amara* L., aurantii amari floris aetheroleum, bitter-orange flower oil, esencia de azahar, essência de flor de laranjeira, oleum neroli, orange flower oil

Pharmacopoeias

In European Pharmacopoeia.

Safety

CHIP details
Xn; R10, 65; 40%; S62 (A26)

RIFM recommended safety of use limits
4% essential oil; 3% absolute (A23)

EU sensitiser total
71.3 (based on citral 0.3%, geraniol 3.5%, farnesol 4%, limonene 18% and linalool 44%) (A27)

GRAS status
Granted (Fenaroli, 1997).

Extraction, source, appearance and odour

Extraction
A volatile oil obtained from steam-distilled flowers of *Citrus aurantium*. The essential oil obtained, neroli bigarade (0.1%), is often mixed with the solvent-extracted orange flower concrete (0.6%) from the orange flower water remaining after distillation (70%). From this, an orange flower absolute (0.3%) is obtained by extracting into alcohol. An orange flower concrete (0.2%) and orange flower absolute (0.1%) is also made from the flowers. Carbon dioxide extractions are also made (Arctander, 1960).

Source
France, Bulgaria, Morocco, Turkey, Italy and Tunisia.

Appearance and odour
A colourless to pale yellow, slightly fluorescent essential oil, becoming reddish-brown on exposure to air and light. It has a powerful, light, fresh, floral, sweet, faintly citrusy odour, with a peculiar sweet-terpeney top-note, but poor tenacity. Keeping qualities are very poor (Arctander, 1960).

The orange flower concrete and absolutes are orange-coloured.

Aromatherapy uses

Neroli is classified by aromatherapists as a hypnotic, aphrodisiac and a euphoric. Uses include: anxiety, depression, stress, hysteria, shock, insomnia; neuralgia, headaches, vertigo; premenstrual tension, menopausal symptoms; palpitations, constricted circulation, phlebitis, varicosities, haemorrhoids; bronchitis, pleurisy and pulmonary disease; chronic diarrhoea, colic, colitis, spasm, liver and pancreas; protecting and regenerating skin cells, improving elasticity, thread veins, scar tissue and stretch marks (Ryman, 1991; Lawless, 1992; Rose, 1992a,b; Price, 1993; Sheppard-Hanger, 1995).

Scientific comment

Neroli essential oil is both sedative (on the smooth muscle of the gut) and stimulant using contingent negative variation studies in human brain (A14). The odour is very pleasant for most people, therefore even if initially stimulating to the CNS, it may also subsequently relax the patient. The massaging of the essential oil/absolute on the skin is not recommended due to the inherent high sensitisation potential, but also due to the widespread adulteration which could introduce photosensitisers as well as sensitisers. It is unlikely that most of the conditions listed above are alleviated by aromatherapy with neroli; however, massage itself can prove of benefit in many of the stress-related and muscular conditions, and the added benefit of the fragrance used separately could be beneficial for some conditions.

Herbal uses

Neroli is considered to be sedative and used for palpitations, reducing heart rate, encouraging sleep, soothing the digestive tract. The distilled flower water is used as an antispasmodic and sedative. Orange flowers were used in bridal bouquets to calm the couple before going to the marriage bed (Lawless, 1992; Chevallier, 1996).

Food and perfumery uses

Food Neroli bigarade oil (FEMA 2771) is used in many different foods and beverages (Fenaroli, 1997).

Perfumery The essential oil and other extracts are used in fine perfumery, especially floral, citrus and oriental blends; it was used in the original eau de Cologne (Arctander, 1960).

Chemistry

Major components

	% (Lawrence, 1976–2001)	Essential oil sensitiser value
Limonene	trace	18
Linalool	24	44
Linalyl acetate	69	
Geraniol	6	3.5
Citral	trace–0.3	0.3
Farnesol	trace–4	4

Minor components

No coumarins and psoralens (bergaptenes) should be present, but see adulteration. Orange flower oil contains an odourless stearopten.

The concentrations of the main constituents of hydrodistilled and CO_2-extracted orange flower oil are compared below (BACIS, 1997):

	Hydrodistilled oil	CO₂ extract
Monoterpene hydrocarbon	38	28
Linalyl acetate	3–5	24
Linalool	38	35
Sesquiterpene alcohols	4	<2

The odour intensity of the CO_2-extracted bitter orange oil was twice that of the hydrodistilled oil because more odour-intense constituents are extracted with CO_2 and fewer compounds decompose during the extraction than in boiling water during hydrodistillation. Just the reverse was true for two rose oils with respect to the odour intensity, due to the fact that much (65%) of the less odour-intense 2-phenylethanol is dissolved in the distillate water and therefore was not present in the hydrodistilled oils (Ohloff, 1978, 1994).

Adulteration

There is seldom a decent neroli oil on the market due to the high cost of production and low yield. Most is either entirely petitgrain oil or this may be mixed in with some of its terpenoids and/or bitter orange oil, synthetic linalool, other citrus oil terpenes, distilled bitter orange/other citrus oils, sweet orange oil, synthetic limonene, linalyl acetate, phenylethylalcohol, decanal, nonanal, isojasmone, nerol, nerolidol, etc. (A8; see Chapter 4). To illustrate the point, on offer on the Internet was a neroli oil/absolute which consists of two-thirds distilled neroli blossom and one-third absolute neroli blossom (because, apparently, the neat absolute has a rather harsh off-note on its own, but it soften downs well in neroli oil to give a much more agreeable bouquet!). A neroli light was also on sale, which is recovered from water distillation and then sharpened up with other natural citrus distillates to give a very good approximation of neroli blossom essential oil, but at a much lower price.

Toxicity

Acute toxicity (A22)

Oral LD$_{50}$ >4.5 g/kg (rat).

Dermal LD$_{50}$ >5 g/kg (rabbit).

Irritation and sensitisation (A22)

Nil at 4% (human). Cutaneous irritation could be produced due to adulteration as reports have increased over the years for all citrus oils and sensitisation is very possible (see essential oil value of over 70% total sensitisers).

Estimated acceptable daily intake of methyl anthranilate (artificial neroli oil) is up to 1.5 mg/kg body weight and of methyl N-methylanthranilate is up to 200 µg (Martindale, 1992).

Phototoxicity

There is a slight chance of phototoxicity after skin massage with the oil followed by sunlight or UV light, if it has been adulterated with orange or other citrus extracts.

Bioactivities

Pharmacological activities *in vitro* and *in vivo*

Smooth muscle   Neroli oil (commercial sample of unknown purity) had a spasmolytic effect on electrically stimulated guinea-pig ileum *in vitro* (A2; Lis-Balchin *et al.*, 1996a).

Uterus   There was a decrease in the spontaneous contractions in the rat (A3; A4; Lis-Balchin and Hart, 1997b).

Other activities   Neroli bigarade oil (10 mg, as a 1:25 solution in olive oil) injected intramuscularly weekly had a slight effect on experimental tuberculosis of the guinea-pig, but it was combined with subeffective doses of dihydrostreptomycin. At 100 µg/mL it had no effect on the tubercle bacilli *in vitro* (A22). Neroli was found to reduce stress and systolic blood pressure in humans (when blood pressure was high) (Warren and Warrenburg, 1993). A sedative effect of neroli oil vapour on mice was noted, giving a 75% decrease in their movement (Jager *et al.*, 1992). A lesser effect was shown by citronellal and phenylethylacetate.

Antimicrobial activities

Antibacterial activity
Relative data: Neroli oil samples showed activity against 20–22/25 different bacterial species and 11–19/20 *Listeria monocytogenes* varieties (A1; Lis-Balchin and Deans, 1997; Lis-Balchin *et al.*, 1998a). Neroli oil was apparently 5.5 times more effective than phenol as a bactericide (Martindale, 1972). It was effective against 5/5 bacteria (Yousef and Tawil, 1980), and the vapour was effective against 1/5 bacteria (Maruzella and Sicurella, 1960).

Antifungal activity
Relative data (% inhibition): *Aspergillus niger* 95%; *A. ochraceus* 94%; *Fusarium culmorum* 74% (A1).

Moderate antifungal action was found against 13/15 fungi (Maruzella, 1960) and 11/12 phytopathogenic fungi (A22).

Use in pregnancy and lactation: contraindications

Due to the widespread adulteration, high sensitisation potential and lack of information on the effects of the neroli essential oil/absolute during pregnancy and parturition, except for *in vitro* studies in the rat which showed a decrease in the spontaneous contractions of the uterus, use in massage is not recommended. The fragrance could be used alone in small doses as a stimulant, as shown in human brain studies (A14), although some people find it relaxing.

Pharmaceutical guidance

The massaging of the essential oil/absolute on the skin is not recommended, due to the inherent high sensitisation potential, but also due to the widespread adulteration which could introduce photosensitisers as well as sensitisers. The massage could be used without the essential oil/absolute, but with the fragrance used separately to provide a pleasant and stimulating environment.

Use in babies and young children

Due to the immaturity and the delicate nature of the skin of babies and young children, it is inadvisable for any essential oils, especially this essential oil with high sensitisation potential, to be used in massage, however much the essential oil has been diluted in the carrier oils. This is also a necessary precaution due to the possibilities of sensitisation of the children at this young age through skin or air-borne odorant effects (see Chapters 5 and 7).

Instillation or administration of essential oils near the baby or young child's nose is not only not recommended, but distinctly inadvisable, as there have been numerous cases reported of severe toxicity and even death from such applications (see Chapter 7).

Nutmeg Oil

CAS numbers

USA: 8008-45-5; EINECS: 84082-68-8

Species/Botanical name

Myristica fragrans Houtt. (Myristicaceae)

Synonyms

East Indian nutmeg oil, West Indian nutmeg oil, *Myristica officinalis*, *M. aromata*, nux moschata, myristica oil, ätherisches muskatöl, esencia de nuez moscada, essência de moscada, essence de muscade, myristica oil, myristicae fragrantis aetheroleum, oleum myristicae

Pharmacopoeias

In European Pharmacopoeia.

Safety

CHIP details
Xn; R10, 65; 85%; S62 (A26)

RIFM recommended safety of use limits
2%; mace oil: 10% (A23)

EU sensitiser total
8.4 (based on eugenol 0.2%, isoeugenol 0.6%, citronellol 0.2%, limonene 7% and linalool 0.4%) (A27)

GRAS status
Granted (Fenaroli, 1997).

Extraction, source, appearance and odour

Extraction
The essential oil is obtained by steam or water distillation of the dried, worm-eaten nutmeg seeds (which are now devoid of protein, fat and carbohydrate). The dried, finger-like orange-brown arils or husks are distilled separately to give mace oil (rather rare). A solvent-extracted mace oleoresin is also produced in small quantities (Arctander, 1960).

Source
East and West Indies, Sri Lanka, Grenada and Indonesia.

Appearance and odour
A colourless to almost colourless or pale yellow essential oil or pale green, with a light fresh, warm-spicy and aromatic odour of nutmeg and a distinctly terpeney top-note and a rich, sweet-spicy, warm body-note. The undertone and dry-out is somewhat woody, but warm and sweet. There is apparently some similarity to sweet marjoram oil (Arctander, 1960).

Aromatherapy uses

Uses for nutmeg essential oil include: calming and relaxing; relieving pain; arthritis, gout, muscular aches, poor circulation; stimulating digestion, indigestion, nausea, flatulence; frigidity, impotence, neuralgia, nervous fatigue; labour pains; debility. A drop of essential oil, applied directly, helps toothache. It is an aphrodisiac and the oil for the Third Eye and helps develop psychic insight (Ryman, 1991; Lawless, 1992; Rose, 1992a,b; Price, 1993; Sheppard-Hanger, 1995).

Scientific comment

Nutmeg essential oil is relatively toxic due mainly to its myristicin content, which can have a profound effect on the CNS, and is also related to the carcinogen safrole. Nutmeg oil/grated seed can cause hallucinations and convulsions in large doses and produce narcotic effects comparable to alcohol intoxication. It is therefore inadvisable to use it for aromatherapy massage. However, massage alone can alleviate stress-related and muscle conditions and the use of nutmeg essential oil as a fragrance could help this.

Herbal uses

Nutmeg essential oil is carminative and rubefacient: it stimulates the digestive and circulatory systems; helps treat digestive tract infections, chronic diarrhoea, bad breath and flatulence and may be beneficial for the heart, menstrual regularity and brain activities; external application may be effective for treatment of rheumatism, sore muscles and lumbago. Nutmeg is favoured by the Chinese as an aphrodisiac. Although it smells spicy, it is a relaxing scent that lowers blood pressure and creates a euphoric feeling, which some describe as intoxicating; it also strengthens and stimulates. In eighteenth-century North America it was popular in nightcaps; in Edwardian England, men used to take a nutmeg to parties and grate it for sniffing, as with cocaine. It is also smoked and eaten as a substitute for marijuana because of its ability to elicit powerful psychedelic effects, thus linking it directly with the brain. It may be helpful when lack of energy, tiredness or depression are present. Nutmeg oil also influences dream activity, making dreams more intense and colourful (Wren, 1988; Rätsch, 1992; Chevallier, 1996).

Food and perfumery uses

Food Nutmeg oil (FEMA 2793) is used in many foods and beverages. Nutmeg masks many odours in the food industry, e.g. boiled cabbage (Fenaroli, 1997).

Perfumery It is used in spicy and masculine perfumes, blending well with lavandin, bay, orange, geranium, clary sage, rosemary, lime, petitgrain, mandarin and coriander (Arctander, 1960).

Conventional uses

Pharmacopoeial: Nutmeg oil and expressed nutmeg oil, a solid fat, are rubefacient (Martindale, 2004). Aromatic ammonia spirit (BP 2003).

Chemistry

Major components

	% (Lawrence, 1976–2001)
α-Pinene	10–27 (East Indian highest)
β-Pinene	7–18 (East Indian highest)
Sabinene	15–51 (West Indian highest)
Myrcene	2–4
Limonene	2–7
Linalool	trace–0.4
Citronellal	trace–0.2
Citronellol	trace–0.2
Eugenol	trace–0.2
1,8-Cineole	1–4
Terpinen-4-ol	2–18 (East Indian highest)
Myristicin	0.5–13.5 (East Indian highest)
Elemicin	0.3–5
Safrole	1–2.1 (East Indian highest)

Minor components

α-Terpineol, α-terpinene, α-phellandrene, *p*-cymene. Myristicin is normally lower in oil distilled from West Indian nutmegs and the recent study found only trace amounts in Jamaican nutmeg oil. Two types of nutmeg oil, West and East Indian, have different compositions in terms of concentration of each component, but due to intermixing, only the ranges are given. The East Indian nutmeg oil is preferred by perfumers to that of West Indian. Terpeneless oil is also produced.

Adulteration

Synthetic components such as pinenes, sabinene, etc. are added; also tea tree oil (A8; see Chapter 4).

Toxicity

Acute toxicity (A22)

Oral LD$_{50}$ 0.6–2.6 g/kg (rat); >5 g/kg (mice and hamsters).

Dermal LD$_{50}$ >10 g/kg (rabbit).

Irritation and sensitisation (A22)

Nil at 2% (human).

Phototoxicity

Untested.

Other toxicities

Nutmeg is toxic due mainly to its myristicin content, which is related to the carcinogen safrole. Nutmeg can cause hallucinations, visual impairments, delirium and prolonged sleep when used orally or via inhalation. It can act as either a stimulant or a depressant of the CNS. Overdosing can cause convulsions, vomiting and delirium.

Myristicin in monkeys caused ataxia and disorientation; also enhanced morphine-induced rage in cats (A22). Myristicin is apparently converted in the body to amphetamine (Buchanan, 1978) and has structural similarity with sympathomimetic amines. It may therefore compete for monoamine oxidase enzymes, thereby exhibiting a monoamine oxidase inhibitor (MAOI)-like action (Cootes, 1982). Several intoxications have been reported after an ingestion of approximately 5 g of nutmeg, corresponding to 1–2 mg myristicin/kg body weight.

Although these intoxications may be ascribed to the actions of myristicin, it is likely that other components of nutmeg may also be involved. The metabolism of myristicin resembles that of safrole (Hallstrom and Thuvander, 1997).

The acute toxicity of myristicin appears to be low. No toxic effects were observed in rats administered myristicin orally at a dose of 10 mg/kg while 6–7 mg/kg may be enough to cause psychopharmacological effects in humans. A weak DNA-binding capacity has been demonstrated, but there are no indications that myristicin exerts carcinogenic activity in short-term assays using mice. Intake estimations indicate that non-alcoholic drinks may be the most important single source of myristicin intake. Based on available data, it seems unlikely that the intake of myristicin from essential oils and spices in food, estimated to be a few milligrams per person and day in this report, would cause adverse effects in humans. It is, however, at present not possible to make a complete risk assessment, as studies regarding genotoxicity and chronic toxicity, including reproductive toxicity and carcinogenicity, are still lacking.

Safrole: In Europe, safrole is categorised as a category 2 carcinogen (i.e. carcinogenic to humans) under the 22nd Commission Directive para 1.7.2 of Labelling guide (annex VI to Commission Directive 93/21/EEC) as oils containing more than 0.1% safrole (i.e. nutmeg, brown camphor (*Cinnamomum camphora*) oil and ylang ylang oil) should all be classified and labelled as such. However this does not apply if safrole is not an impurity (but is a constituent). Similar restrictions apply in the USA. Safrole metabolism proceeds via formation of 1'-hydroxysafrole in rat and mouse liver from the hydroxylation of safrole via the microsomal P_{450} enzymes and has been indicated as the likely carcinogen. However, the major excretion product in humans is 4-allyl catechol and 1'-hydroxysafrole was not detected. 1'-Sulphooxysafrole is the major ultimate electrophilic and tumour-initiating metabolite of 1'-hydroxysafrole (Boberg et al., 1983).

Nutmeg oil may contain 0.1–2% safrole, and mace oil is broadly similar. The effects of safrole and myristicin in producing hepatic DNA adducts from cola drinking have raised concerns (Randerath et al., 1993).

Bioactivities

Pharmacological activities *in vitro* and *in vivo*

Smooth muscle Nutmeg oil had a spasmogenic effect on electrically stimulated smooth muscle of the guinea-pig *in vitro* (A2; Lis-Balchin et al., 1996a). Some of its components had a similar effect.

Uterus There was a decrease in the spontaneous contractions in the rat uterus when nutmeg oil, limonene and some of the other components were added. Mixing several other essential oils with nutmeg oil also had a relaxant effect (A3; A4; Lis-Balchin and Hart, 1997b).

Skeletal muscle There was a contracture and inhibition of the twitch response to nerve stimulation by nutmeg essential oil on the phrenic nerve–diaphragm preparation of the rat *in vitro* (Lis-Balchin and Hart, 1997c).

Other activities Nutmeg has been used as an inhaled expectorant with/without camphene (Boyd and Sheppard, 1970). Myristicin given to monkeys caused ataxia, disorientation and also morphine-induced rage in cats. Nutmeg is a constituent of Vicks VapoRub, an ointment used to relieve decongestion and muscle aches. This product has an association with recreational drug abuse, being used in conjunction with MDMA (methylenedioxymethamfetamine, ecstasy) by clubbers. Myristicin is thought to contribute to the hallucinogenic properties of the extracts.

Antimicrobial activities

Antibacterial activity

Relative data: Nutmeg oil had an effect on 18–19/25 different bacterial species and 0–12/20 *Listeria monocytogenes* varieties (A1; Lis-Balchin and Deans, 1997; Lis-Balchin et al., 1998a). It showed low activity against 5/5 bacteria (Friedman et al., 2002).

Antifungal activity

Relative data (% inhibition): *Aspergillus niger* 95%, *A. ochraceus* 94%, *Fusarium culmorum* 74% (A1).

Antioxidant activity

Nutmeg essential oil has antioxidant activity (Dorman et al., 1995 a,b).

Use in pregnancy and lactation: contraindications

One tablespoonful of grated nutmeg instead of one-eighth teaspoon in cookies resulted in acute anticholinergic hyperstimulation in a pregnant mother (Lavy, 1987). There was also a decrease in the spontaneous contractions in the rat uterus *in vitro*, therefore nutmeg essential oil is not recommended for use in pregnancy, parturition and also lactation due to its toxicity.

Pharmaceutical guidance

Nutmeg essential oil is relatively toxic due mainly to its myristicin content, which can have a profound effect on the CNS, and is also related to the carcinogen safrole. Nutmeg oil/grated seed can cause hallucinations and convulsions in large doses and produce narcotic effects comparable to alcohol intoxication. Nutmeg essential oil should be avoided by people with cancer (Tisserand and Balacs, 1995) and in aromatherapy altogether, according to Ryman (1992), but this is not generally indicated in aromatherapy books. The use of nutmeg as a food additive makes it acceptable for use as an odorant in small doses, although aromatherapy massage with the essential oil is not advised.

Use in babies and young children

Due to the immaturity and the delicate nature of the skin of babies and young children, it is inadvisable for any essential oils, especially in an essential oil containing a carcinogen, to be used in massage, however much the essential oil has been diluted in the carrier oils. This is also a necessary precaution due to the possibilities of sensitisation of the children at this young age through skin or air-borne odorant effects (see Chapters 5 and 7).

Instillation or administration of essential oils near the baby or young child's nose is not only not recommended, but distinctly inadvisable, as there have been numerous cases reported of severe toxicity and even death from such applications (see Chapter 7).

Orange Oil

CAS numbers

USA: 8028-48-6; EINECS: 8028-48-6

Species/Botanical name

Citrus sinensis (L.) Osbeck (Rutaceae)

Synonyms

Sweet orange, *C. aurantium* L. var. *sinensis* L./var. *dulcis* L., oleum aurantii corticis USP, orange oil BP

Other species

Citrus aurantium L. subsp. *amara* (bitter orange), *C. vulgaris* Risso, bigaradier, naranja amarga, pomeranze, Seville orange

Pharmacopoeias

In European, Japanese and Polish Pharmacopoeias.

Safety

CHIP details

Xn; R10, 65; 97%; S62 (A26)

RIFM recommended safety of use limits

Sweet orange: 10%; bitter orange: 8% (A23)

EU sensitiser total

95.5 (based on limonene 95% and linalool 0.4%) (A27)

GRAS status

Granted (Fenaroli, 1997).

Extraction, source, appearance and odour

Extraction

The 'essential oil' is obtained by cold expression from the fresh peel of either the bitter orange, *Citrus vulgaris* Risso, or the sweet orange, *Citrus aurantium* L. The peels can also be steam distilled to give an essential oil of a slightly different composition. Most of the orange oil is obtained as a by-product of the orange juice industry using various processes, including: the extraction with solvents of processed residual waters; the distillation of the concentrated orange juice which has collected significant amounts of the oil; the steam distillation of the pressed cakes of peel remaining after orange juice extraction; the steam distillation of peels after they have been expressed; and the steam distillation of virgin orange peels. All these methods yield different types of orange oil, but admixing yields a satisfactory produce (Arctander, 1960).

Sweet orange oil (Ph. Eur. 4.8) is an essential oil obtained without heating by suitable mechanical treatment from the fresh peel of the fruit of *Citrus sinensis* (*Citrus aurantium* var. *dulcis*). A suitable antioxidant may be added (Martindale, 2004).

Orange oil (USNF 22) contains not less than 1.2% w/v and not more than 2.5% of aldehydes, calculated as decanal ($C_{10}H_{20}O = 156.3$). It may be California-type or Florida-type orange oil (Martindale, 2004).

Terpeneless orange oil (oleum aurantii deterpenatum) is prepared by concentrating the orange oil until most of the terpenes are removed, or by solvent partition. Due to the presence of waxes, concentration is often limited to ×15. As the oil is concentrated it will contain mainly alcohols and aldehydes.

The sweet orange oil is more common (Arctander, 1960). It consists chiefly of the free alcohols (+)-linalol and (+)-terpineol and contains not less than 18% w/w of aldehydes calculated as decanal. It is soluble 1 in 1 of alcohol (90%) (Martindale, 2004).

Source

USA, Brazil, China, the West Indies and Spain.

Appearance and odour

Orange oil is deep yellow to orangey, olive-yellow and even brownish, if expressed, with citrus-like odour reminiscent of the species: fresh and yet bitter, dry-like with a rich and lasting sweet undertone (Arctander, 1960).

The distilled oils are colourless to pale yellow, fresh, sweet and have little odour compared with the expressed oils. They become rancid more quickly, so addition of an antioxidant is imperative as soon as it is produced (Arctander, 1960).

Aromatherapy uses

The distilled sweet orange essential oil or expressed essential oil has many uses including: rejuvenating the skin, eczema, dermatitis, after-sun wrinkles, oily skin; fatigue, menopause, oedema, palpitations, premenstrual tension, stress; obesity, mouth ulcers, colds, flu, bronchitis, dyspepsia, constipation, spasms. Bitter orange is advised for acne, wounds and vertigo and both oils for anxiety and insomnia; it is apparently a good oil for children's first aid kit and for the second chakra (Ryman, 1991; Lawless, 1992; Rose, 1992a,b; Price, 1993; Sheppard-Hanger, 1995).

Scientific comment

The oxidation of the high limonene content to produce sensitisers in a short time of storage and the added problem of phototoxicity, especially when using the expressed essential oil, makes the dermal application of the orange essential oil hazardous. The use of a distilled essential oil or a FCF (furanocoumarin-free) essential oil would greatly improve the chances against phototoxicity, but the problem of the sensitisation potential remains. It is likely that massage itself could alleviate many stress symptoms and the added benefit of the stimulating essential oil used as a fragrance could be of benefit.

Herbal uses

Orange oil is apparently an irritant, and is somewhat narcotic and those who prepare the oil are subject to mental confusion, muscular debility, neuralgia, headaches, disordered digestion, erythema, papules, and vesicles upon the skin (Felter and Lloyd, 1898). In Puerto Rico *Citrus aurantium* is used for sleep disorders, gastrointestinal disorders, respiratory ailments and raised blood pressure. The orange is said to be anti-inflammatory, antimicrobial, carminative, aromatic and stomachic. The juice is best known for its vitamin C content, which is not found in the essential oil. Orange essential oil is used to dissolve the glue when removing stoma bags (Martindale, 1972; Wren, 1988; Chevallier, 1996).

Conventional uses

Orange oil is used in various syrups and infusions, etc. Pharmacopoeial preparations with bitter orange include concentrated compound gentian infusion, concentrated orange peel infusion, orange peel infusion and orange syrup (BP 2003) and bitter-orange-epicarp and mesocarp tincture (Ph. Eur.). Preparations with sweet orange include orange syrup and sweet orange peel tincture (USNF 22). Terpeneless orange (sweet) is used in compound orange spirit (BP 2003).

Food and perfumery uses

Food   Sweet orange oil (FEMA 2825), distilled (FEMA 2821), terpeneless (FEMA 2822), bitter orange (FEMA 2345, 2923) are all used in many foods and beverages (Fenaroli, 1997).

Perfumery   Orange oil is used in many perfumes; it blends well with citrus oils, petitgrain, neroli and orange flower (Arctander, 1960).

Chemistry

Major components

	% (Lawrence, 1976–2001)	
	Sweet	*Bitter*
Limonene	94–98	73–98
Myrcene	1–4	1–11
α-Pinene	0.1–0.4	0.3–1.4
Sabinene	trace–2	0
Octanal	trace–0.2	0?
Decanal	0.1–2.5	0
1,8-Cineole	0	0.7–9

Minor components

Coumarins and psoralens (bergaptenes) are phototoxic. These are not found in distilled oils of FCF redistilled oils. The α- and β-sinensals contribute to the orange aroma, together with e.g. (+)-valencene and (−)-caryophyllene. Cold-pressed orange oil has a limonene content of about 95%, but the 10-fold oil has 80% and the 25-fold oil only 57%; in fact limonene can decrease to 0.2% on total deterpenation, raising other components to extremely high levels, e.g. linalool to 28% and decanal to 17% (Lawrence, 1976–2001).

Adulteration

Deterpenation, amongst other procedures, makes possible a very wide range of orange oil compositions. Adulteration persists by mixing in other citrus oil terpenes, distilled bitter orange/other citrus oils for the sweet orange oil, and addition of synthetic limonene. Terpeneless, sesquiterpeneless and concentrated bitter and sweet orange oils are blended in. Antioxidants such as butylhydroxy anisole (BHA), butylhydroxy toluene (BHT) are frequently added as oxidation occurs very rapidly and reduces shelf-life. Sweet orange is frequently used as a substitute for bergamot oil (A8; see Chapter 4).

Toxicity

Acute toxicity (A22)

Oral LD_{50} Sweet oil: >5 g/kg (rat); bitter oil: >5 g/kg (rat).

Dermal LD_{50} Sweet oil: >10 g/kg (rabbit); bitter oil: >5 g/kg (rabbit).

Irritation and sensitisation (A22)

Nil at 8% (bitter) and 10% (sweet), but 1/200 dermatitis patients were sensitive to sweet and 3/200 to bitter orange oil (Rudzki et al., 1976). Cutaneous irritation was reported for bitter oil and there was a case of severe dermatitis involving the fingers, hands, forearms and face of a girl peeling the fruit. The sensitisation reports have increased over the years to all citrus oils (A27; A28).

Poor storage and degrading oils: d-limonene-high oils (citrus oils) in particular will quickly degrade after opening to produce weak carcinogenic chemicals (Homberger and Boger, 1968) or will increase risk of sensitisation and skin irritation. Therefore the shelf-life of opened bottles, if stored correctly, is recommended to be 1 year, or 2 years if stored in a fridge. Citrus oils will last at least six months if stored correctly (Homberger and Boger, 1968).

Phototoxicity

Slight to very serious phototoxicity has occurred after skin massage with orange oil followed by sunlight or UV light. Natural extracts containing furanocoumarin-like substances may be used in cosmetic products, provided that the total concentration of furanocoumarin-like substances in the finished cosmetic product does not exceed 1 ppm (A30). Distilled orange oils are not phototoxic. See lemon oil monograph.

Bioactivities

Pharmacological activities *in vitro* and *in vivo*

Smooth muscle Sweet orange oil had a spasmogenic effect on electrically stimulated guinea-pig smooth muscle *in vitro*. Limonene had a similar effect (A2; Lis-Balchin et al., 1996a).

Uterus There was a decrease in the spontaneous contractions in the rat for orange oil, limonene and the other components; mixing several other essential oils with orange oil also had a relaxant effect (A3; A4; Lis-Balchin and Hart, 1997b).

Other activities Oils high in d-limonene (citrus oils such as sweet orange, lime, lemon and grapefruit) have been shown to stimulate tumorous growths in mice on the site of topical application (Roe, 1959; Roe and Peirce, 1960; Peirce, 1961; Elegbede et al., 1986).

Antimicrobial activities

Antibacterial activity

Relative data: Sweet orange oil showed good activity against: 19/25 different bacterial species (A1; Lis-Balchin and Deans, 1997; Lis-Balchin et al., 1998a); also against 4/25 bacteria (same set of bacteria but different commercial essential oil) (Deans and Ritchie, 1987); also against 4/5 bacteria (Yousef and Tawil, 1980). 10/20 *Listeria monocytogenes* varieties were affected (A1; Lis-Balchin and Deans, 1997; Lis-Balchin et al., 1998a); no effect was shown, however, on five other *Listeria* species (Aureli et al., 1992). Bitter orange vapour was effective against 1/5 bacteria (Maruzella and Sicurella, 1960).

Antifungal activity

Sweet orange essential oil showed good activity against *Fusarium culmorum* (84% inhibition) but poor activity against *A. ochraceus* (34%) and none against *Aspergillus niger* (A1).

Sweet orange oil was effective against 15/15 fungi (Maruzella and Liguori, 1958); both sweet and bitter were effective against 3/5 fungi (Maruzella, 1960).

Antioxidant effect

No activity was detected for sweet orange oil (Lis-Balchin et al., 1996a).

Clinical studies

In a blind, randomised trial of 120 children undergoing dental extraction under sevoflurane anaesthesia, the effect of the essential oil of sweet orange (*Citrus sinensis*) on induction and recovery characteristics was investigated. The test group had a breathing filter impregnated with four drops of essential oil interposed between the breathing system and the mask. After taking two breaths, the children were asked to grade the odour of the anaesthetic vapour on a scale ranging from 'horrid' to 'pleasant'. The concentration of sevoflurane was then increased and the induction was assessed by the anaesthetist according to the resistance of the children upon application of the facemask. After recovery, the children graded the acceptability of their induction. Compared with the control group, children exposed to the essential oil were more relaxed and cooperative during induction (a smooth induction in 85% of cases) and they also graded the anaesthetic odour more favourably (72% as against 23%) (Mehta et al., 1998). Ambient odour of orange oil in a dental office reduced anxiety and improved mood in female patients (Lehrner et al., 2000).

The perceptional change of fragrance of essential oils was described in relation to type of work, i.e. mental work, physical work, and hearing environmental (natural) sounds using orange, geranium, cypress, bergamot, spearmint, ylang ylang and juniper. For mental work, inhalation of juniper seemed to create a favourable impression after work, whereas geranium and orange both produced an unfavourable impression then (Sugawara et al., 1999).

Use in pregnancy and lactation: contraindications

The sensitisation potential and possible effect on the uterine muscle, as indicated by animal studies in vitro suggest caution in using this essential oil as a massage oil during pregnancy and parturition.

The use of the essential oil as a fragrance in moderate quantities is not considered hazardous.

Pharmaceutical guidance

The risk of oxidation of the limonene to produce sensitisers in a short time when stored and the added problem of phototoxicity, especially when using the expressed essential oil, makes the dermal application of the orange essential oil hazardous. The use of a distilled essential oil or an FCF essential oil would greatly reduce the risk of phototoxicity, but the problem of the sensitisation potential remains unless the essential oil is folded many times to remove as much limonene as possible, which would probably make it unacceptable to aromatherapists. The problem of using the whole essential oil with its potential toxicity should be understood and acknowledged to prevent any hazard. See also lemon oil monograph.

Use in babies and young children

Due to the immaturity and the delicate nature of the skin of babies and young children, it is inadvisable for any essential oils, especially a phototoxic essential oil, to be used in massage, however much the essential oil has been diluted in the carrier oils. This is also a necessary precaution due to the possibilities of sensitisation of the children at this young age through skin or air-borne odorant effects (see Chapters 5 and 7).

Instillation or administration of essential oils near the baby or young child's nose is not only not recommended, but distinctly inadvisable, as there have been numerous cases reported of severe toxicity and even death from such applications (see Chapter 7).

Palmarosa Oil

CAS numbers

USA: 8014-19-5; EINECS: 84649-81-0

Species/Botanical name

Cymbopogon martini var. *martini* (var. *motia*)

Synonyms

Anthropogon martini, Cymbopogon martini (Roxb.) Stapf var. *motia, Cymbopogon martinii* (Roxb.) Wats var. *martinii*

Safety

CHIP details
None

RIFM recommended safety of use limits
8% (A23)

EU sensitiser total
86.7 (based mainly on geraniol, 83; linalool, 3; farnesol, 0.2) (A27)

GRAS status
Granted (Fenaroli, 1997).

Extraction, source, appearance and odour

Extraction
The essential oil is obtained by steam distillation of the fresh or dried grass (Arctander, 1960).

Source
India, Madagascar, Central America and Brazil.

Appearance and odour
A pale yellow to yellow or olive essential oil with a sweet, floral-rosy odour and various types of mainly herbaceous undertones, depending on the quality (Arctander, 1960).

Aromatherapy uses

Uses include: acne, dermatitis, scars, sores, wrinkles, moisturising skin, regenerating cells; anorexia, intestinal infection, stress-related conditions; flu, high temperature, laryngitis, pharyngitis, sinusitis; cardiac stimulation, thrush, cystitis, urethritis, vaginitis; irritability, excitement (Ryman, 1991; Lawless, 1992; Rose, 1992a,b; Price, 1993; Sheppard-Hanger, 1995).

Scientific comment
Palmarosa oil is relatively non-toxic but its sensitisation potential is extremely high and therefore care must be taken in using the essential oil on the skin, especially in sensitive individuals and those with a sensitivity to any geraniol-containing essential oil. Palmarosa essential oil is to be regarded as hazardous for use in aromatherapy massage, but its use as a fragrance can be acceptable in small doses. Massage alone can alleviate many stress-related conditions.

Herbal uses

Palmarosa is an antiseptic, antifungal, febrifuge, stimulant (digestive, circulatory, cardiac), tonic (uterine, nervous) and cools the body. Traditional uses include: insect repellent, skin conditioner, soothing agent, emollient and muscle relaxant (Lawless, 1992; Sheppard-Hanger, 1995).

Food and perfumery uses

Food Palmarosa oil (FEMA 2831) has many food and beverage uses (Fenaroli, 1997).

Perfumery Palmarosa oil has a sweet floral, rose- and geraniol-like odour and is an excellent extender in all floral, rose-like, perfume compounds. It blends well with: geranium, cananga, amyris and guaicawood. It is used in soap perfumes and for bases with geranium odour, as palmarosa was known as geranium palmarosa (Arctander, 1960).

Chemistry

Palmarosa (ISO 4727: 1988):

	Major components %	
	Min	Max
Geraniol		
Indian	74	94
Other	72	86
Limonene	trace–0.5	
Linalool	2–4	
Geranyl acetate	5–11	
Farnesol	0.3–1.5	

Minor components

Other components include: nerol, nerolidol, hexadecanol and sesquiterpenes.

Adulteration

Gingergrass is a common adulterant due to its abundance in the wild and therefore cheapness. Turpentine and citronella are often used together with synthetic geraniol. Palmarosa is a cheap substitute for rose and geranium oils, with slight additions of various components. It is an excellent source of geraniol (A8; see Chapter 4).

Toxicity

Acute toxicity (A22)

Oral LD$_{50}$ >5 g/kg body weight (rat).

Dermal LD$_{50}$ >5 g/kg (rabbit).

Irritation and sensitisation (A22)

Nil at 8% but the new EU sensitisation value is very high, therefore there is the likelihood of sensitisation, especially in sensitive individuals. (See also geraniol sensitisation in Chapter 7.)

Phototoxicity

None reported.

Bioactivities

Pharmacological activities *in vitro* and *in vivo*

Smooth muscle Palmarosa oil had a spasmolytic effect on electrically stimulated smooth muscle of guinea-pig ileum *in vitro* (A2; Lis-Balchin *et al.*, 1996a).

Uterus There was a decrease in the spontaneous contractions in the rat when palmarosa oil, limonene, geraniol and some of the other components were introduced. Mixing several other essential oils with palmarosa oil also had a relaxant effect (A3; A4; Lis-Balchin and Hart, 1997b).

Antimicrobial activities

Antibacterial activity

Relative values: Considerable activity was shown against 21–23/25 different bacterial species and 17–18/20 *Listeria monocytogenes* varieties (A1; Lis-Balchin and Deans, 1997; Lis-Balchin *et al.*, 1998a). There was moderate to good effect on four different bacterial species (Friedman *et al.*, 2002). The vapour had an effect on only 1/5 bacteria (Maruzella, 1960).

Antifungal activity

Relative values (% inhibition): *Aspergillus niger* 73–92%, *A. ochraceus* 55–92%, *Fusarium culmorum* 55–78% (A1).

Antioxidant activity

This was reported as moderate (Baratta *et al.*, 1998b).

Use in pregnancy and lactation: contraindications

Due to the lack of information regarding its safety during this period and the possible decrease in spontaneous contractions of the uterus shown in animal experiments, together with its sensitisation potential, palmarosa oil is not recommended for use on the skin in pregnancy, parturition and lactation. The use as a fragrance could be acceptable in small amounts.

Pharmaceutical guidance

Palmarosa oil is relatively non-toxic and is an effective antimicrobial, but its sensitisation potential is extremely high and therefore care must be taken in using the essential oil on the skin, especially in sensitive individuals and those with a sensitivity to any geraniol-containing essential oil or perfume or plant (which includes geranium oil, citronella and rose). The essential oil is therefore to be regarded as hazardous for use in aromatherapy massage, but its use as a fragrance may be acceptable in small doses. (See also monographs on geranium, citronella and rose oils.)

Use in babies and young children

Due to the immaturity and the delicate nature of the skin of babies and young children, it is inadvisable for any essential oils, especially an essential oil with a high sensitisation potential, to be used in massage, however much the essential oil has been diluted in the carrier oils. This is also a necessary precaution due to the possibilities of sensitisation of the children at this young age through skin or air-borne odorant effects (see Chapters 5 and 7).

Instillation or administration of essential oils near the baby or young child's nose is not only not recommended, but distinctly inadvisable, as there have been numerous cases reported of severe toxicity and even death from such applications (see Chapter 7).

Parsley Oil

CAS numbers

Herb and seed: USA: 8000-68-8; EINECS: 84012-33-9

Species/Botanical name

Petroselinum crispum (Mill.) Nyman (Apiaceae/Umbelliferae)

Synonyms

Apium petroselinum L., *Carum petroselinum* (L.) Benth., *Petroselinum sativum* Hoffm.

Safety

CHIP details

Herb: Xn; R10, 38, 65; 40%; S62; seed: Xn; R10, 21/22, 65; 40%; S36/37, 62 (A26)

RIFM recommended safety of use limits

2% (A23)

EU sensitiser total

3 (based on limonene) (A27)

GRAS status

Granted (Fenaroli, 1997).

Extraction, source, appearance and odour

Extraction

The essential oil is obtained by steam distillation of the herb or seeds (Arctander, 1960).

Source

Europe.

Appearance and odour

Seed oil is a yellow to light/dark brown liquid, with a warm, woody, sweet-herbaceous odour, not like the actual herb. Parsley herb oil is much harsher in odour (Arctander, 1960).

Aromatherapy uses

Very few aromatherapy books mention parsley oil. Uses include: treating women of all ages – a tonic for the nervous system, menstrual cycle problems like flatulence, water retention, pain; also cystitis, (for premenstrual tension the essential oil is massaged or used in the bath water); for beauty – broken capillaries and bruises, psoriasis and varicose veins; removal of toxins, rheumatism, sciatica, haemorrhoids (Ryman, 1991; Lawless, 1992; Sheppard-Hanger, 1995).

Scientific comment

Parsley essential oil is unlikely to alleviate all the conditions mentioned and it is a potent photosensitiser so caution is advised for its use in aromatherapy massage. Massage alone can alleviate many stress-related conditions and it is unlikely that the fragrance of parsley essential oil would assist this therapy.

Herbal uses

Parsley is a carminative, antispasmodic, diuretic, emmenagogue and expectorant, and has antirheumatic and antimicrobial properties. Traditionally, it has been used for flatulent dyspepsia, colic, cystitis, dysuria, bronchitic cough in the elderly, dysmenorrhoea, functional amenorrhoea, myalgia and specifically for flatulent dyspepsia with intestinal colic (Grieve, 1937/1992; Chevallier, 1996; Barnes *et al.*, 2002).

Food and perfumery uses

Food Parsley is commonly used in foods, especially pickles, sauces, meats and drinks. It is used as gripe water for babies (Fenaroli, 1997).

Perfumery The seed oil is used in perfumes especially men's and colognes. It mixes in with spicy-aromatic essential oils and is used for special effects. Also in soaps, detergents and cosmetics (Arctander, 1960).

Chemistry

Major components

| Commercial EO | % (Lawrence, 1976–2001) | |
	Herb	Seed
α-Pinene	5.1	10–18
Myrcene	4.3	0.1–0.2
Limonene	3.6	0.3
β-Phellandrene	12.4	trace–1.5
Terpinolene	2.1	trace–0.2
p-Mentha-1.3,8-triene	9.2	–
α-p-Dimethylstyrene	7.2	
p-Methyl acetophenone	1.9	
Myristicin[a]	20.6	21.6
Apiole[a]	18.3	15–40 (trace–80)

[a] Myristicin can be from 9 to 77%; apiole from 0 to 80% in either herb or seed.

Minor components

Other mono- and sesquiterpenes. Benzyl benzoate has even been found at 25.0% (which is unusual), but could have been due to ageing of the essential oil. Furanocoumarins such as bergapten and oxypeucedanin also occur at up to 0.02% and 0.01% respectively; 8-methoxypsoralen at up to 0.003%. A recent study showed that the essential oil content of a large germplasm collection ranged from 0 to 0.16% (v/fresh weight) and that the oil constituents varied significantly although the major constituent was 1,3,8-p-menthatriene, followed by β-phellandrene, myristicin and myrcene (Simon and Quinn, 1988). In a parallel study evaluating the essential oils of commercially available parsley, curly-leaf types had as high essential oil content as the flat-leaf types, commonly believed to be more flavourful (Simon, 1990).

Adulteration

The essential oils of parsley seed and herb can be grossly mixed and other components, such as benzyl benzoate, added (A8; see Chapter 4).

Toxicity

Acute toxicity (A22)

Oral LD$_{50}$ Parsley herb oil: 3.3 g/kg (rat); seed oil: 3.9 g/kg (rat) and 1.5 g/kg (mice).

Dermal LD$_{50}$ Herb oil >5 g/kg rabbit; seed oil >5 g/kg (guinea-pig).

Dermal LD$_{50}$ values for apiole and myristicin 50 mg/kg and 200 mg/kg body weight, respectively (mice, intravenous injection) (Buchanan, 1978).

The herb is toxic to chickens and at a dose of 17.8 g/kg it caused diarrhoea, convulsions, paralysis and death. In mice, a single dose of 10 mL/kg of parsley seed extract caused anuria, drowsiness, dyspnoea and hyperaemia, with death after 24–60 hours. No toxic effects were seen in dogs at extremely high levels of 60 g/kg. This indicates species specificity (A22).

Irritation and sensitisation (A22)

No irritation or sensitisation at 2% in humans.

Phototoxicity

Furanocoumarins make it potentially phototoxic.

Other toxicities

Myristicin, the toxic principle in parsley essential oil, is related to the carcinogen safrole. It is also abundant in nutmeg oil. Myristicin can cause hallucinations, visual impairments, delirium and prolonged sleep when used orally or via inhalation. It can act as either a stimulant or depressant of the CNS. Overdosing can cause convulsions, vomiting and delirium (see nutmeg oil monograph for further details on myristicin and safrole). However, parsley contains lower concentrations of myristicin (less than 0.05% in parsley leaf, compared with about 0.4–0.89% in nutmeg). Parsley seed oil is potentially more hazardous than the herb due to a higher content of apiole and myristicin. However, there is an immense range of these two components in commercial samples and much admixing, making it difficult to generalise. Apiole may cause irritation of the kidneys during excretion (Barnes et al., 2002).

Chronic and excessive consumption of fresh parsley (170 g daily for 30 years) has been associated with generalised itching and pigmentation and was probably as a result of concomitant chronic liver disease and possibly due to the psoralens in parsley (Cootes, 1982).

Bioactivities

Pharmacological activities *in vitro* and *in vivo*

Smooth muscle Opposing results were obtained for two commercial samples tested: one showed a spasmolytic effect and the other a spasmogenic effect on electrically stimulated smooth muscle of the guinea-pig *in vitro* (A2; Lis-Balchin et al., 1996a,d). These parsley essential oils could have been obtained from seed and herb, but this was not stated and their gas chromatographs were very similar except for the higher monoterpene content in the sample showing spasmogenic activity (New Zealand plants). Parsley extract lowered the blood pressure of cats by more than 40% (Petkov, 1979) and decreased both respiratory movements and blood pressure in anaesthetised dogs (A22). Parsley seed oil stimulated hepatic regeneration (Gershbein, 1977). Parsley seed essential oil had calcium channel blocking activity (Neuhaus-Carlisle *et al.*, 1993).

Uterus   Parsley seed essential oil showed a relaxation effect on the rat uterus *in vitro* (A3; A4; Lis-Balchin and Hart, 1997b). Parsley had a tonic effect on both intestinal and uterine muscle (A22); the effect was attributed to its apiole content (Farnsworth, 1975) but has also been observed with apiole-free aqueous extracts (A22).

Other activities   Parsley seed oil stimulates hepatic regeneration (Buchanan, 1978). An oral dose of 10 g apiole (equivalent to 200 g of parsley) apparently caused acute haemolytic anaemia, thrombocytopenia purpura, nephrosis and hepatic dysfunction. Myristicin is very toxic (see toxicities above and also nutmeg oil monograph), causing hallucinations and, in severe cases, paralysis, followed by fatty degeneration of the liver and kidney (Duke, 1985).

Antimicrobial activities

Antibacterial activity
Relative values: Activity was found against 9–11/25 different bacterial species and 15–16/20 *Listeria monocytogenes* varieties (A1; Lis-Balchin *et al.*, 1996d, 1998a; Lis-Balchin and Deans, 1997).

Antifungal activity
Relative values (% inhibition): *Aspergillus niger* 76–86%, *A. ochraceus* 68–82%, *Fusarium culmorum* 37–52% (Lis-Balchin *et al.*, 1996d).

Antioxidant activity
This was shown in two samples of commercial parsley from New Zealand (Lis-Balchin *et al.*, 1996d).

Other activities
Myristicin and apiole are both effective insecticides (Buchanan, 1978).

Clinical studies

Parsley oil has been included in the diet of pregnant women and is reported to increase diuresis, and plasma protein and plasma calcium concentrations (Buchanan, 1978). The diuretic effect associated with the consumption of parsley is probably due to the pharmacological activities of myristicin (sympathomimetic action) and apiole (irritant effect).

Use in pregnancy and lactation: contraindications

Parsley (oral intake) has been implicated in effects on the menstrual cycle (Zaynoun *et al.*, 1985), various utero activities in humans and animals (Farnsworth, 1975) and there was a loss of spontaneous uterine contractions in animal studies *in vitro*. This suggests caution in using the essential oils, especially as myristicin crosses the placenta and could lead to fetal tachycardia (Lavy, 1987). In view of this, parsley essential oils should not be used during pregnancy, parturition and lactation.

Pharmaceutical guidance

The pharmacological and toxicological properties of parsley are primarily associated with components of the essential oils, particularly apiole, myristicin and furanocoumarins. Parsley essential oils may cause a photoactive reaction, especially following external application and especially in sunlight. They may aggravate existing renal disease, and may potentiate existing monoamine oxidase inhibitor therapy. Myristicin is toxic (see nutmeg oil monograph). It is therefore inadvisable to use the essential oil in aromatherapy massage. It could be used as a fragrance, but the odour is not really pleasing to most people outside the context of cooking.

Use in babies and young children

Due to the immaturity and the delicate nature of the skin of babies and young children, it is inadvisable for any essential oils, especially an essential oil with toxic components, to be used in massage, however much the essential oil has been diluted in the carrier oils. This is also a necessary precaution due to the possibilities of sensitisation of the children at this young age through skin or air-borne odorant effects (see Chapters 5 and 7).

Instillation or administration of essential oils near the baby or young child's nose is not only not recommended, but distinctly inadvisable, as there have been numerous cases reported of severe toxicity and even death from such applications (see Chapter 7).

Patchouli Oil

CAS numbers
USA: 8014-09-3; EINECS: 84238-39-1

Species/Botanical name
Pogostemon cablin (Blanco) Benth. (Labiatae)

Synonyms
P. patchouly Pellet, var. *suavis* Hook. F.

Safety
CHIP details
None; 60% (A26)

RIFM recommended safety of use limits
10% (A23)

EU sensitiser total
0 (A27)

GRAS status
Granted (Fenaroli, 1997).

Extraction, source, appearance and odour
Extraction
The essential oil is obtained by steam distilling the dried leaves and young shoots of the tree (Arctander, 1960).

Source
Sumatra, Indonesia, India, Java, the Seychelles and Brazil.

Appearance and odour
A dark orange or brown viscous oil with a rich, heavy, sweet-herbaceous, aromaticspicy/camphoraceous, woody-balsamic, long-lasting odour. There is a wine-like ethereal-floral sweetness in the initial notes. The odour remains sweet during evaporation. It is very long-lasting, remaining for months on a blotter. Some patchouli oils have a dry cade-like odour. The body odour is very rich, root-like and delicately earthy. The colour of the crude oil is dark, mainly due to the presence of iron; iron-free oils can be obtained which are lighter in colour and odour (Arctander, 1960).

Aromatherapy uses
Patchouli essential oil is supposedly an antidepressant, antiemetic, anti-inflammatory, antiphlogistic, antiseptic, anti-microbial, aphrodisiac, astringent, bactericidal, carminative, cicatrizant, decongestant, deodorant, febrifuge, fungicidal, nervine, prophylactic, nervous stimulant (sedative in low dose, stimulating in high dose) and tonic (digestive stimulant). Its uses include: allergies, herpes, impetigo, burns, cracked skin, haemorrhoids, acne, skin rejuvenator, dandruff; frigidity (Ryman, 1991; Lawless, 1992; Rose, 1992a,b; Price, 1993; Sheppard-Hanger, 1995).

Scientific comment
Patchouli essential oil is one of the safest of the essential oils as regards its toxicology, however there is scant information on its bioactivity, except that it has some antibacterial potential and relatively little antifungal activity. It is therefore unlikely that the essential oil will alleviate all the conditions mentioned. However, massage itself can have a profound effect on stress-related conditions and the fragrance of patchouli can have a beneficial effect. It was reported to be stimulant in human brain studies but is considered by many people to be relaxant.

Herbal uses
It is used in China, Japan and Malaysia for colds, headaches, nausea, vomiting, diarrhoea, halitosis and as an antidote to snakebites. It was known by the 1960s ravers for its ability to obscure the odour of drugs. It was used to treat Indian carpets, preventing insect and fungal deterioration (Lawless, 1992).

Food and perfumery uses
Food Patchouli oil (FEMA 2838) is used in a variety of food and beverages (Fenaroli, 1997).

Perfumery It is used in a great variety of perfumes, including oriental bases, woody bases, fougeres and chypres. It blends well with: labdanum, vetiver, sandalwood, cedarwood, geranium, clove, lavender, rose, neroli, bergamot, myrrh and clary sage (Arctander, 1960).

Chemistry

Major components

	% (Lawrence, 1976–2001)
Patchouli alcohol	31–58
α-Guaiene	10–15
Caryophyllene	2–4
α-Bulnesene	13–17
Seychellene	6–9
α-Patchouline	3–6
β-Patchouline	1–5
Pogostol	0–3

Minor components

Trace components contributing to the aroma include: (+)-norpatchoulenol <0.5% and nortetrapatchoulol at 0.0001%.

Adulteration

Cedarwood, clove oils and their components are frequently used for cutting the oil; also methyl acetate, hydroabietic alcohols, vetiver residues, camphor residues, gurjun balsam oil, cubeb oil, copaiba balsam, castor oil and isobornyl acetate (A8; see Chapter 4).

Toxicity

Acute toxicity (A22)

Oral LD$_{50}$ >5 g/kg (rat).

Dermal LD$_{50}$ >5 g/kg (rabbit).

Irritation and sensitisation (A22)

Nil at 20% (human), but should be reduced to 0.1% in people with dermatoses.

Phototoxicity

None reported.

Bioactivities

Pharmacological activities *in vitro* and *in vivo*

Smooth muscle Patchouli oil had a strong spasmolytic effect on electrically stimulated smooth muscle guinea-pig ileum *in vitro* (A2; Lis-Balchin *et al.*, 1996a).

Uterus There was a decrease in the spontaneous contractions in the rat uterus *in vitro* (A3; A4; Lis-Balchin and Hart, 1997b).

Antimicrobial activities

Antibacterial activity

Relative values: There was slight activity against 6/25 different bacterial species and 15/20 *Listeria monocytogenes* varieties (A1; Lis-Balchin and Deans, 1997; Lis-Balchin *et al.*, 1998a). The vapour affected 2/5 bacteria (Maruzella and Sicurella, 1960). Patchouli had an effect against 5/5 bacteria (Friedman *et al.*, 2002).

Antifungal activity

Relative data: Patchouli essential oil had a poor effect on *Aspergillus niger* 6% inhibition, *A. ochraceus* 29%, *Fusarium culmorum* 27% (A1).

Use in pregnancy and lactation: contraindications

Patchouli essential oil is relatively safe and the main hazard could be its possible spasmolytic effect on uterine muscle, which has been shown to occur *in vitro*. Provided that dosages of the essential oil remain low, aromatherapy massage may be relatively safe if used infrequently.

Pharmaceutical guidance

Patchouli essential oil is one of the safest of the essential oils as regards its toxicology, however there is scant information on its bioactivity, except that it has some antibacterial potential and relatively little antifungal activity. There are few reports on clinical usage and possible effects on different muscles and organs *in vivo*. However, there have been no serious adverse reports and the essential oil poses little hazard when used at low concentration in aromatherapy.

Use in babies and young children

Due to the immaturity and the delicate nature of the skin of babies and young children, it is inadvisable for any essential oils to be used in massage, however much the essential oil has been diluted in the carrier oils. This is also a necessary precaution due to the possibilities of sensitisation of the children at this young age through skin or air-borne odorant effects (see Chapters 5 and 7).

Instillation or administration of essential oils near the baby or young child's nose is not only not recommended, but distinctly inadvisable, as there have been numerous cases reported of severe toxicity and even death from such applications (see Chapter 7).

Pepper Oil

CAS numbers

USA: 8006-82-4; EINECS: 84929-41-9

Species/Botanical name

Piper nigrum L. (Piperaceae)

Synonyms

Black pepper

Safety

CHIP details
Xn; R10, 65; 95%; S62 (A26)

RIFM recommended safety of use limits
4% (A23)

EU sensitiser total
10 (based on limonene 9.5% and linalool 0.5%) (A27)

GRAS status
Granted (Fenaroli, 1997).

Extraction, source, appearance and odour

Extraction
The essential oil is obtained by steam distillation of the ripe dry peppercorns or berries, which have been crushed. An oleoresin is also produced by solvent extraction (Arctander, 1960).

Source
India, Indonesia, China and Madagascar.

Appearance and odour
The essential oil is colourless, pale yellow or pale greenish-grey with a fresh, dry-woody, warm-spicy, pungent odour, reminiscent of peppercorns and also elemi and cubeb (Arctander, 1960).

Aromatherapy uses

Uses include: chilblains, arthritis, anaemia, muscular aches and pains, neuralgia, poor circulation, rheumatic pain, sprains, catarrh, chills, colds and flu, infections and viruses, colic, nausea, constipation, diarrhoea, heartburn, flatulence, increasing flow of saliva, stimulating appetite, expelling wind, restoring tone to the colon muscles; sciatica, nervous conditions; dermatitis, backache, headache; dilating and increasing circulation of local blood vessels – used for muscular aches and stiffness and a prophylactic before physical exertion; rheumatoid arthritis and temporary paralysis of limbs (Ryman, 1991; Lawless, 1992; Rose, 1992a,b; Price, 1993; Sheppard-Hanger, 1995).

Scientific comment

There seem to be no data for any pharmacological bioactivity, and the value of using black pepper essential oil has not been proven scientifically in aromatherapy, so, although there are no data to indicate any great hazard at present, it seems unlikely that the essential oil can alleviate any of the conditions mentioned above. Massage alone, however, can have a profound effect on stress-related symptoms.

Herbal uses

Black pepper is a gastrointestinal stimulant, and is much used as a condiment to improve the flavour of food, and to favour its digestion by stimulating the stomach. It has been advantageously used as a carminative to remove flatulency (Felter and Lloyd, 1898). It promotes urine and stimulates the kidneys. Its warming action also aids respiratory illnesses involving cold, as it is antiseptic to the lungs. It is supposed to bring down high fevers in very small amounts and is useful for treating bruises (Wren, 1988; Chevallier, 1996; Barnes *et al.*, 2002).

Food and perfumery uses

Food   Pepper oil (FEMA 2845) is used in various baked goods, frozen diary, meats, candies and beverages (Fenaroli, 1997).

Perfumery   In perfumery, pepper gives interesting effects with eugenol, e.g. in carnation and rose bases and in oriental fragrances or modern aldehydic bases (Arctander, 1960).

Chemistry

Black pepper, *Piper nigrum* L. (ISO 1984), Sarawak:

Major components

	%
α-Pinene	5.8
β-Pinene	10.4
δ-3-Carene	20.2
Limonene	17
Terpinolene	0.9
δ-Elemene	2.6
α-Copaene	2.4
β-Caryophyllene	28.1
α-Humulene	1.4
δ-Cadinene	0.7

Adulteration

Pepper oil is often adulterated with phellandrene, pinenes, limonene, *Schinus molle* essential oil, elemi essential oil, cedrela essential oil, sesquiterpenes from clove oil, *Eucalyptus dives* oil, copaiba balsam and cubeb oil. Falsification of the whole pepper fruit is of rare occurrence, but it may be found admixed with the fruit of cubebs, allspice, *Piper longum*, etc. giving rise to a different essential oil (A8; see Chapter 4).

Toxicity

Acute toxicity (A22)

Oral LD$_{50}$ >5 g/kg (rat).

Dermal LD$_{50}$ >5 g/kg (rabbit).

Irritation and sensitisation (A22)

Nil at 4%, human.

Phototoxicity (A22)

Insignificant, very low photoxicity when used alone, but this increases if mixed with other phototoxic essential oils.

Bioactivities

Pharmacological activities *in vitro* and *in vivo*

Smooth muscle No reports found in the literature.

Uterus No reports found in the literature.

Antimicrobial activities

Antibacterial activity

Antibacterial effect was moderately low against 10/25 species of bacteria (Deans and Ritchie, 1987) and also against four bacteria (Friedman *et al.*, 2002).

Antifungal activity

Mycelial growth of aflatoxin-producing *Aspergillus parasiticus* is stopped by 0.2–1% black pepper essential oils (Tantaoui-Elaraki and Beraoud, 1994).

Use during pregnancy and lactation: contraindications

In the absence of any data on pharmacological effects on any tissue, the use of black pepper essential oil in aromatherapy massage during these times is not recommended.

Pharmaceutical guidance

There seems to be no evidence of any pharmacological bioactivity, but a few papers indicated moderate antimicrobial activity and limited toxicological evaluations show low risk in acute studies, though there are no subacute or chronic data. Sensitisation potential is low and dermatitis absent up to 4% dermal application in humans. The use of black pepper essential oil therefore does not indicate any great hazard at present when used in aromatherapy, although its value has not been proven.

Use in babies and young children

Due to the immaturity and the delicate nature of the skin of babies and young children, it is inadvisable for any essential oils to be used in massage, however much the essential oil has been diluted in the carrier oils. This is also a necessary precaution due to the possibilities of sensitisation of the children at this young age through skin or air-borne odorant effects (see Chapters 5 and 7).

Instillation or administration of essential oils near the baby or young child's nose is not only not recommended, but distinctly inadvisable, as there have been numerous cases reported of severe toxicity and even death from such applications (see Chapter 7).

Note: Pepper powder has been implicated in numerous murders of young children in India.

Peppermint Oil

CAS numbers

USA: 8006-90-4; EINECS: 98306-02-6

Species/Botanical name

Mentha × piperita L. (Lamiaceae). Hybrid of *M. spicata × M. aquatica* L.

Synonyms

Mitcham mint, balm mint, brandy mint

Other species

Mentha spicata L. (spearmint), *Mentha arvensis* var. *piperascens* Holmes (cornmint)

Safety

CHIP details
None (A26)

RIFM recommended safety of use limits
8% (23)

EU sensitiser total
2.2 for peppermint (A2)

GRAS status
Granted.
Note: FEMA classifies menthol as GRAS and the US FDA has approved menthol for food use (A22; Fenaroli, 1997).

Extraction, source, appearance and odour

Extraction
A volatile oil is obtained by steam distillation of freshly harvested, flowering sprigs. Peppermint essential oil is often rectified. It is characterised by the presence of menthofuran (Arctander, 1960).

Source
USA, China, India, South America, Italy and Japan.

Appearance and odour
Peppermint oil is a colourless to pale yellow oil with a strong, grassy-minty odour with a deep balsamic undertone and a sweet dry-out (Arctander, 1960).

Aromatherapy uses

It is considered one of the most important essential oils in aromatherapy as it apparently stimulates, refreshes, cools, restores and uplifts mind and body. Other uses include: acne, dermatitis, scabies, toothache; neuralgia, palpitations, muscular pain; asthma, bronchitis, halitosis, sinusitis, and when inhaled in steam, it relieves head colds, and bronchitis; aids the digestive system, e.g. dyspepsia, colic, cramp, flatulence, nausea; tired head and feet, nervous stress (Ryman, 1991; Lawless, 1992; Rose, 1992a,b; Price, 1993; Sheppard-Hanger, 1995).

Scientific comment

Peppermint is a stimulant for the nervous system and a relaxant for the smooth muscle of the gut (A14) and uterus *in vitro*, however it is irritant to the skin and can cause hypersensitive reactions. High doses can be fatal and peppermint essential oil should never be used even near babies and young children. Peppermint essential oil is best used as an inhalant for colds in adults, with and without eucalyptus essential oil (as in Vicks VapoRub and Olbas oil, etc.) and can be massaged all over the body, unless there is danger of sensitive skin and mucosal areas being involved (see Chapter 7). There is no scientific proof of its aromatherapeutic efficacy to date. However, massage itself can alleviate many conditions induced by stress and also muscular pain.

Herbal uses

The essential oil was said to be analgesic, anesthetic, anti-inflammatory, antimicrobial, antispasmodic, antiseptic, decongestant, emmenagogue, expectorant; mucolytic; tonic and stimulant. It apparently relieves muscle spasm, increases sweating and stimulates bile. It is used nowadays for digestive purposes, pain relief (e.g. headaches and migraines) and to reduce sensitivity on the skin; also as an inhalant and chest rub for respiratory complaints (Wren, 1988; Chevallier, 1996).

Conventional uses

Inhalants and various cough lozenges, etc. contain menthol (Martindale, 2004).

Internal uses include spastic discomfort of the upper gastrointestinal tract and bile ducts, irritable colon, catarrhs of the respiratory tract, inflammation of the oral mucosa. External uses include myalgia and neuralgia.

Peppermint oil or its menthol component is in several licensed medicinal product in the UK, used for dyspepsia, bronchitis and irritable bowel syndrome (Somerville *et al.*, 1984) although there is controversial evidence for the latter (Nash *et al.*, 1986). Enterically coated tablets (e.g. Colpermin or Mintec) deliver the peppermint oil to the colon without causing upper respiratory and digestive system irritation. Peppermint oil can also reduce colonic spasm during endoscopy when introduced with the endoscope. It is a good local anaesthetic and counterirritant for muscular pains and aches (Martindale, 2004).

Mint oil is used in a cream (Uddermint) to prevent and treat mastitis in cows (Teisen).

Pharmacopoeial preparations include menthol and benzoin inhalation (BP 2003); benzocaine and menthol topical aerosol, menthol lozenges, tetracaine and menthol ointment (USP 27).

Food and perfumery uses

Food Peppermint (FEMA 2848) is used in various baked goods, frozen diary, meats, candies, beverages, toothpastes and chewing gum. Pulegone (high in pennyroyal) is restricted to 25 mg/kg in general foods, but mint confectionary can contain 350 mg/kg, mint and spearmint drinks 250 mg/kg and other drinks 100 mg/kg. All mints have a cool feeling on the mucous membranes in the nose and mouth and on the skin (Fenaroli, 1997).

Perfumery Peppermint is used to a limited extent in perfumery. It blends well with bergamot, geranium, lavender, marjoram, rosemary, sandalwood and is used in chypres and fougeres, etc. (Arctander, 1960).

Chemistry

Major components

Comparison between the three main mints:

	% (Lawrence, 1976–2001)		
	Peppermint	Spearmint	Cornmint
Menthol	27–50	0.1–0.3	65–80 (38)
Menthone	13–32	0.7–2	3–15 (31)
Isomenthone	2–10	trace	1.9–4.8 (12)
1,8-Cineole	5–14	1–2	0.1–0.3 (0.2–0.8)
Limonene	1–3	8–12	0.7–6.2 (10)
Carvone	0	58–70	0

Brackets indicate values for dementholised cornmint oil (Martindale, 1973).

Minor components

Menthofuran (0.3–12%) occurs only in peppermint and is generally removed by rectification to improve the taste of the oil. It is used as guidance for the essential oil purity. Piperitone is found in minute concentration. Pulegone is found at trace to >4%, although it should be under 4%.

ISO for Peppermint 856:1981 Steam-distilled extremities of *Mentha* × *piperita* L. var. *piperita* growing in France, Italy, UK, USA. Ester value (menthyl acetate) min/max: 14/19 Fr; 14/34 It; 11/26 UK; 14/19 USA. Carbonyl value (menthol) min/max: 54/108 Fr; 68/108 It; 54/115 UK; 68/115 USA. Miscibility with 70% EtOH: 1:5 Fr; 1:3.5 It; 1:4 UK; 1:5 USA. Opalescence may be seen on further addition of solvent.

BP (1993) Esters: 4.5–10%; no less than 44% free alcohols (as menthol). Ketones (15–32%) as menthone. The 1995 Addendum replaces this with gas chromatographic profile: limonene 1–5%; cineole 3.5–14%; menthone 14–32%; menthofuran 1–9%; isomenthone 1.5–10%; menthyl acetate 2.8–10%; menthol 30–55%; pulegone under >4%; carvone >1%. Ratio of cineole: limonene exceeds 2. Dementholised mint oil: The British Pharmacopoeia describes Brazilian oil containing between 3 and 10% esters calculated as menthyl acetate and 35–55% free alcohols calculated as menthol.

Adulteration

Peppermint oil is one of the most widely produced and also one of the most commonly adulterated.

Cornmint is cheaper as it grows wild and is frequently used to dilute or even be a substitute for the oil. Adulteration with this oil is difficult to detect even when it is added at 85% to pure peppermint oil, as the colour test for menthofuran remains constant, even when it is diluted. Cornmint can also be mixed with inferior fore-runs of peppermint oil, which also give a positive menthofuran test. Identification of adulteration: small quantities of viridiflorol is a useful identification in peppermint (see cornmint oil) (A8; see Chapter 4).

Toxicity

Acute toxicity (A22)

Oral LD$_{50}$ 4.4 g/kg (rat); >5 g/kg (mouse and hamster).
Menthol: 2.9 g/kg (rat); 3.1 g/kg (mouse).

Dermal LD$_{50}$ >5 g/kg (rabbit).
Menthol may irritate the eyes and may be harmful if ingested in quantity.

Irritation and sensitisation (A22)

Peppermint oil can be irritating on the skin. It is generally considered safe at 4%, but 0.1% is recommended for peppermint in sensitive people, as 1/200 patients showed response to peppermint. Peppermint oil is an irritant and can cause hypersensitivity reactions (Martindale, 1993). Reported reactions include erythematous skin rash, headache, bradycardia, muscle tremor and ataxia. Idiopathic atrial fibrillation and exacerbation of asthma have occurred. It is very dangerous taken internally if undiluted or very concentrated, as even a few drops can cause a feeling of asphyxiation due to the sharpness of the odour and burning effect on the nose and throat, and it can be fatal in a young child (see below). Peppermint and spearmint oils can cause heartburn and gastritis and medicinal products are used only in the form of enteric-coated capsules.

Massive intakes of peppermint sweets have caused allergic reactions: idiopathic auricular fibrillation occurred in two patients addicted to mint sweets and the symptoms subsided after they stopped indulging in mints. There was also an acute allergic response in the mouth, neck and throat of a sensitive individual using toothpastes flavoured with peppermint and spearmint (A22; Martindale, 1982).

Hypersensitivity reactions have been reported in adults: symptoms included headache, flush, rash, dizziness and hypertension from contact with menthol in a variety of forms, e.g. toothpaste, cigarette smoke, candies and medications (Larkin and Castellano, 1967). Ingestion of menthol can cause severe abdominal pain, nausea, vomiting, vertigo, ataxia, drowsiness and coma (Martindale, 1993). Overdose of menthol, particularly over long periods, for example through overuse of mentholated cigarettes (Luke, 1962), can result in gastrointestinal distress, ataxia, stupor and convulsions – even blood dyscrasias have been reported (Dukes, 1996).

Twelve cases of contact sensitivity to menthol and peppermint oil were reported in patients presenting with intra-oral symptoms in association with burning mouth syndrome, recurrent oral ulceration or a lichenoid reaction (interlacing network of white lines – a spider web pattern on the mouth cavity mucosa). Five patients with burning mouth syndrome demonstrated contact sensitivity to menthol and/or peppermint, with one sensitive to both agents, three positive to menthol only and one to peppermint only. Four cases with recurrent intra-oral ulceration were sensitive to both menthol and peppermint. Three patients with an oral lichenoid reaction were positive to menthol on patch testing, with two also sensitive to peppermint. After a mean follow-up of 32.7 months (range 9–48 months), of the nine patients that could be contacted, six patients described clearance or improvement of their symptoms as a consequence of avoidance of menthol/peppermint (Morton *et al.*, 1995).

A case of contact cheilitis (inflammation of the lip) due to peppermint oil and menthol in toothpaste has been reported. A 70-year-old man with a 10-year history of whitish eruption on his lower lip developed erosion and pain on the same area. Results of allergic tests showed positive reactions to cobalt chloride, balsam of Peru, fragrance mix, toothpaste and to captopril. He stopped taking the captopril for four months but the cheilitis did not improve. Further allergic testing with the ingredients of the toothpaste he used revealed that he had a positive reaction to fragrance. Looking at the ingredients of the toothpaste a positive reaction was seen with peppermint oil and menthol (1% petroleum spirit and 5% petroleum spirit respectively). After these tests he began to use toothpaste without peppermint oil and menthol and his cheilitis improved within one month (Nishioka, 1997).

Phototoxicity

None reported.

Other toxicities

Mint tea poisoned two infants: one who died was found to have a menthofuran level of 10 ng/mL serum. The other had 41 ng/mL plus 25 ng/mL of pulegone (Bakerink *et al.*, 1996). The estimated acceptable daily intake of menthol is up to 200 µg/kg body weight (Martindale, 1993). Ingested pure menthol can be poisonous – as little as a teaspoonful (1 g/kg body weight) can be fatal.

A number of reports have appeared suggesting toxicity to menthol in small infants. Because of respiratory tract infections of unknown severity, these patients received home treatments which included menthol-containing ointments (Martindale, 1993, 2004; Dukes, 1996; Leung and Foster, 1996, Medical Economics, 2000) and went on to develop severe respiratory distress in most cases and cyanosis in a few. Symptoms persisted for one or more days in many infants and was thought to be due to the inhalation of menthol (Larkin and Castellano, 1967). The contraindications for some menthol-containing products caution against their use in infants and young children, specifying that menthol-containing preparations should not be used on areas of the face, especially the nose (Barnes *et al.*, 2002).

Several examples of toxic reactions have been reported:

- A six-week-old boy who had developed a slight cold with a little rhinitis had mentholated ointment applied to his chest. He became dyspnoeic and in a short while stopped breathing, becoming cyanotic and stiff with very slow movements of the limbs. A relative turned him upside down and slapped him slightly on the back and the boy produced a little mucus and started breathing again and recovered uneventfully. The story was repeated on three consecutive days before the family realised that it was ointment causing the toxic reaction (Wilken-Jensen, 1967).
- Ataxia, confusion, euphoria, nystagmus and diplopia developed in a 13-year-old boy following the inhalation of 5 mL of Olbas oil instead of the recommended few drops. Olbas oil contains menthol 4.1%, oil of cajuput 18.5%, clove 0.1%, eucalyptus 35.5%, juniper berry 2.7%, peppermint 35.5% and wintergreen oil (methyl salicylate) 3.7%. Possibly the menthol in the preparation was responsible for the symptoms as the amount inhaled was approximately 200 mg and the amount of methyl salicylate was too low to cause salicylate toxicity (O'Mullane *et al.*, 1982).
- A 63-year-old woman with a past history of alcoholism and ongoing nicotine dependence was hospitalised on three occasions in a one-year period secondary to episodes of euphoria, confusion, lethargy, agitation, odd behaviour and auditory and visual hallucinations, which were found to be related to the oral ingestion of mentholatum, containing menthol and methyl salicylate (Huntimer and Bean, 2000).
- A 58-year-old woman became addicted to mentholated cigarettes and developed toxic exhaustive psychosis from which she recovered once she stopped smoking. It was believed that due to the excessive use and craving for mentholated cigarettes, the bradycardia, ataxia, confusion and mental irritability could be correlated with the inhalation of volatile menthol (Luke, 1962).
- A case of non-thrombocytopenic purpura caused by mentholated cigarettes was described by Highstein and Zeligman (1951).
- Two cases of idiopathic auricular fibrillation were reported, both of which were investigated in hospital. The patients later admitted to being excessive peppermint addicts (Thomas, 1962).
- Genotoxicities of dill, peppermint and pine essential oils have been reported using chromosome aberration and sister-chromatid exchange tests in human lymphocytes *in vitro* and *Drosophila melanogaster* somatic mutation and recombination tests *in vivo* (Lazutka *et al.*, 2001).

Note: The final safety report on *Mentha piperita* (peppermint) oil, which is currently used in cosmetic formulations as a fragrance component, should be of value to aromatherapists (Nair, 2001a). Peppermint essential oil is used at a concentration of 3% in rinse-off formulations and 0.2% in leave-on cosmetic formulations, which would be roughly the aromatherapeutic concentration. It was found to be minimally toxic in acute oral studies, whilst short-term and subchronic oral studies reported cyst-like lesions in the cerebellum in rats given doses of peppermint oil containing pulegone, pulegone alone, or large amounts (>200 mg/kg/day) of menthone. Repeated intradermal dosing with peppermint oil produced moderate and severe reactions in rabbits, although it was not phototoxic. It was negative in the Ames test and a mouse lymphoma mutagenesis assay but gave equivocal results in a Chinese hamster fibroblast cell chromosome aberration assay. Carcinogenicity study of toothpaste and its components showed no apparent differences between mice treated with peppermint oil and those treated with the toothpaste base. Isolated clinical cases of irritation and/or sensitisation to peppermint oil and/or its constituents have been reported, but peppermint oil (8%) was not a sensitiser when tested using a maximisation protocol. It was expected that dermal absorption of peppermint oil would be rapid, as is menthol, but no greater than absorption through the gastrointestinal tract. Because of evidence that menthol can enhance penetration of other agents, formulators must be cautioned that this enhanced penetration can affect the use of other ingredients whose safety assessment was based on their lack of absorption (this applied to perhaps other essential oils in the mixture applied by aromatherapists). With the limitation that the concentration of pulegone should not exceed 1%, it was concluded that *Mentha piperita* essential oil is safe as used in cosmetic formulations (Nair, 2001a).

Bioactivities

Pharmacological activities *in vitro* and *in vivo*

Smooth muscle Peppermint oil had a spasmolytic effect on guinea-pig ileum *in vitro* (A2; Taddei *et al.*, 1988; Lis-Balchin *et al.*, 1996a). The mode of action seemed to be via cAMP rather than calcium or potassium channels (Lis-Balchin and Hart, 1999b). Calcium antagonist action of menthol on gastrointestinal smooth muscle, however, was shown by other workers in a different study (Taylor *et al.*, 1985). In rat and guinea-pig atrial and papillary muscle, both menthol and peppermint demonstrated calcium channel blocking properties (Hawthorn *et al.*, 1988). Peppermint was also antispasmodic in the mouse intestine (Haginiwa *et al.*, 1963). Both peppermint and spearmint in a watery dilution caused relaxation of the gastric wall and a decrease in contractions in the ileum and colon of dogs (Plant and Miller, 1926). There was a relaxant effect on tracheal muscle in guinea-pig (Reiter and Brandt, 1986).

Uterus There was a decrease in the spontaneous contractions in the rat for peppermint oil, and the other major components. Mixing several other essential oils with other essential oil also had a relaxant effect (A3; A4; Lis-Balchin and Hart, 1997b). Pregnancy was unaffected by pennyroyal (containing pulegone) usage (Black DR, 1985).

Other activities Anti-inflammatory effects of L-menthol were greater than mint oil using human monocytes *in vitro* (Juergens *et al.*, 1998). The authors suggest that these data support the use of clinical trials to investigate L-menthol for treatment of chronic inflammatory problems such as bronchial asthma, colitis and allergic rhinitis. A study investigating the effect of peppermint oil on intestinal transport processes in the rat small intestine reasoned that it alleviates symptoms of irritable bowel syndrome by reducing the availability of calcium to the tissue (Beesley *et al.*, 1996).

The most potent essential oils towards oral bacteria were peppermint oil, Australian tea tree oil and sage oil (Shapiro *et al.*, 1994). *Mentha piperita* was found to have significant anti-inflammatory and analgesic effects when used against induced, localised acute and chronic inflammation in rodents. The effects were dose-dependent. The authors concluded that the study affirmed the traditional use of peppermint for these conditions of pain and inflammation (Atta and Alkofahi, 1998).

A study on excised rat skin showed that peppermint oils caused a 48-fold increase in penetration of 5-fluorouracil through the skin (Abdullah *et al.*, 1996).

Pulegone, a very minor component of peppermint oil induced atonia, decreased blood creatinine content, lowered terminal body weight and caused histopathological changes in the liver and in the white matter of cerebellum in rats at 80 or 160 mg/kg per day, with no effect at 20 mg/kg per day (Thorup *et al.*, 1983).

People exposed for 5 minutes to camphor, eucalyptus or menthol vapor showed no effect on nasal resistance to airflow, but a majority of subjects reported a cold sensation in the nose and a feeling of improved airflow (Burrow *et al.*, 1983).

There was a risk of jaundice in glucose-6-phosphate dehydrogenase deficient babies exposed to menthol (Olowe and Ransome-Kuti, 1980).

Pulegone is discussed in Chapter 5.

Antimicrobial activities

Antibacterial activity

Peppermint oils (18 samples) were effective against 12–15/25 different bacterial species and 13–20/20 *Listeria monocytogenes* varieties (A1; Lis-Balchin and Deans, 1997; Lis-Balchin *et al.*, 1998a); 19/25 different bacteria were affected in another test (Deans and Ritchie, 1987) and 3/5 bacteria (Maruzella, 1960); and 5/5 *Listeria monocytogenes* varieties were limited by a peppermint oil from Piedmont (Aureli *et al.*, 1992). Spearmint and peppermint were strongly active against five bacteria tested *in vitro* (Friedman *et al.*, 2002), as was menthol.

The peppermint vapour affected 3/5 bacteria and the rectified vapour 2/5; spearmint vapour was active against 1/5 bacteria (Maruzella and Sicurella, 1960). Peppermint vapour had a good effect against 5/6 respiratory tract pathogens but not an *Escherichia coli* variant (Inouye *et al.*,

2001). Menthol showed the same trend but menthone was less active.

Antifungal activity

Relative data (% inhibition) (18 samples): *Aspergillus niger* 81–98%, *A. ochraceus* 70–94%, *Fusarium culmorum* 47–86% (A1). Peppermint oil affected 3/5 fungi (Maruzella, 1960) and low activity was found against 15/15 fungi (Maruzella and Liguori, 1958). Peppermint oil was effective against all 22 bacterial strains and 11 fungi strains (Pattnaik *et al.*, 1996). The essential oils of three species of mint (*Mentha* spp.) showed strong antibacterial and antifungal activity against 10 bacterial strains and a fungus, *Candida albicans* (Sow *et al.*, 1995). Essential oils from peppermint, eucalyptus, lemongrass and palmarosa were tested against a strain of *E. coli*. All four oils killed the strain at very low dilutions (Pattnaik *et al.*, 1998). A strain of *Pseudomonas aeruginosa* harbouring a plasmid was not inhibited by large concentrations of essential oils of eucalyptus, lemongrass, palmarosa or peppermint. Resistance to the bactericidal effects of the oils was thus demonstrated (Pattnaik *et al.*, 1995a).

The effects of peppermint (*Mentha piperita* L.) essential oil and four of its major constituents on the proliferation of *Helicobacter pylori*, *Salmonella enteritidis*, *E. coli* O157:H7, methicillin-resistant *Staphylococcus aureus* (MRSA) and methicillin-sensitive *S. aureus* (MSSA) showed that the essential oils and the various constituents inhibited the proliferation of each strain and the effects were almost the same against antibiotic-resistant and antibiotic-sensitive strains of *H. pylori* and *S. aureus* (Imai *et al.*, 2001).

Clinical studies

The following clinical studies used the peppermint oil orally and therefore cannot be regarded as supporting normal aromatherapy usage. A randomised, double-blind, placebo-controlled study of 110 outpatients with symptoms of irritable bowel syndrome showed that symptoms improved significantly better in the group taking peppermint oil capsules (Colpermin) than in the group taking the placebo. Symptoms addressed were alleviation of abdominal pain, less abdominal distention, reduced stool frequency, less intestinal rumbling and less flatulence (Liu *et al.*, 1997). A double-blind, placebo-controlled trial using 45 patients with non-ulcer dyspepsia studied the efficacy and safety of Enteroplant, a standardised preparation consisting of peppermint oil and caraway oil in an enteric coated capsule. After four weeks of treatment, the peppermint/caraway capsule was significantly superior to the placebo in terms of relief of pain severity and frequency. Similar favourable findings occurred with other gastrointestinal symptoms as well (May *et al.*, 1996). A review of eight randomised clinical trials of peppermint extracts (*Mentha* × *piperita*) as a treatment for symptoms for irritable bowel syndrome indicated that peppermint oil seemed to help relieve symptoms, but the efficacy of peppermint has not been established beyond a reasonable doubt (Pittler and Ernst, 1998).

Another study used a control (placebo) and an experimental group of gynaecological patients to test for postoperative nausea relief using peppermint oil. The experimental group required less nausea medication following surgery than the placebo group and this was statistically significant (Tate, 1997).

Other clinical trials used external application of the peppermint essential oil. In a randomised, controlled clinical trial, 20 healthy subjects inhaled 75% menthol in eucalyptus oil or one of two placebos prior to having a cough induced. Results showed that menthol inhalation caused a significant reduction in induced cough, and can be considered an effective antitussive agent for induced cough (Morice *et al.*, 1994). Using a randomised, placebo-controlled, double-blind study, a locally applied, diluted peppermint oil preparation was tested on 41 patients for relief of headaches. The peppermint oil preparation was applied across the forehead three times at 15-minute intervals, and showed a significant reduction in headache compared with the placebo, and a reduction in pain intensity similar to that achieved with 1000 mg acetaminophen. No adverse effects were reported. The researchers concluded that the peppermint oil preparation is efficient at alleviating tension-type headaches, and is well-tolerated and cost-effective (Gobel *et al.*, 1996). In a double-blind, placebo-controlled, randomised cross-over study involving 32 healthy subjects, four test preparations were applied to large areas of the forehead and temples. A reduction in sensitivity to headache with a significant analgesic effect was found with a combination of peppermint oil and ethanol. The researchers concluded that essential oil preparations can have significant effects on the pathophysiology of headache (Gobel *et al.*, 1994).

Use in pregnancy and lactation: contraindications

There was a loss of spontaneous contractions in the uterus when the essential oil was administered *in vitro*; although there are no data to suggest that peppermint essential oil is an abortifacient, pulegone, which can occur in small concentrations, has traditionally had this effect. Peppermint oil should only be used with caution in small amounts on the skin, as it can be irritant and a sensitiser. Some aromatherapists advise that peppermint essential oil should not be used when pregnant; however if diluted to 1% and not more than three drops are used in the bath it may be safe even for sensitive skins (Tisserand and Balacs, 1995).

Pharmaceutical guidance

Peppermint oil is useful for many illnesses when taken internally, and for respiratory conditions when used with other volatiles. Its usefulness in aromatherapy has to be judged against its possible sensitisation when applied on the skin and possible fibrillation or asthmatic symptoms when used as a volatile. Reported adverse reactions include erythematous skin rash, headache, bradycardia, muscle tremor and ataxia. Idiopathic atrial fibrillation and exacerbation of asthma have occurred.

Peppermint oil should be avoided in cases of obstruction of bile ducts, gallbladder inflammation and severe liver damage. It should be avoided in cardiac disease (Tisserand and Balacs, 1995). The essential oil should only be used for gallstones after consultation with a physician (Blumenthal *et al.*, 2000).

Use in babies and young children

Due to the immaturity and the delicate nature of the skin of babies and young children, it is inadvisable for any essential oils to be used in massage, however much the essential oil has been diluted in the carrier oils. This is also a necessary precaution due to the possibilities of sensitisation of the children at this young age through skin or air-borne odorant effects (see Chapters 5 and 7).

Instillation or administration of essential oils, especially peppermint or menthol-containing products, near the baby or young child's nose is not only not recommended, but distinctly inadvisable, as there have been numerous cases reported of severe toxicity and even death from such applications (Blumenthal *et al.*, 2000; see Chapter 7). Even mint water, wrongly prepared by a pharmacist, caused a baby's death recently (Bunyan, 1998; *Evening Standard*, 1998).

Peru Balsam

CAS numbers

USA: 8007-00-9; EINECS: 8007-00-9

Species/Botanical name

Myroxylon balsamum var. *pereirae* Royle (Leguminosae)

Synonyms

Baume de Pérou, *Toluifera pareirae* (Royle) Baillon, myrospermum of sonsonate, pareira, *Myrospermum pareirae* Royle, *Myroxylon pereirae* Klotzsch, *Toluifera balsamum* var. Baillon, *Balsamum peruvianum*, black balsam, China oil, Honduras balsam, Indian balsam, Peruvian balsam, Surinam balsam, Baume du San Salvador

Related species

Myroxylon peruiferum L. f. (*Myroxylon pedicellatum* Klotzsch, *Toluifera peruifera* Baillon)

Pharmacopoeias

In European Pharmacopoeia.

Safety

CHIP details
Xi; R43; S24, 37 (A26)

RIFM/IFRA recommended safety of use limits
Balsam: do not use; essential oil: 8% (A23)

EU sensitiser total
Peru oil: 91.5 based on benzyl benzoate, 78%; benzyl cinnamate, 9% and benzyl alcohol, 4.5% (A27)

Extraction, source, appearance and odour

Extraction
The balsam is obtained from exposed lacerated wood, after strips of the bark have been removed. It is a 'true' balsam, which is collected in the form of a dark brown or amber semi-solid mass. The essential oil is distilled from the balsam using high vacuum dry distillation. An inferior quality wood oil is also produced by steam distillation (Arctander, 1960; Evans, 1996), The 'Peru' part of balsam of Peru originates from when it was first named, El Salvador then being part of a Peruvian colony.

Source
El Salvador, South America.

Appearance and odour
The balsam is a syrupy liquid, free from stringiness or stickiness, of a brownish-black colour in bulk, reddish-brown and transparent in thin layers (Arctander, 1960). It has an agreeable vanilla-like, somewhat smoky odour, and a bitter taste, leaving a persistent after-taste. Balsam of Peru smells of vanilla and cinnamon because it contains 60–70% cinnamein (a combination of cinnamic acid, cinnamyl cinnamate, benzyl benzoate, benzoic acid and vanillin). The other 30–40% comprises resins of unknown composition (Arctander, 1960).

Aromatherapy uses

Although the balsam is banned by the IFRA, the essential oil is still used in aromatherapy although the sensitisation value is extremely high. It is considered by some aromatherapists as non-toxic and non-irritant. Uses include: skincare for dry and chapped skin, eczema, rashes, sores and wounds; low blood pressure, rheumatism; asthma, bronchitis, coughs, colds; nervous tension, stress (Ryman, 1991; Lawless, 1992; Rose, 1992a,b; Price, 1993; Sheppard-Hanger, 1995).

Scientific comment

Although still used in numerous medicinal products both externally and internally, Peru balsam has a very high sensitisation potential when applied to the skin. Its uses for treatment of skin complaints are therefore rather dangerous and none of the other uses quoted above have been proven as being alleviated by Peru balsam applied in aromatherapy massage. Massage itself alleviates many stress-related conditions, however.

Herbal uses

Balsam of Peru apparently possesses expectorant and stimulating properties acting more especially on mucous tissues, lessening their secretions when profuse. It was used in the past for all chronic affections of mucous tissues, catarrh, gonorrhoea, mucous inflammation of the stomach and bowels, chronic diarrhoea, dysentery, leucorrhoea, etc. It was used externally for obstinate ulcers, wounds, ringworm of the scalp, eczema and other cutaneous conditions. It is considered antiseptic and able to readily heal wounds, chilblains, sore nipples and pruritus vulvae (Felter and Lloyd, 1898). It stimulates the heart, increases blood pressure, lessens mucous secretions, and is useful for respiratory disorders such as asthma, chronic coughs and bronchitis. Used in scabies and skin diseases; it destroys the itch acarus and its eggs, and is much to be preferred to sulphur ointment, also of value in prurigo, pruritus and in later stages of acute eczema. It is applied externally to sore nipples and discharges from the ear (Lawless, 1992) also for infected and poorly healing wounds, for burns, decubitus ulcers, frostbite, ulcus cruris, bruises caused by prostheses and haemorrhoids (Blumenthal *et al.*, 2000).

Conventional uses

Peru balsam is used in haemorrhoidal suppositories, rectal ointment, tincture of benzoin, wound spray, calamine lotion, dental cement, cough medicine, lozenges, lip preparations, insect repellents, surgical dressings, toothpaste and mouthwash.

Anugesic suppositories contain 51.65 mg of Peru balsam, as does the wound care spray Granulex aerosol (Bertek) (each 0.82 mL of medication delivered to the wound site contains trypsin crystallised 0.1 mg, balsam Peru 72.5 mg, castor oil 650.0 mg and an emulsifier). The balsam is an effective capillary bed stimulant used to increase circulation in the wound site area and has a mildly bactericidal action. Diluted with an equal part of castor oil, it has been used as an application to bedsores and chronic ulcers. It has also been used in topical preparations for the treatment of superficial skin lesions and pruritus. It is an ingredient of some rectal preparations used for the symptomatic relief of haemorrhoids (Martindale, 2004) and of some preparations used in the treatment of respiratory congestion.

Food and perfumery uses

Food It is used in citrus fruit peel, artificially baked goods and confectionery, cola and other soft drinks, aperitifs (e.g. vermouth, bitters) and mixed spices (Fenaroli, 1997).

Perfumery Peru balsam is used in deodorants, aftershaves, cosmetics, medicinal creams and ointments, sunscreens, suntan lotions, shampoos and conditioners, perfumed tea and coffee, and tobacco. It blends well with ylang ylang, patchouli, petitgrain, sandalwood, rose, spices, and floral and oriental bases. It is used as a fixative and fragrance component in soaps, detergents, creams, lotions. The oil is often used in perfumery since this avoids any resin deposits or discoloration (Arctander, 1960).

Chemistry
Major components
The percentage composition is variable (Lawrence, 1976–2001; Evans, 1996), consisting of 45–70% esters, including benzyl cinnamate (known as cinnamein), cinnamyl cinnamate, benzyl benzoate and benzyl acetate, also benzoyl alcohol; benzoic acid and vanillin.

Minor components
Present in lesser concentrations in the resin (30% of balsam) are cinnamic acid, cinnamic alcohol, cinnamic aldehyde, eugenol, isoeugenol, nerolidol and farnesol.

The balsam is almost insoluble in water; it is soluble in 1 volume 90% alcohol, but becomes turbid on further addition (Trease and Evans, 1996). The British Pharmacopoeia includes tests for absence of artificial balsams, fixed oils and turpentine.

Peru balsam (Ph. Eur. 4.8) is obtained from the scorched and wounded trunk of *Myroxylon balsamum* var. *pereirae*. It contains not less than 45.0% w/w and not more than 70.0% w/w of esters, mainly benzyl benzoate and benzyl cinnamate (Martindale, 2004).

Adulteration
The commercial balsam as well as the essential oil is often diluted with benzyl alcohol or another solvent. Tolu and other balsams are added as well as

the major and minor synthetic components (A8; see Chapter 4).

Toxicity

Acute toxicity

Oral LD$_{50}$ Balsam >5 g/kg (rat); essential oil 2.4–3 mL/kg.

Dermal LD$_{50}$ Balsam >10 g/kg (rabbit); essential oil 2–5 g/kg.

Irritation and sensitisation

Both the essential oil and balsam are non-irritant and non-sensitising on animal and normal human skin, but contain potential sensitisers. Flare-up of eczema of the hands is common in sensitive individuals if they use products containing balsam of Peru or related allergens. Oral exposure may cause sore mouth (tongue) and rash of the lips or angles of the mouth. Sensitivity to a perfume or cream is usually the first indicator of an allergy to balsam of Peru and is confirmed by patch testing using 10% balsam of Peru in petrolatum: a positive result is seen in 50% of fragrance allergy cases. The individual may also have problems with flavourings (both artificial and natural), some medications and other perfumed products.

Note: Most people tested for fragrance allergy will be patch tested with balsam of Peru and a fragrance mix (a mixture of eight commonly used individual fragrances), which detects approximately 75% of fragrance allergy cases.

Cross-reactions occur with: balsam of tolu, beeswax, benzaldehyde, benzoates, benzoin, benzylsalicylate, coniferyl alcohol, coumarin, eugenol, farnesol, isoeugenol, propolis, styrax, tiger balm, clove and cinnamon essential oils, pimento, nutmeg, camphor, rose, carnation, hyacinth and violet essential oils and absolutes as well as the plant material; also rosin (colophony), citrus fruit peel and vanilla. Allergy to balsam of Peru may therefore make one sensitive to spices and flavourings used in daily cooking.

Extracts and distillates of Peru balsam (the exudation from *Myroxylon pereirae* (Royle) Klotzsch) should not be used such that the total level exceeds 0.4% in cosmetic products, based on a wide variety of test results on the sensitising potential of Peru balsam and its derivatives (European Union (EU) 2001).

Phototoxicity

None reported.

Other toxicities

The Cosmetic Ingredient Review Expert Panel, USA reviewed benzyl alcohol (used in a wide variety of cosmetic formulations as a fragrance component, preservative, solvent, and viscosity-decreasing agent) and benzoic acid (used in a wide variety of cosmetics as a pH adjuster and preservative). Sodium benzoate is the sodium salt of benzoic acid used as a preservative, also in a wide range of cosmetic product types; benzyl alcohol is metabolised to benzoic acid, which reacts with glycine and is excreted as hippuric acid in the human body. Acceptable daily intakes were established by the World Health Organization at 5 mg/kg for benzyl alcohol, benzoic acid and sodium benzoate. Benzoic acid and sodium benzoate have GRAS status. No adverse effects of benzyl alcohol were seen in chronic exposure animal studies using rats and mice and the effects of benzoic acid and sodium benzoate in chronic exposure animal studies were limited to reduced feed intake and reduced growth. Some small differences were noted in some reproductive toxicity studies but not in others. Genotoxicity tests for these ingredients were mostly negative. Carcinogenicity studies were negative. Clinical data indicated that these ingredients can produce non-immunologic contact urticaria and non-immunologic immediate contact reactions, characterised by the appearance of wheals, erythema and pruritus. In one study, 5% benzyl alcohol elicited a reaction, and in another study, 2% benzoic acid did likewise. Benzyl alcohol, however, was not a sensitiser at 10%, nor was benzoic acid at 2%. Recognising that the non-immunologic reactions are strictly cutaneous, likely involving a cholinergic mechanism, it was concluded that these ingredients could be used safely at concentrations up to 5%, but that manufacturers should consider the non-immunologic phenomena when using these ingredients in cosmetic formulations designed for infants and children. Additionally, benzyl alcohol was considered safe up to 10% for use in hair dyes. The limited body exposure, the duration of use and the frequency of use were considered in concluding that the non-immunologic reactions would not be a concern. Because of the wide variety of product types in which these ingredients may be used, it is likely that inhalation may be a route of exposure. The available safety tests are not considered sufficient to support the safety of these ingredients in formulations where inhalation is a route of exposure. Inhalation toxicity data are needed to complete the safety assessment of these ingredients where inhalation can occur (Nair, 2001b).

Bioactivities

Pharmacological activities *in vitro* and *in vivo*

Smooth muscle No data found.

Uterus No data found.

Other activities The positive efficacy of a low-balsam diet was found in about 50% of patients who had a positive patch test to either balsam of Peru, the perfume mixture or both substances. Food items most commonly mentioned by patients as causing aggravation of their symptoms on at least three different occasions were wine, candy, chocolate, cinnamon, curry, citrus fruit and flavourings (Veien *et al.*, 1985).

Antimicrobial activities

Antibacterial activity

Moderate activity was shown against 5/5 different bacteria including two *Listeria monocytogenes* varieties (Friedman *et al.*, 2002).

Antifungal activity

None found.

Use in pregnancy and lactation: contraindications

The use of Peru balsam on the skin is not recommended in pregnancy and lactation due to the possible sensitisation reaction and also lack of pharmacological data. The essential oil is likewise not recommended.

Pharmaceutical guidance

There is scant pharmacological information available for the bioactivity of Peru balsam other than the sensitisation potential of the balsam and its components and also the cross-sensitisations. In view of this, dermal application is unwise and has been banned by fragrance organisations. The essential oil has similar sensitisation components and is likewise undesirable on the skin. However, the fragrance can be used as such for relaxation.

Use in babies and young children

Due to the immaturity and the delicate nature of the skin of babies and young children, it is inadvisable for any essential oils to be used in massage, however much the essential oil has been diluted in the carrier oils. This is also a necessary precaution due to the possibilities of sensitisation of the children at this young age through skin or air-borne odorant effects (see Chapters 5 and 7).

Instillation or administration of essential oils near the baby or young child's nose is not only not recommended, but distinctly inadvisable, as there have been numerous cases reported of severe toxicity and even death from such applications (see Chapter 7).

Petitgrain Oil

CAS numbers

USA: 8014-17-3; EINECS: 72968-50-4

Species/Botanical name

Citrus aurantium L. subsp. *amara* (Rutaceae)

Synonyms

Bigarade, bitter orange

Other species

C. limonum (lemon), *C. reticulata* (mandarin/tangerine), *C. aurantifolia* (lime)

Safety

CHIP details
None

RIFM recommended safety of use limits
Bigarade: 8%; lemon: 10% (A23)

EU sensitiser total
31.4 (based on citral 0.3%, geraniol 3%, limonene 1%, linalool 27%) (A27)

GRAS status
Granted (Fenaroli, 1997).

Extraction, source, appearance and odour

Extraction
The essential oil is obtained by steam distillation of the leaves and twiglets of various citrus trees, mainly the orange or lemon, to give an essential oil of a different composition for each species. The commonest is petitgrain bigarade oil, distilled from the bitter orange tree (see neroli oil monograph). The water remaining after distillation is known as eau de brout, and this yields eau de brout concrete by solvent extraction and eau de brout absolute. Solvent extraction of the twiglets directly yields bigaradier concrete and thence bigaradier absolute (Arctander, 1960).

Source
Paraguay, other South American countries, and the USA.

Appearance and odour
Bigarade petitgrain essential oil is a pale yellow or amber-coloured liquid with a pleasant, fresh-floral, sweet odour reminiscent of orange flowers with a slightly woody-herbaceous undertone and very faint, sweet-floral dry-out notes. There is a bitter top-note as is its taste (Arctander, 1960).

Orange, sweet petitgrain is an olive-green to green-orange liquid with a peculiar dry, almost bitter undertone after a brief fresh top-note; tenacity is poor and the odour changes rapidly during evaporation (Arctander, 1960).

Aromatherapy uses

This is another oil from the same trees as neroli/orange blossom, though petitgrain is distilled from the leaves rather than the petals. Like neroli essential oil, it relaxes, restores, cleanses and uplifts the spirit; it has deodorant properties and helps to relieve anxiety and stress. It is also used for palpitations, rhematism, to improve appetite and for sluggish liver (Ryman, 1991; Lawless, 1992; Rose, 1992a,b; Price, 1993; Sheppard-Hanger, 1995).

Scientific comment

Although petitgrain essential oil has a pleasant smell, there is no scientific data to prove its effectiveness in any aromatherapy usage. However, massage alone can alleviate many stress-related conditions, therefore the pleasant fragrance could possibly add to the relaxation and thereby add to the relief of stress.

Herbal uses

The petitgrain essential oils were produced for the fragrance trade so there are no herbal uses.

Food and perfumery uses

Food Used in some foods (Fenaroli, 1997).

Perfumery All petitgrain oils are used in perfumes, especially for floral bases, citrus colognes and light aldehydic perfumes and as a neroli perfume. Petitgrain blends well with citrus oils, lavender, clary sage, rosemary and olibanum (Arctander, 1960).

Chemistry

Major components

	% (Lawrence, 1976–2001)
Linalool	19–27
Linalyl acetate	46–55
Neryl acetate	2–3
α-Terpineol	4–8
Geraniol	2–4
Myrcene	1–6

The main components of bergamot petitgrain (ISO 8900: 1987) (amber colour) are limonene, linalool, α-terpineol, nerol, linalyl acetate, neryl acetate, geranyl acetate. The main components of lemon petitgrain (8899 1991) (pale-yellow to greenish yellow) are limonene, linalool, neral, geranial, neryl acetate and geranyl acetate. The main components of mandarin petitgrain (ISO 8898: 1991) (amber to reddish-orange with violet fluorescence) are α-pinene, β-pinene, *p*-cymene, limonene, γ-terpinene, terpinolene, linalool, terpinen-4-ol, α-terpineol, linalyl acetate and *N*-methyl anthranilate.

Minor components
There are over 400 known minor components, many of which can contribute to the odour, e.g. β-damascenone (also in rose oil); β-ionone, 2-isopropyl-3-methoxypyrazine; α- and β-sinensal, α-terpinyl acetate. Mandarin leaf oil has 10–15% methyl anthranilate.

Adulteration
Lemongrass is frequently used to adulterate petitgrain oil, or substitute for it with the addition of citral, lemon oil, *Leptospermum citratum*, orange oil fractions, etc. Various mandarin/tangerine petitgrain oils are often fraudulent and some examples include: addition of synthetic methyl anthranilate to a mandarin oil; acetylated linalool and methyl anthranilate to mandarin oil; distillation of a mixture of leaves from different species like mandarin, sweet and bitter orange or clementine; the mixed petitgrain could then also be adulterated further

with linalool, oil of orange and other citruses, etc. Petitgrain itself is used as a cheap substitute for the expensive flower oil neroli (A8; see Chapter 4).

Toxicity

Acute toxicity (A22)
Oral LD_{50} 5 g/kg (rat).
Dermal LD_{50} >5 g/kg (rabbit).

Irritation and sensitisation (A22)
Nil at 7% (bigarade) and 10% (lemon petitgrain). Sensitisation was rare and 1/200 dermatitis patients were affected (Rudzki, *et al.*, 1976).

Phototoxicity
None reported: The essential oil is distilled from leaves not the rind of citrus, therefore does not contain furanocoumarins unless adulterated (A22).

Bioactivities

Pharmacological activities *in vitro* and *in vivo*

Smooth muscle A commercial petitgrain oil had an initial spasmogenic effect on electrically stimulated smooth muscle guinea-pig ileum *in vitro*, followed by spasmolysis (A2; Lis-Balchin *et al.*, 1996a).

Uterus There was a decrease in the spontaneous contractions in the rat for petitgrain oil, and the other components *in vitro*. Mixing several other essential oils with petitgrain oil also had a relaxant effect on the uterus (A3; A4; Lis-Balchin, Hart, 1997b).

Antimicrobial activities

Antibacterial activity
There was generally a strong antibacterial effect. Relative data: There was a strong effect against 21/25 different bacterial species and 16/20 *Listeria monocytogenes* varieties (A1; Lis-Balchin and Deans, 1997; Lis-Balchin *et al.*, 1998a). Other reports showed effect against 5/5 bacteria (Maruzella, 1960). The vapour, however, was only active against 1/5 bacteria (Maruzella and Sicurella, 1960). In another study 21/25 bacteria were affected (Deans and Ritchie, 1987). No activity was shown against five *Listeria* species (Aureli *et al.*, 1992). There was moderate to good activity against five species including *Listeria* (Friedman *et al.*, 2002).

Antifungal activity

Relative data (% inhibition): *Aspergillus niger* 61%, *A. ochraceus* 69%, *Fusarium culmorum* 78% (A1). Antifungal effect was shown against 5/5 fungi (Maruzella, 1960); low to moderate effect on 15/15 fungi (Maruzella and Liguori, 1958).

Antioxidant activity

Slight activity was found (Lis-Balchin *et al.*, 1996a).

Use in pregnancy and lactation: contraindications

There was a loss of spontaneous contractions in the uterus when the essential oil was applied *in vitro*, but no studies in the human uterus have been found. The sensitisation potential is moderate and the limited toxicity studies show no hazards, therefore the essential oil could possibly be used sparingly during pregnancy and lactation.

Pharmaceutical guidance

There is scant pharmacological information available for petitgrain essential oils, but the limited toxicological data show little potential hazard apart from moderate potential sensitisation. Careful use in aromatherapy should not prove hazardous, but there is no proof for its effectiveness for any of the uses mentioned in aromatherapy books.

Use in babies and young children

Due to the immaturity and the delicate nature of the skin of babies and young children, it is inadvisable for any essential oils to be used in massage, however much the essential oil has been diluted in the carrier oils. This is also a necessary precaution due to the possibilities of sensitisation of the children at this young age through skin or air-borne odorant effects (see Chapters 5 and 7).

Instillation or administration of essential oils near the baby or young child's nose is not only not recommended, but distinctly inadvisable, as there have been numerous cases reported of severe toxicity and even death from such applications (see Chapter 7).

Pine Oil

CAS numbers
USA: 8021-29-2; EINECS: 84012-35-1

Species/Botanical name
Pinus sylvestris L. (Pinaceae)

Synonyms
Scotch pine, fir leaf oil, oleum folii pini sylvestris

Other species
Pinus mugo var. *pumilio* (pumilio, pumilio pine oil: dwarf pine needle oil, essence de pin de montagne, latschenöl, oleum pini pumilionis, olio di mugo, pumilio pine oil), *Pinus palustris* (southern yellow pine or pitch pine). See below under Other toxicities for information about other species of Pinaceae and Abietaceae.

Safety
CHIP details
Xn; R10, 65; 95%; S62 (A26)

RIFM recommended safety of use limits
10% (A23)

EU sensitiser total
4 (A27)

GRAS status
Granted (Fenaroli, 1997).

Extraction, source, appearance and odour
Extraction
A volatile oil is obtained by steam distillation of the needles of the pine tree (Arctander, 1960). Sometimes the sawdust from the hardwood is used.

Source
USA and Hungary.

Appearance and odour
A colourless to pale yellow essential oil with a strong, dry, balsamic, turpentine-like odour (Arctander, 1960).

Aromatherapy uses
Sometimes the species are lumped together or else treated separately. Mainly the *P. sylvestris* essential oil is indicated and used for cuts, lice, excessive perspiration, scabies, sores on the skin; muscles, joints, arthritis, gout, muscular aches and pains, rheumatism, poor circulation; respiratory system (asthma, bronchitis, catarrh, coughs, sinusitis, sore throat), the genito-urinary system (cystitis, urinary infection) and the immune system (colds and flu), as well as the nervous system (fatigue, nervous exhaustion), and stress-related conditions as neuralgia (Ryman, 1991; Lawless, 1992; Rose, 1992a,b; Price, 1993; Sheppard-Hanger, 1995).

Scientific comment
Pine essential oil is relatively safe (except for some sensitisation reactions) and has been used in many medicinal preparations without harm, but the value of inhalation in concentrated form or its local rubefacient effect may not provide the same results as that using very dilute concentrations in aromatherapy. Massage itself can have a positive effect on many stress-related and muscular conditions.

Herbal uses
Scotch pine properties are stated to be: antimicrobial, antineuralgic, antirheumatic, antiseptic (pulmonary, urinary), decongestant, expectorant and rubefacient. Pine oils are used as remedies for coughs and colds, particularly as inhalants and as rubefacients for muscular stiffness and rheumatism and also for relaxation when added to the bath (Wren, 1988).

Food and perfumery uses
Food Pine oil, *Pinus sylvestris* (FEMA 2906) is used in a number of foods and beverages (Fenaroli, 1997).

Perfumery Pine essential oil is used mainly to perfume household (cheap) products, such as detergents, soaps, disinfectants and veterinary products. Its use in perfumes is also widespread: it blends with rosemary, cedarwood, citronella, ho leaf, coumarin and oakmoss (Arctander, 1960).

Chemistry

Major components

	% (Lawrence, 1976–2001)
α-Pinene	14–58
β-Pinene	4–36
Limonene	1–8
Myrcene	0.5–7
Bornyl acetate	trace–21

Minor components
Monoterpenes: α-terpineol, *p*-cymene, δ-3-carene, terpinolene, camphene, 1, 8-cineole and sesquiterpenes: caryophyllene, γ-cadinene, muurolene.

Adulteration
Different varieties of pine can be substituted; mixtures of camphene, pinenes and isobornyl acetate, limonene and other components are used (A8; see Chapter 4).

Toxicity

Acute toxicity (A22)
Oral LD50 >5 g/kg body weight (rat).
Dermal LD50 >5 g/kg (rabbit).

Irritation and sensitisation (A22)
No irritation or sensitisation effect at 12% (human) but possible sensitisation as it appears that pine oils high in δ-3-carene or oils that are oxidised could contain more potent sensitising agents, causing dermatitis and eczema type reactions. Therefore oils for use on the skin should be fresh. Cross-sensitisation reactions are possible to pine balsam, spruce, and Peru and tolu balsam.

Phototoxicity
None reported.

Other toxicities
Certain other pine oil fragrances may be used subject to certain restrictions (Issued 25 September 2001, see also A27; A28). Essential oils and isolates derived from the pine trees (Pinaceae family),

including *Pinus* and *Abies* genera, should only be used when the level of peroxides is kept to the lowest practicable level, for instance by adding antioxidants at the time of production. Such products should have a peroxide value of less than 10 mmol peroxide per litre (based on the published literature mentioning sensitising properties when containing peroxides). The following are listed:

- Abies alba oil from cones (*Abies Alba* Mill.)
- Abies alba oil from needles (*Abies Alba* Mill.)
- *Abies sachalinensis* oil
- Fir balsam (*Abies balsamea* (L.) Mill.)
- Fir needle oil (*Abies sibirica*)
- Fir needle oil, Canadian (*Abies balsamea*)
- Pine needle, dwarf, oil (*Pinus mugo turra* var. *pumilio* (Haenke) Zenari)
- Pine needle oil (*Abies* spp.)
- Scots pine oil (*Pinus sylvestris* L.)
- *Pinus nigra* oil
- Turpentine gum (*Pinus* spp.)
- Turpentine oil
- Turpentine oil rectified
- Turpentine, steam distilled (*Pinus* spp.).

Bioactivities

Pharmacological activities *in vitro* and *in vivo*

Smooth muscle and other tissues Pine oil activity has not been reported.

Other activities Pine oil, at 10 mg as a 2% solution in olive oil when injected i.m. once weekly in combination with subeffective doses of dihydrostreptomycin had a therapeutic effect on experimental tuberculosis in the guinea-pig. Genotoxicity of pine essential oil has been reported using chromosome aberration and sister-chromatid exchange tests in human lymphocytes *in vitro* and *Drosophila melanogaster* somatic mutation and recombination tests *in vivo* (Lazutka *et al.*, 2001).

Antimicrobial activities

Antibacterial activity
There was moderate action against 4/5 different bacterial species and addition of pine oil to other oils decreased their activity (Maruzella and Henry, 1958). There was both activity and no activity exhibited against the tubercle bacillus (A22).

Antifungal activity

Moderate action was shown against 4/5 fungi (Maruzella, 1960) and against 15/15 fungi (Maruzella and Liguori, 1958).

Use during pregnancy and lactation: contraindications

There have been no studies on the effect of pine essential oil during pregnancy, parturition and lactation, therefore it should be used in moderation for massage and as a fragrance.

Pharmaceutical guidance

Pine essential oil is relatively safe, except for some sensitisation reactions, but there are a large number of species used for the production of pine essential oil and therefore adulteration is rampant. Pine essential oil has been used in many medicinal preparations without harm, but there is no proof that the value of inhalation in concentrated form or its local rubefacient effect provides the same results as that using very dilute concentrations in aromatherapy. Pine essential oil should be avoided in people with allergenic conditions as sensitisation reactions are possible and should also be avoided in people with prostate cancer (Tisserand and Balacs, 1995). Pine essential oil can otherwise be used both in massage and as an inhalant and in the bath.

Use in babies and young children

Due to the immaturity and the delicate nature of the skin of babies and young children, it is inadvisable for any essential oils to be used in massage, however much the essential oil has been diluted in the carrier oils. This is also a necessary precaution due to the possibilities of sensitisation of the children at this young age through skin or air-borne odorant effects (see Chapters 5 and 7).

Instillation or administration of essential oils near the baby or young child's nose is not only not recommended, but distinctly inadvisable, as there have been numerous cases reported of severe toxicity and even death from such applications (see Chapter 7).

Rose Oil

CAS numbers

Rose oil and absolute: USA: 8007-01-0; EINECS: 90106-38-0

Species/Botanical name

Rosa damascena Mill. (Rosaceae)

Synonyms

Rose otto, bulgarian rose oil, turkish rose oil, attar of rose, esencia de rosa, oleum rosae, otto of rose

Other species

Rosa centifolia L. (French or Moroccan rose oil), *Rosa gallica* L., *Rosa alba* L.

Pharmacopoeias

In United States National Formulary.

Safety

CHIP details
None

RIFM recommended safety of use limits
2% (A23)

EU sensitiser total
Rose oil: 76.3. (based on citral 0.6%, eugenol 1.5%, geraniol 23%, citronellol 49%, farnesol 0.8%, linalool 1.4%) (A27)

GRAS status
Granted (Fenaroli, 1997).

Extraction, source, appearance and odour

Extraction
Steam distillation of freshly picked flowers gives the essential oil; solvent or CO_2 extraction gives a concrete and then an absolute can be obtained: different methods (also different species of rose) give an essential oil of a different composition. Rose otto water is frequently redistilled (cohabation) to retrieve some of the water-soluble components like phenylethyl alcohol, and the distillates are then bulked (Arctander, 1960). USNF 22 describes a volatile oil distilled with steam from the fresh flowers of *Rosa gallica*, *R. damascena*, *R. alba*, *R. centifolia*, and varieties of these species (Rosaceae) (Martindale, 2004).

Source
Bulgaria, France, Morocco, Turkey and Italy.

Appearance and odour
Moroccan rose oil is a colourless to pale yellow essential oil with a deep-sweet, rich and tenacious floral rose-like odour (Arctander, 1960). Rose otto is a pale yellow to slightly olive-green essential oil which separates white or colourless crystals of stearopten below 21°C. It becomes a crystalline solid below this temperature, the crystals growing from the surface due to their lower specific gravity, but can easily be liquefied by gentle warming (e.g. by holding the bottle in the hands). It has a warm, deep-floral, slightly spicy, intensely rich odour, reminiscent of roses with nuances of spicy and honey-like notes (Arctander, 1960). *Rosa centifolia* absolute (known as Rose de Mai absolute) is an orange yellow to orange-brown liquid with a rich and sweet, deep-rosy, very tenacious odour (Arctander, 1960). Bulgarian rose absolute is an orange-yellow, orange-red or even slightly olive tinted liquid with an extremely rich, warm, spicy-floral and very deep rose odour with a pronounced honey-like undertone (Arctander, 1960).

Aromatherapy uses

There are hundreds of uses given for rose essential oil and absolute. Rose absolute, *Rosa damascena*, is known as the queen of oils and its 'feminine' properties make it emotionally soothing. It tones, cleanses, uplifts the spirit and helps maintain self-confidence; it is sensual and even aphrodisiac; excellent skincare oil, perfect for dry/mature, ageing or thread-veined skin. *Rosa centifolia* absolute has a soothing effect on the emotions and in particular, depression, melancholy, apathy, grief, jealousy and resentment. It is used for: insomnia, migraine, headache, nervous tension and stress-related emotions.

Rose essential oil apparently brings joy and happiness; a feeling of well-being and reportedly aids poor memory. It is excellent for babies and when used as a tonic for the female reproductive system, calming premenstrual tension, promoting vaginal secretions and regulating the menstrual cycle. It also aids semen production in men and can be used for sexual difficulties resulting from frigidity. It is also used for palpitations, poor circulation, relieving cardiac congestion, toning capillaries; digestive problems due to emotional upset, inflamed gallbladder and liver, jaundice, hangovers, nausea; asthma, coughs, hay fever and sore throats (Ryman, 1991; Lawless, 1992; Rose, 1992a,b; Price, 1993; Sheppard-Hanger, 1995).

Scientific comment

There is no direct scientific evidence for rose oil alleviating any of the conditions above. However, due to its very pleasant nature, rose essential oil and absolutes offer a pleasant, usually relaxing ambiance. Rose essential oil has also been shown to have a stimulating effect on the human brain (A14), which suggests that differing effects are possible.

Herbal uses

It is antidepressant, antiseptic, antispasmodic, aphrodisiac, astringent, bactericidal, choleric, cicatrizant, emmenagogue, haemostatic, hepatic, laxative, a regulator of appetite, nervous sedative, stomachic, and tonic for heart, liver and uterus. During the Middle Ages the rose was a remedy for depression (Chevallier, 1996). There are no herbal uses at present.

Food and perfumery uses

Food Bulgarian, *R. damascena* oil, rose otto (FEMA 2989) and rose absolute (FEMA 2988) are used in many baked goods, gelatines, soft candies and beverages (Fenaroli, 1997). Rose absolute, centifolia, used at very low concentration, is used to round-off and lift many flavours. Bulgarian rose absolute offers special effects in trace amounts especially in raspberry, strawberry, apricot and bitter almond products.

Perfumery Rose otto is used extensively in high-class perfumes, where even traces can do wonders

for florals, especially carnation or jasmine-type perfumes (Arctander, 1960). Moroccan rose oil (*Rosa centifolia*) is used in high-quality perfumes to give life, depth and warm naturalness to countless floral and non-floral perfumes, rose bases and similar. Rose absolute, *R. centifolia*, is used both in high-price and medium-priced perfumes, particularly in floral bases, chypres, fougeres, oriental bases and in minute amounts to round off synthetic compositions. Its excellent tenacity makes it economical to use (Arctander, 1960). Bulgarian rose absolute is very potent even when used almost in trace amounts. It is used extensively in high-class perfumes such as rosy florals, rose-jasmines, carnation bases, chypres, oriental bases and fantasy bouquets.

Chemistry
Major components

	% (Lawrence, 1976–2001)	
	Rose oil	*Absolute*
(–)-Citronellol	18–55	18–22
Geraniol	12–40	10–15
Nerol	3–9	3–9
Linalool	1.4	1.4
Phenylethyl alcohol	1–3	60–65

The two rose extractives differ with respect to the odour intensity, due to the fact that much (65%) of the less odour-intense 2-phenylethanol is dissolved in the distillate water and therefore is not present in the hydrodistilled oils (unless cohabated).

Minor components
There are at least 300 minor components in rose oil and absolute. For example:

Rose oxides	0.1–0.5
Farnesol	0.8
β-Damascenone	0.14
β-Damascone	0.01
β-Ionone	trace–0.03

These impart the rose-like odour: β-damascenone at 0.14% provides 70% of the perceived odour, compared with citronellol which provides only 4.3% (Ohloff, 1978, 1994). β-Ionone gives 19% of the odour units, while nerol gives 0.1% and geraniol 0.8% and citronellol only 4% (but constitutes around 40% of the essential oil).

Adulteration

Rose oils are very expensive and therefore sophisticated cutting and adulteration is rampant. Many rose oils sold are completely synthetic; others are cut with synthetic phenylethyl alcohol, diethylphthalate, citronellol, geraniol, isoeugenol, heliotropine, cyclamal, amyl salicylate and fractions from geranium oil, such as rhodinol, etc. The absolute is frequently diluted with synthetic palmarosa fractions, peru balsam, costus oil or clove bud oil. Rose otto is often a combination of the distillate plus cohabation water (containing further dissolved components from the oil) and this contributes most of the phenylethyl alcohol. Rose absolutes are also adulterated (e.g. with phenylethyl alcohol, rhodinol from geranium oil, costus oil, clove bud absolute, palmarosa oil fractions, Peru balsam, synthetic citronellol, etc.). The Bulgarian absolute is frequently adulterated with the cheaper *R. centifolia* absolute (Arctander, 1960; A8; see Chapter 4).

Toxicity

An estimated acceptable daily intake of the main components is up to 500 µg/kg body weight, but note the sensitisation possibility on the skin.

Acute toxicity (A22)

Oral LD_{50} *R. damascena* and *R. centifolia*: >5 g/kg (rat); rose absolute (French): >5 g/kg (rat).

Dermal LD_{50} *R. damascena* and *R. centifolia*: >2.5 g/kg (rabbit); rose absolute (French): uncertain in rabbit.

Irritation and sensitisation (A22)

Nil at 2% (human) but adulteration could change this. Furthermore, sensitisers are present totalling 76% (see above). Damascones and related compounds should not be used as fragrance ingredients such that the total level in finished cosmetic products exceeds 0.02%, individually or in combination, based on test data showing sensitising potential for these materials and on evidence of cross-reactivity. These chemicals are: *cis*-α-damascone; *trans*-β-damascone and isodamascone.

Phototoxicity
None reported.

Bioactivities

Pharmacological activities *in vitro* and *in vivo*

Smooth muscle Rose oil and absolute had a spasmolytic effect on guinea-pig ileum *in vitro*. Citronellol, geraniol and the other components had a similar effect (A2; Lis-Balchin *et al.*, 1996a).

Uterus There was a decrease in the spontaneous contractions in the rat for the rose oil and its major and minor components. Mixing several other essential oils with rose oil also had a relaxant effect (A3; A4; Lis-Balchin and Hart, 1997b).

Other activities The pharmacological actions of four different plant-derived essential oils (rose, ylang ylang, chamomile, orange) in two types of conflict tests using ICR (Institute of Cancer Research) mice showed that in the Vogel Conflict Test, in which any drinking behaviour of the mice was punished by an electric shock, the benzodiazepine agonist diazepam increased the number of electric shocks the mice received and this number increased after administration of rose oil. In contrast, ylang ylang, chamomile and orange oil did not produce such an effect. In the Geller Conflict Test, in which lever-pressing of mice was reinforced by food pellets and then punished by electric shock, response (lever-pressing) rate during the alarm period was increased by the positive control drug diazepam, and again the response rate during the alarm period increased after administration of rose oil. Ylang ylang, chamomile and orange oils again did not produce an anticonflict effect. The effects with rose oil are not mediated by the benzodiazepine binding site of the $GABA_A$ receptor complex (Umezu, 1999).

Rosa damascena essential oil had a spasmolytic effect on smooth muscle at higher concentrations of 50–100 µ/mL. Guinea-pigs given *R. damascena* essential oil in doses of 35 mg/kg i.p. after preliminary sensitisation with egg albumen went into anaphylactic shock. The spasmolytic effect is considered to be chiefly myotropic (Shipochliev, 1968).

Antimicrobial activities

Antibacterial activity
The essential oil had moderate activity against 19/25 different bacteria (Deans and Ritchie, 1987). The vapour had activity against 1/5 different bacterial species (Maruzella and Sicurella, 1960). Rose damask and French both had moderate effect on 5/5 bacteria, which included two *Listeria monocytogenes* varieties (Friedman *et al.*, 2003).

Rosa damascena essential oil was tested for antimicrobial activity against *Staphylococcus aureus*, *Escherichia coli*, *Pseudomonas aeruginosa* and the yeast *Candida albicans*. Some antimicrobial activity was shown against *Staph. aureus*, *E. coli* and *C. albicans* but not against *Ps. aeruginosa* (Lisin, 1999).

Antifungal activity

None reported for the oil, except for the yeast above (see geranium oil monograph for activity of components).

Other activities

Rose oil had no effect on the activity of mice and either had no effect on contingent negative variation tests or a stimulating effect (A14).

Use in pregnancy and lactation: contraindications

There seem to be no adverse effects apart from the sensitisation potential and the fact that geranium oil, which has most of the same components, decreased the spontaneous contractions in the rat uterus *in vitro*, suggesting caution during pregnancy and parturition regarding excessive usage. However, the concentrations used in aromatherapy massage are too dilute to cause concern if the rose essential oil is pure. Use of the fragrance can be either stimulating or relaxing.

Pharmaceutical guidance

Apart from the sensitisation potential, which is very high, there are no adverse effects found for rose essential oil. However, the absolute could cause a dermatitic effect, especially in sensitive people and if it was adulterated.

Use in babies and young children

Due to the immaturity and the delicate nature of the skin of babies and young children, it is inadvisable for any essential oils to be used in massage, however much the essential oil has been diluted in the carrier oils. This is also a necessary precaution due to the possibilities of sensitisation of the children at this young age through skin or air-borne odorant effects (see Chapters 5 and 7).

Instillation or administration of essential oils near the baby or young child's nose is not only not recommended, but distinctly inadvisable, as there have been numerous cases reported of severe toxicity and even death from such applications (see Chapter 7).

Rosemary Oil

CAS numbers

USA: 8000-25-7; EINECS: 84604-14-8

Species/Botanical name

Rosmarinus officinalis L. (Labiatae)

Synonyms

R. coronarium, incebsier, oleum rosmarini, esencia de romero, essência de alecrim, essence de romarin, oleum roris marini, rosmarinöl, rosmarini aetheroleum

Pharmacopoeias

In European Pharmacopoeia.

Safety

CHIP details

Xn; R10, 65; 50%; S62 (A26)

RIFM recommended safety of use limits

10% (A23)

EU sensitiser total

6.3 (based on limonene 5.5% and linalool 0.8%) (A27)

GRAS status

Granted (Fenaroli, 1997).

Extraction, source, appearance and odour

Extraction

A volatile oil is obtained by steam distillation of the herb (Arctander, 1960). It is available as Spanish type rosemary oil (Ph. Eur. 4.8) and Moroccan and Tunisian type rosemary oil (Ph. Eur. 4.8) (Martindale, 2004).

Source

Spain, France, Tunisia, Morocco, Yugoslavia and Italy.

Appearance and odour

A pale yellow or almost colourless essential oil with a strong, fresh, woody-herbaceous, somewhat forest-like odour. The high notes vanish rapidly and yield a clean, woody-balsamic body note which tones out into a dry herbaceous odour, pleasant, tenacious and bitter-sweet. Many inferior grades of the essential oil have a harsh camphoraceous odour (Arctander, 1960).

Aromatherapy uses

Rosemary has a multitude of uses: it is said to be stimulating and clears the head; is a good pick-me-up and may improve memory; used for mental strain or dullness and lethargy or exhaustion; chronic fatigue and multiple sclerosis; all respiratory infections and congestion (otitis, sinusitis, bronchitis), and chills; colitis, dyspepsia, sour stomach and slow elimination; oily hair and dandruff; muscular pain, rheumatism, arteriosclerosis, poor circulation, palpitations, gout, dysmenorrhoea, leucorrhoea, seborrhoea; anosmia, asthma, bacache, bursitis, cuts and wounds, menopause, shingles (Ryman, 1991; Lawless, 1992; Rose, 1992a,b; Price, 1993; Sheppard-Hanger, 1995).

Scientific comment

Rosemary essential oil has been shown to have both stimulant and relaxant properties in humans (A14), although its camphoraceous content tends to make it stimulating. There is no scientific evidence that many of the conditions listed above would be alleviated by rosemary essential oil, however, massage itself can remedy many stress-related conditions and the use of the stimulating rosemary essential oil could be of some benefit in addition.

Herbal uses

Culpeper states that the virtues of the oil are more powerful than that of cinnamon, nutmeg, caraway and juniper berries: 'strengthening the brain and memory, fortifying the heart, resisting poison, and curing all sorts of agues; it is absolutely the greatest strengthener of the sight, and restorer of it also, if lost: it makes the heart merry and takes away all foolish phantasms out of the brain. It cleanseth the blood, cures the toothache, easeth all pains, and takes away the causes which hinder conception.' Traditionally rosemary is indicated for flatulent dyspepsia, headache, and topically for myalgia, sciatica and intercostal neuralgia. The rubefacient properties of the essential oil were well-known: it was used as a component in liniments and also Hungary water, which was used to renovate vitality of paralysed limbs (Grieve, 1937/1992). It was also used as a hair lotion to stimulate hair-bulbs and prevent baldness. Nowadays, rosemary oil is stated to be carminative, spasmolytic, thymoleptic, sedative, diuretic and antimicrobial. Applied topically, it is rubefacient, mildly analgesic, a parasiticide and mildly irritant. It is approved for internal use for dyspeptic complaints and external use as supporting therapy for rheumatic diseases and circulatory problems (Martindale, 1982; Wren, 1988; Chevallier, 1996; Blumenthal *et al.*, 2000; Barnes *et al.*, 2002).

Food and perfumery uses

Food Rosemary oil (FEMA 2992) is used in many foods and beverages (Fenaroli, 1997).

Perfumery Rosemary oil is used extensively in perfumery for various citrus colognes, lavender waters, fougeres and pine needle fragrances and oriental perfumes. It is used in room deodorants, insecticides and disinfectants (Arctander, 1960). It was a component of the original Hungary water and eau de Cologne. It blends well with olibanum, lavender, lavandin, citronella, thyme, basil, peppermint, labdanum, elemi, cedarwood, petitgrain and cinnamon.

Chemistry

Major components

	% (*Lawrence, 1976–2001*)
1,8-Cineole	7–60
Camphor	3–50
Myrcene	0–10
α-Pinene	3–24
β-Pinenes	1–8
Borneol	1–2
Limonene	1–5.5
Linalool	trace–0.8

Components vary according to chemotype: Spanish type rosemary oil (Ph. Eur. 4.8) contains: 2.0–4.5%

borneol, 0.5–2.5% bornyl acetate, 8.0–12.0% camphene, 13.0–21.0% camphor, 16.0–25.0% cineole, 1.0–2.2% *p*-cymene, 2.5–5.0% limonene, 1.5–5.0% β-myrcene, 18–26% α-pinene, 2.0–6.0% β-pinene, 1.0–3.5% α-terpineol and 0.7–2.5% verbenone. Moroccan and Tunisian type rosemary oil contains: 1.5–5.0% borneol, 0.1–1.5% bornyl acetate, 2.5–6.0% camphene, 5.0–15.0% camphor, 38.0–55.0% cineole, 0.8–2.5% *p*-cymene, 1.5–4.0% limonene, 1.0–2.0% β-myrcene, 9.0–14.0% α-pinene, 4.0–9.0% β-pinene, 1.0–2.6% α-terpineol, and a maximum of 0.4% verbenone (Martindale, 2004).

Adulteration

Rosemary oil is adulterated with camphor oil, fractions from *Eucalyptus* (*globulus* and *radiata*) and turpentine oils, light cedarwood fractions and fractions from synthetic terpineol production. It can be contaminated by *Salvia lavandulaefolia* (Spanish sage). Otherwise, numerous synthetic components are added. Flower oil from low-grade Spanish rosemary is often deterpenised to give a good quality oil (A8; see Chapter 4).

Toxicity

Acute toxicity (A22)

Oral LD50 >5 g/kg (rat).

Dermal LD50 >5 g/kg (rabbit).

Irritation and sensitisation (A22)

Rosemary oil is stated to be non-irritating and non-sensitising when applied at 10% to human skin (A22) but irritant when applied to rabbit skin undiluted (Leung, 1980). Bath preparations, cosmetics and toiletries containing rosemary oil may cause erythema and dermatitis in hypersensitive individuals (Mitchell and Rook, 1979).

Phototoxicity

Untested in animals, but photosensitivity has been associated with the oil (Mitchell and Rook, 1979).

Bioactivities

Pharmacological activities *in vitro* and *in vivo*

Smooth muscle Rosemary oil had a strong initial spasmogenic effect on electrically stimulated smooth muscle of the guinea-pig ileum *in vitro*, which was followed by a lesser spasmolytic action (A2; Lis-Balchin *et al.*, 1996a). However, in contrast, rosemary was said to be spasmolytic, but at lower doses, showed an initial spasmogenic action due to the low spasmogenic effect of pinene (Taddei et al., 1988). α-Pinene and β-pinene have a spasmogenic action on smooth muscle (A2; Lis-Balchin et al., 1996a), with no effect on cardiac muscle (Hof and Ammon, 1989). Rosemary oil, 1,8-cineole and bornyl acetate have a spasmolytic action in both smooth muscle (guinea-pig ileum) and cardiac muscle (guinea-pig atria) preparations (A2; Hof and Ammon, 1989; Lis-Balchin et al., 1996a). In smooth muscle this spasmolytic effect has been attributed to antagonism of acetylcholine, borneol being the most active component (Hof and Ammon, 1989).

Rosemary essential oil inhibited contractions of rabbit tracheal smooth muscle induced by acetylcholine, and inhibited contraction of guinea-pig tracheal smooth muscle induced by histamine (Aqel, 1992) and also inhibited contractions induced by high potassium concentrations. Contractions of rabbit and guinea-pig tracheal smooth muscle induced by both acetylcholine and histamine were inhibited by rosemary essential oil in a calcium-free solution, suggesting that it is a calcium channel blocker (Aqel, 1991). 1,8-Cineole showed a rise in tone, rather than a contraction (A2; Lis-Balchin et al., 1996a). Noradrenaline (norephinephrine) and potassium ion-induced contractions of rabbit aortic rings were significantly reduced by rosemary oil, possibly by a direct vascular smooth muscle action (Aqel, 1992).

Spasmolytic action *in vivo* (guinea-pigs) was shown by rosemary essential oil (administered intravenously) via a relaxant action on Oddi's sphincter, previously contracted by morphine. The maximum dose for immediate unblocking was 25 mg/kg and increasing the dose gave a delayed response time (Giachetti et al., 1988).

Uterus There was a decrease in the spontaneous contractions in the rat when rosemary oil was applied, and this was also shown by some of its components. Mixing several other essential oils with rosemary also had a relaxant effect (A3; A4; Lis-Balchin and Hart, 1997b).

Other activities A hyperglycaemic effect was observed in glucose-loaded rats treated after an intramuscular dose of 925 mg/kg of rosemary essential oil (Al-Hader et al., 1994). In rabbits with alloxan-induced diabetes given 25 mg/kg intramuscular rosemary essential oil 6 hours after fasting, plasma glucose concentrations increased by 17% 6 hours later. The essential oil was toxic to L-1210 leukaemia cells (Ilarionova et al., 1992). Benzo(a)pyrene- and DMBA-induced tumours are inhibited by rosemary oil applied to mouse skin. Carnosol or ursolic acid inhibited TPA-induced ear inflammation, ornithine decarboxylase activity and tumour promotion (Huang et al., 1994). A stimulating effect was observed for rosemary oil by the increase in locomotor activity in mice (Kovar et al., 1987) after both inhalation or oral administration of rosemary essential oil. This was accompanied by a dose-related increase in serum 1,8-cineole level. There was a stimulating effect on the contingent negative variation brain waves in humans (Kubota et al., 1992). Anticholinesterase activity was absent (Perry et al., 1996). 1,8-Cineole was one of the best acetylcholine inhibitors and best antidistonics of monoterpenes studied (Gracza, 1984). Actions of the essential oils of rosemary and certain of its constituents (eucalyptol and camphor) have an effect on the cerebral cortex of the rat *in vitro* (Steinmetz et al., 1987).

Analysis of performance in 144 participants randomly assigned to one of three independent groups showed that whereas lavender produced a significant decrement in performance of working memory, and impaired reaction times for both memory and attention-based tasks compared with controls, in contrast, rosemary produced a significant enhancement of performance for overall quality of memory and secondary memory factors, but also produced an impairment of speed of memory compared with controls. With regard to mood, both the control and lavender groups were significantly less alert than the rosemary condition; however, the control group was significantly less content than either the rosemary or the lavender group. These findings indicate that the olfactory properties of these essential oils can produce objective effects on cognitive performance, as well as subjective effects on mood (Moss et al., 2003). Three minutes of aromatherapy to 40 adults decreased frontal alpha and beta power, suggesting increased alertness. They also had lower anxiety scores, and were faster, but not more accurate, at completing math computations (Diego et al., 1998).

Rubbing oils (thyme, rosemary, lavender and cedarwood) into the scalp helped with alopecia in 44% of patients compared with 15% of controls in a seven-month, double-blind study of 86 patients (Hay et al., 1998). Lowering of plasma levels of dienic conjugates and ketones, and activation of catalase in red cells characteristic of antioxidant effect were observed in exposure of 150 bronchitis patients to essential oils of rosemary as well as basil, fir and eucalyptus (Siurin, 1997).

In the 1700s rosemary oil was given internally by doctors to control epilepsy. However, it is now continually stated in aromatherapy books to provoke epilepsy, especially in epileptics. There is the possible effect of a conditioned response to the smell. Also apprehension about using a 'dangerous' oil might be enough to trigger a seizure.

Antimicrobial activities

Antibacterial activity

Relative data: There was moderate activity against 21/25 different bacterial species (A1; Lis-Balchin and Deans, 1997; Lis-Balchin et al., 1998a), which was confirmed by other workers using the same species (Deans and Ritchie, 1997). There was also moderate activity against 16/20 Listeria monocytogenes varieties (A1; Lis-Balchin and Deans, 1997; Lis-Balchin et al., 1998a) but no activity was shown against five Listeria varieties in other studies (Aureli et al., 1992). Moderately good activity was shown against four different bacteria (Friedman et al., 2002); good activity against 5/5 bacteria (Maruzella, 1960); and poor activity against respiratory tract pathogens (Inouye et al., 2001).

Antifungal activity

Relative data (% inhibition): Aspergillus niger 12%, A. ochraceus 14%, Fusarium culmorum 0% (A1). In other studies 5/5 fungi were affected (Maruzella and Sicurella, 1960) and low to moderate activity was shown against 15/15 fungi (Maruzella and Liguori, 1958). Mycelial growth of aflatoxin-producing Aspergillus parasiticus is stopped by 0.2–1% rosemary essential oil (also coriander, black pepper and bay) (Tantaoui-Elaraki, Beraoud, 1994).

Other activity

Antiviral activity was shown only in a dried 95% ethanol extract of rosemary containing no essential oil (Barnes et al., 2002). Antioxidant activity was also apparent in extracts not the essential oil (Baratta et al., 1998b).

Use in pregnancy and lactation: contraindications

Rosemary is stated to be an abortifacient (Farnsworth, 1974) and to affect the menstrual cycle (i.e. an emmenagogue). It also has a spasmolytic effect on the uterine muscle in vitro and therefore use of rosemary essential oil in aromatherapy massage is not recommended in pregnancy and parturition, nor advised during lactation.

Pharmaceutical guidance

As it has possible epilepsy-inducing properties (probably due to camphor, which can be as high as 50%), rosemary essential oil should not be used in epileptics as high doses could cause epileptiform convulsions, as found when taken orally (Tisserand and Balacs, 1995; see also Chapter 7). It should not be used in aromatherapy massage or inhalation in children under five. Rosemary essential oil can otherwise be used in aromatherapy massage, except in sensitive people, and also as a fragrance; its stimulating properties could be of some benefit alone or in addition to massage.

Use in babies and young children

Due to the immaturity and the delicate nature of the skin of babies and young children, it is inadvisable for any essential oils, especially this essential oil high in camphor, to be used in massage, however much the essential oil has been diluted in the carrier oils. This is also a necessary precaution due to the possibilities of sensitisation of the children at this young age through skin or air-borne odorant effects (see Chapters 5 and 7).

Instillation or administration of essential oils near the baby or young child's nose is not only not recommended, but distinctly inadvisable, as there have been numerous cases reported of severe toxicity and even death from such applications (see Chapter 7).

Rosewood Oil

CAS numbers

USA: 8015-77-8; EINECS: 83863-32-5

Species/Botanical name

Aniba roseadora var. *amazonica* Ducke (Lauraceae)

Synonyms

Bois de rose, *Aniba parviflora* Mez., *Ocotea caudata* Mez.

Other species

Bois de rose refers only to the *Aniba roseadora* oil, but other species of tree are used as rosewood, including: *Acacia excelsia* (Australian), *Amyris balsamifera* (West Indian), *Dicypellium caryophyllatum* (Brazilian), *Myrospermum erythroxylon* (Japanese), *Pterocarpus erinaceus* (African), *Thespesia populaca* (Polynesian) and *Louro nhamuy* (Brazilian). See also ho leaf oil monograph.

Safety

CHIP details
None

RIFM recommended safety of use limits
10% (A23)

EU sensitiser total
92.5 (based on linalool 90%, limonene 1% and geraniol 1.5%) (A27)

GRAS status
Granted (Fenaroli, 1997).

Extraction, source, appearance and odour

Extraction
A volatile oil is obtained by steam distillation or water distillation of comminuted wood of the tree (Arctander, 1960).

Source
Brazil, Peru and French Guiana.

Appearance and odour
A colourless to pale yellow, sweet-smelling, slightly woody, somewhat floral-spicy essential oil; the top-note sometimes has a peppery-camphoraceous note reminiscent of cineole and nutmeg terpenes. There is often a drop-out of water, which is dissolved in the essential oil during distillation, after shipment, especially if the drums are exposed to cold (Arctander, 1960).

Aromatherapy uses

Rosewood essential oil, like Moroccan chamomile, citronella, clary sage, geranium, vetiver and ylang ylang, was originally produced solely for the perfumery and fragrance trades. However, aromatherapy uses include: acne, wrinkles; immune system (colds, fever); nervous system (frigidity, headaches), stress-related disorders; urinogenital (vaginal *Candida*), sexual abuse victims, aphrodisiac; nervous depression, low energy via overwork, jet-lag, calming during meditation (Ryman, 1991; Lawless, 1992; Rose, 1992a,b; Price, 1993; Sheppard-Hanger, 1995).

Scientific comment

Rosewood essential oil has a pleasant fragrance and should be used as such, as the sensitisation potential when massaged into the skin may prove detrimental, especially to people with existing skin problems. Massage itself can alleviate many stress-related conditions and in combination with the fragrance should prove beneficial as rosewood essential oil has relaxant effects on the human brain (A14).

Herbal uses

No traditional essential oil uses have been documented as the essential oil was originally produced solely for the perfumery and fragrance trades; the wood is used for furniture and figurines.

Food and perfumery uses

Food   Rosewood (FEMA 2156) is used in various baked goods, frozen diary, meats, candies, beverages and chewing gum (Fenaroli, 1997).

Perfumery   Rosewood is used in perfumery where linalool notes are needed. Due to ecological considerations, it is not favoured greatly and is often replaced nowadays by ho leaf oil and synthetic linalool (Arctander, 1960).

Chemistry

Major components

	% (*Lawrence, 1976–2001*)
Linalool	85.3
1,8-Cineole	0–1.6
Limonene	0–1.5
Geraniol	trace–1.5
α-Terpineol	1–3.5

Rosewood Brazil ISO 3761 (1976) gives the following data: min. 84% linalool (alcohol) max 93% after acetylation; the 1990 draft gives: linalool****; methyl benzoate**; α-terpineol**; geraniol*; cis-linalool oxide, *trans*-linalool oxide, pinenes. The number of asterisks denotes relative concentrations.

The small amount of genuine rosewood oil that is around is probably illegal. This is because the rosewood species that have been used for logging and oil are classified as endangered species under international agreements. To get round this, traders sometimes label the essential oil from the leaves of the trees as 'rosewood oil'.

Adulteration

Ho leaf oil is more often produced these days, because of the ecological reasons mentioned above. Rosewood is often made of synthetic linalool with other synthetic components such as terpineol and myrcene and also various fractions of pine oil, added for 'authenticity' (A8; see Chapter 4).

Toxicity

Acute toxicity (A22)

Oral LD$_{50}$ >5 g/kg (rat).

Dermal LD$_{50}$ >5 g/kg (rabbit).

Irritation and sensitisation (A22)

It is reported as non-irritant and non-sensitising on animal and human skin but contains potential sensitisers. Acetylated essential oil nil at 12%.

Phototoxicity

None reported.

Bioactivities

Pharmacological activities *in vitro* and *in vivo*

Smooth muscle   Rosewood oil had a spasmolytic effect on the electrically stimulated smooth muscle of the guinea-pig ileum *in vitro* (A2; Lis-Balchin *et al.*, 1996a). Linalool had a similar effect and also relaxed tracheal muscle (Brandt, 1988).

Uterus   There was a decrease in the spontaneous contractions in the rat for rosewood oil, linalool and limonene; mixing several other essential oils with rosewood oil also had a relaxant effect (A3; A4; Lis-Balchin and Hart, 1997b).

Skeletal muscle   Linalyl acetate caused a decrease in the twitch and a delayed increase in resting tone in the rat phrenic nerve–diaphragm; linalool caused a decrease in the twitch only (Lis-Balchin and Hart, 1997c).

Other activities   Linalool is a general relaxant (see lavender oil monograph). Evidence for the sedative properties of linalool after inhalation in animals was provided as it significantly decreased the motility of 'normal' test mice as well as that of animals rendered hyperactive or 'stressed' by an intraperitoneal dose of caffeine (Buchbauer *et al.*, 1991, 1993b). The dose-dependent, sedative effect of linalool on the CNS of rats (Elisabetsky *et al.*, 1995) may be caused by its inhibitory activity on glutamate binding in the cortex (Elisabetsky *et al.*, 1995). There are many psychological, physiological and biochemical effects of linalool and lavender, with linalool as its main component (see lavender oil monograph). The effect of linalool and lavender on guinea-pig ileum correlated with its chemical profile and the relaxant effect shown in aromatherapy (A11; A12; A13).

Antimicrobial activities

Antibacterial activity

Relative effect: Rosewood oil was effective against 24/25 different bacterial species and 12/20 *Listeria monocytogenes* varieties (A1; Lis-Balchin and Deans, 1997; Lis-Balchin *et al.*, 1998a). Good effect was noted against four different bacteria (Friedman *et al.*, 2002).

Antifungal activity (A1)

Relative effect (% inhibition): *Aspergillus niger* 72%, *A. ochraceus* 63%, *Fusarium culmorum* 71%.

Poor to good activity was shown against 4/5 fungi (Maruzella and Sicurella, 1960).

Use in pregnancy and lactation: contraindications

There was a loss of spontaneous contractions in the uterus when the essential oil was applied to the rat *in vitro*, and as there are no further data available and the sensitisation potential is so high, rosewood essential oil should not be massaged into the skin during pregnancy, parturition and lactation. The fragrance should be harmless in moderation.

Pharmaceutical guidance

Many species of the so-called 'rosewoods' are on the CITES (Convention on International Trade in Endangered Species) lists which prohibit importation of the wood into all signatory countries, including the USA. One such species, *Aniba rosaeodora*, which is found in Brazil, Colombia, Ecuador, French Guiana, Peru and Surinam, is endangered in all these countries and is in the global threat category. Severe ecological harm was being caused by the 'mining' of wild forest trees (Ohashi *et al.*, 1997), especially in Brazil.

The essential oil is non-toxic except for its strong sensitisation potential. It should not be used in aromatherapy massage due to the sensitisation risk and because of the ecological reasons outlined above. Ho leaf essential oil is readily available as a replacement (see ho leaf oil monograph).

Use in babies and young children

Due to the immaturity and the delicate nature of the skin of babies and young children, it is inadvisable for any essential oils to be used in massage, however much the essential oil has been diluted in the carrier oils. This is also a necessary precaution due to the possibilities of sensitisation of the children at this young age through skin or air-borne odorant effects (see Chapters 5 and 7).

Instillation or administration of essential oils near the baby or young child's nose is not only not recommended, but distinctly inadvisable, as there have been numerous cases reported of severe toxicity and even death from such applications (see Chapter 7).

Sage Oil

CAS numbers

Dalmatian: USA: 84082-79-1; EINECS: 97952-71-1
Spanish: USA: 8016-65-7; EINECS: 93384-40-8

Species/Botanical name

Salvia officinalis L. (Labiatae/Lamiaceae)

Synonyms

Dalmatian sage, garden sage, true sage.

Other species

Other sages used for the production of essential oils are *S. lavandulaefolia* Vahl. (Spanish sage) and *S. sclarea* L. (clary sage) (see separate clary sage monograph).

Safety

CHIP details
Dalmation: Xn; R10, 65; 30%; S62 (A26)
Spanish: Xn; R10, 65; 30%; S62 (A26)

RIFM recommended safety of use limits
Dalmatian and Spanish: 8% (A23)

EU sensitiser total
Dalmatian sage oil: 0.9 (based on geraniol 0.4% and linalool 0.5%)
Spanish sage oil: 4 (based on geraniol 0.4%, limonene 1% and linalool 2.6%) (A27)

GRAS status
For both Dalmatian and Spanish sage oils (Fenaroli, 1997).

Extraction, source, appearance and odour

Extraction
Steam distillation of the tops of herb (Arctander, 1960).

Source
Yugoslavia, Hungary and Spain.

Appearance and odour
Dalmatian sage oil is a pale yellow liquid and has a fresh herbaceous, warm spicy, somewhat camphoraceous odour and flavour, reminiscent of *Artemisia vulgaris* oil. The fade-out is sweetly-herbaceous and pleasant (Arctander, 1960).

Spanish sage is a pale yellow liquid and has a fresh-herbaceous odour, with cineole and camphor notes. It has a sharp pine-like top-note and little or no sweetness on dry-out (Arctander, 1960).

Aromatherapy uses

Some aromatherapy books do not advise the use of Dalmatian sage or ignore it (Tisserand and Balacs, 1985; Ryman, 1991; Lawless, 1992), but others give many uses including: external use as an astringent, mouth rinse, vaginal or anal rinse; insect bites, stings, bruises, burns, wounds, herpes, laryngitis, flu, catarrh, toothache; inhaled for depression, although it may be too strong for some; activating adrenals; asthma, menopause, painful periods, thrush, epilepsy, giddiness. It is also said to act on the psyche and emotions to soothe nerves (Rose, 1992a,b; Price, 1993; Sheppard-Hanger, 1995).

Scientific comment

It is unlikely that most of the uses above could be alleviated by massage with a dilute sage essential oil, however massage itself can prove beneficial in symptoms of stress and muscular aches and pains. The use of sage essential oil to enhance memory is only now beginning to be re-examined after many centuries of herbal use.

Herbal uses

Sage is considered to be carminative, antispasmodic, antiseptic, astringent and to have antihidrotic properties (Martindale, 1992). It is used with other essential oils in treating respiratory tract disorders; also in mouthwashes and gargles for disorders of the mouth and throat; also in homeopathic medicine. Traditionally, it has been used to treat flatulent dyspepsia, pharyngitis, uvulitis, stomatitis, gingivitis, glossitis (internally or as a gargle/mouthwash), hyperhidrosis and galactorrhoea. The herbals of Gerard, Culpeper and Hill credit sage with the ability to enhance memory and this is now being researched further (Perry *et al.*, 1998). Presently, sage herb, taken orally, is approved for dyspeptic symptoms and excessive perspiration, and external use for inflammation of mucous membranes of mouth and throat (Wren, 1988; Chevallier, 1996; Blumenthal *et al.*, 2000; Barnes *et al.*, 2002).

Food and perfumery use

Food Dalmatian sage essential oil (FEMA 3001), category N2, is found in many foods and beverages: this category (Flavourings and Food Regulation, 1992) indicates that the concentration of thujones (α and β) present in the final product 'does not exceed 0.5 mg/kg, with the exceptions of alcoholic beverages (10 mg/kg), bitters, vermouth and absinth (35 mg/kg), food containing sage (25 mg/kg) and sage stuffing (250 mg/kg)'. Spanish sage (FEMA 3003) is also used in foods and beverages (Fenaroli, 1997).

Perfumery Dalmatian sage oil is used in perfumery partly as a top-note and partly for its tenacity. The oil blends well with lavandin, rosemary, citrus, and bois de rose oil. It is used in fougeres, chypres, aldehydic perfume bases, colognes and spicy men's fragrances and aftershaves (Arctander, 1960).

Spanish sage oil is used in soap perfumery and reconstitution of other essential oils like spike lavender, as the latter is very similar (Arctander, 1960).

Chemistry

Major components

	% (Lawrence, 1976–2001)	
	Dalmatian	Spanish
1,8-Cineole	8–24	18–54
α-Thujone	15–48	0
β-Thujone	2–25	0
Camphor	2–27	1–36
Linalool	0–32	0–9
α-Pinene	trace	4–20
β-Pinene	trace	6–19
Camphene	trace	4–30
p-Cymene	trace	1–5

Sage (ISO 526: 1991): *Salvia lavandulaefolia* Spanish sage:

	%	
	Min	Max
α-Pinene	4	11
Sabinene	0.1	3
Limonene	2	5
1,8-Cineole	11	25
Thujone α- β-	less than 0.5, usually zero	
Camphor	11	36
Linalool	0.5	9
Linalyl acetate		less than 5
Terpinen-4-ol		less than 2
Borneol	1	8

Adulteration

Commercial sage oil is often substituted with *Salvia triloba* whose main component is 1,8-cineole (42–64%), with α-thujone only accounting for 1–5%. Compared with *S. officinalis*, the volatile oil yield of various *Salvia* species is lower, with lower total ketone content and higher total alcohol content (Ivanic and Savin, 1976). Thujone from American cedarwood is also added to the Dalmatian sage or even Greek sage. Palmarosa oil is also added (A8; see Chapter 4).

Toxicity

Acute toxicity (A22)

Oral LD$_{50}$ Dalmatian and Spanish: 5 g/kg (rat).

Dermal LD$_{50}$ Dalmatian and Spanish: >5 g/kg (rabbit).
Greek oil is untested.

Irritation and sensitisation (A22)

Both nil at 8% (human). But sage oil has been reported as a moderate skin irritant (A22).

Phototoxicity

Nil for Spanish oil; Dalmatian untested.

Other toxicities

A case of human poisoning has been documented following ingestion of sage oil for acne (Centini *et al.*, 1987). Convulsant activity in both humans and animals has been reported for sage oil (Millet, 1980; Millet *et al.*, 1981). In rats, the subclinical, clinical and lethal doses for convulsant action of sage oil were estimated as 0.3, 0.5 and 3.2 g/kg when studied in 65 male and female rats intra-peritoneally at progressively increasing doses. The thujone and pinocamphone components were also tested (Millet *et al.*, 1981). Convulsions were shown for thujone and pinocamphone at lower doses: thujone at 0.2 g/kg and pinocamphone at 0.05 g/kg, suggesting that small doses repeated every day for a short time could produce convulsions (Millet *et al.*, 1981; see also Chapter 7). This toxicity is largely due to the ketones camphor and thujone in the essential oil. Camphor readily produces convulsions at high doses (Craig, 1953). Poisoning by the essential oil showed a period of latency, then the patients vomited and had convulsions, resembling epileptic fits, sometimes with cyanosis (Millet *et al.*, 1981). Three case studies associated with epileptic seizures in normal people, including a child, were reported due to sage and other essential oils. One adult had taken 'a mouthful' of sage essential oil daily for hyperlipaemia over several years, but after a larger dose she had had tonic seizures and became unconscious for an hour. She recovered afterwards. A person, 'feeling tired', was given a dozen drops of sage by a friend and started epileptic fits within 20 minutes (see also Chapter 7).

Salvia officinalis has no mutagenic or DNA-damaging activity using the Ames test or *Bacillus* rec-assay (*Monographs on the Medicinal Uses of Plant Drugs*, 1996).

Bioactivities

Pharmacological activities *in vitro* and *in vivo*

Smooth muscle Dalmatian sage oil had a spasmolytic effect on the electrically stimulated smooth muscle of the guinea-pig ileum *in vitro* (A2; Taddei *et al.*, 1988; Lis-Balchin *et al.*, 1996a). Antispasmodic action *in vitro* (guinea-pig ileum) has been reported for a sage extract (Todorov *et al.*, 1984). Antispasmodic activity *in vivo* (guinea-pig) was shown for sage oil given intravenously, and the contraction of Oddi's sphincter induced by intra-venous morphine was relaxed (Giachetti *et al.*, 1988).

Uterus Dalmatian sage essential oil and some of its components caused a decrease in the spontaneous contractions of rat uterus (A3; A4; Lis-Balchin and Hart, 1997b).

Other activities Hypotensive activity in anaesthetised cats and CNS-depressant action (prolonged barbiturate sleep) in anaesthetised mice were reported (Taddei *et al.*, 1988). The latest research for novel drugs for the treatment of Alzheimer's disease has concentrated on the anticholinesterase activity of sage as it was noted in old herbals that sage enhances the memory (Perry *et al.*, 2001). Anticholinesterase was inhibited *in vitro* by the essential oils of *S. officinalis* (52%) and *S. lavandulaefolia* (63%) (Perry *et al.*, 2001). The IC_{50} value of *S. lavandulaefolia* oil was very low at 0.03 µg/mL and the components 1,8-cineole and α-pinene were also shown to be acetylcholinesterase inhibitors with low IC_{50} values of 0.67 and 0.63 mmol/L, respectively (Perry *et al.*, 2000). These findings suggest that if the inhibitory activity of the essential oil is primarily due to the main inhibitory terpenoid constituents identified, *S. lavandulaefolia* essential oil showed a selective decrease in acetylcholinesterase activity in different parts of the brain at lower and higher doses (Barnes *et al.*, 2002).

Hypoglycaemic activity *in vivo* (rabbits) was shown for *S. lavandulaefolia* (herb) (Jimenez *et al.*, 1986) and various extracts of *Salvia* species, including *S. officinalis* (Cabo *et al.*, 1985).

Antimicrobial activities

Antibacterial activity

Relative data for Dalmatian sage oil: there was activity against 16/25 different bacteria and 6/20 *Listeria monocytogenes* varieties (A1; Lis-Balchin and Deans, 1997; Lis-Balchin *et al.*, 1998a); no activity was shown against five *Listeria* varieties (Aureli *et al.*, 1992) and 3/25 different bacteria were affected (Deans and Ritchie, 1987). The vapour affected 2/5 bacteria (Maruzella and Sicurella, 1960) and moderate to good activity was shown against 5/5 bacteria (Friedman *et al.*, 2002).

Spanish sage oil inhibited the growth of only 1/10 different bacteria (A22).

Antifungal activity

Relative data for Dalmatian sage (% inhibition): *Aspergillus niger* 0%, *A. ochraceus* 53%, *Fusarium culmorum* 33% (A1). Both Dalmatian and Spanish sage oils had an effect on 5/5 fungi; Grecian sage oil had an effect on 14/15 fungi and Spanish oil on 15/15 (Maruzella and Ligouri, 1958).

The antimicrobial activity of the essential oil was attributed to thujone using gelatin-acacia capsules of sage essential oil which exhibited a lag-time for antibacterial activity and inhibited antifungal activity (Jalsenjak *et al.*, 1987).

Clinical studies

A double-blind, placebo-controlled, crossover study involving 20 healthy volunteers compared the effects of *S. lavandulaefolia* oil and sunflower oil and the results showed some effects of sage oil in modulating mood and cognition (Barnes *et al.*, 2002).

Use in pregnancy and lactation: contraindications

Sage oil (especially Dalmatian) is contraindicated during pregnancy as traditionally it is considered to be an abortifacient and to affect the menstrual cycle (Farnsworth, 1975). This is due to the high proportion of α- and β-thujones, which are known to be abortifacient and emmenagogic. In recent studies *in vitro*, there was a loss of spontaneous contractions in the uterus when the essential oil was applied, which also occurs with other essential oils. The essential oil could possibly be used sparingly as a fragrance.

Pharmaceutical guidance

Sage (Dalmatian) oil is toxic (due to the thujone content) and therefore should not be ingested, however, it is commonly used as a culinary ingredient in processed foods and presents no hazard when ingested in small amounts.

As there is a suspicion of toxic effects associated with Dalmatian sage essential oil (which at high doses may cause convulsions and seizures) even at low repeated doses, it is not recommended for aromatherapy massage (Tisserand and Balacs, 1996), but it could be used sparingly as a fragrance.

S. lavandulaefolia oil is being investigated for symptomatic treatment of Alzheimer's disease and it has been shown to have bioactive properties related to the pinene and 1,8-cineole content.

Use in babies and young children

Due to the immaturity and the delicate nature of the skin of babies and young children, it is inadvisable for any essential oils to be used in massage, however much the essential oil has been diluted in the carrier oils. This is also a necessary precaution due to the possibilities of sensitisation of the children at this young age through skin or air-borne odorant effects (see Chapters 5 and 7).

Instillation or administration of essential oils near the baby or young child's nose is not only not recommended, but distinctly inadvisable, as there have been numerous cases reported of severe toxicity and even death from such applications (see Chapter 7).

Sandalwood Oil

CAS numbers

East Indian only: USA: 8006-87-9; EINECS: 84757-70-2

Species/Botanical name

Santalum album L. (Santalaceae)

Synonyms

East Indian sandalwood, oleum santali (USP), santal oil

Other species

Eucaria spicata (Australian sandalwood), syn. *Fusanus spicatus* R. Brown, *Santalum spicatum* A. De Candolle, *S. cygnorum* Miquel, muhuhu wood (*Brachyleana hutchensii*) or African sandalwood.

Pterocarpus santalius or *Santalum rubrum* (red sandalwood, red saunders) is solely used for colouring and dyeing. Other varieties come from the Sandwich Islands, Western Australia and New Caledonia. West Indian sandalwood or amyris (*Amyris balsamifera*) is a poor imitation and bears no botanical relation to the East Indian sandalwood. Indonesian sandalwood is a poor imitation of the real *Santalum album*, but is at present the only one available legally.

Safety

CHIP details
None

RIFM recommended safety of use limits
Sandalwood, East Indian: 10% (A23)

EU sensitiser total
0 (A27)

GRAS status
Granted (Fenaroli, 1997).

Extraction, source, appearance and odour

Extraction
The essential oil is obtained by steam distillation of comminuted dried wood chips of the tree (Arctander, 1960). The true sandalwood, *S. album*, is an evergreen, semi-parasitic tree native to southern Asia, the other varieties growing in the Pacific and Australasia. The tree is medium sized (12–15 m) and matures at 40–50 years old, which is when the centre of the slender trunk (the heartwood) has achieved its greatest oil content. The heartwood and roots are fragrant and contain the oil; the bark and sapwood are odourless as are the branches (Arctander, 1960). It grows in the mountainous districts in the Nilgherry Hills, lying mainly in Mysore and Coimbatore, which yield the most valuable wood. By the provisions of a treaty made in 1770 with Hyder Ali, the cutting of the trees in Mysore is entirely under the control of the East India Company, whose officers see to the felling of the trees.

Source
Mysore (India), Indonesia and Australia.

Appearance and odour
A pale yellow to yellow viscous essential oil with a soft, sweet-woody, warm, animal-balsamic odour, of great tenacity. It has no top-note and remains the same during evaporation, having a lingering aroma (Arctander, 1960).

Aromatherapy uses

Uses include: calming, antidepressing, sedating; insomnia, nervous tension, neuralgia (sciatica, lumbago), stress problems; aphrodisiac; chest infections, bronchitis, catarrh, dry cough, laryngitis, sore throat; stimulating the immune system; heart tonic, haemorrhoids, varicosities; decongestion of the lymph and venous systems; digestive and genito-urinary problems, including diarrhoea, nausea, vomiting, heartburn, constipation; cystitis, kidney or bladder inflammation or congestion, pelvic and prostate congestion; stimulates the sex hormones and reproductive cells; infected wounds, acne, oily skin, dry aged, cracked and chapped skin; a moisturiser; fungal infections (athlete's foot, ringworm and *Candida*); sunburn, dry skin, bacterial skin infection, impetigo, acne, folliculitis; upper respiratory tract infection and inflammatory symptoms from psoriasis, menstrual cramp and arthritis.

Note: Amyris wood (*Amyris balsamifera*) is relaxing to nervous tension. It contains a large percentage of sesquiterpenes, similar to sandalwood, and is used similarly as soothing sedative base note, as antispasmodic to ease coughs and high blood pressure, and as an aphrodisiac (Ryman, 1991; Lawless, 1992; Rose, 1992a,b; Price, 1993; Sheppard-Hanger, 1995).

Scientific comment

It is unlikely that most of the aromatherapy uses are alleviated as there is no scientific evidence apparent. However, sandalwood (Mysore variety) has been shown to be relaxing on human brain waves (A14) and this together with massage, which itself can alleviate many stress symptoms, should prove a useful combination.

Herbal uses

Sandalwood has an uninterrupted sacred 4000-year history. It is mentioned in Sanskrit and Chinese manuscripts. The oil was used in religious ritual, and many deities and temples were carved from its wood. The Ancient Egyptians imported the wood and used it in medicine, embalming and ritual burning to venerate the gods.

In India it is largely consumed in the celebration of sepulchral rites, wealthy Hindus showing their respect for a departed relative by adding sticks of sandalwood to the funeral pile. The powder of the wood, made into a paste with water, is used for making the caste mark, and also for medicinal purposes. The consumption of sandalwood in China appears to be principally for the incense used in the temples. Sandalwood is used for: treatment of subacute and chronic infections of mucous tissues, particularly gonorrhoea; chronic bronchitis, with fetid expectoration, chronic mucous diarrhoea, chronic inflammation of the bladder and pyelitis. It was formerly used as a urinary antiseptic (Martindale, 1982; Wren, 1988; Chevallier, 1996).

Food and perfumery uses

Food East Indian sandalwood oil (FEMA 3005) is used in a variety of food and beverages, but has no great importance (Fenaroli, 1997).

Perfumery It is used as a blender in numerous perfumes like woody-orientals, chypres, fougeres, carnation and numerous floral perfumes. It blends well with: rose, violet, clove, lavender, black pepper, bergamot, geranium, labdanum, vetiver, patchouli, mimosa, myrrh and jasmine (Arctander, 1960).

Chemistry

Major components

	% (*Lawrence, 1976–2001*)
α-Santalol	45–60
β-Santanol	17–30
epi-β-Santalol	4–5
trans-β-Santalol	1–2
α-Santalene	5–7
cis-Lanceol	1–3

The essential oil from *S. spicatum* contains santalols but at a lower level than that of *S. album*. It contains bisabolols and farnesol in significant amounts and it contains significantly higher levels of nuciferols. *S. album* is being grown in Australia too, but will take 15 years to mature.

Adulteration

East Indian sandalwood oil is often adulterated with Australian sandalwood oil, auracaria oil, copaiba oil, Atlas cedar fractions, amyris oils and various other woody oils, e.g. muhuhu. It is diluted with solvents such as benzyl alcohol, benzyl benzene and dipropyl glycol.

Sandela, sandalore, santal and other synthetic sandalwood-smelling components are used as much cheaper substitutes (A8; see Chapter 4).

Toxicity

Acute toxicity (A22)

Oral LD$_{50}$ >5 g/kg (rat).

Dermal LD$_{50}$ >5 g/kg (rabbit).

Irritation and sensitisation (A22)

None at 10%; rare dermatitis and allergic reactions in hypersensitive individuals.

Phototoxicity

None reported.

Other toxicities

Acute oral and dermal toxicity studies for the Australian sandalwood essential oil found no signs of toxicity (Kaaber, 2000) and repeat insult patch testing assayed to ascertain allergenic/sensitivity potential showed that the oil is not a primary irritant nor primary sensitiser to the skin.

Bioactivities

Pharmacological activities *in vitro* and *in vivo*

Smooth muscle   No data found.

Other activities   Anti-inflammatory activities of Australian sandalwood oil were significant against UV-induced inflammation, similar to that of the positive control, indometacin, a known anti-inflammatory agent (Greenoak, 2000). The research involved testing the ability of the essential oil to inhibit the enzymes responsible for the inflammatory reaction at a cellular level, including the enzyme 12-lipoxygenase. 12-Hydroxyeicosatetraenoic acid (12(*S*) HETE) plays a role in the growth-promoting effects of angiotensin II in vascular smooth muscle and adrenal cells and the chemotactic effects of platelet-derived growth factor (Ask, 2000). These were largely commissioned studies and not published in peer-reviewed journals.

The sedative action of sandalwood essential oil has been shown using contingent negative variation studies in humans, motility in mice and smooth muscle *in vitro* (A14).

Antimicrobial activities

Antibacterial activity

Only 1/5 different bacteria were affected by the vapour (Maruzella and Sicurella, 1960). Australian sandalwood oil demonstrated the greatest degree of antimicrobial efficacy of 10 essential oils studied (Beylier and Givaudan, 1979). The bacteriostatic effect against *Staphylococcus aureus* was 25 times greater than that of tea tree oil and demonstrated the greatest degree of bacteriostatic activity against the yeast *Candida albicans*. European research (Ask, 2000) confirmed that Australian sandalwood oil is biocidal, *in vitro*, against many Gram-positive organisms, including *Staph. aureus* and methicillin-resistant *Staph. aureus* (MRSA) in addition to the organisms responsible for acne, thrush and tinea (Athlete's foot and ringworm). The diptheroid organism implicated in the manifestation of body odour, *Corynebacterium xerosis*,

was also strongly inhibited. With all bacteria except the Enterobacteriaceae, sandalwood oil demonstrated significantly greater antimicrobial efficacy than terpinen-4-ol, the main component of tea tree oil. Australian sandalwood oil also inhibits the growth of *Herpes simplex virus 1*, the causative agent of cold sores and genital herpes.

Antifungal activity

Only 3/15 different fungi were slightly affected by the essential oil (Maruzella and Liguori, 1958).

Use in pregnancy and lactation: contraindications

There are no grounds for restricting the use of this essential oil, provided that it is genuine.

Pharmaceutical guidance

The toxicity of the essential oil is low and the biological activity is largely unknown except for its microbiological action and anti-inflammatory effects. It does not offer any serious contraindications for usage, if the genuine *S. album* essential oil is used or the Australian, *S. spicatum*. It is unlikely that most of the aromatherapy conditions are alleviated and there is no scientific evidence apparent; however, sandalwood (Mysore variety) has been shown to be relaxing, and this together with massage, which itself can alleviate many stress symptoms, should prove a useful combination.

Use in babies and young children

Due to the immaturity and the delicate nature of the skin of babies and young children, it is inadvisable for any essential oils to be used in massage, however much the essential oil has been diluted in the carrier oils. This is also a necessary precaution due to the possibilities of sensitisation of the children at this young age through skin or air-borne odorant effects (see Chapters 5 and 7).

Instillation or administration of essential oils near the baby or young child's nose is not only not recommended, but distinctly inadvisable, as there have been numerous cases reported of severe toxicity and even death from such applications (see Chapter 7).

Savory Oil

CAS numbers

USA: 8016-68-0; EINECS: 84775-98-4

Species/Botanical name

Satureja hortensis L. (Labiatae)

Synonyms

Summer savory, garden savory, *Calamintha hortensis*

Other species

Winter savory, *Satureya montana*, syn. *S. obovata*, *Calamintha montana*

Safety

CHIP details
T; R24, 38, 65; 70%; S28, 36/37, 45, 62 (A26)

RIFM recommended safety of use limits
0.5% (A23)

EU sensitiser total
Not given (A27)

GRAS status
Granted (Fenaroli, 1997).

Extraction, source, appearance and odour

Extraction
A volatile oil is obtained by steam distilling the tops and leaves of the herb (Arctander, 1960).

Source
France and Eastern Europe.

Appearance and odour
A light yellow to dark brown essential oil, with a spicy, aromatic odour resembling thyme and origanum (Arctander, 1960).

Aromatherapy uses

Uses include: cuts, bites, abcesses, burns, ulcers; acne, asthma, cold sores, flatulence, sexual problems, arthritis, lumbago, rheumatism; vaginal thrush, cystitis; agitation, frigidity, impotence, depression, nervous exhaustion (Lawless, 1992; Rose, 1992a,b; Price, 1993). Some aromatherapy books do not advise the use of savory essential oil in aromatherapy (e.g. Ryman, 1991).

Scientific comment
There is no scientific proof that any of the conditions listed are alleviated by massage with the diluted savory essential oil, and the herbal uses on which all the uses are based mainly involve the water-soluble tea. Massage itself can alleviate many stress and muscular conditions.

Herbal uses

Satureja hortensis L. (Lamiaceae) is a medicinal plant that has been used since the times of Ancient Greece. It is named after the satyr, due to its aphrodisiac properties. In the Middle Ages the great Hildegard of Bingen advised the use of savory for gout and it has been in the German and French Pharmacopoeiae since 1582 as a stomachic and stimulant. It is used in Iranian folk medicine as a muscle and bone pain reliever. It has also been used, mainly as a tea, for nausea, indigestion, menstrual disorders, asthma, catarrh, insect bites, externally (Wren, 1988; Lawless, 1992; Chevallier, 1996).

Food and perfumery uses

Food Summer savory (FEMA 3013) and winter savory (FEMA 3017) are used in many foods and beverages (Fenaroli, 1997).

Perfumery Savory is sometimes used in herbaceous types of perfumery (Arctander, 1960).

Chemistry

Major components

	% *(Lawrence, 1976–2001)*
Carvacrol	18–75
γ-Terpinene	34–63
p-Cymene	3–5

Myrcene	0.5–3
α-Pinene	tr–1
Myrtenol	tr–0.5
Camphene	tr–6
Linalool	tr–0.4

Adulteration

The usual adulteration with similar essential oils, such as high carvacrol marjoram, is found, as well as the use of synthetic components (A8; see Chapter 4).

Toxicity

Acute toxicity (A22)

Oral LD$_{50}$ 1.4 g/kg (rat).

Dermal LD$_{50}$ 0.34 g/kg (rabbit); >2.5 g/kg (guinea-pig).

Irritation and sensitisation (A22)

No effect when tested at 6% on humans. It was strongly irritating to rabbit and guinea-pig skin undiluted and caused excoriation to mouse skin in 48 hours after application and 50% died. At 10% oedema occurred, but it was non-irritating at 1%.

Phototoxicity

None reported.

Bioactivities

Pharmacological activities *in vitro* and *in vivo*

Smooth muscle None found.

Other activities Antinociceptive and anti-inflammatory effects of *Satureja hortensis* L. extracts and essential oil have been described (Hajhashemi *et al.*, 2002). The analgesic activity of savory essential oil was assessed using light tail flick, formalin and acetic acid-induced writhing in mice and the anti-inflammatory effects were assessed using carrageenan-induced paw oedema in rats. The essential oil (200 mg/kg, p.o.) inhibited the mice writhing responses caused by acetic acid and in the formalin test the essential oil (50–200 mg/kg, p.o.) showed analgesic activity. Pretreatment with naloxone (1 mg/kg, i.p.) or caffeine (20 mg/kg, i.p.) failed to reverse this antinociceptive activity. The essential oil (200 mg/kg) reduced oedema caused by carrageenan. These results suggested to the authors that *S. hortensis* has antinociceptive and anti-inflammatory effects without involvement of opioid and adenosine receptors mediating the antinociception.

Antispasmodic and antidiarrhoeal effects of *S. hortensis* essential oil were also shown (Hajhashemi *et al.*, 2000).

Antimicrobial activities

Antibacterial activity

There was a strong effect against different bacterial species (Deans and Svoboda, 1989) by the essential oil and its constituents: the best were carvacrol, eugenol, thymol, cineole and linalool.

Antifungal activity

None found.

Use in pregnancy and lactation: contraindications

Very little is known about the bioactivity of savory essential oil, especially during pregnancy, etc. and as it has substantial irritant properties, the essential oil cannot be recommended for dermal usage in pregnancy, parturition or lactation. The essential oil can be used as a fragrance in moderation.

Pharmaceutical guidance

There is no scientific proof that any of the conditions treated by aromatherapy are alleviated by massage with the diluted savory essential oil, and the herbal uses, on which all the uses are based, mainly involve the water-soluble tea. Massage itself can alleviate many stress-related and muscular conditions and the fragrance can be used as an accessory for its antimicrobial effect, but should not be used dermally in aromatherapy massage due to its irritant nature.

Use in babies and young children

Due to the immaturity and the delicate nature of the skin of babies and young children, it is inadvisable for any essential oils, especially an irritant essential oil, to be used in massage, however much the essential oil has been diluted in the carrier oils. This is also a necessary precaution due to the possibilities of sensitisation of the children at this young age through skin or air-borne odorant effects (see Chapters 5 and 7).

Instillation or administration of essential oils near the baby or young child's nose is not only not recommended, but distinctly inadvisable, as there have been numerous cases reported of severe toxicity and even death from such applications (see Chapter 7).

Spearmint Oil

CAS numbers

USA: 8008-79-5; EINECS: 84696-51-51

Species/Botanical name

Mentha spicata L.

Synonyms

Mentha viridis L., *Mentha × cardiaca*, green mint, lamb mint, huile essentielle de menthe crépue, oleum menthae crispae, oleum menthae viridis

Pharmacopoeias

In British and French Pharmacopoeias (Martindale, 2004).

Other species

Mentha arvensis var. *piperascens* Holmes (cornmint), *Mentha × piperita* L. (Lamiaceae), hybrid of *M. spicata × M. aquatica* L. (peppermint)

Safety

CHIP details
Xn; R65; 20%; S62 (A26)

RIFM recommended safety of use limits
4% (A23)

EU sensitiser total
20.2 (based on limonene 20% and linalool 0.2%) (A27)

GRAS status
Granted (Fenaroli, 1997).

Extraction, source, appearance and odour

Extraction
A volatile oil is obtained by steam distillation of freshly harvested, flowering sprigs (Arctander, 1960).

Source
USA, China, India, South America, Italy and Japan.

Appearance and odour
Spearmint is a pale yellow/pale olive essential oil with a very warm, slightly green-herbaceous odour penetrating and powerful, just like the crushed herb (Arctander, 1960). It is similar to peppermint, but sweeter and lighter and spicy.

Aromatherapy uses

Despite this essential oil having not being used in herbal medicine and designated as a flavour ingredient, aromatherapy books offer many uses for spearmint oil, probably based on mints generally. These include: fatigue, headache, migraine, nervous strain, and stress (exhaustion); digestion (e.g. vomiting, flatulence, constipation and diarrhoea), colic, dyspepsia and hepato-biliary disorders, stimulates the appetite, aids bad breath and sore gums; controls abundance of breast milk and accompanying hardness of breasts, menstrual complaints, eases labour; cystitis, retention of urine; asthma, bronchitis, catarrh, sinusitis; severe itching of the skin, acne, dermatitis, wounds, sores, scabs and healing in general and acts as a local anaesthetic (Lawless, 1992; Sheppard-Hanger, 1995).

Scientific comment

As the chemical composition of spearmint essential oil is totally different to that of the other common mints, peppermint and cornmint, it seems illogical to equate its properties and uses to that of the latter, especially as there is no scientific evidence for alleviation of conditions quoted above. The use of spearmint essential oil in massage is not recommended; the fragrance, used sparingly, could be acceptable but is unlikely to benefit the patient any more than just a massage, which can alleviate many stress and muscular conditions.

Herbal uses

No traditional essential oil uses have been documented. The essential oil is used in flavour trade products; however, properties of spearmint include: local anaesthetic, anti-inflammative, anti-septic, antispasmodic, astringent, carminative, cephalic, cholagogue, choleretic, cicatrizant, decongestant, digestive, diuretic, expectorant, febrifuge, hepatic, nervine, stimulant, stomachic and sedative (Wren, 1988; Sheppard-Hanger, 1995). This is almost identical as for peppermint.

Food and perfumery uses

Food Spearmint (FEMA 3032) is used in various baked goods, frozen diary, meats, candies, beverages and chewing gum (Fenaroli, 1997).

Perfumery Spearmint oil is used in chypres and fougeres (Arctander, 1960). It blends well with bergamot, jasmine, lavender and sandalwood.

Chemistry

Comparison between the three main mints.

Major components

	% (Lawrence, 1976–2001)		
	Peppermint	Spearmint	Cornmint
Menthol	27–50	0.1–0.3	65–80 (38)
Menthone	13–32	0.7–2	3–15 (31)
Isomenthone	2–10	trace	1.9–4.8 (12)
1,8-Cineole	5–14	1–2	0.1–0.3 (0.2–0.8)
(−)-Limonene	1–3	8–12	0.7–6.2 (10)
(−)-Carvone	0	58–70	0
cis-Dihydrocarvone	0	trace–22	0
trans-Dihydrocarvone	0	trace–22	0

Brackets indicate values for dementholised cornmint oil.

ISO for spearmint 3033: (1988) includes the following: species include *M. spicata* L. and *M. viridis* Linn.; *M. x cardiaca* and the essential oil is obtained by steam distillation. Both the BP and ISO state that the oil has not less than 55% carvone. Main components in these are given as: (−)-carvone, dihydrocarvone, menthone, (−)-limonene, phellandrene which is not given in chemical compositions (Lawrence, 1976–2001) and esters.

Adulteration

Addition of (−)-carvone is common but otherwise it is a cheap essential oil, therefore not worth adulterating.

Toxicity

Acute toxicity (A22)

Oral LD$_{50}$ 5 g/kg (rat).
Dermal LD$_{50}$ >5 g/kg (rabbit); 2 g/kg (guinea-pig).

Irritation and sensitisation (A22)

Spearmint has been shown to be safe at 4%, but should be reduced to 0.1% in sensitive people as spearmint oil in toothpaste has caused allergic stomatitis and dermatitis. The acceptable daily intake of carvone (+) and (−) is up to 1.0 m g/kg body weight (Martindale, 1990).

Phototoxicity

None reported.

Bioactivities

Pharmacological activities *in vitro* and *in vivo*

Smooth muscle Both peppermint and spearmint in a watery dilution caused relaxation of the gastric wall and decrease in contractions in the ileum and colon of dogs (Plant and Miller, 1926).

Antimicrobial activities

Antibacterial activity

The effects of the essential oils of spearmint (*Mentha spicata* L.) and of its three major constituents was assessed on the proliferation of *Helicobacter pylori*, *Salmonella enteritidis*, *Escherichia coli* O157:H7, methicillin-resistant *Staphylococcus aureus* (MRSA) and methicillin-sensitive *Staphylococcus aureus* (MSSA). These studies showed that the essential oil and its constituents inhibited the proliferation of each strain and the effects were almost the same against antibiotic-resistant and antibiotic-sensitive strains of *H. pylori* and *Staph. aureus* (Imai *et al.*, 2001). Spearmint oil had inhibitory activity against *Aspergillus flavus*, *A. parasiticus*, *A. ochraceus* and *Fusarium moniliforme* at 3000 ppm (a high concentration) (Soliman and Badeaa, 2002).

Spearmint and peppermint were strongly active against five bacteria tested *in vitro* (Friedman *et al.*, 2002), as was menthol.

Use in pregnancy and lactation: contraindications

As there are few data as to the toxicology and bioactivity of spearmint essential oil, it is not recommended for use in massage during pregnancy and parturition and lactation. It could possibly be used sparingly as a fragrance.

Pharmaceutical guidance

There is scant toxicological, pharmacological or other information available for spearmint essential oil, and as the chemical composition of spearmint essential oil is totally different to that of the other common mints, peppermint and cornmint, it seems illogical to equate its properties and uses to that of the latter. Therefore spearmint essential oil is not recommended for general use in aromatherapy. The use of the occasional fragrance is probably without hazard.

Use in babies and young children

Due to the immaturity and the delicate nature of the skin of babies and young children, it is inadvisable for any essential oils to be used in massage, however much the essential oil has been diluted in the carrier oils. This is also a necessary precaution due to the possibilities of sensitisation of the children at this young age through skin or air-borne odorant effects (see Chapters 5 and 7).

Instillation or administration of essential oils near the baby or young child's nose is not only not recommended, but distinctly inadvisable, as there have been numerous cases reported of severe toxicity and even death from such applications (see Chapter 7).

Spike Lavender Oil

CAS numbers

USA; 8016-78-2; EINECS: 84837-04-7

Species/Botanical name

Lavandula latifolia (L.) Medikus (Labiatae)

Synonyms

Lavandula spica (D.C.), spike lavender; ol. lavand. spic., huile essentielle d'aspic, oleum lavandulae spicatae, spicae actheroleum, spike lavender oil, spike oil

Pharmacopoeias

In French Pharmacopoeia (Martindale, 2004).

Safety

CHIP details
None; R10 (A26)

RIFM recommended safety of use limits
8% (A23)

EU sensitiser total
47 (linalool, 46%; limonene, 1%; coumarin: below 0.1%; geraniol, below 0.1%) (A27)

GRAS status
Granted (Fenaroli, 1997).

Extraction, source, appearance and odour

Extraction
Steam distillation of the herbal tops and flowers gives the essential oil. The different parts of the plant give an essential oil of totally different composition (Arctander, 1960).

Source
Spain and France.

Appearance and odour
A colourless to pale yellow essential oil with a camphoric, eucalyptus-like, fresh, herbaceous, sweet odour, reminiscent of lavandin and rosemary oils and with a dry-woody undertone (Arctander, 1960).

Aromatherapy uses

Spike lavender essential oil is usually merged together with *L. angustifolia*, although it is very different in chemistry and odour. Uses include: calming yet making one more alert; asthenia, neuritis, neuralgia, debility; depressive headaches; upper respiratory and throat infections; bronchitis, laryngitis, rhinitis, sore throat, coughs, tonsillitis, ear infections; rheumatic and muscle pain and paralysis plus rheumatoid arthritis; immune response, influenza and viral infections; digestive disturbances such as flatulence, dyspepsia, colic, colitis due to virus, teething pain when diluted; induces menstruation and eases cramps when used with sages. Used in topical applications for severe burns and wound healing, fungal infections (e.g. ringworm), acne and scar tissue healing; insect stings and bites (Sheppard-Hanger, 1995).

Scientific comment

The aromatherapy uses are taken directly from the old herbals and none of the conditions have been proven to be alleviated using the diluted essential oil. Massage itself can aid many stress and muscular problems and the fragrance of the essential oil, undiluted, with its high camphor content, could alleviate some respiratory problems when inhaled.

Herbal uses

Nardus was the name given to lavender, from Naarda, a city of Syria near the Euphrates; St Mark mentions it as spikenard. 'The chemical oil drawn from Lavender, usually called Oil of Spike, is of so fierce and piercing a quality, that it is cautiously to be used, some few drops being sufficient to be given with other things, either for inward or outward griefs' (Culpeper, 1653). In Spain and Portugal it was only used for strewing the floors of churches and houses on festive occasions. The flowers of this species were used medicinally in England until about the middle of the eighteenth century, the plant being called 'sticadore'. It was one of the ingredients of the 'Four Thieves' Vinegar' famous in the Middle Ages. It was not used for distillation, although in France and Spain country folk extracted an oil, used for dressing wounds, by hanging the flowers downwards in a closed bottle in the sunshine. The Arabs make use of the flowers as an expectorant and antispasmodic (Fernie, 1914). The essential oil, or a spirit of lavender made from it, proves restorative and tonic against faintness, palpitations of a nervous sort, weak giddiness, spasms and colic. It is agreeable to the taste and smell, provokes appetite, raises the spirits and dispels flatulence. A few drops of the essence of lavender in a hot footbath has a marked influence in relieving fatigue. Outwardly applied, it relieves toothache, neuralgia, sprains and rheumatism; used in hysteria, palsy and similar disorders of debility and lack of nerve power, as a powerful stimulant (Gerard, 1597; Culpeper, 1653). It is 'good also against the bitings of serpents, mad-dogs and other venomous creature, being given inwardly and applied poultice-wise to the parts wounded. The spirituous tincture of the dried leaves or seeds, if prudently given, cures hysterick fits' (Salmon, 1710, quoted by Festing, 1989).

Lavender oil was rubbed externally for stimulating paralysed limbs. Mixed with 3/4 spirit of turpentine or spirit of wine it made the famous oleum spicae, formerly much celebrated for curing old sprains and stiff joints. Fomentations with lavender in bags, applied hot, will speedily relieve local pains. An infusion taken too freely, will, however, cause griping and colic, and lavender oil in too large doses is a narcotic poison and causes death by convulsions (Grieve, 1937; Culpeper, 1653).

Results of pharmacological experiments using various lavender species and extracts (see lavender oil monograph) support the findings (Lis-Balchin, 2002b, chs 1, 3, 23) that the information on lavender has been mistakenly transcribed from early herbals, like those of Culpeper (1653), where *L. spica*, the more camphoric lavender was used medicinally and not the very floral *L. angustifolia*. The spasmolytic results shown for the water-soluble extracts of the more camphoraceous *L. stoechas* again support the well-quoted action of the camphoraceous spike lavender over the centuries, emphasising the confusion.

Paramedical uses appear in many modern books (Wren, 1988), where *L. angustifolia* is stated to be a carminative, spasmolytic, tonic and antidepressant. Numerous uses for *L. angustifolia* have been suggested (Bertram, 1995) that are identical to those suggested in the old herbals by Culpeper (1653) and Gerard (1597) for a different species! These

include: nervous headache, neuralgia, rheumatism, depression, insomnia, windy colic, fainting, toothache, sprains, sinusitis, stress and migraine (see also Chapters 2 and 5).

Chemistry

Major components

Lavandula latifolia (L. Medikus) (ISO 4719: 1992) or spike lavender, the spike oil of commerce, has a high yield, 0.8–1.2% and variable composition (Lawrence, 1976–2001). More than 300 components have been identified, the main ones being linalool (19–48%), 1,8-cineole (21–42%) and camphor (5–17%).

	% composition	
	Boelens (1986)	Naef and Morris (1992)
Linalool	41.7	27.6
Linalyl acetate	1.1	1.1
Camphor	12.8	16.3
1, 8-Cineole	26.3	22.9
Terpinen-4-ol	0.6	0.4
β-Caryophyllene	1.4	2.2
Lavandulol	0.6	0.5
Borneol	0.8	1.7
Myrcene	0.2	0.8
β-Farnesene	0	0.3
Limonene	1.1	3.1

Adulteration

Camphor (synthetic) may be added to lavandin oils or synthetic linalool, linalyl acetate etc. It is also cut with Spanish sage oil, rosemary oil, lavandin oils, eucalyptus oils or their fractions; also terpineol production fractions, Chinese camphor oil fractions, etc. Formerly adulteration used to be with oil of turpentine, often mixed with coconut oil, but this has given place to various artificial esters prepared chemically, which are practically odourless and only added to make the oil appear to have a higher ester percentage than it really has. Petitgrain oil has also been mixed in (Lawrence, 1976–2001; A8; see Chapter 4).

Food and perfumery use

Food Spike oil (FEMA 3033) is used in a variety of foods and beverages (Fenaroli, 1997).

Perfumery It has limited use in perfumery (Arctander, 1960), but is used in cheap soaps, etc.

Toxicity

Acute toxicity (A22)

Oral LD$_{50}$ >2 g/kg (rat).
Dermal LD$_{50}$ >4 g/kg (rabbit).

Irritation and sensitisation

Nil at 8%: non-irritant and non-sensitising on animal and human skin but contains potential sensitisers.

Phototoxicity (A22)

Nil, but see lavender oil monograph.

Bioactivities

Pharmacological activities *in vitro* and *in vivo*

Smooth muscle Spike lavender had a spasmolytic action on electrically stimulated smooth muscle of the guinea-pig ileum *in vitro*, as did linalool (A2; Lis-Balchin *et al.*, 1996a). Linalool was reported to relax the small intestine of the mouse (Imaseki and Kitabatake, 1962). A spasmolytic action on rabbit and guinea-pig gut by the essential oil of lavender (*L. spica* L.) has been reported (Shipochliev, 1968). Linalool relaxed the longitudinal muscle of guinea-pig ileum (Reiter and Brandt, 1985).

Uterus There was a decrease in the spontaneous contractions in the rat for spike lavender oil, linalool, limonene and the other components; mixing several other essential oils with spike lavender also had a relaxant effect (A3; A4; Lis-Balchin and Hart, 1997b).

Skeletal muscle Action on skeletal muscle of linalool and linalyl acetate produced a reduction in the size of the contraction in response to stimulation of the phrenic nerve and also when the muscle was stimulated directly (Lis-Balchin and Hart 1997a) (see lavender oil monograph).

Other activities The use of *L. latifolia*, with its high camphoric content was recently suggested as an expectorant (Charron, 1997). (For other physiological, pharmacological and biochemical effects see lavender oil monograph.)

Antimicrobial activities

Antibacterial activity

Antibacterial effect was shown against 19/25 different bacterial species and 12/20 *Listeria*

monocytogenes varieties (A1; Lis-Balchin and Deans, 1997; Lis-Balchin *et al.*, 1998a).

Antifungal activity

Relative values (% inhibition) (A1): *Aspergillus niger* 93%, *A. ochraceus* 58%, *Fusarium culmorum* 31% (see also lavender oil monograph).

Other activities

Spike lavender is included in some veterinary shampoos and other products as an insect repellent, especially for fleas (Wren, 1988).

Use in pregnancy and lactation: contraindications

Spike lavender essential oil is not recommended in aromatherapy massage during pregnancy, parturition and lactation due to its possible deleterious action on the uterus and other muscles. Its high camphoric content and sensitiser value also suggest caution in massage and the use of the fragrance should also be restricted.

Pharmaceutical guidance

Spike lavender essential oil is a very powerful oil, which has been used for centuries in herbal medicine, but its species was misinterpreted by the original aromatherapists and substituted by *L. angustifolia*, which is much less strong. Due to the high camphor content of this essential oil it is unwise to use it frequently in aromatherapy massage or for inhalation (undiluted). There is also a possible deleterious effect in epilepsy and fever (Tisserand and Balacs, 1995; see also rosemary oil monograph).

Use in babies and young children

Due to the immaturity and the delicate nature of the skin of babies and young children, it is inadvisable for any essential oils, especially an essential oil with such a high camphor content, to be used in massage, however much the essential oil has been diluted in the carrier oils. This is also a necessary precaution due to the possibilities of sensitisation of the children at this young age through skin or airborne odorant effects (see Chapters 5 and 7).

Instillation or administration of essential oils near the baby or young child's nose is not only not recommended, but distinctly inadvisable, as there have been numerous cases reported of severe toxicity and even death from such applications (see Chapter 7).

Tea Tree Oil

CAS numbers

USA: 68647-73-4; EINECS: 85085-48-9 8022-72-8

Species/Botanical name

Melaleuca alternifolia (Maiden & Betche) Cheel (Myrtaceae)

Synonyms

Ti-tree, narrow-leaved paperback tea tree, melasol, Australian tea tree oil, melaleucae aetheroleum, oleum melaleucae

Note: The name Ti-tree is also applied to a species of *Cordyline* (Liliaceae) indigenous to New Zealand.

Other species

Melaleuca linariifolia, *M. dissitiflora* and other species. Related species include manuka (*Leptospermum scoparium*) and kanuka (*Kunzea ericoides*). Also cajuput (*Melaleuca leucadendron*). (See separate monographs).

Note: There is a substantial difference between these 'tea-tree' genera and *Melaleuca* (see monographs). Although all three essential oils are used by aromatherapists, only *Melaleuca* has been tested for toxicity, and its antimicrobial activity studied (except for unpublished data by a commercial New Zealand firm).

Safety

CHIP details
Xn; R10, 22, 38, 65; 50%; S62 (A26)

RIFM recommended safety of use limits
1% (A23)

EU sensitiser total
19% (4% limonene, 15% linalool) although linalool is usually under 1%, but seems to increase in some adulterated commercial oils (A27)

GRAS status
Not given.

Extraction, source, appearance and odour

Extraction
A volatile oil is obtained by steam distillation of the leaves and twiglets of the trees (Arctander, 1960).

Source
Australia and Indonesia.

Appearance and odour
A white to pale-yellow, yellow-green liquid with an acrid odour (which can be described as spicy camphoraceous by those that like it) with an occasional whiff of citrus, if fresh (Arctander, 1960).

Aromatherapy uses

Uses include: colds, flu, fever, infections such as *Candida*, chicken pox; sweating out toxins; haemorrhoids, varicosities, phlebitis, stimulating lymphatic circulation; asthma, bronchitis, emphysema, catarrh coughs, tuberculosis, sinusitis, whooping cough, tonsillitis, plus ear, nose and throat infections; thrush, vaginitis, cystitis, and genital infections; mouth ulcers, gingivitis, oral mucosa inflammation, thrush, dental abscesses and ulcers, pyorrhoea, sore throat, and bacterial and parasitic infestation; disinfecting skin, infected wounds, boils, carbuncles; sunburn, abscess and wound healing, acne, ringworm, warts, tinea, impetigo, herpes, rashes, insect bites, nappy rash, burns, cold sores, dandruff (Ryman, 1991; Lawless, 1992; Rose, 1992a,b; Price, 1993; Sheppard-Hanger, 1995).

Scientific comment
There is ample scientific evidence for the antimicrobial potential of tea tree essential oil, but there is a wide variation in the commercial essential oils available and therefore massage with a given tea tree essential oil could not guarantee any effect. Topical applications of tea tree essential oil, including vaginal inserts, etc., do not constitute true aromatherapy application as this is a clinical/medical application and should not be undertaken by non-medically qualified aromatherapists. The use of massage alone can benefit many stress and muscular

conditions and the fragrance in addition could be of antimicrobial significance (see also Chapters 5 and 8).

Herbal uses

The whole plant extract was used originally by aboriginals and the essential oils themselves were used during World War II as a general antimicrobial agent and insect repellant and provided in the first aid kits of serving Australian soldiers. The Australian tea tree oil from *M. alternifolia* and other *Melaleuca* species has strong antimicrobial potential (Carson and Riley, 1993, 1994, 1995b; Lis-Balchin *et al.*, 1996a, 1999; Lis-Balchin and Hart, 2000). It is said to be anti-inflammatory, antiseptic, antiviral, bactericidal, antiparasitic, antifungal, decongestant, expectorant, immune stimulant and insecticidal. It is used for various skin infections including athlete's foot, ringworm, corns, boils, wounds, insect bites. It is also taken internally for chronic infections like cystitis, glandular fever, chronic fatigue syndrome. It is also used in mouthwashes for oral infections and sore throats as a gargle. One of the major novel uses has become the treatment of vaginal infections including thrush (Wren, 1988; Chevallier, 1996; Blumenthal *et al.*, 2000; Barnes *et al.*, 2002).

Food and perfumery uses

Food Tea tree is granted temporary acceptability in foods (Fenaroli, 1997).

Perfumery Not used (Arctander, 1960) or its use in perfumery is marginal; it blends well with lavandin, lavender, clary sage, rosemary, cananga, geranium, marjoram, clove and nutmeg.

Chemistry

Major components

Melaleuca terpinen-4-ol type tea tree (ISO 4730: 1996) (*M. alternifolia*, *M. linariifolia*, *M. dissitiflora* and other species, miscible in 85% EtOH 1:2):

	%	
	Min	Max
Terpinolene	1.5	5
1,8-Cineole	0	15*
α-Terpinene	5	13
γ-Terpinene	10	28
p-Cymene	0.5	12
Terpinen-4-ol	30	30*
α-Terpineol	1.5	8
Limonene	0.5	4
Sabinene	0.5	3.5
Aromadendrene	tr	7
δ-Cadinene	tr	8
Globulol	tr	3
Viridiflorol	tr	1.5
α-Pinene	1	6

*High-grade oil contains less than 10% 1,8-cineole and 45% terpinen-4-ol.

Different *Melaleuca* trees are used and there are a wide variety of grades of seedlings produced; there are even differences between leaves on different branches of the same tree.

Tea tree oil (Ph. Eur. 4.8) is described as the essential oil obtained by steam distillation from the foliage and terminal branchlets of *M. alternifolia*, *M. linariifolia*, *M. dissitiflora*, and/or other species of *Melaleuca*. It contains less than 7.0% aromadendrene, less than 15% cineole, 0.5–12.0% *p*-cymene, 0.5–4.0% limonene, 1.0–6.0% α-pinene, less than 3.5% sabinene, 5.0–13.0% α-terpinene, 10.0–28.0% γ-terpinene, minimum of 30% terpinen-4-ol, 1.5–8.0% α-terpineol and 1.5–5.0% terpinolene (Martindale, 2004).

Adulteration

The oil is relatively cheap and getting cheaper, so adulteration would probably be uneconomical. However, the level of the high-activity terpinen-4-ol and γ-terpinene may be low due to low-quality production and import from Indonesia (this makes the oil less effective, if at all, against microbes), so terpinen-4-ol is added, plus other components. Blending occurs to a large extent using tea tree oils from different species and localities (Perry *et al.*, 1997a,b; Porter *et al.*, 1998; Porter and Wilkins, 1999).

Toxicity

Acute toxicity (A22)

Oral LD$_{50}$ 1.9 g/kg (rat).

Dermal LD$_{50}$ >5 g/kg (rabbit).

Irritation and sensitisation

Tea tree oil is non-irritant at 1% (human), and non-sensitising on animal and human skin (A22) but sensitisation is common (see below) and 1,8-cineole is the main cause, hence its percentage is reduced by the Australian Standards. The essential oil also contains potential sensitisers.

Over 30 cases of allergic sensitivity to tea tree essential oil have been documented and a recent study found that fresh tea tree oil was a very weak allergen. When the oil was exposed to light for 4 days on a windowsill it deteriorated, or photo-oxidised, changing the chemistry of the oil and tripling the allergenic property: peroxides in the deteriorated oil increased by more than ten times compared to that in the fresh oil. It appears that the degradation products from tea tree oil caused by photo-oxidation must be considered responsible for the development of allergic contact dermatitis (Hausen et al., 1999).

A 23-month-old boy became confused and was unable to walk 30 minutes after ingesting less than 10 mL of T36-C7, a commercial product containing 100% melaleuca oil. The child was referred to a nearby hospital. His condition improved and he was asymptomatic within 5 hours of ingestion. He was discharged home the following day (Jacobs and Hornfeldt, 1994).

A 17-month-old boy who ingested less than 10 mL of the oil developed ataxia and drowsiness (Del Beccaro, 1995). A 60-year-old man ingested half a teaspoonful of tea tree oil and developed a dramatic rash, malaise and neutrophil leukocytosis (Elliott, 1993). Some tea tree oils containing a high concentration of 1, 8-cineole have a toxicity similar to that of eucalyptus oil. Toxic doses of eucalyptus oil range from 5 to 30 mL in humans, with symptoms including respiratory depression, coma and death (Seawright, 1993).

A report in a human showed that this toxic reaction was caused by the allergin cineol present in the tea tree oil (De Groot and Weyland, 1992).

Phototoxicity
None reported.

Note: Cases of *Melaleuca* oil toxicosis in cats and dogs have been reported by veterinarians to the National Animal Poison Control Center when the oil was applied dermally. In most cases, the oil was used to treat dermatologic conditions at inappropriately high doses. The typical signs observed were depression, weakness, incoordination and muscle tremors (Villar et al., 1994). Paralysis of the hind legs and also quadriplegia have been reported. Personal experience with tea tree oil applied directly to a cut on the tail of a dog resulted in a 24-hour quadriplegia. Many cases of toxicity to cats were subsequently reported (Florida Vet Scene, 1995).

Bioactivities

Pharmacological activities *in vitro* and *in vivo*

Smooth muscle   Tea tree oil had an initial spasmogenic effect followed by spasmolysis on electrically stimulated guinea-pig ileum *in vitro*. α-Terpinene, γ-terpinene and α-terpineol showed the same effect. Limonene showed only a contraction as did the two pinenes, and 1,8-cineole produced only a rise in tone, not a true contraction (Lis-Balchin and Hart, 2000; Table 1).

Uterus   *Melaleuca* oil caused a decrease in the force of the spontaneous contractions in the rat

Table 1   Pharmacological activity of tea tree oils and their major components on guinea-pig ileum (smooth muscle) (conc. 5×10^{-5} v/v)

Essential oil/component	Pharmacological action (%)	
	Spasmogenesis	*Spasmolysis*
Melaleuca oil	15 (3.5) initially	46.8 (4.6)
Manuka		38.1 (1.4)
Kanuka	28.6 (3.1) initially	59.7 (4.6)
1,8-Cineole	25 (4.5) rise in tone	
α-Pinene (+)	7 (4.6)	
β-Pinene (−)	98 (4.7)	23.5 (3.5)
γ-Terpineol		86 (2.5)
α-Terpinene	78 (3.2)	87 (2.5)
γ-Terpinene	3.8 (0.5)	73 (2.2)
Terpinen-4-ol	93 (3.5)	

Table 2 Pharmacological activity of *Melaleuca* oil, manuka and kanuka and some of their components on rat uterine muscle. Rat uterus at 1×10^{-5} dilution

Essential oil/component	Pharmacological effect
Melaleuca	26.0 (1.5) decrease in force*
Manuka (at 1×10^{-6})	100% decrease in force, quick recovery
Kanuka (at 1×10^{-6})	100% decrease in force, quick recovery
1,8-Cineole	51.0 (2.5) decrease in force
α-Pinene	21.0 (1.7) decrease in force
β-Pinene	25.0 (2.5) decrease in force
α-Terpineol	100% decrease in force and loss of contractions
α-Terpinene	100% decrease in force and frequency, quick recovery
p-Cymene	25 (0.5) decrease in force
Terpinen-4-ol	100% decrease in force

*Decrease in force of spontaneous contractions.

uterus *in vitro* (Lis-Balchin and Hart, 1997a; Table 2).

Skeletal muscle   Using both chick biventer muscle and rat phrenic nerve–diaphragm, *Melaleuca* decreased the tension and caused a delayed contracture (Lis-Balchin and Hart, 1997c; Table 3).

Other activities   A study of tea tree oil on human white blood cells showed that the crude oil and the purified 'active' component caused an increase in the activation of white blood cells in the blood serum (Budhiraja *et al.*, 1999). Using human epidermis, 26 different terpenes were tested to enhance the permeability of 5-fluorouracil, a chemotherapy agent, through skin. 1,8-Cineole enhanced the effect of 5-fluorouracil much more than limonene (Moghimi *et al.*, 1998).

In studies comparing the effects of manuka and kanuka tea tree oils with those of *Melaleuca* oils on guinea-pig ileum, skeletal muscle (chick biventer

Table 3 Pharmacological activity of *Melaleuca* oil and components in skeletal muscle

	Increase in resting tone	Decrease in tension
1. Rat phrenic nerve–diaphragm at 2.5×10^{-3}		
Melaleuca		87.5 (4.8)
	+delayed increase to 100%	
Manuka		82.5 (2.5)
	+delayed increase to 100%	
Kanuka		nil effect
α-Pinene (+)		85 (4.0)
	+delayed increase to 56%	
β-Pinene (−)		18 (2.4)
2. Rat diaphragm direct at 2.5×10^{-3}		
Melaleuca		66.7 (3.8)
	+delayed increase to 100%	
Manuka		65.0 (8.8)
	+delayed increase to 100%	
Kanuka		nil effect
3. Chick biventer muscle at 1×10^{-3}		
Melaleuca		71.0 (5.8)
Manuka		27.8 (4.7)
Kanuka		24.0 (2.5)
α-Pinene	15% rise in resting tone	
β-Pinene	10% rise in resting tone	
p-Cymene	20% increased twitch, +14% increase in resting tone	

Numbers indicate mean (SEM) %.

muscle and the rat phrenic nerve–diaphragm) and also rat uterus *in vitro*, the results showed considerable differences between the three essential oils. This was especially in their action on smooth muscle: manuka had a spasmolytic action, while kanuka and *Melaleuca* had an initial spasmogenic action as well. Differences in the mode of action in guinea-pig ileum had previously been shown between manuka and kanuka (Lis-Balchin and Hart, 1998b) and there was some evidence for the involvement of cAMP in the mechanism of action of manuka, but not kanuka. Neither used cGMP, and they did not seem to behave like calcium channel blockers or potassium channel openers. The activity of *Melaleuca* oils resembles kanuka to some extent as the oil has an initial spasmogenic action followed by a potent spasmolytic action; the mechanism of the latter action was apparently neither via cAMP, or cGMP nor acting as potassium channel openers at low concentrations, but some evidence was obtained for action as calcium channel blockers at higher concentrations (Lis-Balchin *et al.*, 2000).

Results in one type of skeletal muscle, using the diaphragm, showed that manuka and *Melaleuca* decreased the tension and caused a delayed contracture; kanuka had no activity at the same concentration. The action on chick biventer muscle was however similar for all three oils, as was the action on the uterus, where they all caused a decrease in the force of the spontaneous contractions. The latter action suggests caution in the use of these essential oils during childbirth, as cessation of contractions could put the baby and mother at risk (Lis-Balchin and Hart, 1998b). See also manuka and kanuka monographs.

Antimicrobial activities

The activity of the tea tree essential oil largely depends on the tea tree oil composition, with different grades of essential oil giving different results (Table 4). 1,8-Cineole has low antimicrobial activity (see A1 and Table 4). There is an inverse correlation between its content and antifungal (and antibacterial) activity, so tea tree oils with a high cineole content will have low activity. Terpinen-4-ol is very effective as an antibacterial agent, but *p*-cymene is even stronger (though it is found at low concentrations in the oil). The antibacterial activity against 25 different bacterial species and 20 *Listeria monocytogenes* varieties was strongest for *Melaleuca* oils compared with manuka and kanuka oils from different sites in New Zealand (Table 4). Different samples of the New Zealand manuka and kanuka oils showed considerable variation, whilst *Melaleuca* oils from different sites remained more constant.

The actual activity of two samples of *M. alternifolia* oil and some of their components against individual bacteria (Table 4) showed some variation, with γ-terpinene exhibiting very low activities on all five out of 25 bacteria and α-terpinene showing only one high antibacterial

Table 4 Summary of the activity of samples of three different 'tea tree' oils and their components against 25 different bacterial species and 20 different *Listeria monocytogenes* strains

	No. affected	
	25 bacterial species	20 Listeria strains
Melaleuca alternifolia Austr.	24	20
Melaleuca alternifolia NZ	24	15
Manuka NI	15	20
Manuka SI	11	0
Kanuka NI	12	19
Kanuka SI	16	20
Kanuka/manuka NI	18	18
1,8-Cineole	16	0
p-Cymene	6	0
Terpinen-4-ol	24	20
α-Terpinene	14	8
γ-Terpinene	5	0
α-Pinene	23	9

activity. The activities were generally low for all the components, with γ-terpinene exhibiting no activity at all. The results are in agreement with studies by Carson and Riley (1994), who studied the antibacterial effect of eight *Melaleuca* components against ten different bacteria. The results against 20 *Listeria monocytogenes* varieties show that γ-terpinene and 1,8-cineole have zero effect, whilst α-pinene has a low effect against only eight varieties (Table 4). γ-Terpineol is slightly more effective than terpinen-4-ol against most of the *Listeria* varieties, which shows that generalisations cannot be made as to the effectiveness of individual essential oils or components against all bacteria.

The essential oil is nowadays used as a strong antimicrobial and antifungal agent in creams, soaps, toothpastes and other preparations and has been used both externally and internally by herbalists and aromatherapists for many years (Blackwell, 1991; Lis-Balchin, 1997).

Antibacterial activity

Relative data: 23/25 different bacteria and 20/20 *Listeria monocytogenes* varieties were affected (A2; Lis-Balchin *et al.*, 1996a; Table 4).

Terpinen-4-ol was the most active out of eight components of tea tree oil against a wide range of test organisms (Carson and Riley, 1995b). Since tea tree oil high in terpinen-4-ol is desirable for use in therapeutic formulations (e.g. for vaginal thrush), the production of clones that produce tea tree oil high in terpinen-4-ol has been initiated (Williams, 1998). Four major components of two tea tree oil samples were tested against bacteria common to skin problems, including acne: terpinen-4-ol, α-terpineol and α-pinene were active against all three bacterial strains, whilst 1,8-cineole showed no activity (Raman *et al.*, 1995). Minimal inhibitory concentrations (MICs) and minimal bactericidal concentrations (MBCs) of essential oils were determined against anaerobic oral bacteria: the most potent essential oils were Australian tea tree oil, peppermint oil, sage oil, also thymol and eugenol (Shapiro *et al.*, 1994). Australian tea tree oil and other oils from the family Myrtaceae, tested against 12 common strains of bacteria, including *Escherichia coli*, *Staphylococcus aureus* and *Salmonella choleraesuis* showed that tea tree had the highest antibacterial activity, and was effective against all bacteria except *Pseudomonas aeruginosa*.

Both tea tree and manuka oil had significant antibacterial effects on various strains of antibiotic-resistant *Staphylococcus* species (Harkenthal *et al.*, 1999). Sixty-four out of 66 varieties of *Staph. aureus* were susceptible to tree oil; 64 of the isolates were methicillin-resistant *Staph. aureus* (MRSA) and 33 were mupirocin-resistant. The MICs were between 0.25% and 0.50% (Carson *et al.*, 1995b).

Staph. aureus and most of the Gram-negative bacteria tested were more susceptible to tea tree oil than the coagulase-negative staphylococci and micrococci, suggesting that tea tree oil may be useful in removing transient skin flora while suppressing but maintaining resident flora (Hammer *et al.*, 1996).

The mechanism of action of *M. alternifolia* oil on *Staph. aureus* was recently determined by time-kill, lysis, leakage, and salt tolerance assays and electron microscopy (Carson *et al.*, 2002). Tea tree oil was reviewed as an alternative topical decolonisation agent for MRSA, but statistical significance of its benefits was not reached (Caelli *et al.*, 2000). The safety, efficacy and provenance of *M. alternifolia* oil was recently reviewed (Carson and Riley, 2001).

Antifungal activity

Relative data (%inhibition): Results against *Aspergillus niger* 85%, *A. ochraceus* 91%, *Fusarium culmorum* 76% (A1; Table 5). Tea tree oil inhibited the growth of over 100 different strains of fungi, including 32 strains of *Candida albicans* at concentrations of 0.5–0.44%, however tea tree is often used in commercial products at much higher concentrations of 5–10% (Nenoff *et al.*, 1996). Tea tree oil was also investigated by a different team against 81 varieties of *Candida albicans* and 33 non-*albicans* isolates. The minimum concentration of oil inhibiting 90% of all isolates was 0.25% in broth. Three tea tree oil products for intravaginal (topical) use showed anticandidal activity (Hammer *et al.*, 1998).

The *in vitro* activity of tea tree oil against dermatophytes ($n = 106$) and filamentous fungi ($n = 78$) has been determined (Hammer *et al.*, 2003). Tea tree oil MICs for all fungi ranged from 0.004% to 0.25% and minimum fungicidal concentrations (MFCs) ranged from <0.03% to 8.0%. Time-kill experiments with 1–4 × MFC demonstrated that three of the four test organisms were still detected after 8 hours of treatment, but not after 24 hours. Comparison of the susceptibility to tea tree oil of germinated and non-germinated *Aspergillus niger* conidia showed germinated conidia to be more susceptible than

Table 5 Antifungal activity of *Melaleuca alternifolia* oil compared with manuka and kanuka samples

	Antifungal activity						
	NZ Mel	*Austr* Mel	*Man1*	*Man2*	M/K	*Kan1*	*Kan2*
Aspergillus niger	94	85	64	68	30	1	0
Aspergillus ochraceus	89	91	49	87	13	10	27
Fusarium culmorum	78	76	25	57	0	0	16

Numbers approaching 100 indicate most potent antifungal activity.
Mel = *Melaleuca*; Man1 = manuka from North Island; Man2 = manuka from South Island; Man/Kan = manuka/kanuka mix; Kan1 = kanuka from North Island; Kan2 = kanuka from South Island.

non-germinated conidia showing that tea tree oil has both inhibitory and fungicidal activity.

Melaleuca alternifolia oil inhibited germ tube formation (GTF) by *Candida albicans*. It is affected by the presence of or pre-exposure to subinhibitory concentrations of tea tree essential oil (Hammer *et al.*, 2000).

Antioxidant activity
See Table 6.

Table 6 Antioxidant activity of *Melaleuca alternifolia* oil compared with manuka and kanuka samples and components

	Zone in mm	Intensity+
Mel Australian	0	
Man1	11.1	+
Man2	8.2	+
Kan/Man	0	
Kan1	17.7	
Kan2	0	
α-Pinene	0	
α-Terpinene	7.1	+
γ-Terpinene	0	
Terpinen-4-ol	9.1	+
α-Terpineol	0	

+ indicates a faint intensity.
Mel = *Melaleuca*; Man1 = manuka from North Island; Man2 = manuka from South Island; Man/Kan = manuka/kanuka mix; Kan1 = kanuka from North Island; Kan2 = kanuka from South Island.

Other activities
Terpinen-4-ol, the main component of the essential oil of *M. alternifolia* oil, suppresses inflammatory mediator production by activated human monocytes; however, the water-soluble components were much more active (Hart *et al.*, 2000).

Melaleuca alternifolia oil gel (6%) was partly beneficial in the treatment of recurrent herpes labialis, but statistical significance was not reached (Carson *et al.*, 2001).

Organic matter and surfactants compromise the antimicrobial activity of tea tree oil, although these effects vary between organisms (Hammer *et al.*, 1999c).

Clinical studies

Clinical studies on tea tree oil to date have involved mainly tinea pedis. In a randomised, double-blind trial 104 patients with tinea pedis (athlete's foot) tested the efficacy of tea tree oil cream (10%) against a standard pharmaceutical cream (tolnaftate 1%) and a placebo cream. Similar improvement in scaling, inflammation, itching, and burning was shown, but in contrast to tolnaftate, tea tree was no better than the placebo at eradicating the fungus completely (Tong *et al.*, 1992).

In a double-blind, multicentre, randomised controlled trial, 117 patients with toenail onychomycosis received either 1% clotrimazole solution or 100% tea tree oil applied twice daily to the infection for six months. The two treatment groups were comparable after six months of therapy, 60% reporting full or partial resolution of the condition and showing improvement in nail appearance and symptoms (Buck *et al.*, 1994).

In a single-blind, randomised clinical trial, 124 patients with mild to moderate acne were given either topical 5% tea tree oil gel or 5% benzoyl peroxide lotion. Both significantly reduced the number of lesions. Although tea tree showed fewer side-effects than the benzoyl peroxide, benzoyl peroxide acted faster (Bassett *et al.*, 1990).

Use in pregnancy and lactation: contraindications

As there are no studies on the effect of the *Melaleuca* essential oil on the uterus other than the *in vitro* studies in rat, which showed a decrease in the spontaneous contractions and because this essential oil has also not been properly assessed toxicologically, it cannot be recommended for use in pregnancy, parturition or during lactation.

Pharmaceutical guidance

Tea tree essential oil (*Melaleuca*) is relatively non-toxic, but has a sensitisation potential which has affected many people. There is a possible danger of a toxic effect transmitted via the spinal cord in young children and babies who are massaged with this essential oil, as there are numerous such cases in cats and dogs, which have even resulted in reversible but long-lasting quadriplegia.

Many medically non-qualified aromatherapists now practise 'clinical aromatherapy', where they prescribe internal usage of essential oils which involves oral, rectal and vaginal intake. However, the use of tampons soaked in various potentially toxic essential oils, like the various 'tea-tree' oils with variable biological potential, could have a possible harmful effect on the delicate internal mucosal membranes. The possibility of misdiagnosis of a urino-genital condition by a medically unqualified aromatherapist or by the patients themselves could also result in serious consequencies.

Note: The problem with many Myrtaceae is that they display wide genetic variation and the production of spontaneous chemotypes, giving many different essential oil compositions with differing bioactivities. The quality of commercial Australian tea tree oil has now been generally stabilised, mainly by the selection of clones and the blending of different essential oils from different species of *Melaleuca* to conform with the Australian Standards. However, the problem of diversity remains in other parts of the world where *Melaleuca* species grow (e.g. Zimbabwe, New Zealand, Indonesia). The diversity of manuka and kanuka oils is even more pronounced and the use of these New Zealand oils, especially in aromatherapy, may therefore be premature, unless their quality can be assured and toxicological studies (which have been done for all essential oils used in the food and cosmetics industry) are undertaken.

Use in babies and young children

Due to the immaturity and the delicate nature of the skin of babies and young children, it is inadvisable for any essential oils to be used in massage, however much the essential oil has been diluted in the carrier oils. This is also a necessary precaution due to the possibilities of sensitisation of the children at this young age through skin or air-borne odorant effects (see Chapters 5 and 7).

Instillation or administration of essential oils near the baby or young child's nose is not only not recommended, but distinctly inadvisable, as there have been numerous cases reported of severe toxicity and even death from such applications (see Chapter 7).

Thyme Oil

CAS numbers

USA: 8007-46-3; EINECS: 84929-51-1

Species/Botanical name

Thymus vulgaris L., *Thymus zygis* L. (Labiatae)

Synonyms

Red thyme, white thyme (Spanish thyme), sweet thyme, ol. thym., esencia de tomillo, essência de tomilho, oleum thymi

Pharmacopoeias

In European and Polish Pharmacopoeias. Thyme oil (Ph. Eur. 4.8) contains 36–55% thymol (Martindale, 2004).

Safety

CHIP details
Xn; R10, 38, 65; 40%; S62 (A26)

RIFM recommended safety of use limits
8% tentative (A23)

EU sensitiser total
2.5%

GRAS status
(Fenaroli, 1997).

Extraction, source, appearance and odour

Extraction
A volatile oil is obtained by steam distillation of the flowering tops and leaves of the herb to give an essential oil of a different composition depending on cultivar and species (Arctander, 1960).

Source
Spain, France, Italy, Turkey, Eastern Europe and USA.

Appearance and odour
Red thyme, crude, white thyme oil and rectified red thyme have a medicinal, herbal odour. Sweet thyme oil is colourless and has a slightly sweeter odour (Arctander, 1960).

Aromatherapy uses

Uses include: stimulation of the brain aiding in memory and concentration; general fatigue, depression, exhaustion; gout, oedema, urinary infection, clearing mucus in the urinary and reproductive systems, cystitis; an emmenagogue inducing menstruation and aiding leucorrhoea; sluggish digestion, wind, intestinal infection, upset stomach, parasites; poor circulation and to raise low blood pressure; arthritis, sciatica, rheumatism, gout pain, muscular aches, pains, sprains, swelling, inflammation, sports injuries, and to restore mobility; asthma, spasm, bronchitis, pneumonia, colds, coughs, sore throat, whooping cough, flu, bronchitis, clearing the lungs and sinuses.

Thyme oil is an irritant and must be diluted for use against abscesses, insect bites, lice, scalp tonic, dandruff, acne, boils, infectious inflammations, gum infections, hair loss, increasing capillary circulation, skin gland malfunctions such as seborrhoea, acne, blackheads, and sweat gland abscess (Ryman, 1991; Lawless, 1992; Rose, 1992a,b; Price, 1993; Sheppard-Hanger, 1995).

Scientific comment

Although thyme essential oil is an excellent antimicrobial agent and rubefacient at high concentrations, it is not scientifically proven that the essential oil in dilute concentrations will alleviate many of the conditions listed above. There is also the problem of different types (chemotypes or species) of thyme essential oil on the market, and some of these are not very bioactive. Note: Thyme linalool chemotype and other chemotypes have had no formal testing and should not be used. Massage itself can alleviate many muscular and stress conditions.

Herbal uses

Thyme (herb) is stated to possess carminative, antispasmodic, antitussive, expectorant, secretomotor, bactericidal, anthelmintic and astringent properties. Traditionally, it has been used for dyspepsia, chronic gastritis, asthma, diarrhoea in children, enuresis in children, laryngitis, tonsillitis (as a gargle), and specifically for pertussis and bronchitis. It is approved for internal use for treating symptoms of bronchitis, whooping cough and catarrh of the upper respiratory tract. Thyme is used in various combinations with anise oil, eucalyptus oil, fennel oil, fennel fruit, Iceland moss, lime flower, liquorice root, marshmallow root, primrose root and star anise fruit for catarrh and diseases of the upper respiratory tract. Thymol is used in Listerine, Vicks VapoRub and various other medicinal products (Wren, 1988; Chevallier, 1996; Blumenthal *et al.*, 2000; Barnes *et al.*, 2002).

Food and perfumery uses

Food   Thyme is used in numerous foods (Fenaroli, 1997).

Perfumery   Used in cheap perfumes (Arctander, 1960); blends well with bergamot, lemon, rosemary, lavender, lavandin and marjoram.

Chemistry

Major components

Commercial oils	% (Lawrence, 1976–2001)	
	Red	Sweet
Thymol	45–48	0
Carvacrol	2.5–3.5	0.7
Geraniol	0	30
Geranyl acetate	0	50
β-Caryophyllene	1.3–8	4
α-Pinene	0.5–6	0
p-Cymene	18.5–21.5	0
1,8-Cineole	3.6–15	0
Terpinolene	1.8–6	0

Variation in the chemical composition of thyme oils occurs more in wild populations, due to the numerous chemotypes of this unstable species. Several main chemotypes have been reported, but there is confusion regarding the nomenclature and taxonomy of the thyme, oregano and marjoram group.

The main commercial thyme oils are: red (unrectified); white (rectified) (both thymol/carvacrol chemotypes) and the sweet, geraniol-rich chemotype. The white oil should contain over 60% of thymol, but it is frequently an origanum oil with 60% carvacrol.

Wild thyme oil according to ISO 4728: (1992) is given as light yellow with the following composition: 1,8-cineole apparent after 40 min. max. 65%; α-pinene; camphor; β-pinene*; sabinene; myrcene; limonene*; 1,8-cineole***; γ-terpinene; *p*-cymene; linalool***; α-terpineol.

The essential oil distilled from *Thymus serpyllum* L. is a colourless or golden-yellow, laevogyrate oil of specific gravity 0.905–0.930. The odour is slightly like thyme, but more like melissa.

Adulteration

Oregano and various Spanish thyme or other oils are frequently used. Ajowan is often added or substituted, if the price is lower than thyme. White thyme oil is often a compounded mixture of pine oil fractions, terpineol, rosemary, eucalyptus and red thyme fractions, with or without synthetic *p*-cymene, pinenes, limonene, caryophyllene and oregano added. The presence of oil of turpentine in oil of thyme may be recognised by the specific gravity being lower than 0.900, or by the diminished solubility in alcohol, and the deficiency in the phenol contents of the oil (A8; Chapter 4).

Toxicity

Acute toxicity (A22)

Oral LD$_{50}$ 4.7 g/kg (rat).

Dermal LD$_{50}$ 2.8 g/kg (rat); >5 g/kg (rabbit).

Irritation and sensitisation (A22)

Red thyme oil at 8% had nil effect, but applied undiluted to animal skin it proved severely irritating.

Phototoxicity

Nil reported.

Other toxicities

Thyme oil is a dermal and mucous membrane irritant (A22) and toxic symptoms mainly for thymol include: nausea, vomiting, gastric pain, headache, dizziness, convulsions, coma, and cardiac and respiratory arrest (Duke, 1985). Thymol, present in some toothpaste preparations caused cheilitis and glossitis; hyperaemia and severe inflammation was caused by thyme oil in bath preparations (Mitchell and Rook, 1979). An individual with allergy to oral oregano and thyme was reported (Benito *et al.*, 1996). Patch tests with 100 patients with ulcus cruris found positive results with thyme oil (5%), Peru balsam (14%), wool-wax alcohols (10%) and neomycin (5%) (Le Roy *et al.*, 1981).

Extracts of thyme decreased locomotor activity and caused a slight slowing down of respiration in mice following oral administration and a concentrated ethanol extract of the herb in subacute toxicity tests caused increased weights of liver and testes. Thyme oil had no mutagenic or DNA-damaging activity in either the Ames test or *Bacillus subtilis* rec-assay (Barnes *et al.*, 2002). Kochi thyme essential oil, a related species, produced hypotensive and cardiotonic effects in rabbits but no toxic effects were seen in mice or guinea-pigs (Guseinov *et al.*, 1987).

Bioactivities

Pharmacological activities *in vitro* and *in vivo*

Smooth muscle Thyme oil, red and white and sweet had a spasmolytic effect on electrically stimulated smooth muscle of the guinea-pig ileum *in vitro*. Carvacrol and thymol had a similar effect (A2; Lis-Balchin *et al.*, 1996a). Relaxation of tracheal smooth muscle was found with the volatile oils of 22 plants, including thyme oil. Phasic contractions of the ileal myenteric plexus–longitudinal muscle preparation were inhibited by thyme, balm leaves, angelica root oil, clove, etc. (Reiter and Brandt, 1985).

Uterus There was a decrease in the spontaneous contractions in the rat using thyme oils, including red and sweet essential oils (A3; A4; Lis-Balchin and Hart, 1997b).

Skeletal muscle Skeletal muscle is contracted by thyme oil without a change in the twitch response (Lis-Balchin and Hart, 1997c).

Other activities The antitussive, expectorant and antispasmodic actions are associated with the volatile oils (e.g. thymol, carvacrol) as well as flavonoid constituents. Thyme oil has produced hypotensive and respiratory stimulant effects in rabbits following oral or intramuscular administration, and in cats following intravenous injection; an increase in rhythmic heart contraction was also observed in rabbits (Leung, 1980).

In vitro antispasmodic activity of thyme apparently involves calcium channel blockage and analgesic and antipyretic properties in mice were seen with a thyme extract. Thyme oil also inhibits prostaglandin synthesis (Barnes *et al.*, 2002).

Fast wave bursts of about 20 Hz in the rat pyriform cortex are induced by benzyl alcohol, carvacrol, eucalyptol and salicylaldehyde and volatile organic solvents (Zibrowski 1998) but there was no evidence that the bursts of 20 Hz activity seen in the rat rhinencephalon were kindling-induced seizure-like reactions of the olfactory brain to the vapours of toxic chemicals.

Ames test revertants were increased 1.5- to 1.7-fold by carvacrol and thymol. The IC_{50} was 0.3 mmol/L (cinnamaldehyde) to 0.7 mmol/L (thymol) in the Hep-2 viability test and 0.2 mmol/L (carvacrol) to 0.9 mmol/L (carvone) in the Hep-2 proliferation test (Stammati *et al.*, 1999). The age-associated decrease of 22:6 (*n*-3) fatty acids in brain, kidney and heart is countered by thyme oil or thymol at 42.5 mg/kg/day, while the age-related increase in liver is not affected. 20:4 (*n*-6) fatty acids are also kept higher in tissues by thyme (Youdim *et al.*, 1999).

Antimicrobial activities

Hundreds of papers mention thyme oil and it is generally recognised as being extremely active against numerous microbial species *in vitro*. Some of the data are presented here.

Antibacterial activity

Relative data: Red and white thyme oils were active against 25/25 different bacterial species; sweet thyme oil only against 14/25. Red thyme was active against 6–20/20 *Listeria monocytogenes* varieties; sweet thyme against 8/20 (A1; Lis-Balchin and Deans, 1997; Lis-Balchin *et al.*, 1998a). An unidentified thyme oil was active against 22/25 bacteria (Deans and Ritchie, 1987). Red and white thyme vapours were active against 5/5 bacteria (Maruzella and Sicurella, 1960). A thyme oil was very active against four bacteria (Friedman *et al.*, 2002) and the vapour against four respiratory pathogens (Inouye *et al.*, 2001). The antibacterial action of eugenol, thyme oil and related essential oils used in dentistry was assessed (Meeker and Linke, 1988). Sardinian thyme oil was assessed against a panel of standard reference strains and multiple strains of food-derived spoilage and pathogenic bacteria and shown to be similar to other thyme oils, as was the thymol and carvacrol (Cosentino *et al.*, 1999). Thyme oil was better than *Pelargonium* oil against *Salmonella enteritidis* and comparable against *Saccharomyces ludwigii*, *Zygosaccharomyces bailii* and *Listeria innocua* (Lis-Balchin *et al.*, 1998d).

Essential oils from *Thymus vulgaris* and *Calamintha nepeta* showed high antibacterial and antifungal activity compared with *Satureja montana* and *Rosmarinus officinalis* (Pannizzi et al., 1993). Out of 52 plant extracts tested against ten microbes, thyme oil was the most effective for *Candida albicans* and *Escherichia coli* (Hammer et al., 1999a). *Bacillus cereus* viability was reduced exponentially by 30 minutes of treatment with 1–3 mmol/L carvacrol. Permeability of the cytoplasmic membrane for H^+ and K^+ was increased and the intracellular ATP pool was depleted (Ultee et al., 1999). *Bacillus cereus* is inhibited by carvacrol (thyme, oregano) dose-dependently and inhibition is total at 0.75 mmol/L; spores are a third as sensitive. Membrane fluidity appears to be an important factor (Ultee et al., 1998).

Salmonella typhimurium is inhibited by essential oil of thyme or its constituent thymol whereas the chemically related terpenes *p*-cymene and γ-terpinene had no effect (Juven et al., 1994). Oils of bay, cinnamon, clove and thyme were the most antimicrobial against *Campylobacter*, *Salmonella*, *E. coli*, *Staph. aureus* and *Listeria* (Smith-Palmer et al., 1998). Thyme essential oil had good activity against 5/5 bacteria (Friedman et al., 2002).

Antifungal activity

Relative data (% inhibition) (A1):

	Red	Sweet
Aspergillus niger	91–96	95
A. ochraceus	61–92	88
Fusarium culmorum	75–86	83

Red and white thyme oils were active against 5/5 fungi (Yousef and Tawil, 1980); red thyme against 18/18 fungi (Maruzella and Ligouri, 1958); mycelial growth of aflatoxin-producing *Aspergillus parasiticus* is stopped by 0.1% thyme (Tantaoui-Elaraki and Beraoud, 1994).

Antioxidant activity

High activity was found for all thyme essential oils studied (Dorman et al., 1995a,b; Lis-Balchin et al., 1996a).

Other activities

Thymol has anthelmintic properties, especially against hookworms (Leung, 1980).

Headlice are effectively treated by essential oils (in alcoholic solution) of aniseed, cinnamon leaf, red thyme, tea tree, peppermint or nutmeg, followed by a rinse the following morning with an essential oil/vinegar/water mixture (Veal, 1996).

Clinical studies

Thyme oil has been used for the treatment of enuresis in children (Martindale, 1982).

Rubbing oils (thyme, rosemary, lavender and cedarwood) into the scalp helped with alopecia for 44% of patients versus 15% of controls in a seven-month, double-blind study of 86 patients (Hay et al., 1998).

Use in pregnancy and lactation: contraindications

Traditionally, thyme is said to affect the menstrual cycle, and experiments *in vitro* showed that thyme essential oils caused a decrease and cessation of spontaneous contractions in the rat uterus, therefore, thyme oil should be restricted in aromatherapy massage during pregnancy, parturition and lactation.

Pharmaceutical guidance

Thyme essential oil (*Thymus vulgaris*) is very active, especially antimicrobially, but is also toxic and should not be ingested in any great concentrations, although used in small amounts in many foods. It should only be applied externally if diluted in a suitable carrier oil and used with considerable caution. Many thyme essential oils are on the market, some of which have very poor bioactivity due to source or adulteration or are chemotypes, which have not been toxicologically evaluated and should therefore not be used.

Use in babies and young children

Due to the immaturity and the delicate nature of the skin of babies and young children, it is inadvisable for any essential oils, especially a potentially irritant essential oil, to be used in massage, however much the essential oil has been diluted in the carrier oils. This is also a necessary precaution due to the possibilities of sensitisation of the children at this young age through skin or air-borne odorant effects (see Chapters 5 and 7).

Instillation or administration of essential oils near the baby or young child's nose is not only not recommended, but distinctly inadvisable, as there have been numerous cases reported of severe toxicity and even death from such applications (see Chapter 7).

Valerian Oil

CAS numbers
USA: 8008-88-6; EINECS: 8057-49-6

Species/Botanical name
Valeriana officinalis L.s.l. (Valerianaceae)

Synonyms
All-Heal, common valerian, fragrant valerian, garden valerian

Other species
Valeriana wallichi, Valeriana jatmansi

Safety
CHIP details
Xn; R65; 25%; S62 (A26)

EU sensitiser total
1.3% (A27)

GRAS status
Granted (Fenaroli, 1997).

Extraction, source, appearance and odour
Extraction
A volatile oil is obtained by steam distillation of the rhizome/root (Arctander, 1960).

Source
Eastern Europe and China.

Appearance and odour
Valerian essential oil is deep olive-green to brown with distinctive odour described as warm, woody, balsamic, root-like, with animal musky undertones and great tenacity. When aged, it becomes darker and more viscous and obtains an objectionable odour of isovaleric acid. Valerian absolute is an ether-extracted fraction, a by-product of the pharmaceutical extraction of valerian, and is not generally available.

Valeriana wallichii essential oil is a pale brown/amber liquid with a balsamic-woody, slightly spicy, root-like and distinct valerian acid odour; it has characteristic musk-like and camphoraceous notes (Arctander, 1960).

Aromatherapy uses
This essential oil is not mentioned in many aromatherapy books. However, uses include: insomnia, nervous indigestion, migraine, restlessness, tension states; haemorrhoids, cramp, palpitations, varicose veins, agitation and anxiety debility (Lawless, 1992; Price, 1993; Sheppard-Hanger, 1995).

Scientific comment
The safety of valerian essential oil usage in aromatherapy massage has not been established and, due to lack of toxicity data, caution is required, especially as it has either a sedative or stimulant action on the human brain (A14). Massage itself can alleviate many of the stress-related problems mentioned and the use of valerian essential oil as an inhalant (e.g. a drop of valerian essential oil on the pillow at night) would probably be beneficial for sleep.

Herbal uses
Valerian was known as 'all-heal' during the Middle Ages and used for numerous conditions, especially for controlling epilepsy. Valerian is a sedative, mild anodyne, hypnotic, antispasmodic, carminative and has hypotensive properties. Uses include: hysterical states, excitability, insomnia, hypochondriasis, migraine, cramp, intestinal colic, irritable bowel syndrome, rheumatic pains, dysmenorrhoea, nervous excitability, high blood pressure, asthma, shoulder and neck tension (Wren, 1988; Chevallier, 1996; Barnes *et al.*, 2002).

Food and perfumery uses
Food Valerian root oil (FEMA 3100) is used in many foods and beverages, giving interesting effects with apple, beer, tobacco and liqueur flavours (Fenaroli, 1997).

Perfumery Valerian is used seldom but combines well with oakmoss, patchouli, rosemary, lavender, pine and provides specials effects in chypres, fougeres and forest notes.

Chemistry

Major components

	% *(Lawrence, 1976–2001)*
α-Pinene	3–10
Camphene	7–15
β-Pinene	trace–1
β-Caryophyllene	trace–3
Limonene	trace–1.5
Elemol	2–12
Valeranone	0–18
Valeranal	3–16
Bornyl acetate	0.5–3.5

V. jatmansi has a similar composition and both are rather variable.

Adulteration

Valerian extracts can be mixed in and different valerian essential oils are sometimes admixed. Spikenard oil may also be added (A8; see Chapter 4).

Toxicity

Acute toxicity

Oral and dermal LD₅₀ These have not been determined recently as an RIFM monograph. Toxicological studies in older literature reported an LD_{50} of 3.3 mg/kg for an ethanolic extract of valerian administered intraperitoneally in rats.

Short-term oral daily doses of 400–600 mg/kg, administered intraperitoneally for 45 days in rats, showed no changes in weight, blood or urine measurements (Upton, 1999). Valerenic acid administered to mice at 150 mg/kg, by intraperitoneal injection, caused muscle spasms and 400 mg/kg caused heavy convulsions (Hendriks *et al.*, 1985) and was lethal to 86%. *In vitro* cytotoxicity and mutagenicity have been studied for the valepotriates (Barnes *et al.*, 2002), but these are not present in the essential oil, which is not considered likely to present any hazard in aromatherapy (Kneibel and Burchard, 1988).

Irritation and sensitisation

No data found.

Phototoxicity

No data found.

Other toxicities

The safety of valerian root extracts, mainly water-soluble, have been reviewed and overdoses of valerian have shown serious transient effects which could be reversed using activated charcoal (Barnes *et al.*, 2002).

Bioactivities

Pharmacological activities *in vitro* and *in vivo*

Smooth muscle Valerian oil had a very strong spasmolytic effect on electrically stimulated smooth muscle of the guinea-pig ileum *in vitro* (A2; Lis-Balchin *et al.*, 1996a) and the mode of action was through calcium channels. Antispasmodic activity on intact and isolated guinea-pig ileum was shown for valeranone (Hazelhoff *et al.*, 1982), which was apparently due to a direct action on the smooth muscle receptors rather than ganglion receptors.

Uterus There was a decrease in the spontaneous contractions in the rat when valerian oil was added *in vitro* (A3; A4; Lis-Balchin and Hart, 1997b). Mixing several other essential oils with valerian oil also had a relaxant effect (A5). Valerian oil has shown antispasmodic activity on isolated guinea-pig uterine muscle in older studies (Pilcher *et al.*, 1916), but proved inactive when tested *in vivo* (Pilcher and Mauer, 1918).

Other activities It remains unclear precisely which of the constituents of valerian are responsible for its sedative properties (Houghton, 1997) as both the essential oil and then the valepotriates and their degradation products have been shown to be responsible. However, the effects of the volatile oil could not account for the whole action of the drug which is probably due to several different groups of constituents (Houghton, 1997). The constituents bornyl acetate and the sesquiterpene valerenic acid (characteristic of the species), in addition to other sesquiterpenes, have shown a direct action on the amygdaloid body of the brain and valerenic acid has been shown to inhibit enzyme-induced breakdown of gamma-aminobutyric acid (GABA) in the brain, resulting in sedation. As increased concentrations of GABA are associated with a decrease in CNS activity, this may cause the sedative activity. Valerenic acid also inhibits the enzyme system responsible for the central catabolism of GABA (Riedel *et al.*, 1982). Further experiments on

GABA have been described in detail (Barnes *et al.*, 2002).

Valerenal and valerenic acid were shown to be the most active compounds causing ataxia in mice (by intraperitoneal injection): valerenic acid acted as a general CNS depressant, like pentobarbitone, requiring high doses for activity (Hendricks *et al.*, 1985) and a four-fold dose resulted in muscle spasms, convulsions and death; valerenic acid also prolonged pentobarbitone-induced sleep in mice.

Antimicrobial activities

Antibacterial activity

No data found.

Antifungal activity

No data found.

Clinical studies

Valerian essential oil reduced stress and systolic blood pressure in humans (when blood pressure was high to start with) (Warren and Warrenburg, 1993). Numerous other studies have investigated the effects of valerian preparations, often water-soluble extracts, on subjective and/or objective sleep parameters, but conclusions were difficult as so many different parameters were used, including valerian preparations, different dosages, healthy volunteers or patients with diagnosed sleep disorders, etc. (Barnes *et al.*, 2002). A systematic review of randomised, double-blind, placebo-controlled trials of valerian preparations included nine studies (Stevinson and Ernst, 2000) and concluded that the evidence for valerian as a treatment for insomnia is unproven.

Oral valerian extracts, in combination with hops (*Humulus lupulus*) and/or melissa (*Melissa officinalis*), were studied in relation to sleep and showed improvement in sleep quality but it was not significantly greater from the control using different analysis criteria (Barnes *et al.*, 2002).

Use in pregnancy and lactation: contraindications

The safety of valerian essential oil usage in aromatherapy massage during pregnancy and lactation has not been established but a decrease in the spontaneous contractions in the rat uterus when valerian oil was added *in vitro* suggests that the essential oil should be avoided in pregnancy, parturition and due to lack of toxicity data also during lactation. However, many oral preparations containing valerian are used for sedation and sleep without apparent hazard, suggesting that a drop of valerian essential oil on the pillow at night would not be detrimental to health.

Pharmaceutical guidance

The sedative action of valerian is due to both the essential oil and iridoid valepotriate fractions plus other components in valerian. Studies have compared valerian with certain benzodiazepines and the CNS-depressant activity may potentiate existing sedative therapy. Valerian oil should not be used for several hours before driving a car or operating machinery and greater care should be taken if alcohol is also consumed, as the effect of valerian oil may be enhanced, as it is for other valerian products. In conclusion, valerian essential oil should be used with great caution in aromatherapy, and massage with the essential oil is not advised.

Use in babies and young children

Due to the immaturity and the delicate nature of the skin of babies and young children, it is inadvisable for any essential oils to be used in massage, however much the essential oil has been diluted in the carrier oils. This is also a necessary precaution due to the possibilities of sensitisation of the children at this young age through skin or air-borne odorant effects (see Chapters 5 and 7).

Instillation or administration of essential oils near the baby or young child's nose is not only not recommended, but distinctly inadvisable, as there have been numerous cases reported of severe toxicity and even death from such applications (see Chapter 7).

Vanilla Tincture/Absolute

CAS numbers

USA: 8024-06-4; EINECS: 84650-63-5

Species/Botanical name

Vanilla plantifolia (Orchidaceae)

Synonyms

V. fragrans, common vanilla, Bourbon or Reunion vanilla

Other species

V. tahitense (Tahiti vanilla)

Safety

CHIP details
None

RIFM recommended safety of use limits
Tincture: 3% (A23)

GRAS status
Granted (Fenaroli, 1997).

Extraction, source, appearance and odour

Extraction
A volatile oil is obtained by steam distillation of the ripe pods frosted with vanillin crystals (see also Chapter 5). This essential oil is produced in small amounts, as the absolute, resinoid and tincture are preferred. Vanilla absolute is obtained after vanilla is first extracted with petroleum ether and dichloromethane; different concentrations of ethanol in water are used, ending up with water itself and the fractions are pooled. Vanilla tincture is the most commonly used perfume and flavour vanilla and is made up as 125 g vanilla fruit pods to 1000 g 95% ethanol and is therefore akin to an absolute, but then diluted 1:10 in ethanol (Arctander, 1960). According to US Food and Drug Administration standards, vanilla tincture contains no less than 35% alcohol.

Source
Madagascar, Réunion, Mexico, Tahiti, Comoro Islands, East Africa and Indonesia.

Appearance and odour
The oil is a viscous dark brown liquid with a rich, sweet, balsamic, and characteristic vanilla-like odour of great tenacity (Arctander, 1960).

Aromatherapy uses

Vanilla pods chopped and infused in oil apparently make a dynamic massage oil for the impotent, frigid or sterile patient due to its warming, soothing and aphrodisiac nature. It can be used to lubricate the vaginal area. Inhalation of the aroma reminds one of home, mother, sweet baked goods and is very calming, and stimulates the third chakra; induces menstruation, calms emotions, anger, frustration, brings back warm memories (Rose, 1992; Sheppard-Hanger, 1995). No uses are given in most aromatherapy books.

Scientific comment

The use of massage alone can have beneficial effects on stress and muscular problems and the fragrance/aroma of vanilla can prove very soothing and relaxing, either alone or in conjunction with other essential oils. Massage with the tincture or 'essential oil' is not recommended.

Herbal uses

Vanilla is apparently an aromatic stimulant and said to exhilarate the brain, prevent sleep, increase muscular energy, and stimulate the sexual propensities. It is useful in infusion for hysteria, rheumatism, and low forms of fever. It is also considered an aphrodisiac, powerfully exciting the generative system (Felter and Lloyd, 1898). Vanillin BP is available as a substitute.

Food and perfumery uses

Food Vanilla oleoresin (FEMA 3106) has many uses in foods, especially cakes and ice-creams, and beverages and to flavour tinctures, syrups, ointments and confectionery (Fenaroli, 1997).

Perfumery Vanilla is much used in perfumery, in sweet, floral, heavy amber and oriental perfumes (Arctander, 1960).

Chemistry

Major components

	% (Lawrence, 1976–2001)
Vanillin (vanillic aldehyde)	26–97
Vanillic acid	0.5–1.6
p-Hydroxybenzaldehyde	0.9–1.7
Anisyl alcohol	trace–>1
Anisaldehyde	trace–>1
Anisyl ethers	trace–>1
Anisic acid esters	trace–>1

Minor components

β-Phenylethyl alcohol, guaiacol, creosol, octanoic acid, γ-nonalactone, p-cresol, *trans*-methyl cinnamate, *cis*-methyl cinnamate, furfural.

Adulteration

Coumarin can be added or vanillin added in bulk or even substituted (A8; see Chapter 4).

Vanillin is also a constituent of many other plant products, such as Siam benzoin and balsam of Peru.

Toxicity

Acute toxicity (A22)

Oral LD_{50} >5 g/kg (rat).
Dermal LD_{50} >10 g/kg (rabbit).

Irritation and sensitisation (A22)

No primary irritation was produced when applied neat to 31 human volunteers. Vanilla is a cross-sensitiser in 34/75 patients sensitive to Peru balsam, but it did not work the other way round, indicating that it is not a strong sensitiser.

Phototoxicity

None reported.

Bioactivities

Pharmacological activities *in vitro* and *in vivo*

Smooth muscle   None found.

Antimicrobial activities

Antibacterial activity

Antibacterial effect of vanilla oleoresin was low in 5/5 bacteria (Friedman *et al.*, 2002).

Antifungal activity

None found.

Uses in pregnancy and lactation: contraindications

Due to the lack of knowledge about possible hazards associated with the use of this tincture and its sensitisation potential, aromatherapy massage during pregnancy, parturition and lactation is not advised. However, use of the fragrance simply by inhalation can be very calming and relaxing.

Pharmaceutical guidance

Massage with the tincture or 'essential oil' is not recommended as so little is known of the bioactivity and possible hazards. The use of massage alone can have a beneficial effects on stress and muscular problems and the aroma of vanilla, used as a fragrance, can prove very soothing and relaxing if inhaled with the massage or used alone.

Use in babies and young children

Due to the immaturity and the delicate nature of the skin of babies and young children, it is inadvisable for any essential oils/tinctures to be used in massage, however much the essential oil has been diluted in the carrier oils. This is also a necessary precaution due to the possibilities of sensitisation of the children at this young age through skin or air-borne odorant effects (see Chapters 5 and 7).

Instillation or administration of essential oils near the baby or young child's nose is not only not recommended, but distinctly inadvisable, as there have been numerous cases reported of severe toxicity and even death from such applications (see Chapter 7).

Wintergreen Oil

CAS numbers
USA: 68917-75-9; EINECS: 90045-28-6

Species/Botanical name
Gaultheria procumbens L. (Ericaceae)

Synonyms
Oil of wintergreen, teaberry, checkerberry

Safety

CHIP details
Xn; R22, 36; 0%; S26 (A26)

GRAS status
Granted (Fenaroli, 1997).

Extraction, source, appearance and odour

Extraction
A volatile oil is obtained by water distillation from the leaves of the small creeping plant. The effect of the water allows its enzymes to liberate the essential oil (Arctander, 1960).

Source
Europe, Nepal and the USA.

Appearance and odour
It is a pale yellow to pinkish essential oil with an intense sweet, woody, antiseptic odour (Arctander, 1960). Its odour distinctly differs from that of synthetic methyl salicylate. The only physical difference between the oils of *Gaultheria* and sweet birch is in the optical inactivity of the latter.

Aromatherapy uses
Most aromatherapy books do not recommend the use of wintergreen essential oil in aromatherapy. However, uses include: rheumatic conditions, gout, sciatica, stiffness of old age, muscular pains – especially for athletes (using six drops of essential oil in the bath water). It is also used for various skin problems (e.g. eczema, acne, blemishes), but some people are allergic to it. When inhaled it brings back memories of youth. The essential oil stimulates the liver, induces menstruation and is effective for heart disease and prevention of hypertension (Ryman, 1991; Rose, 1992a,b; Sheppard-Hanger, 1995).

Scientific comment
Wintergreen essential oil has high potential toxicity and is a severe skin and eye irritant (National Toxicology Program) and it has not been proven to be effective for any of the aromatherapy conditions listed above. It could be toxic if used in patients taking aspirin or warfarin. It is therefore not recommended in aromatherapy massage.

Herbal uses
The wintergreen essence, or the oil dissolved in alcohol, is effectual in curing intermittent fever and was largely used in gonorrhoea, and in gonorrheal and other forms of rheumatism, in trigeminal neuralgia, and in subacute and chronic cystitis. As large doses as can be borne should be given in rheumatic disorders, but like salicylic acid and the salicylates its action upon the heart must be closely watched. Locally used, it relieves pain. The dose of the oil is from 5 to 30 drops on sugar, in capsules, or in emulsion (Felter and Lloyd, 1898). Wintergreen essential oil is used nowadays in liniments and ointments for the relief of pain of lumbago, sciatica and rheumatic conditions. It is also used on horses for overexertion-related stiffness and soreness. It is sometimes used as a UV absorber in sun lotions (Wren, 1988; Chevallier, 1996).

Food and perfumery uses
Food Wintergreen oil (FEMA 3113) is used in many foods and beverages and in candies, also toothpastes (Fenaroli, 1997).

Perfumery Not widely used except in forest-type or woody perfumes (Arctander, 1960).

Chemistry

Major components

	% (Lawrence, 1976–2001)
Methyl salicylate	up to 98

Minor components
Gaultheriline, formaldehyde, benzyl benzoate, bornyl acetate, phenol, eugenol, hexanal, benzaldehyde, cinnamaldehyde and linalool.

Adulteration
As this volatile oil is not peculiar to *Gaultheria* alone, but has been derived also from the bark of *Betula lenta*, the root of *Polygala paucifolia*, and the stems and roots of *Spiraea ulmaria*, *Spiraea lobata*, the leaves of *Gaultheria hispidula*, *Gaultheria leucocarpa*, *Gaultheria punctata* and from *Monotropa hypopity*, adulterations are common. Often just the synthetic methyl salicylate is given as the essential oil (A8; see Chapter 4).

Toxicity

Acute toxicity (A22)

Oral LD$_{50}$ 0.9 g/kg (rat); 1 g/kg (guinea-pig); 1.3 g/kg (rabbit); 2.1 g/kg (dog). LD$_{Lo}$ (lowest published lethal dose) oral for humans is 0.1 g/kg (men); 0.3 g/kg (women); 0.2–0.7 g/kg (children); 1.5 g/kg (infants).

Dermal LD$_{50}$ Unrecorded; subcutaneous 4.2 g/kg (rabbit).

Irritation and sensitisation
Methyl salicylate at 8% applied to human skin for 48 hours produced nil effect. When incorporated into liniments, it has some irritant effect at 1%. Sensitivity to methyl salicylate has been shown in some people.

Skin and eye irritation data: skin (rabbit) = 500 mg/24-hour: moderate; eye (rabbit) = 500 mg/24-hour: mild; skin (guinea-pig) = 100%: severe; eye (guinea-pig) = 100%: severe.

Phototoxicity
None reported.

Other toxicities
Oil of wintergreen possesses decidedly active properties, and in 1/2 oz doses has produced death. It acts much like salicylic acid, but death is preceded by coma. Congestion of the kidneys, stomach and duodenum, and black fluid blood are revealed upon autopsy. The symptoms produced are drowsiness, cerebral congestion with throbbing of the arteries, delirium, visual impairment with contracted or dilated pupils, tinnitus, paresis, somnolence and coma (Felter and Lloyd, 1898). Other symptoms include burning, tearing, reddening and swelling of the eyes and surrounding tissue; itching, irritation of the mucous membranes, coughing, sore throat, severe gastrointestinal lesions, kidney and brain damage and dermatitis. Symptoms of exposure to this compound include CNS stimulation, hyperpnoea, metabolic derangement, accumulation of organic acids, prolonged bleeding time, mild burning pain in the mouth, throat and abdomen, lethargy, vomiting, tinnitus, hearing loss, dizziness, excitability, delirium, fever, sweating, dehydration, incoordination, restlessness, ecchymoses, coma, convulsions, cyanosis, oliguria, uraemia, pulmonary oedema, respiratory failure, hypoglycaemia, rhinorrhoea, bronchiolar constriction, abnormal bleeding, gastric ulcer, weight loss, mental deterioration, skin eruptions and liver damage. Death from respiratory failure has occurred after convulsions and unconsciousness. It can cause flaccid paralysis, general anaesthesia and dyspnoea (Sax and Lewis, 1989; Health and Safety, NIEHS and NIH websites).

Bioactivities

Pharmacological activities *in vitro* and *in vivo*
Smooth muscle No data found.

Antimicrobial activities

Antibacterial activity
No recent data found except for low activity in five bacterial species (Friedman *et al.*, 2002).

Antifungal activity
No recent data found.

Uses in pregnancy and lactation: contraindications

Due to its toxicity and the lack of data during human pregnancy and only some experimental reproductive effects reported, wintergreen essential oil is not recommended for use in aromatherapy during these periods.

Pharmaceutical guidance

Wintergreen essential oil is a severe skin and eye irritant (National Toxicology Program) and has high potential toxicity, reacts with aspirin and warfarin and therefore is not recommended in aromatherapy massage. It is banned by IFRA (A30).

Use in babies and young children

Due to the immaturity and the delicate nature of the skin of babies and young children, it is inadvisable for any essential oils, especially the highly toxic wintergreen essential oil, to be used in massage, however much the essential oil has been diluted in the carrier oils. This is also a necessary precaution due to the possibilities of sensitisation of the children at this young age through skin or air-borne odorant effects (see Chapters 5 and 7).

Instillation or administration of essential oils near the baby or young child's nose is not only not recommended, but distinctly inadvisable, as there have been numerous cases reported of severe toxicity and even death from such applications (see Chapter 7).

Yarrow Root Oil

Species/Botanical name

Achillea millefolium L. (Asteraceae/Compositae)

Synonyms

Milfoil, millefolium

Safety

CHIP details
Not listed

GRAS status
Not given (Council of Europe category 4, with limits on camphor, eucalyptol and thujone).

Extraction, source, appearance and odour

Extraction
The essential oil is obtained by steam distillation of the root (Arctander, 1960).

Source
Eastern Europe.

Appearance and odour
The essential oil is dark blue when fresh, ageing to yellowish-green (Arctander, 1960). It can also be almost colourless.

Aromatherapy uses

Although untested for toxicity, yarrow is considered safe in many aromatherapy books and is often used by aromatherapists as a cheap substitute for the very expensive German chamomile essential oil and also inadvertently where the German chamomile oil has been adulterated by yarrow oil. Uses include: skin, hair, nails, wounds, warts, ulcers, varicose veins; sinus congestions, catarrh; rheumatism, backache; high blood pressure, thrombosis; digestion, diarrhoea, drug detoxication, urogenital disorders (menopausal, menstruation, breast fibroids,

prostates); neuralgia, insomnia and stress (Ryman, 1991; Lawless, 1992; Rose, 1992a,b; Price, 1993; Sheppard-Hanger, 1995).

Scientific comment
Yarrow essential oil, with its unknown toxicity and possible allergic reaction in sensitive individuals, especially those with an existing hypersensitivity to other members of the Asteraceae/Compositae, cannot be recommended for use in aromatherapy, although it has many traditional herbal uses. It is however, often found as an adulterant in German chamomile essential oil and this raises the problem of possible toxicity for the latter, though no adverse reports have been reported to date.

Herbal uses

Yarrow is an 'Approved Herb' (Blumenthal *et al.*, 2000). Internal uses include loss of appetite, dyspeptic ailments, such as mild, spastic discomforts of the gastrointestinal tract. Added to a sitz bath it is used for painful, cramp-like conditions of psychosomatic origin (in the lower part of the female pelvis). Traditionally, yarrow was used as an astringent, diaphoretic, digestive stimulant, antispasmodic, menstrual regulator, wound herb, fever management; anti-inflammatory; for intestinal colic, stomach and other cramps, nervous dyspepsia, palpitations, painful periods, asthma and convulsions, especially in children; high blood pressure, haemorrhoids and varicose veins; gynaecological conditions, especially heavy or painful menstruation (Chandler *et al.*, 1982; Wren, 1988; Chevallier, 1996; Barnes *et al.*, 2002).

Food and perfumery uses

Food   Yarrow oil is not used in many foods but in alcoholic beverages (Fenaroli, 1997). In the USA, yarrow is only approved for use in alcoholic beverages, and the finished product must be thujone-free (Leung, 1980).

Perfumery   Not used.

Chemistry

Major components

	% (Lawrence, 1976–2001)
α-Pinene	1–9
Camphene	trace–6.0
β-Pinene	7.0
Sabinene	trace–15
p-Cymene	trace–8
1,8-Cineole	trace–29
Limonene	trace–4
γ-Terpinene	trace–6
trans-Sabinene hydrate	trace–10
cis-Sabinene hydrate	trace–5
Camphor	trace–8
Terpinen-4-ol	trace–6
cis-Chrysanthenyl acetate	trace–3
Germacrene-D	trace–65
α-Thujone	trace–1.4
β-Thujone	trace–35
Chamazulene	trace–51

There are immense variations in the chemical composition of yarrows from different countries and during different stages of development as well as differences between the leaves and the flowers (Lawrence, 1976–2001; Figuereido et al., 1992). Chamazulenes are not present in the fresh herb: they are formed as artefacts during steam distillation of the oil, from unstable precursors called proazulenes (e.g. achillin and achillicin) (Sticher, 1977).

Adulteration

Yarrow is frequently used as a substitute wholly or partly of the expensive German chamomile oil, as both are blue and rather similar in odour. A drop or two added to an old yellowish chamomile turns it into a 'fresh oil'!

Toxicity

Acute toxicity

Neither the oral or dermal LD_{50} have been done for the essential oil. However, for the herb, the oral LD_{50} for mice is 3.65 g/kg; 3.1 g/kg i.p.; >1 g/kg s.c. In rats an LD_{50} (s.c.) was given as 16.86 g/kg (Barnes et al., 2002).

Irritation and sensitisation

No formal testing recorded.

Phototoxicity

No formal testing recorded.

Other toxicities

Allergic reactions to the yarrow (e.g. dermatitis) and positive patch tests in sensitised people have been reported, but there is no concrete reason for allergenic properties nor the photosensitisation shown (Barnes et al., 2002). Terpinen-4-ol and thujone are usually present at very low concentrations in the essential oil – too low to cause toxicity. A compositae mixture of ether extracts of arnica, German chamomile, feverfew, tansy and yarrow elicited an allergic response in 118 of 3851 people (3.1%) (Hausen, 1996) and 31 out of 686 patients (4.5%) had a positive patch test to a compositae mix (Paulson, 1993) but this has not been linked to essential oil components.

Yarrow (Achillea millefolium) extract in polypropylene glycol is reported to function as a 'biological additive' in 65 cosmetic products. Historically, it was reported to be used at concentrations of <25%, but recent data indicate it is 0.5–10%. Only limited toxicity data are available. Guinea-pigs were sensitised to crude extracts of the whole plant and the flowers of A. millefolium; the tea was weakly genotoxic in a somatic mutation and recombination test using Drosophila melanogaster (Barnes et al., 2002).

In clinical testing, product formulations containing 0.1–0.5% of ingredient that actually contained 2% of yarrow extract were generally not irritating. In provocative testing, patients reacted to a compositae mix that contained yarrow, as well as to yarrow itself (Final Report, 2001a). Also in clinical testing, a formulation containing 0.1% yarrow (A. millefolium) extract (2% yarrow in propylene glycol and water) was not a sensitiser in a maximisation test and alcoholic extracts of dried leaves and stalks of A. millefolium did not produce a phototoxic response (Final Report, 2001a). These data were not considered sufficient to support the safety of this ingredient in cosmetics and UV absorption data were required. If absorption occurs in the UVA or UVB range, photosensitisation data, gross pathology and histopathology in skin and other major organ systems associated with repeated exposures, reproductive and developmental toxicity data, two genotoxicity studies (one using a mammalian system) may be required. Then if positive, a two-year dermal carcinogenicity assay performed using National Toxicology Program (NTP) methods may be needed, plus clinical sensitisation testing at maximum concentration of use. In the absence of these data, it was concluded that the available data are insufficient to support the safety of yarrow extract for use in cosmetic products (Final Report, 2001a).

Bioactivities

Pharmacological activities *in vitro* and *in vivo*
Some activities quoted for yarrow are associated with the chamazulene component (see German chamomile), especially the anti-inflammatory properties, but most are using aqueous extracts which do not contain the essential oil (Barnes *et al.*, 2002). The essential oil has CNS-depressant activity: a dose of 300 mg/kg decreased the spontaneous activity of mice and lowered the body temperature of rats. At higher doses, the essential oil inhibited pentetrazole-induced convulsions and prolonged sleep induced by a barbiturate preparation (Kudrzycka-Bieloszabska and Glowniak, 1966). Antispasmodic activity, which has been associated with chamazulene, has not been verified for yarrow essential oil, but the aqueous fraction was quite active (Barnes *et al.*, 2002).

The wound-healing properties of the essential oils of yarrow and Yakut wormwood and khamazulen have been studied in napalm burns (Taran *et al.*, 1989).

Antimicrobial activities

Antibacterial activity
No essential oil activities were found, but moderate activity was shown for an ethanolic extract of yarrow against six organisms (Barnes *et al.*, 2002).

Use in pregnancy and lactation: contraindications

The essential oil of yarrow is virtually untested for any toxicity. The trace amounts (0.3%) of thujone, which is an abortifacient component, can be disregarded, but there is the danger of allergic reactions and the use of yarrow essential oil should therefore be contraindicated during pregnancy and lactation.

Note: As yarrow is often used to adulterate German chamomile, the latter essential oil should also be restricted, unless the exact source and history is known.

Pharmaceutical guidance

Yarrow essential oil has unknown toxicity so cannot be recommended for use in aromatherapy massage. It may cause an allergic reaction in sensitive individuals, especially those with an existing hypersensitivity to other members of the Asteraceae/Compositae. Excessive doses may interfere with existing anticoagulant and hypo- and hypertensive therapies, and may have sedative and diuretic effects (as with the herb). The herbal usage was apparently discarded officially in 1781 (Grieve, 1937/1992) and the present usage is not greatly supported by scientific evidence.

Use in babies and young children

Due to the immaturity and the delicate nature of the skin of babies and young children, it is inadvisable for any essential oils to be used in massage, however much the essential oil has been diluted in the carrier oils. This is also a necessary precaution due to the possibilities of sensitisation of the children at this young age through skin or air-borne odorant effects (see Chapters 5 and 7).

Instillation or administration of essential oils near the baby or young child's nose is not only not recommended, but distinctly inadvisable, as there have been numerous cases reported of severe toxicity and even death from such applications (see Chapter 7).

Ylang Ylang Oil

CAS numbers

USA: 8006-81-3; EINECS: 83863-30-3

Species/Botanical name

Cananga odorata Hook. f. et Thomson (Anonaceae)

Synonyms

Cananga odorata var. *genuina*, *Unona odoratissimum*

Other species

Cananga, *C. odorata* var. *macrophylla*

Safety

CHIP details
Xn; R65; 50%; S62 (A26)

RIFM recommended safety of use limits
10% and also for *Cananga* essential oil (A23)
On IFRA list as banned (A30)

EU sensitiser total
37.6 (based on benzyl alcohol, 0.5%; benzyl salicylate, 4%; eugenol, 1%; isoeugenol, 1%; geraniol, 3%; benzyl benzoate, 12.5%; farnesol, 0.6% and linalool, 15%) (A27)

GRAS status
Granted (Fenaroli, 1997).

Extraction, source, appearance and odour

Extraction
A volatile oil obtained from fresh, early-morning-picked flowers of the tree, which are steam distilled for different times to give several essential oils of a different composition (Arctander, 1960).

Source
Comores, Réunion, the Phillipines and Indonesia.

Appearance and odour
'Extra', the most expensive first grade to come off from the distillation, is a pale yellow essential oil with a floral, sweet odour and a creosylic and benzoate top-note of limited tenacity. The fade-out is more pleasant, soft and sweet, slightly spicy and balsamic-floral. A good extra resembles the absolute and has a peculiar creamy-sweet note (Arctander, 1960). The 'third' grade is a yellowish oily liquid of sweet-floral and balsamic-woody odour with a tenacious and very sweet-balsamic undertone. It is useful in soaps and a cheaper floral material for hyacinth, lilac and other floral bases. The 'first' and 'second' grades are in between and are colourless to yellowish essential oils with an exotic, floral, sweet, lingering aroma; they are used for cutting the 'extra' and the lower grades and frequently take the place of the most expensive grade (Arctander, 1960).

Note: Cananga oil is water distilled from the flowers of *Cananga odorata* in the northern and western parts of Java (Indonesia). The oil is a yellow to orange-yellow or slightly greenish-yellow somewhat viscous liquid of sweet floral, balsamic and tenacious odour. The first notes are woody to leathery with a floral undertone. This odour profile appears to be much heavier than that of ylang and cananga oil is used in soap perfumery and for popular notes in men's/women's fragrances where it combines well with castoreum, calamus, birch tar oil rectified, copaiba oil, etc. (Arctander, 1960).

Aromatherapy uses

Although ylang ylang was originally produced solely for the perfumery and fragrance trades, it has found wide usage in aromatherapy. The essential oil (all grades) is apparently relaxing to the CNS and regulates adrenaline flow. It is therefore used for anger, rage, anxiety, shock, panic and fear; insomnia, nervous tension, stress, low self-esteem; hyperpnoea, palpitations, tachycardia, lowering blood pressure, balancing hormones; firming breasts; aphrodisiac, antidepressant; impotence; frigidity; intestinal infection, diarrhoea; balancing sebum production: both oily and dry skin, acne, insect bites (Ryman, 1991; Lawless, 1992; Rose, 1992a,b; Price, 1993; Sheppard-Hanger, 1995).

Scientific comment

Ylang ylang essential oil has a stimulant, not relaxant effect on the human CNS, so may possibly help to alleviate depression when used as a fragrance (inhalation), but at low concentrations it may also relax. Massage itself alleviates numerous stress-related and muscular conditions (see Chapter 3) and thereby the essential oil can add a positive, stimulant effect to the therapy.

Herbal uses

Although ylang ylang (like Moroccan chamomile, citronella, clary sage, geranium, rosewood and vetiver) was originally produced solely for the perfumery and fragrance trades, some herbal uses have emerged. The flowers are used in an ointment (in coconut oil) for cosmetic and hair care, skin disease, prevention of fever and for infection in the Molucca Islands (Lawless, 1992). The essential oil was apparently used in macassar oil for hair growth on the scalp and for insect bites and for regulation of cardiac and respiratory rhythm.

Food and perfumery uses

Food Ylang ylang oil (FEMA 3119) is used in many foods and beverages (Fenaroli, 1997).

Perfumery Ylang ylang absolute is one of the most floral of any essential oil and is used in high-class muguet perfumes (e.g. Diorissimo), blending well with jasmine, rose, Peru balsam oil, sandalwood oil, cassie, mimosa and floral components. It is used in many floral bases (e.g. carnation, lilac, narcissus, gardenia, violet, honeysuckle, freesia and sweet pea). Ylang ylang oil is known as the poor man's jasmine. The 'extra' is used mainly in high-class floral and heavy-oriental type perfumes and mere traces of the essential oil improve medium-priced floral bases. The essential oil blends well with virtually every other essential oil and component (Arctander, 1960). The other grades are used in less expensive perfumes, soaps, etc. and as substitutes for the more expensive grade or to make the lower grades more 'classy'. It blends well with: bergamot, lavender, lemon, narcissus, neroli, palmarosa, sandalwood and vetiver.

Chemistry

Major components

	% (Lawrence, 1976–2001)	
	Range	*EU sensitisers*
Benzyl alcohol	trace–1	0.5
Benzyl salicylate	1–5	4
Eugenol	trace–1	1
Geraniol	0.2–3	3
Isoeugenol	trace–1	1
Benzyl benzoate	2–10	12.5
Farnesol	1–3	0.6
Linalool	1–19	15
Total		37.6

Minor components

p-Cresylmethyl ether	0.5–16.5
Germacrene D	5–10
β-Caryophyllene	1–10
Geranyl acetate	3–10
Benzyl acetate	3–25
Methyl benzoate	2.2–5.3
Farnesene	trace–18

The extra grade has more benzyl acetate and *p*-cresylmethyl ether than the other three grades, with a high proportion of linalool and low proportion of sesquiterpenes. The composition of this and the other grades is very variable and it is impossible to correlate the different grades between different suppliers and at different times. The extra grade is distilled for 15 minutes in some cases, the next, grade 1, is distilled for half an hour (or longer) and the following grades 2–3 of inferior quality are distilled over an hour to 22 hours. The best fraction is the most expensive and is produced only in small amounts (Arctander, 1960).

Adulteration

Cananga oil is often used as a substitute or adulterant. Gurjum balsam oil is also often used, but can be detected by the α-gurjunene content. The extra grade, in small volume, is mixed with larger volumes of the lower grades. Adulteration is also effected with synthetic vanillin, *p*-cresylmethyl ether, methyl benzoate, geraniol, isoeugenol, isosafrole, benzyl alcohol, benzyl benzoate, benzyl propionate and cinnamate, anisyl acetate, anisyl alcohol; also with copaiba oil, Peru balsam and other pure oils and synthetic components (A8; see Chapter 4).

Toxicity

Acute toxicity (A22)
Oral LD$_{50}$ >5 g/kg (rat).

Dermal LD$_{50}$ >5 g/kg (rabbit).

Irritation and sensitisation
Older reports showed nil at 10% (human); 4/200 patients with dermatitis showed a sensitisation reaction at 2% (Rudzki *et al.*, 1976) and ylang ylang is now considered to be a sensitiser. This may often be due to cananga oil, used as adulterant, which is a sensitiser and irritant to the rabbit skin when applied undiluted.

It is advised not to use the essential oil on inflamed skin or if dermatitis is apparent; excess may lead to nausea and headache (Sheppard-Hanger, 1995).

Phototoxicity
None reported.

Bioactivities

Pharmacological activities *in vitro* and *in vivo*
Smooth muscle Ylang ylang oil (all fractions) had a spasmolytic effect on guinea-pig ileum *in vitro* (A2; Lis-Balchin *et al.*, 1996a).

Uterus There was a decrease in the spontaneous contractions in the rat for ylang ylang and some of its components (A3; A4; Lis-Balchin and Hart, 1997b).

Other activities Ylang ylang showed a stimulant action according to CNV studies in human (A14) and mice motility (A14). Spraying depressed patients with ylang ylang, in uncontrolled studies, apparently stimulated them (Rovesti and Colombo, 1973).

Antimicrobial activities

Antibacterial activity
The vapour was effective against 1/5 different bacterial species (Maruzella and Sicurella, 1960). The essential oil showed mainly very low activity against only 15/25 different bacteria (Baratta *et al.*, 1998b) and poor activity against 5/5 bacteria (Friedman *et al.*, 2002).

Antifungal activity
Moderate activity was shown by an unspecified ylang ylang oil against 5/5 fungi (Maruzella, 1960) and a mainly fungistatic action against 11/15 fungal species (Maruzella and Ligouri, 1958). There was considerable activity against *Aspergillus niger* (Baratta *et al.*, 1998b).

Antioxidant activity
Ylang ylang essential oil has some antioxidant potential (Baratta *et al.*, 1998a).

Use in pregnancy and lactation: contraindications
Due to considerable adulteration, which could affect its toxicity and bioactivity, and a decrease in the spontaneous contractions noted in the rat uterus *in vitro*, ylang ylang should be avoided in pregnancy and parturition. Ylang ylang also has a high sensitisation potential and therefore it should not be massaged into the skin during these times or during lactation. The fragrance could be used sparingly for its brain stimulant activity.

Pharmaceutical guidance
Ylang ylang essential oil is a very well-used essential oil in aromatherapy. However, its chemical composition is very changeable in commerce, due to methods of production and widespread adulteration, making its actual toxicity and bioactivity suspect. It is a potent fragrance, which can bring on nausea and headaches in some people. The essential oil should be used with caution on the skin, especially if sensitive, as it has a high sensitisation potential, but otherwise it can be used as a fragrance essential oil for overall stimulation or even relaxation in some people, diluted alone or in a mixture with other essential oils. Banned (A30).

Use in babies and young children
Due to the immaturity and the delicate nature of the skin of babies and young children, it is inadvisable for any essential oils to be used in massage, however much the essential oil has been diluted in the carrier oils. This is also a necessary precaution due to the possibilities of sensitisation of the children at this young age through skin or air-borne odorant effects (see Chapters 5 and 7).

Instillation or administration of essential oils near the baby or young child's nose is not only not recommended, but distinctly inadvisable, as there have been numerous cases reported of severe toxicity and even death from such applications (see Chapter 7).

Floral Absolutes and Essential Oils (other than Jasmine, Rose, Lavender, Neroli)

CAS numbers

CAS numbers are indicated in the species list below.

Species/Botanical names

		CAS numbers
Boronia	Boronia megastigma	8053-33-6
Broom	Spartium junceum	8025-80-1
Carnation	Dianthus caryophyllus	8021-43-0
Cassie	Acacia farnesiana	8023-82-3
Champaca	Michelia champaca	Essential oil: 8006-76-6
Frangipani	Plumeria alba	No CAS
Gardenia	Gardenia jasminoides syn. G. grandiflorum	68916-47-2
Honeysuckle absolute	Lonicera caprifolium	8023-93-6
Hops	Humulus lupulus	Essential oil: 8007-04-3
Hyacinth absolute	Hyacinthus orientalis	8023-94-7
Immortelle	Helichrysum angustifolium	8023-95-8
Jonquil absolute	Narcissus jonquilla	8023-75-4
Lilac	Syringa vulgaris	68916-92-7
Lily of the valley, muguet	Convallaria majalis	68916-82-5
Linden blossom or lime	Tilia europoea, T. vulgaris	No CAS
Lotus	Nymphea alba	No CAS
Magnolia	Magnolia glauca	No CAS
Mimosa absolute	Acacia dealbata, A. decurrens	8031-03-6
Narcissus absolute	Narcissus poeticus	68917-12-4
Orris absolute	Iris pallida	8002-73-1
Osmanthus	Osmanthus fragrans	68917-05-5
Tuberose absolute	Polianthes tuberosa	8024-05-3
Violet leaf absolute	Viola odorata	8024-08-6

Safety

CHIP details

None for most or not available, except: helichrysum essential oil (Xn; R10, 65; 70%, S62) and hop (Xn; R10, 65; 55%, S62).

RIFM recommended safety of use limits

RIFM limits not provided for most, except:

Honeysuckle absolute *Lonicera caprifolium*	3%
Hyacinth absolute, *Hyacinthus orientalis*	8%
Immortelle, *Helichrysum angustifolium*	abs 2%; oil 4%
Jonquil absolute, *Narcissus jonquilla*	2%
Orris absolute, *Iris pallida*	3%
Violet leaf absolute	2%

EU sensitiser total

Sensitiser values not given for most, except hops (1.8%) and *Helichrysum* essential oil (10%).

GRAS status

Not applicable.

Extraction, source, appearance and odour

Extraction

Floral absolutes are usually extracted in hexane, hexene and petroleum ether (benzene has now been banned due to carcinogenicity) to give the concretes and thence redissolved in alcohol to give the absolutes (see Chapter 5).

Source

Some of the authentic absolutes come from Egypt, China, Bulgaria, Morocco, Tunisia, India and Tahiti, but they are mainly produced in France. They are extremely expensive and rare, hence most of the florals on the market are perfumes, rather than absolutes (i.e. they have been composed from natural essential oils, natural fractions and a variety of synthetic components or are entirely synthetic).

Appearance and odour

The authentic absolutes are usually very thick and difficult to dispense from the bottles and, unless diluted appropriately, have a different odour to that of the flower itself. Most people prefer the 'synthetic' versions and these come under different names from different perfumery wholesalers (e.g. Charabot sells them as 'Floralines'). They could be in dipropyl glycol or even an alcoholic base, and when used in perfumery the concentration ranges from 3 to 30% oil as in: extrait perfumes, containing 15–30% of perfume oil; eau de parfum, 15–20% perfume oil; eau de toilette or toilet water, 5–10%; and eau de Colognes or toilet waters, 3–5% of perfume oil in a 70% alcohol/water. These are more like the concentrations of essential oils used in aromatherapy massage, whilst the higher concentrations could be used as scents or inhalants.

Floral absolutes and synthetics can be diluted very substantially and still retain their odour. The most common essential oils are often sold as 10% dilutions to make them economical. These are also a good idea as the originals are often difficult to dispense without incurring an extra drop or two in the diluent (fixed oil or alcohol) in the process. Many florals are middle notes.

All the florals have individual odours. The exact odours are presented for a few examples in the profiles section below.

Aromatherapy uses

Floral absolutes are not generally used apart from the well-known rose, jasmine, lavender and neroli, except for the few examples given below (Ryman, 1991; Lawless, 1992; Rose, 1992a,b; Price, 1993; Sheppard-Hanger, 1995).

Scientific comment

The most useful usage is by inhalation of the scent, rather than skin application in massage, as dermatitis and sensitisation can occur. The pleasant odour gives a feeling of relaxation and happiness, which can contribute to the relief of stress-related disorders.

Herbal uses

No herbal usage exists for these floral absolutes. However, some flower extracts (e.g. linden or lime blossom) have had successful folk-medicinal usage in teas for sedation and sleep (Barnes *et al.*, 2002). Narcissus flowers were formerly used in France for hysteria and epilepsy, but could be too overpowering, causing headaches and nausea. Immortelle is used as a decoction for headaches, migraines and liver ailments; it is said to have a strong psychological effect, including relaxation, increased dream activities and awareness, and is thus useful for meditation (Lawless, 1994).

Hops are renowned for their relaxation and sleep-inducing effects. *Humulus* belongs to the same plant family as cannabis and has some of the latter's qualities, including its narcotic and also hypnotic properties. It is used in modern herbal medicine as a general nerve tonic and sedative (Barnes *et al.*, 2002).

Some local usage is made of the erotic nature of some flowers, especially for seduction and the bridal bed (Aftel, 2001; Lawless, 1994).

See also individual floral profiles below.

Food and perfumery uses

Food Very few floral absolutes are used in foods and drinks due to their exhorbitant cost and the preference for synthetic equivalents (Fenaroli, 1997).

Perfumery Most of the floral absolutes are only used in a very few expensive perfumes, although they were used extensively in the past. Individual uses are given for a few examples below (Arctander, 1960).

Chemistry

Major components

The main components of many florals include chemicals with a fresh, floral odour and character, found in tertiary monoterpene alcohols and their lower esters. The compounds are branched chain and have methyl groups on the 2-, 3-, 6- or 7-positions. The presence of one or two double bonds increases their freshness and naturalness (BACIS, 1997).

They include:

Linalool and linalyl acetate Tetrahydrolinalool and acetate	More or less fresh floral olfactive properties, however with a slightly fatty and earthy undertone
Myrcenol (2-methyl-6-methylene-7-octen-2-ol) and its acetate	Natural, fresh, floral odours, even more delicate than those of linalool and its acetate
Ocimenol (2,6-dimethyl-5,7-octadien-2-ol) and its acetate	Very freshly floral olfactive qualities and are preferred to myrcenol and its acetate
Dihydromyrcenol (2,6-dimethyl-7-octen-2-ol) and its acetate	Dihydromyrcenol is olfactively somewhat reminiscent of linalool. It is often used to replace linalool. Its acetate is used as replacer for linalool and in detergent compounds
Tetrahydromyrcenol (2,6-dimethyloctan-2-ol) and its acetate	Sometimes used instead of tetrahydrolinalool and its acetate because they have a less earthy note and are also stable in all media. The compounds have fresh floral, slightly fatty, odours

Other components shown by headspace analysis of different flowers (Surburg *et al.*, 1993) include the following:

- Lily-of-the-valley flowers: citronellyl acetate, benzyl acetate, benzyl alcohol, farnesol, geraniol, cinnamic alcohol
- Lilac flowers: (*E*)-ocimene, 1,4-dimethoxybenzene, indole.

Cryogenic vacuum trapping (headspace) of some temperate and tropical flowers (Joulain, 1993) showed:

- Jonquil: (*E*)-β-ocimene, methyl benzoate, linalool, indole, methyl (*E*)-cinnamate, benzyl benzoate
- Jasminum sambac: linalool, (*E*)(*E*)-a-farnesene, indole, 1(10),5-germacradien-4-ol, benzyl alcohol, 1,3,7,11, tetraene
- Gardenia: methyl benzoate, 3(*Z*)-hexeny-1-yl benzoate, linalool, benzyl benzoate, jasmine lactone; the Tahitian species had a high percentage of methyl salicylate as well
- Mimosa: benzyldehyde, 3(*Z*)-hexen-1-yl acetate, (*E*)-β-ocimene, benzyl alcohol, linalool, anisaldehyde, pentacecane and a very high percentage of heptadecene.

Perfumes are constructed from about 17 to hundreds of different components, both natural and synthetic (Calkin and Jellinek, 1994). Some basic compositions of floral accords include:

- Carnation: ylang extra, geraniol, eugenol, cinnamic alcohol, benzyl salicylate, vanillin, heliotropin
- Violet: methyl ionone, α-ionone, phenylethyl alcohol (PEA), anisaldehyde, amyl cinnamic aldehyde, heliotropin, sandalwood, benzyl benzoate
- Hyacinth: PEA, benzyl acetate, galbanum essential oil, rosatol, cinnamic alcohol, phenylpropyl alcohol, amyl salicylate, eugenol, indol
- Lilac: PEA, terpineol, ylang ylang, hydroxy-citronellol, phenylacetaldehyde, anisaldehyde, heliotropin, cinnamic alcohol, isoeugenol, indol.

Variants, both natural essential oils and mainly synthetic components, are added in other compositions or else modify the basic formula. It is surprising how several of the same main components are used for such different fragrances, but they are mixed together in different proportions for each floral accord or perfume.

Adulteration

Most of the floral absolutes are nowadays replaced by synthetic or semi-synthetic substitutes (e.g. floralines from Charabot) (see below; also A8; Chapter 4).

Toxicity

Acute toxicity

There are no scientific data for most of these floral absolutes and if studies on toxicity have been done in the past, they would be irrelevant today due to the changes in the methods of production of the genuine floral absolutes and also the use of synthetic formulations.

Boronia absolute is considered to be possibly toxic if taken orally (Watts, 1997).

Irritation and sensitisation

In recent years there has been an increase worldwide in the incidence of allergic contact dermatitis and many studies have shown that this is due partly to the increase in use of perfumes (see Chapter 7). Many absolutes are possibly irritant and sensitising on human skin due to the presence of other components in the absolutes, and because of residual extractant solvents and synthetic components (see also Chapters 4 and 7). Extreme caution in use of carnation, tuberose and immortelle absolutes is advised and very low concentrations should be used on the skin due to possible cutaneous irritation (Watts, 1997). Mimosa, tuberose and violet absolutes may cause dermatitis in hypersensitive people. Hops are known to cause dermatitis and also sensitisation in pickers and processors and also in animal experiments (Barnes *et al.*, 2002).

There is a general problem of possible sensitisation when using absolutes (Chapter 7) due to the extraction of other non-volatile components etc. There are also numerous studies indicating that there has been a dramatic rise in the incidence of sensitisation due to more widespread use of perfumes (see Chapter 7). There is also the list of sensitising components issued by the EU in the 7th Amendment (2002), which are included in many floral absolutes and perfumes. Suspected floral sensitisers include hyacinth and violet absolutes, the two most commonly used florals (Watts, 1997).

Phototoxicity

The possibility of photosensitisation exists for some extracts (e.g. honeysuckle absolute) (Watts, 1997).

Bioactivities

Pharmacological activities *in vitro* and *in vivo*

No data found for these absolutes.

Other activities

Floral scents are very pleasant and relaxing. Many of the common florals already described in the monographs have been given aphrodisiac properties (e.g. jasmine, neroli, ylang ylang, rose); tuberose and narcissus are also considered very sensual. Jasmine, ylang ylang, rose, tuberose and narcissus all have euphoric properties, which may lower sexual inhibitions. Some florals have an apparent effect on the heart (e.g. neroli and ylang ylang). Some florals act on the emotions, for example rose, jasmine and neroli stimulate feelings of love as well as sexual desire. Some of the floral essential oils help heal emotional issues that may prevent us from giving and receiving love, for example immortelle (*Helichrysum angustifolium, H. italicum, H. orientale*), ormenis flower (*Ormenis monticules*) and linden blossom (*Tilia vulgaris*). Carnation (*Dianthus caryophyllus*) is apparently known for counteracting detachment and emotional solitude, while encouraging tenderness, nurturing, openness and self-worth. Hyacinth (*Hyacinthus orientalis*) and jasmine also nurture self-esteem (Lawless, 1994; Worwood, 1996).

The heavy florals have an intensely narcotic effect (Aftel, 2001) and apparently may induce receptivity and surrender, rather like being ravished. Many have a faecal undertone (which has the yin-yang appeal), which is due to indole, found also in faeces which also provides the aphrodisiac quality (Jellinek, 1956). Rose oil does not contain indole and yet also has the aphrodisiac quality.

The psychological and emotional effects of several florals have been discussed in Chapter 6. Other effects are described by Lawless (1994). In most studies, perfumes have probably been used (see A16; Rovesti and Colombo, 1973).

Antimicrobial activities

No data found for these absolutes.

Profiles of selected florals

Boronia absolute

Boronia flowers are very pervasive with a lemon and rose odour. There are two varieties of absolute: a green, viscous liquid with a rich fresh, fruity and tea-like odour and a bright yellow-orange absolute from Tasmania with a powerful scent of cassis, violet, apricot and freesia (Aftel, 2001). It contains ionones, which is unique for floral absolutes (Arctander, 1960). The green viscous absolute is also described as fresh, fruity-green, tea-like, spicy-herbaceous, like cinnamon and tobacco-leaf and the main body is warm and woody-sweet (Arctander, 1960). It has been used in expensive perfumes, mixing well with numerous bases like violet, mimosa, cassie, honeysuckle, sweet pea, bergamot, sandalwood, helichrysum, linalool, salicylates, etc. It has also been incorporated into a few flavours like raspberry, strawberry, plum and artificial blackcurrant flavour.

Broom absolute
This is obtained from a small, decorative shrub that grows wild in the south of France, Spain and Italy and is a semi-solid pasty dark red to brown product with a mild herbaceous-honeylike-hay and dry fruits top-note with animalic undertones (Charabot et Cie information). It is used in rose bases, tuberose, cassie, mimosa, violet, ionones, vetiver, castoreum etc. and is useful in aldehydic perfumes (Arctander, 1960).

Carnation absolute
The absolute is an olive green or orangey-brown, viscous liquid of very sweet, honey-like, herbaceous, heavy and tenacious fragrance, reminiscent of the odour of the live carnation flowers only when very diluted to 5% and below. There is frequent adulteration with synthetic components like eugenol, methyl eugenol, benzyl benzoate, clove bud absolute, etc. It is used sparingly in some perfumes, blending well with lavender, ylang ylang, clary sage, etc. (Arctander, 1960). It can irritate sensitive skins, so should be used sparingly. The main components are benzyl benzoate, eugenol, phenylethyl alcohol, benzyl salicylate, methyl salicylate, many of which are known sensitisers (A26).

Cassie absolute
Commercial production occurs in India, although the tree grows all over Europe and in the USA, Australia, etc. The absolute is dark-yellow to pale brown viscous liquid usually much darker than mimosa. It has a warm, powdery-spicy odour with herbaceous and floral qualities and has tenacious cinnamic-balsamic undertones (Arctander, 1960). It is used in expensive perfumes to give warmth and a woody-floral note and blends well with ionones, methyl ionones, heliotropine, cyclamal, orris, bergamot and amber bases.

Champaca absolute
Champaca flowers (yellow to deep red in colour) are worn by Indian women to contrast and adorn their black hair, and are often inserted as buds, which open during the evening, giving out the scent

of orange blossom/tea and ylang ylang. Champaca is a tree related to magnolia. The absolute used to be produced in Madagascar but nowadays more in India and is dark-yellow to brownish-orange viscous liquid with a unique dry-floral, orange-flower, ylang ylang, carnation and tea rose odour, with notes of clary sage, methyl eugenol and guaiacwood oil, the latter being a frequent adulterant. Ylang ylang flowers are frequently co-extracted with champaca flowers (Arctander, 1960). Recently the odour was described as fresh, grassy top-note which evolves into a delicately sweet, tea-like fragrance with leafy undertones (Aftel, 2001) and as a heavy floral honey-like fragrance, with various flowery undertones (Charabot et Cie information). Champaca absolute is used in some expensive perfumes to give a unique, warm, floral-leafy note often compared to a fine grade tea (Arctander, 1960). It blends well with lily-of-the-valley bases, carnation, rose, violet, sandalwood, etc.

Frangipani absolute
In India, the *Plumeria* tree is sacred and bears fragrant flowers. The 'temple flower' originates from Central and South America, Central Asia, South Africa and the Philippines. In India, it is given as an offering to the Hindu gods and has a heavy floral fragrance, with various flowery undertone (Charabot et Cie information).

Gardenia absolute
Gardenia flowers were originally produced in Réunion Island, also in Tahiti and China, possibly from a different species. The true absolute is no longer produced and has been replaced by synthetics (Arctander, 1960).

Honeysuckle absolute
This is an orange-green to dark-green or brownish, viscous fluid with an intensely sweet, fatty-floral odour, reminiscent of jasmine absolute from chassis and of orange flower absolute. The sweetness is similar to that of tuberose (Arctander, 1960). Artificial honeysuckle perfumes have become the norm and used as such or blended in perfumes.

Jonquil absolute
This is a viscous dark brown to dark orange to olive-brown liquid with a heavy, honey-like, deep-sweet floral odour with a strong green undertone and a somewhat bitter and very tenacious dry-out note. It resembles tuberose and hyacinth. It blends well with other floral absolutes and many of their components. It is frequently adulterated with

narcissus, ylang ylang absolutes and also benzoin Siam, Peru balsam, vanilla absolute and many synthetics and is frequently replaced entirely by synthetics (Arctander, 1960).

Lilac and lily-of-the-valley (muguet) absolutes

These are now entirely perfumes or bases (Arctander, 1960). Lilac absolute has no place in perfumery. Muguet is extremely difficult to compound to resemble the actual flower odour but the real absolute cannot be prepared with the intensity and also to resemble the excellent artificial versions. Muguet is a very useful ingredient of many perfumes (e.g. Diorissimo) and is also sold as a perfume in its own right by many perfume houses.

Lotus absolute

The lotus became a symbol of Buddhism as it originates in dirty ponds and breaks through the water to blossom. It has a floral, daffodil, leather, animal, slightly fruity odour, reminiscent of *Osmanthus* (Charabot et Cie information). There are other sources of lotus absolute (e.g. *Nelumbo nucifera*, which is known both as the blue lotus and pink lotus).

Mimosa absolute

This is from the yellow flowers of an evergreen tree growing wild in Australia and cultivated in the south of France and in India. It is a yellow-orange to orange liquid, with a rich, floral, slightly green odour (Charabot et Cie information). It resembles the consistency of honey (Arctander, 1960) and has a similar odour to cassie, but is less spicy. It blends with similar components and absolutes to that of cassie (see above) as well as numerous others. This absolute is very much less expensive than the other floral absolutes and is used in numerous perfumes.

Narcissus absolute

Narcissus poeticus originated in the Middle East or the eastern Mediterranean countries but now grows wild in the south of France. It is a dark green to orange viscous liquid with a hay, earthy, honey-like, spicy-animalic odour (Charabot et Cie information). The odour is described as strongly foliage-green, very sweet-herbaceous, over a faint but pervasive floral note (Arctander, 1960). There are two main types of absolutes with distinctive odours, one of which is known as 'des montagnes' and the other 'des plaines': the former is greener and has a violet-leaf-like odour which is more earthy (Arctander, 1960). It is not widely used in perfumery. Nowadays

it is grossly adulterated with other absolutes and components or purely synthetic.

Orris absolute

Iris pallida is a perennial plant with nice blue flowers although only the rhizomes are used. These are washed, husked and dried, then stored for about 3 years. Orris is obtained mainly from Italy and Morocco. The concrete is washed in alkaline ethyl ether to remove myristic acid accounting for 85% of the concrete, or produced from petroleum ether-extracted concrete. It is a watery-white to pale yellow oily liquid of extremely delicate, sweet floral yet somewhat woody odour, which on dilution displays the full strength and diffusion (Arctander, 1960). It has been used in peach, strawberry and raspberry food flavours in minute amounts (0.0010 mg%) (Arctander, 1960). It has been used in expensive perfumes, blending with muguet materials, ylang ylang, mimosa, cassie, linalool, sandalwood essential oil, nerol, geraniol, heliotropine, amber bases, lilac, violet, etc.

Orris Floraline 80 (Charabot et Cie information) is a synthetic reconstitution with a woody, fatty, sweet-floral, warm and tenacious odour.

Osmanthus absolute

This is not commercially available and is produced and used in small amounts in certain local areas. The flowers are used to perfume some tea in China (Arctander, 1960).

Tuberose absolute

The absolute is obtained from the perennial plant, which has long stems and white, very odorous flowers. A native of Central America and imported into France in the sixteenth century, tuberose is now cultivated mainly in India. The tuberose is one of the few flowers which continues to produce odour after picking, hence it was used in enfleurage extraction in the past. It is a soft paste or semi-liquid mass of orange to brown colour with a heavy-sweet, floral, honey-like odour with oily-fatty undertones (Arctander, 1960). Recently it has been described as a light brown to dark brown viscous liquid, with a strong floral, honey-like, spicy odour (Charabot et Cie information). Other descriptions indicate that it has a spicy, green, floral note with undertones of orange and ylang ylang, thus showing that different extractions have different appearances and odours. It is composed mainly of benzyl alcohol, tuberose, methyl and benzyl benzoate, methyl salicylate, and methyl anthranilate. Aromatherapy use is given as perfume (Lawless, 1992).

Tuberose Floraline 75 (CAS no. 94334-35-7) has the same characteristics as above (Charabot et Cie information).

Violet leaves absolute

This originates from plants grown in the south of France and Egypt and is considered to represent Spring. It is semi-solid intensely dark-green liquid with a strong green-earthy-fruity note (Charabot et Cie information). Its odour is very peculiar and powerful and truly green-leaf like (Arctander, 1960). It is used extensively in perfumery due to its tremendous diffusiveness, which allows its use in very small proportions. It appears in certain floral bases like hyacinth, muguet, and high-class chypres, many aldehydic perfumes. It blends well with numerous other floral absolutes and components, including the little-used estragon, cumin and basil as well as boronia, tuberose, narcissus and tea-leaf. It is frequently adulterated with numerous components and is now produced mainly as a synthetic perfume. Aromatherapy uses include: acne, wounds, fibrosis, poor circulation, rheumatism, bronchitis, mouth and throat infections, dizziness, headaches, insomnia and exhaustion (Lawless, 1992).

Use in pregnancy and lactation: contraindications

Due to the consistent loss of spontaneous contractions in the uterus of the rat *in vitro* with essential oils and absolutes and the lack of formal assessment of their safety, there is insufficient evidence to justify their usage on the skin, but the use of the scent for inhalation alone can prove beneficial for relaxation and a happy outlook.

Pharmaceutical guidance

There is scant pharmacological information available for these floral absolutes and due to the widespread substitution by synthetics they should have restricted use. These florals are best used as fragrances for inhalation rather than application to the skin, as they may cause dermatitis or sensitisation (see also Chapters 5 and 7).

Use in babies and young children

Due to the immaturity and the delicate nature of the skin of babies and young children, it is inadvisable for any floral absolutes to be used in massage, however much the absolute has been diluted in the carrier oils. This is also a necessary precaution due to the possibilities of sensitisation of the children at this young age through skin or air-borne odorant effects (see Chapters 5 and 7).

Instillation or administration of essential oils near the baby or young child's nose is not only not recommended, but distinctly inadvisable, as there have been numerous cases reported of severe toxicity and even death from such applications (see Chapter 7).

Bibliography

Abbott DD, *et al.* (1961). Chronic oral toxicity of oils of sassafras and safrole. *Pharmacologist* 3: 62.

Abdullah D, *et al.* (1996). Enhancing effect of essential oils on the penetration of 5-fluorouracil through rat skin. *Yao Hsueh Hsueh Pao* 31: 214–221.

Abebe W (2002). Herbal medication: potential for adverse interactions with analgesic drugs. *J Clin Pharm Ther* 27: 391–401.

Abraham M, *et al.* (1979). Inhibiting effects of jasmine flowers on lactation. *Indian J Med Res* 69: 88–92.

Abraham SK (2001). Anti-genotoxicity of *trans*-anethole and eugenol in mice. *Food Chem Toxicol* 39: 493–498.

Abrahams HJ (1980). Onycha, ingredient of the ancient Jewish incense: an attempt at identification. *Econ Bot* 33: 233–236.

Abramovici A, *et al.* (1985). Benign hyperplasia of ventral prostate in rats induced by a monoterpene (preliminary report). *The Prostate* 7: 389–394.

Achterrath-Tuckermann U, *et al.* (1980). Pharmacological investigations with compounds of chamomile. V. Investigations on the spasmolytic effect of compounds of chamomile and Kamillosan on the isolated guinea pig ileum. *Planta Med* 39: 38–50.

Ackerman D (1991). *A Natural History of the Senses*. New York: Vintage Books, Random House.

Adams O (1945). Maori medicinal plants. *Auckland Botanical Society Bulletin*.

Adams TB, *et al.* (1996). The FEMA GRAS assessment of alicyclic substances used as flavour ingredients. *Food Chem Toxicol* 34: 763–828.

Afifi FU, *et al.* (1997). Evaluation of the gastroprotective effect of *Laurus nobilis* seeds on ethanol induced gastric ulcer in rats. *J Ethnopharmacol* 58: 9–14.

Aftel M (2001). *Essence and Alchemy: A Book of Perfume*. London: Bloomsbury.

Agarwal L, *et al.* (1980). Chemical study and antimicrobial properties of essential oil of *Cymbopogon citratus* Linn. *Bull Med Ethnobot Res* 1: 401–407.

Agarwal OP, *et al.* (1980). Antifertility effects of fruits of *Juniperus communis*. *Planta Med* 40: 98–101.

Agarwal P, *et al.* (1996). Randomized placebo-controlled, single blind trial of holy basil leaves in patients with noninsulin-dependent diabetes mellitus. *Int J Clin Pharmacol Ther* 34: 406–409.

Agricultural Research Service (1998). Phytochemical database (PhytochemDB). http://www.ars-grin.gov/duke (accessed 9 May 2005).

Akgul A, Kivanc M (1988). Inhibitory effects of selected Turkish spices and oregano components on some foodborne fungi. *Int J Food Microbiol* 6: 263–268.

Albert-Puleo M (1980). Fennel and anise as estrogenic agents. *J Ethnopharmacol* 2: 337–344.

Albuquerque AA, *et al.* (1995). Effects of essential oil of *Croton zehntneri*, and of anethole and estragole on skeletal muscles. *J Ethnopharmacol* 49: 41–49.

Alexander M (2001). Aromatherapy and immunity: How the use of essential oils aid immune potentiality. *Int J Aromather* 11: 152–156.

Al-Hader AA, *et al.* (1994). Hyperglycemic and insulin release inhibitory effects of *Rosmarinus officinalis*. *J Ethnopharmacol* 43: 217–221.

Allahverdiyev A, *et al.* (2004). Antiviral activity of the volatile oils of *Melissa officinalis* L. against *Herpes simplex* virus type-2. *Phytomedicine* 11: 657–661.

Allen KL, *et al.* (1991). A survey of the antibacterial activity of some New Zealand honeys. *J Pharm Pharmacol* 43: 817–822.

Aloisi AM, *et al.* (2002). Effects of the essential oil from citrus lemon in male and female rats exposed to a persistent painful stimulation. *Behav Brain Res* 136: 127–135.

Ammon HPT (1989). Phytotherapeutika in der Kneipp-therapie. *Therapiewoche* 39: 117–127.

Ammon HP (1996). Salai guggal – *Boswellia serrata*: from a herbal medicine to a non-redox inhibitor of leukotriene biosynthesis. *Eur J Med Res* 1: 369–370.

Anderson C, *et al.* (2000). Evaluation of massage with essential oils on childhood atopic eczema. *Phytother Res* 14: 452–456.

Anderson IB, *et al.* (1996). Pennyroyal toxicity: measurement of toxic metabolite levels in two cases and review of the literature. *Ann Intern Med* 124: 726–734.

Anderson JW (1923). Geranium dermatitis. *Arch Dermatol Syphilology* 7: 510–511.

Anderson RC, Anderson JH (1998). Acute toxic effects of fragrance products. *Arch Environ Health* 53: 138–146.

Andriantsiferana (1995). Chemical analysis of essential oils of Malagasy endemic species: *Piper* sp. *Ravensara anisata* Danguy & *Ravensara aromatica* Sonnerat. Paper presented at the American Society of Pharmacognosy Conference, 23–27 July.

Anon (1986). *Essential Oils and Oleoresins: A Study of Selected Producers and Major Markets*. Geneva: UNCTAD/GATT.

Aoshima H, Hamamoto K (1999). Potentiation of GABAa receptors expressed in *Xenopus* oocytes by perfume and phytoncid. *Biosci Biotechnol Biochem* 63: 743–748.

Api AM, *et al.* (1996). An evaluation of genotoxicity tests with Musk ketone. *Food Chem Toxicol* 34: 633–638.

Aqel MB (1992). A vascular smooth muscle relaxant effect of *Rosmarinus officinalis*. *Int J Pharmacognosy* 30: 281–288.

Aqel TMBJ (1991). Relaxant effect of the volatile oil of *Rosmarinus officinalis* on tracheal smooth muscle. *Ethnopharmacology* 33: 57–62.

Arctander S (1960). *Perfume and Flavor Materials of Natural Origin*. Elizabeth, NJ: S Arctander.

Armstrong F, Heidingsfeld V (2000). Aromatherapy for deaf and deafblind people living in residential accommodation. *Complement Ther Nurs Midwifery* 6: 180–188.

Arnould-Taylor WE (1981). *A Textbook of Holistic Aromatherapy*. London: Stanley Thornes.

Ashwood-Smith MJ, *et al.* (1985). Mechanisms of photosensitivity reactions to diseased celery. *BMJ* 290: 1249.

Ask E (2000). *Sandalwood Oil, A Study of Antimicrobial Effect*. Skien, Norway: Telelab.

Asre S (1994). Chemical composition and antimicrobial activity of some essential oils. MSc thesis, McQuarie University, Sydney, Australia.

Atanassova-Shopova S, Roussinov KS (1970a). On certain central neurotropic effects of lavender essential oil. *Izvest Inst Fiziol Sofiia* 13: 69–77.

Atanassova-Shopova S, Roussinov KS (1970b). Effects of *Salvia sclarea* essential oil on the central nervous system. *Izvest Inst Fiziol Sofiia* 13, 89–93.

Atanassova-Shopova S, *et al.* (1973). On certain central neurotropic effects of lavender essential oil. II. communication: Studies on the effects of linalool and of terpineol. *Izvest Inst Fiziol Bulg Akad Nauk* 15: 149–156.

Atchley EG, Cuthbert F (1909). *A History of the Use of Incense in Divine Worship*. London: Longmans, Green and Co.

Atta AH, Alkofahi A (1998). Anti-nociceptive and anti-inflammatory effects of some Jordanian medicinal plant extracts. *J Ethnopharmacol* 60: 117–124.

Aureli P, *et al.* (1992). Antimicrobial activity of some plant essential oils against *Listeria monocytogenes*. *J Food Protection* 55: 344–348.

Austad J, Kavli G (1983). Phototoxic dermatitis caused by celery infected by *Sclerotinia sclerotiorum*. *Contact Dermatitis* 9: 448–451.

Avery MD, Burket BA (1986). Effect of perineal massage on incidence of episiotomy and perineal laceration in a nurse-midwifery service. *J Nurse-Midwifery* 31: 128–134.

BACIS (Boelens Aroma Chemical Information Service) (1997). Olfactive properties and chemical identities of jasmine compounds. *BACIS Archives* BNB-99041 www.xs4all.nl/~bacis/bnb99041.html (accessed May 2005).

BACIS Archives [POM-98021]. Some aspects of the adulteration of natural isolates. www.xs4all.nl/~bacis/bacisarc.html (accessed June 2005).

Badia P (1991). Olfactory sensitivity in sleep: The effects of fragrances on the quality of sleep: a summary of research conducted for the fragrance research fund. *Perfumer and Flavorist* 16: 33–34.

Baker JR (1974). *Race*. London: Oxford University Press.

Bakerink JA, *et al.* (1996). Multiple organ failure after ingestion of pennyroyal oil from herbal tea in two infants. *Pediatrics* 98: 944–947.

Balachandran B, Sivaramkrishnan VM (1995). Induction of tumours by Indian dietary constituents. *Indian J Cancer* 32: 104–109.

Balachandran B, et al. (1991). Genotoxic effects of some foods and food components in Swiss mice. *Indian J Med Res* 94: 378–383.

Baldwin CM, et al. (1999). Odor sensitivity and respiratory complaint profiles in a community-based sample with asthma, hay fever, and chemical intolerance. *Toxicol Ind Health* 15: 403–409.

Balk F, Ford RA (1999). Environmental risk assessment for the polycyclic musks, AHTN and HHCB. Ll. Effect assessment and risk characterization. *Toxicol Lett* 111: 81–94.

Ballabeni V, et al. (2004). Novel antiplatelet and antithrombotic activities of essential oils from *Lavandula hybrida* Reverchon 'Grosso'. *Phytomedicine* 11: 596–601.

Ballard C, et al. (2002). Aromatherapy as a safe and effective treatment for the management of agitation in severe dementia: the results of a double-blind, placebo-controlled trial with *Melissa. J Clin Psychiatry* 63: 553–558.

Banner KH, et al. (1995). The effect of selective phosphodiesterase inhibitors in comparison with other anti-asthmatic drugs on allergen-induced eosinophilia in guinea-pig airways. *Pulm Pharmacol Ther* 8: 37–42.

Baratta MT, et al. (1998a). Chemical composition, antibacterial and antioxidative activity of laurel, sage, rosemary, oregano and coriander essential oils. *J Essential Oil Res* 10: 618–627.

Baratta MT, et al. (1998b). Antimicrobial and antioxidant properties of some commercial essential oils, *Flavour Fragrance J* 13: 235–244.

Barber P (1986). *Understanding Archaeological Excavation*. London: Batsford.

Barker A (1994). Aromatherapy and multiple sclerosis. *Aromather Q* 4–6.

Barker A (1995). Bowel care. *Aromather Q* 44: 7–10.

Barnes J, et al. (2002). *Herbal Medicines: A Guide for Healthcare Professionals*. London: Pharmaceutical Press.

Barocelli E, et al. (2004). Antinociceptive and gastroprotective effects of inhaled and orally-administered *Lavandula hybrida* Reverchon 'Grosso'. *Life Sci* 76: 213–223.

Baron RA (1983). 'Sweet smell of success'? The impact of pleasant artificial scents on evaluations of job applicants. *J Appl Psychol* 68: 709–713.

Baron R (1990). Environmentally induced positive affect: its impact on self-efficacy, task performance, negotiation, and conflict. *J Appl Soc Psychol* 16: 16–28.

Barrett S (2000). Aromatherapy company sued for false advertising. *Quackwatch* 25 September.

Barrett S (2001). Aromatherapy: making dollars out of scents. *Quackwatch* 22 August.

Baser KHC (1995). Analysis and quality assessment of essential oils. In: Tuley De Silva K, ed. *A Manual on the Essential Oil Industry*. Vienna: United Nations Industrial Development Organization, pp. 155–177.

Basketter DA, Allenby CF (1991). Studies of the quenching phenomenon in delayed contact hypersensitivity reactions. *Contact Dermatitis* 25: 160–171.

Basketter D, et al. (2000). Quenching: fact or fiction? *Contact Dermatitis* 43: 253–258.

Basketter DA, et al. (2002). Investigation of the skin sensitizing activity of linalool. *Contact Dermatitis* 47: 161–164.

Basnyet J (1999). Tibetan essential oils. *IFA J* 43: 12–13.

Bassett IB, et al. (1990). A comparative study of tea tree oil versus benzoylperoxide in the treatment of acne. *Med J Austr* 153: 455–458.

Battaglia S (1997). *The Complete Guide to Aromatherapy*. Brisbane: The Perfect Potion.

Battaglia S (1999). Aromatherapy and the immune system. *Aromatherapy Today, Austr Aromather J* 10: 26–30.

Baumann JU (1996). Effect of manual medicine in the treatment of cerebral palsy. *Manuelle Med (Berlin)* 34: 127–133.

Baur X, et al. (1999). Occupational asthma to perfume. *Allergy* 54: 1334–1335.

Beasley V ed. (1999) Toxicants that cause central nervous system depression. Veterinary Toxicology. Ithaca NY: International Veterinary Information Service (www.ivis.org), A2608.0899.

Bedini SA (1963). *The Scent of Time. A Study of the Use of Fire and Incense for Time Measurement in Oriental Countries. Transactions of the American Philosophical Society* Vol 53, Part 5. Philadelphia: American Philosophical Society.

Beecher HK (1955). The powerful placebo. *JAMA* 159: 1602–1606.

Beesley A, et al. (1996). Influence of peppermint oil on absorptive and secretory processes in rat small intestine. *Gut* 39: 214–219.

Belaiche P (1985). Treatment of vaginal infections of *Candida albicans* with the essential oil of *Melaleuca alternifolia*. *Phytotherapy* 15: 15–16.

Bell GD, *et al.* (1980). Plant essential oils – candidate treatments for atheroma. *Br J Clin Pharmacol* 3: 309–310.

Bell IR, *et al.* (1993). Self-reported illness from chemical odors in young adults without clinical syndromes or occupational exposures. *Arch Environ Health* 48: 6–13.

Bellanger JT (1998). Perillyl alcohol: application in oncology. *Altern Med Rev* 3: 448–457.

Benito M, *et al.* (1996). Labiatae allergy: systemic reactions due to ingestion of oregano and thyme. *Ann Allergy Asthma Immunol* 76: 416–418.

Benner MH, Lee HJ (1973). Anaphylactic reaction to chamomile tea. *J Allergy Clin Immunol* 52: 307–308.

Benoni H, *et al.* (1996). Studies on the essential oil from guarana. *Z Lebensm Unters Forsch* 203: 95–98.

Benor DJ (1993). *Healing Research – Holistic Energy Medicine and Spirituality*. Deddington, Oxfordshire: Helix Editions.

Benson H, Stark M (1996). *Timeless Healing. The Power and Biology of Belief*. London: Simon and Schuster.

Berghard A, *et al.* (1996). Evidence for distinct signaling mechanisms in two mammalian olfactory sense organs. *Proc Natl Acad Sci USA* 93: 2365–2369.

Berkley SF, *et al.* (1986). Dermatitis in grocery workers associated with high natural concentrations of furanocoumarins in celery. *Ann Intern Med* 105: 351–355.

Berliner DL, *et al.* (1991). The human skin: Fragrance and pheromones. *J Steroid Biochem Mol Biol* 39: 671–679.

Bernath J (1986). Production ecology of secondary plant products, In: Craker LE and Simon JE, eds. *Herbs, Spices, and Medicinal Plants: Recent Advances in Botany, Horticulture and Pharmacology*, Vol 1. Phoenix, AZ: Oryx Press, pp. 185–234.

Bertram T (1995). *Encyclopaedia of Herbal Medicine*. Dorset: Grace Publishers.

Berwick A (1994). *Holistic Aromatherapy*. Minnesota: Llewellyn Publications.

Betts T (2003). Use of aromatherapy (with or without hypnosis) in the treatment of intractable epilepsy – a two-year follow-up study. *Seizure* 12: 534–538.

Betts T, *et al.* (1995). An olfactory countermeasure treatment for epileptic seizures using a conditioned arousal response to specific aromatherapy oils. *Epilepsia* 36 (Suppl 3): S130.

Beylier MF, Givaudan SA (1979). Bacteriostatic activity of some Australian essential oils. *Perfumer and Flavorist* 4.

Bezard M, *et al.* (1997). Skin sensitization to linalyl hydroperoxide: support for radical intermediates. *Chem Res Toxicol* 10: 987–993.

Bhargava AK, *et al.* (1967). Pharmacological investigation of the essential oil of *Daucus carota* Linn. var. *sativa* DC. *Indian J Pharm* 29: 127–129.

BHP (1960). *British Herbal Pharmacopoeia*, published as a private edition by the Nigerian College.

Billany MR, *et al.* (1995). Topical antirheumatic agents as hydroxyl radical scavengers. *Int J Pharm* 124: 279–283.

Bilsland D, Strong A (1990). Allergic contact dermatitis from the essential oil of French Marigold (*Tagetes patula*) in an aromatherapist. *Contact Dermatitis* 23: 55–56.

Bishop CD (1995). Antiviral activity of the essential oil of *Melaleuca alternifolia* (Maiden and Betche) Cheel (tea tree) against tobacco mosaic virus. *J Essent Oil Res* 7: 641–644.

Black DR (1985). Pregnancy unaffected by pennyroyal usage. *J Am Osteopath Assoc* 85: 282.

Black M (1985). *Food and Cooking in Medieval Britain*. London: Historic Buildings and Monument Commission for England.

Blackwell R (1991). An insight into aromatic oils: lavender and tea tree. *Br J Phytother* 2: 26–30.

Blázquez MA, *et al.* (1989). Effects of *Thymus* species extracts on rat duodenum isolated smooth muscle contraction. *Phytother Res* 3: 41–42.

Blinne K (1999). Essential oil profile – *Leptospermum scoparium*. *Scensitivity* 9: 8.

Bloor SJ (1992). Antiviral phloroglucinols from New Zealand *Kunzea* species. *J Nat Prod* 55: 43–47.

Blumenthal M, *et al.* eds (2000). *Herbal Medicine*. Expanded Commission E Monographs. Austin, TX: American Botanical Council.

Boberg EW, *et al.* (1983). Strong evidence from studies with brachymorphic mice and pentachlorophenol that 1′-sulfooxysafrole is the major ultimate electrophilic and carcinogenic metabolite of 1′-hydroxysafrole in mouse liver. *Cancer Res* 43: 5163–5173.

Boelens MH (1986). The essential oil of spike lavender, *Lavandula latifolia* Vill (L spica DC). *Perfumer and Flavorist* 11: 43–63.

Boelens MH (1995). Chemical and sensory evaluation of *Lavandula* oils. *Perfumer and Flavorist* 20: 23–51.

Boelens MH, *et al.* (1993). Sensory properties of optical isomers. *Perfumer and Flavorist* 18: 2–16.

Boffa MJ, *et al.* (1996). Celery soup causes severe phototoxicity during PUVA therapy. *Br J Dermatol* 135: 334.

Bonkovsky HL, *et al.* (1992). Porphyrogenic properties of the terpenes camphor, pinene and thujone (with a note on historic implications for absinthe and the illness of Vincent van Gogh). *Biochem Pharmacol* 43: 2359–2368.

Booth DA (1979). Preference as motive. In: Kroeze JHA, ed. *Preference and Chemoreception.* Oxford: IRL Press.

Born J, *et al.* (2002). Sniffing neuropeptides: a transnasal approach to the human brain. *Nature Neurosci* 5: 514–516.

Bos R, *et al.* (1986). Composition of the volatile oils from the roots, leaves and fruits of different taxa of *Apium graveolens*. *Planta Med* 52: 531.

Boskabady MH, Ramazani-Assari M (2001). Relaxant effect of *Pimpinella anisum* on isolated guinea pig tracheal chains and its possible mechanism(s). *J Ethnopharmacol* 74: 83–88.

Botsoglou NA, *et al.* (2002). The effect of dietary oregano essential oil on lipid oxidation in raw and cooked chicken during refrigerated storage. *Meat Sci* 62: 259–265.

Bowles-Dilys EJ, *et al.* (2002). Effects of essential oils and touch on resistance to nursing care procedures and other dementia-related behaviours in a residential care facility. *Int J Aromather* 12: 1–8.

Boyce E, *et al.* (1987). Behaviour and the major histocompatibility complex of the mouse. In: Ader R, Felten DL and Cohen N, eds. *Psychoneuroimmunology*, 2nd edn. London: Academic Press, pp. 831–846.

Boyd EM, Sheppard EP (1970). Nutmeg oil and camphene as inhaled expectorants. *Arch Otolaryngol* 92: 372–378.

Bradshaw RM, *et al.* (1998). Effects of lavender straw on stress and travel sickness in pigs. *J Altern Complement Med* 4: 271–275.

Brandao FM (1986). Occupational allergy to lavender. *Contact Dermatitis* 15: 249–250.

Brandt W (1988). Spasmolytic effect of essential oils and components [Spasmolytische wirkung atherische ole]. *Z Phytother* 9: 33–39.

Breinlich VJ, Scharnagel K (1968). Pharmakologische Eigenschaften des EN-IN-dicycloäthers aus *Matricaria chamomilla*. *Arzneimittelforschung* 18: 429–431.

Brennan MJ, Weitz J (1992). Lymphedema 30 years after radical mastectomy. *Am J Phys Med Rehabil* 71: 12–14.

Bridges B (2001). Fragrances and allergic reactions. *J Am Board Fam Pract* 14: 400–401.

Brinker F (1997). *Herb Contraindications and Drug Interactions*. Sandy, OR: Eclectic Institute, pp. 46–47.

British Herbal Medicine Association (1983). *British Herbal Pharmacopoeia, 1983*. Keighley: British Herbal Medicine Association.

British Herbal Medicine Association (1990). *British Herbal Pharmacopoeia, 1990*, Vol 1. Bournemouth: British Herbal Medicine Association.

British Herbal Medicine Association (1996). *British Herbal Pharmacopoeia, 1996*. Exeter: British Herbal Medicine Association.

British Pharmacopoeia (2001). London: The Stationery Office.

Brohn P (1986). *Gentle Giants: The Powerful Story of One Woman's Unconventional Struggle Against Cancer*. London: Century Hutchinson.

Bronaugh RL, *et al.* (1985). Comparison of percutaneous absorption of fragrances by humans and monkeys. *Food Chem Toxicol* 23: 111–114.

Bronaugh RL, *et al.* (1990). In vivo percutaneous absorption of fragrance ingredients in rhesus monkey and humans. *Food Chem Toxicol* 28: 369–374.

Brooker DJR, *et al.* (1997). Single case evaluation of the effects of aromatherapy and massage on disturbed behaviour in severe dementia. *Br J Clin Psychol* 36: 287–296.

Brooker SG, *et al.* (1987). *New Zealand Medicinal Plants*, 3rd edn. Auckland: Reed Books.

Bruneton J (1995). *Pharmacognosy, Phytochemistry, Medicinal Plants*. Paris: Lavoisier Publishing.

Brunn EZ, Epiney-Burgard G (1989). *Women Mystics in Medieval Europe*. New York: Paragon House.

Buchanan RL (1978). Toxicity of spices containing methylenedioxybenzene derivatives: A review. *J Food Safety* 1: 275–293.

Buchbauer G (1992). Biological effects of fragrances and essential oils. *Perfumer and Flavorist* 18: 19–24.

Buchbauer G (1993). Molecular interaction: Biological effects and modes of action of essential oils. *Int J Aromather* 5: 11–14.

Buchbauer G (1996). Methods in aromatherapy research. *Perfumer and Flavorist* 21: 31–36.

Buchbauer G, Jirovetz L (1994). Aromatherapy – use of fragrances and essential oils as medicaments. *Flavour Fragrance J* 9: 217–222.

Buchbauer G, et al. (1991). Aromatherapy: Evidence for sedative effects of the essential oil of lavender. *Z Naturforschung* 46c: 1067–1072.

Buchbauer G, et al. (1992). Passiflora and limeblossom: Motility effects after inhalation of the essential oils and of some of the main constituents in animal experiments. *Arch Pharm (Weinheim)* 325: 247–248.

Buchbauer G, et al. (1993a). Fragrance compounds and essential oils with sedative effects upon inhalation. *J Pharm Sci* 82: 660–664.

Buchbauer G, et al. (1993b). Therapeutic properties of essential oils and fragrances. In: Teranishi R, Buttery RG and Sugisawa H, eds. *Bioactive Volatile Compounds from Plants*. Washington DC: American Chemical Society, pp. 159–165.

Buchbauer G, et al. (1993c). New results in aromatherapy research. Paper presented at the 24th International Symposium on Essential Oils, Berlin.

Buchbauer G, et al. (1994). The biology of essential oils and fragrance compounds. *Proceedings from the Aromatherapy Symposium Essential Oils, Health & Medicine, New York*. NAHA, pp. 69–76.

Buck DS, et al. (1994). Comparison of two topical preparations for the treatment of onychomycosis: *Melaleuca alternifolia* (tea tree) oil and clotrimazole. *J Fam Pract* 38: 601–605.

Buck LB (1992). The olfactory multigene family. *Curr Opin Neurobiol* 2: 282–288.

Buck LB (1996). Information coding in the vertebrate olfactory system. *Annu Rev Neurosci* 19: 517–544.

Buck LB (2000). The molecular architecture of odor and pheromone sensing in mammals. *Cell* 100: 611–618.

Buck L, Axel R (1991). A novel multigene family may encode odorant receptors: A molecular basis for odor recognition. *Cell* 65: 175–187.

Buckle J (1993). Does it matter which lavender oil is used? *Nurs Times* 89: 32–35.

Buckle J (1997). *Clinical Aromatherapy in Nursing*. San Diego, CA: Singular Publishing Group.

Buckle J (1999). Use of aromatherapy as a complementary treatment for chronic pain. *Altern Ther* 5: 42–45.

Buckley DA, et al. (2000). The frequency of fragrance allergy in a patch-test population over a 17-year period. *Br J Dermatol* 142: 279–283.

Buckman R, Sabbagh K (1993). *Magic or Medicine: An Investigation into Healing*. London: Macmillan.

Budge EA Wallis (1899/1988). *Egyptian Magic*. Arkana.

Budhiraja SS, et al. (1999). Biological activity of *Melaleuca alternifola* (tea tree) oil component, terpinen-4-ol, in human myelocytic cell line HL-60. *J Manipulative Physiol Ther* 22: 447–453.

Buechel DW, et al. (1983). Pennyroyal oil ingestion: report of a case. *J Am Osteopath Assoc* 82: 793–794.

Bulbring E (1946). Observations on the isolated phrenic nerve diaphragm. *Br J Pharmacol* 1: 38–61.

Bunny S (1984). *Illustrated Book of Herbs*. London: Octopus.

Bunyan N (1998). Baby died after taking mint water for wind. *Daily Telegraph* 21 May.

Burfield T (2003). The adulteration of essential oils – and the consequencies to aromatherapy and natural perfumery practice. Paper presented at the International Federation of Aromatherapists Annual AGM, October 2003.

Burkey JL, et al. (1999). The in vivo disposition and metabolism of methyleugenol in the Fischer 344 rat and the B6C3F1 mouse. *Toxicologist* 48(1-S), 224.

Burkhard PR, et al. (1998). Topical eucalyptus oil poisoning. *Australas J Dermatol* 39: 265–267.

Burkhard PR, et al. (1999). Plant-induced seizures: reappearance of an old problem. *J Neurol* 246: 667–760.

Burkhardt G, et al. (1986). Terpene hydrocarbons in *Pimpinella anisum* L. *Pharmac Weekbl (Sci)* 8: 190–193.

Burnett KM, et al. (2004). Scent and mood state following an anxiety-provoking task. *Psychol Reports* 95: 707–722.

Burns A, et al. (2002). Sensory stimulation in dementia: An effective option for managing behavioural problems. *BMJ* 325: 1312–1313.

Burns E, Blaney C (1994). Using aromatherapy in childbirth. *Nurs Times* 90: 54–58.

Burns E, et al. (2000). An investigation into the use of aromatherapy in intrapartum midwifery practice. *J Altern Complement Med* 6: 141–147.

Burrow A, *et al.* (1983). The effects of camphor, eucalyptus and menthol vapour on nasal resistance to airflow and nasal sensation. *Acta Otolaryngol* 96: 157–161.

Cabo J, *et al.* (1985). Accion hipoglucemiante de preparados fitoterapicos que contienen especies del genero salvia. *Ars Pharmac* 26: 239–249.

Cabo J, *et al.* (1986). The spasmolytic activity of various aromatic plants from the province of Granada. The activity of the major components of their essential oils. *Plant Med Phytother* 20: 213–218.

Caccioni DR, *et al.* (1998). Relationship between volatile components of citrus fruit essential oils and antimicrobial action on *Penicillium digitatum* and *Penicillium italicum*. *Int J Food Microbiol* 40: 73–79.

Caddy R (1997). *Essential Oils in Colour*. Surrey: Amberwood Publishing.

Cady SH, Jones GE (1997). Massage therapy as a workplace intervention for reduction of stress. *Percept Motor Skills* 84: 157–158.

Caelli M, *et al.* (2000). Tea tree oil as an alternative topical decolonization agent for methicillin-resistant *Staphylococcus aureus*. *J Hosp Infect* 46: 236–237.

Cai L, Wu CD (1996). Compounds from *Syzygium aromaticum* possessing growth inhibitory activity against oral pathogens. *J Nat Prod* 59: 987–990.

Calkin RR, Jellinek JS (1994). *Perfumery: Practice and Principles*. Chichester: Wiley, pp. 22–23 and 138–140.

Camarasa JG (1995). New allergens. *J Eur Acad Dermatol Venereol* 5: 15.

Cannard G (1996). The effect of aromatherapy in promoting relaxation and stress reduction in a general hospital. *Complement Ther Nurs Midwifery* 2: 38–40.

Carlson RJ (1975). *The End of Medicine*. Chichester: John Wiley and Son.

Carson CF, Riley TV (1993). Antimicrobial activity of the essential oil of *Melaleuca alternifolia*. *Lett Appl Microbiol* 16: 49–55.

Carson CF, Riley TV (1994). Susceptibility of *Propionibacterium acnes* to the essential oil of *Melaleuca alternifolia*. *Lett Appl Microbiol* 19: 24–25.

Carson CF, Riley TV (1995a). Toxicity of the essential oil of *Melaleuca alternifolia* or tea tree oil. *J Toxicol Clin Toxicol* 33: 193–194.

Carson CF, Riley TV (1995b). Antimicrobial activity of the major components of the essential oil of *Melaleuca alternifolia*. *J Appl Bacteriol* 78: 264–269.

Carson CF, Riley TV (2001). Safety, efficacy and provenance of tea tree (*Melaleuca alternifolia*) oil. *Contact Dermatitis* 45: 65–67.

Carson CF, *et al.* (1995a). Susceptibility of methicillin-resistant *Staphylococcus aureus* to the essential oil of *Melaleuca alternifolia*. *J Antimicrob Chemother* 35: 421–424.

Carson CF, *et al.* (1995b). Broth micro-dilution method for determining the susceptibility of *Escherichia coli* and *Staphylococcus aureus* to the essential oil of *Melaleuca alternifolia* (tea tree oil). *Microbios* 82: 181–185.

Carson CF, *et al.* (1996). In-vitro activity of the essential oil of *Melaleuca alternifolia* against *Streptococcus* spp. *J Antimicrob Chemother* 37: 1177–1178.

Carson CF, *et al.* (1997). Use of the essential oil of *Melaleuca alternifolia* (tea tree oil) in cutaneous fungal infections. *J Br Podiatr Med* 52: iv–v.

Carson CF, *et al.* (1998). Efficacy and safety of tea tree oil as a topical antimicrobial agent. *J Hosp Infect* 40: 175–178.

Carson CF, *et al.* (2000). A randomised, placebo-controlled, single-blind pilot study to evaluate the efficacy of tea tree oil gel (6%) in the treatment of herpes labialis. Poster presented at European Virology 2000, 17–21 September, Glasgow, Scotland.

Carson CF, *et al.* (2001). *Melaleuca alternifolia* (tea tree) oil gel (6%) for the treatment of recurrent herpes labialis. *J Antimicrob Chemother* 48: 450–451.

Carson CF, *et al.* (2002). Mechanism of action of *Melaleuca alternifolia* (tea tree) oil on *Staphylococcus aureus* determined by time-kill, lysis, leakage, and salt tolerance assays and electron microscopy. *Antimicrob Agents Chemother* 46: 1914–1920.

Carter R (1998). *Mapping the Mind*. London: Weidenfeld and Nicolson.

Carvalho-Freitas MI, Costa M (2002). Anxiolytic and sedative effects of extracts and essential oil from *Citrus aurantium* L. *Biol Pharm Bull* 25: 1629–1633.

Casterline CL (1980). Allergy to chamomile tea. *JAMA* 4: 330–331.

Caujolle F, Meynier D (1958). Toxicite de l'estragol et des anetholes (cis et trans). *CR Hebd Seanc Acad Sci Paris* 246: 1465–1468.

Cavanagh HMA, Wilkinson JM (2002). Biological activities of lavender essential oil. *Phytother Res* 16: 301–308.

Cavendish R (1970). *Man, Myth and Magic*, Vol 9. New York: Marshall Cavendish.

Ceccarelli L, *et al.* (2002). Sex differences in the citrus lemon essential oil-induced increase of hippocampal acetylcholine release in rats exposed to a persistent painful stimulation. *Neurosci Lett* 330: 25–28.

Centini F, *et al.* (1987). A case of sage oil poisoning. *Zacchia* 60: 263–274.

Ceska O, *et al.* (1986). Furocoumarins in the cultivated carrot, *Daucus carota*. *Phytochemistry* 25: 81–83.

Chadba A, Madyastha KM (1984). Metabolism of geraniol and linalool in the rat and effects on liver and lung microsomal enzymes. *Xenobiotica* 14: 365–374.

Chaisse E, Blanc M (1990). Les ravageurs de la lavande et du lavandin. *Phytoma* 419: 45–46.

Chaitow L (1998). *Aromatherapy for Back Pain*. New York: Bramley Quadrillion.

Chan VSW, *et al.* (1992). Comparative induction of unscheduled DNA synthesis in cultured rat hepatocytes by allylbenzenes and their 1'-hydroxy metabolites. *Food Chem Toxicol* 30: 831–836.

Chana JS (1993). A review of East Indian sandalwood oil. Paper presented at a Meeting of Forum Essential Augsburg, Germany.

Chana JS (1994). Exotic oils of India. Paper presented at the Aromatherapy Symposium – Essential Oils, Health and Medicine, New York.

Chandler RF, Hawkes D (1984). Aniseed – a spice, a flavor, a drug. *Can Pharm J* 117: 28–29.

Chandler RF, *et al.* (1982). Ethnobotany and phytochemistry of yarrow, *Achillea millefolium*, Compositae. *Econ Bot* 36: 203–223.

Chang Ya-Ching, *et al.* (1997). Allergic contact dermatitis from oxidised d-limonene. *Contact Dermatitis* 37: 308–309.

Chappell R (1991). New sensory dimensions for the deaf and blind. *Int J Aromather* 3: 10–12.

Charabot et Cie. www.charabot.com/mp/mp.

Charabot SA (1999). La vanille: une orchideé dans votre vie. 200th Anniversary presentation pack. Arco Ocean Indien SA.

Charles DJ, Simon J (1999). Lavender: is it real or synthetic? *J NORA* 4.

Charron JM (1997). Use of *Lavandula latifolia* as an expectorant [Letter]. *J Altern Complement Med* 3: 211.

Chaudhary SK, *et al.* (1985). Increased furocoumarin content of celery during storage. *J Agric Food Chem* 33: 1153–1157.

Chaudhary SK, *et al.* (1986). Oxypeucedanin, a major furocoumarin in parsley, *Petroselinum crispum*. *Planta Med* 52: 462–464.

Chen CL, *et al.* (1999). Safrole-like DNA adducts in oral tissue from oral cancer patients with a betel quid chewing history. *Carcinogenesis* 20: 2331–2334.

Chevallier A (1996). *Encyclopaedia of Medicinal Plants*. London: Dorling Kindersley.

Chou YJ, Dietrich DR (1999). Toxicity of nitromusks in early life-stages of South African clawed frog, *Xenopus laevis* and zebra-fish, *Danio rerio*. *Toxicol Lett* 111: 17–25.

Christian MS, *et al.* (1999). Developmental toxicity studies of four fragrances in rats. *Toxicol Lett* 111: 169–174.

Cimanga K, *et al.* (2002). Correlation between chemical composition and antibacterial activity of essential oils of some aromatic medicinal plants growing in the Democratic Republic of Congo. *J Ethnopharmacol* 79: 213–20.

Classen C, *et al.* (1994). *Aroma*. London: Routledge.

Clifford Frances R (1997). *Aromatherapy during your Pregnancy*. Saffron Walden: CW Daniel Co.

Cockayne S, Gawkrodger J (1997). Occupational contact dermatitis in an aromatherapist. *Contact Dermatitis* 37: 306.

Cohen BM, Dressler WE (1982). Acute aromatics inhalation modifies the airways. Effects of the common cold. *Respiration* 43: 285–293.

Coleta M, *et al.* (2001). Comparative evaluation of *Melissa officinalis* L., *Tilia europaea* L., *Passiflora edulis* Sims and *Hypericum perforatum* L. in the elevated plus maze anxiety test. *Pharmacopsychiatry* 34 (Suppl 1): S20–21.

Combe A (1905). *Influences des parfums et des odeurs sur les néuropathes et les hystériques*. Paris.

Cone JE, Shusterman D (1991). Health effects of indoor odorants. *Environ Health Perspect* 95: 53–59.

Connell FEA, *et al.* (2001). Can aromatherapy promote sleep in elderly hospitalized patients? *J Can Geriatr Soc* 4: 191–195.

Conner DE, Beuchat LR (1984). Sensitivity of heat-stressed yeasts to essential oils of plants. *Appl Environ Microbiol* 47: 229–233.

Conti V (1992). Ostoearthritis and diverticulitis. *Int J Aromather* 4: 16.

Cook J (1777). *A Voyage Towards the South Pole and Round the World*. London: Strahan and Cadell.

Cooke A, Cooke MD (1991). *An Investigation into Antimicrobial Properties of Manuka and Kanuka Oil*. Cawthron Institute Report. February.

Cooke B, Ernst E (2000). Aromatherapy: a systematic review. *Br J Gen Pract* 50: 493–496.

Cooper SD, *et al.* (1995). The identification of polar organic compounds found in consumer products and their toxicological properties. *J Exp Anal Environ Epidemiol* 5: 57–75.

Cootes P (1982). Clinical curio: liver disease and parsley. *BMJ* 285: 1719.

Corbin A (1986). *The Foul and the Fragrant*. Cambridge, MA: Harvard University Press.

Corner J, *et al.* (1995). An evaluation of the use of massage and essential oils on the well-being of cancer patients. *Int J Palliat Nurs* 1: 67–73.

Cornwell PA, Barry BW (1994). Sesquiterpene components of volatile oils as skin penetration enhancers for the hydrophilic permeant 5-fluorouracil. *J Pharm Pharmacol* 46: 261–269.

Cornwell S, Dale A (1995). Lavender oil and perineal repair. *Modern Midwife* 5: 31–33.

Cosentino S, *et al.* (1999). In-vitro antimicrobial activity and chemical composition of Sardinian thymus essential oils. *Lett Appl Microbiol* 29: 130–135.

Coulson IH, Khan AS (1999). Facial 'pillow' dermatitis due to lavender oil allergy. *Contact Dermatitis* 41: 111.

Council of Europe (1981). *Flavouring Substances and Natural Sources of Flavourings*, 3rd edn. Strasbourg: Maisonneuve.

Cousins N (1979). *Anatomy of an Illness*. New York: WW Norton.

Craig C (1994). Introduction to CNS pharmacology. In: Craig C and Stitzel R, eds. *Modern Pharmacology*, 4th edn. Boston, MA: Little, Brown and Co, pp. 329–336.

Craig JO (1953). Poisoning by the volatile oils in childhood. *Arch Dis Child* 28: 475–483.

Cramer GM, *et al.* (1978). Estimation of toxic hazard – a decision tree approach. *Food Cosmet Toxicol* 16: 255–276.

Crawford GH, *et al.* (2004). Use of aromatherapy products and increased risk of hand dermatitis in massage therapists. *Arch Dermatol* 140: 991–996.

Crowell PL (1999). Prevention and therapy of cancer by dietary monoterpenes. *J Nutr* 129: 775S–778S.

Cruz T, *et al.* (1989). The spasmolytic activity of the essential oil of *Thymus baeticus* Boiss in rats. *Phytother Res* 3: 106–108.

Culpeper N (1653). *The English Physician Enlarged*. London: printed by Peter Cole.

Culpeper N (1653/1995). *Culpeper's Complete Herbal and The English Physician and Family Dispensatory* (facsimile: Wordsworth editions, 1995).

Culpeper N (1826/1981). *Culpeper's Complete Herbal and English Physician* (facsimile: Pitman Press Ltd, Bath, 1981).

Culpeper N (1835). *The Complete Herbal*. London: Th. Kelly.

Culpepper-Richards K (1998). Effect of a back massage and relaxation intervention on sleep in critically ill patients. *Am J Crit Care* 7: 288–299.

Cunningham S (1989). *Magical Aromatherapy*. Minnesota: Llewellyn Publications.

Curtis T, Williams DG (1996). *Introduction to Perfumery*. London: Ellis Horwood.

Cutler WB, *et al.* (1998). Pheromonal influences on sociosexual behavior in men. *Arch Sex Behav* 27: 1–13.

Cutter K (1989). Cancer of the cervix. *Int J Aromather* 1: 7.

Daferera DJ, *et al.* (2000). GC-MS analysis of essential oils from some Greek aromatic plants and their fungitoxicity on *Penicillium digitatum*. *J Agric Food Chem* 48: 2576–2581.

Dale A, Cornwell S (1994). The role of lavender oil in relieving perineal discomfort following childbirth: a blind randomized clinical trial. *J Adv Nursing* 19: 89–96.

Damian P, Damian K (1995). *Aromatherapy Scent and Psyche*. Rochester, VT: Healing Arts Press.

Darvay A, *et al.* (2001). Photoallergic contact dermatitis is uncommon. *Br J Dermatol* 145: 597–601.

Daughton CG, Ternes TA (1999). Pharmaceuticals and personal care products in the environment: agents of subtle change? *Environ Health Perspect* 107 (Suppl 6): 907–938.

Davis P (1988). *Aromatherapy an A–Z*. Saffron Walden: CW Daniel Co.

Davis P (1991). *Subtle Aromatherapy*. Saffron Walden: CW Daniel Co.

Dawood NJ (1973). *Tales from the Thousand and One Nights*. Harmondsworth: Penguin Classics.

Day LM, *et al.* (1997). Eucalyptus oil poisoning among young children: mechanisms of access and the potential for prevention. *Aust N Z J Public Health* 21: 297–302.

Deans SG (2002). Antimicrobial properties of lavender volatile oil. In: Lis-Balchin M, ed. *Genus Lavandula, Aromatic and Medicinal Plants – Industrial Profiles*. London: Taylor and Francis.

Deans SG, Ritchie G (1987). Antibacterial properties of plant essential oils. *Int J Food Microbiol* 5: 165–180.

Deans SG, Svoboda KP (1989). Antibacterial activity of summer savory (*Satureja hortensis* L.) essential oil and its constituents. *J Horticult Sci* 64: 205–210.

Deans SG, et al. (1994a). Antimicrobial activities of the volatile oil of *Heteromorpha trifoliata* [Wendl.] Eckl. & Zeyh. [Apiaceae]. *Flavour Fragrance J* 9: 245–248.

Deans SG, et al. (1994b). Antimicrobial and antioxidant properties of *Syzygium aromaticum* [L.] Merr. & Perry: Impact upon bacteria, fungi and fatty acid levels in ageing mice. *Flavour Fragrance J* 10: 323–328.

Déchamp C, et al. (1984). Choc anaphylactique au céleri et sensibilisation á l'ambroisie et á l'armoise. Allergie croisée ou allergie concomitante? *Presse Med* 13: 871–874.

Degel J, Koster EP (1999). Odors: implicit memory and performance effects. *Chem Senses* 24: 317–325.

De Groot AC, Frosch PJ (1997). Adverse reactions to fragrances. A clinical review. *Contact Dermatitis* 36: 57–86.

De Groot AC, Liem DH (1983). Facial psoriasis caused by contact allergy to linalool and hydroxycitronellal in an aftershave. *Contact Dermatitis* 9: 230–232.

De Groot AC, Weyland JW (1992). Systemic contact dermatitis from tea tree oil. *Contact Dermatitis* 27: 279–280.

De Groot AC, et al. (1987). Adverse effects of cosmetics: a retrospective study in the general population. *Int J Cosmet Sci* 9: 255–259.

De Hoghton Charles (1970). *Man, Myth and Magic*, Vol 11. London: BPC Publishing.

Deighton N, et al. (1994). The chemical fate of the endogenous plant antioxidants carvacrol and thymol during oxidative stress. *R Soc Edin Proc Section B (Biol Sci)* 102: 247–252.

Dejeans M (Antoine de Hornot) (1764). *Traité des Odeurs*. Paris: Nyon/Guillyn/Saugrain.

Delaveau P, et al. (1989). Sur les proprietes neurodepressives de l'huile essentielle de Lavande. *CR Soc Biol* 183: 342–348.

Delgado IF, et al. (1993). Peri- and post-natal developmental toxicity of beta-myrcene in the rat. *Food Chem Toxicol* 31: 623–628.

Del Beccaro MA (1995). Melaleuca oil poisoning in a 17-month-old. *Vet Human Toxicol* 37: 557–558.

Della Loggia R, et al. (1981). [Evaluation of the activity on the mouse CNS of several plant extracts and a combination of them]. *Riv Neurol* 51: 297–310.

Demarne F, van der Walt JJA (1989). Origin of the rose-scented *Pelargonium* grown on Reunion Island. *S Afr J Bot* 55: 184–191.

Dember WN, Warm JS (1991). Effects of fragrance on performance and mood in a sustained attention task. Lecture at the American Association for the Advancement of Science, 19 February, Washington DC, USA.

Denny EFK (2002). Distillation of the lavender type oils. In: Lis-Balchin M, ed. *Genus Lavandula: Medicinal and Aromatic Plants – Industrial Profiles*. London: Taylor and Francis, ch 10.

Denyer CV, et al. (1994). Isolation of antirhinoviral sesquiterpenes from ginger (*Zingiber officinale*). *J Nat Prod* 57: 658–662.

De-Oliveira CAX, et al. (1997). In vitro inhibition of CYP2B1 monooxygenase by beta-myrcene and other monoterpenoid compounds. *Toxicol Lett* 92: 39–46.

De Smet PAGM, et al., eds (1992). *Adverse Effects of Herbal Drugs*, Vol 1. Berlin: Springer-Verlag.

De Smet PAGM, et al., eds (1993). *Adverse Effects of Herbal Drugs*, Vol 2. Berlin: Springer-Verlag.

De Smet PAGM, et al., eds (1997). *Adverse Effects of Herbal Drugs*, Vol 3. Berlin: Springer-Verlag.

Devereux C, Kirk-Smith M (2000). Why research? *NORA Newsletter* 5.

Devereux P (1991). *Earth Memory*. Slough, Berks: W. Foulsham and Co.

Devereux P (1997). *The Long Trip*. New York: Penguin.

Dhar SK (1995). Anti-fertility activity and hormonal profile of trans-anethole in rats. *Indian J Physiol Pharmacol* 39: 63–67.

Dhondt W, et al. (1999). Pain threshold in patients with rheumatoid arthritis and effect of manual oscillations. *Scand J Rheumatol* 28: 88–93.

Diego MA, et al. (1998). Aromatherapy positively affects mood, EEG patterns of alertness and math computations. *Int J Neurosci* 96: 217–224.

Dimond EG, et al. (1960). Comparison of internal mammary artery ligation and sham operation for angina pectoris. *Am J Cardiol* 5: 483–486.

Dioscorides (1655/1933). *The Greek Herbal of Dioscorides*, translated by John Goodyer and edited by RT Gunther. New York: Hafner Publishing.

Dodd GH (1991). The molecular dimension in perfumery. In: Toller S and Dodd GH, eds. *Perfumery: The Psychology and Biology of Fragrance.* New York: Chapman and Hall.

Doimo L, *et al.* (1999). Chiral excess: measuring the chirality of geographically and seasonally different Geranium oils. *J Essent Oil Res* 11: 291–299.

Dorman HJD (1999). Phytochemistry and bioactive properties of plant volatile oils: Antibacterial, antifungal and antioxidant activities. PhD thesis, Strathclyde Institute of Biomedical Sciences, University of Strathclyde, Glasgow.

Dorman HJD, Deans SG (2000). Antimicrobial agents from plants: Antibacterial activity of plant volatile oils. *J Appl Microbiol* 88: 308–316.

Dorman HJD, *et al.* (1995a). Antioxidant-rich plant volatile oils: in vitro assessment of activity. Paper presented at the 26th International Symposium on Essential Oils, Hamburg, Germany, 10–13 September.

Dorman HJD, *et al.* (1995b). Evaluation in vitro of plant essential oils as natural antioxidants. *J Essent Oil Res* 7: 645–651.

Dossey L (1993). *Healing Words.* San Francisco, CA: Harper Collins.

Dr Phyto. www.doctorphyto.com/Products/Essential_Oils.htm.

Drake TE, Maibach HI (1976). Allergic contact dermatitis and stomatitis caused by a cinnamic aldehyde-flavoured toothpaste. *Arch Dermatol* 112: 202–203.

Drinkwater NR, *et al.* (1976). Hepatocarcinogenicity of estragole(1′-allyl-4-methoxybenzene) and 1′-hydroxyestragole in the mouse and mutagenicity of 1′-acetoxyestragole in bacteria. *J Natl Cancer Inst* 57: 1323–1331.

Duke JA (1985). *Handbook of Medicinal Herbs.* Boca Raton, FL: CRC Press.

Dukes MNG (1996). *Meyler's Side Effects of Drugs*, 13th edn. Amsterdam: Elsevier.

Dundee JW, *et al.* (1988). P6 Acupressure reduces morning sickness. *J R Soc Med* 81: 456–457.

Dunn C, *et al.* (1995). Sensing an improvement: an experimental study to evaluate the use of aromatherapy, massage and periods of rest in an intensive care unit. *J Adv Nurs* 21: 34–40.

Edge J (2003). A pilot study addressing the effect of aromatherapy massage on mood, anxiety and relaxation in adult mental health. *Complement Ther Nurs Midwifery* 9: 90–97.

Ehrlichman H, Halpern JN (1988). Affect and memory: Effects of pleasant and unpleasant odours on retrieval of happy and unhappy memories. *J Pers Soc Psychol* 55: 769–779.

Elegbede JA, *et al.* (1986). Mouse skin tumour activity of orange peel oil and d-limonene: a re-evaluation. *Carcinogenesis* 7: 2047–2049.

Elisabetsky E, *et al.* (1995). Effects of linalool on glutamatergic system in the rat cerebral cortex. *Neurochem Res* 20: 461–465.

Elisabetsky E, *et al.* (1999). Anticonvulsant properties of linalool in glutamate-related seizure models. *Phytomedicine* 6: 107–113.

El-Kattan AF, *et al.* (2001). The effects of terpene enhancers on the percutaneous permeation of drugs with different lipophilicities. *Int J Pharmaceut* 215: 229–240.

Elkins EC, *et al.* (1953). Effects of various procedures on the flow of lymph. *Arch Phys Med* 34: 31.

Elliott C (1993). Tea tree oil poisoning. *Med J Aust* 159: 830–831.

Ellis A (1960). *The Essence of Beauty.* London: Secker and Warburg.

El Mahdy C (1989). *Mummies, Myth and Magic.* London: Thames and Hudson.

Elson CE, *et al.* (1989). Impact of lemongrass oil, an essential oil, on serum cholesterol. *Lipids* 24: 677–679.

Endroczi E, *et al.* (1956). Studies on sexual behaviour and its effects on the conditioned alimentary reflex activity. *Acta Physiol Acad Sci Hung* 9: 153–160.

Engelstein D, *et al.* (1996). Citral and testosterone interactions in inducing benign and atypical prostatic hyperplasia in rats. *Comp Biochem Physiol C Pharmacol Toxicol Endocrinol* 115: 169–177.

Engelstein E, *et al.* (1992). Rowatinex for the treatment of ureterolithiasis. *J Urol* 98: 98–100.

Engen T, *et al.* (1963). Olfactory responses and adaptation in the human neonate – I. *Comp Physiol Psychol* 56: 73–77.

Ericksson NE, *et al.* (1987). Flowers and other trigger factors in asthma and rhinitis – an inquiry study. *Allergy* 42: 374–381.

Ernst E (1994). Clinical effectiveness of massage – a critical review. *Forsch Komplementärmed* 1: 226–232.

Ernst E (1998). Does post-exercise massage treatment reduce delayed onset muscle soreness? *Br J Sports Med* 32: 212–214.

Ernst E (1999a). Abdominal massage for chronic constipation: A systematic review of controlled clinical trials. *Forsch Komplementärmed* 6: 149–151.

Ernst E (1999b). Massage therapy for low back pain: A systematic review. *J Pain Sympt Manage* 17: 56–69.

Ernst E (2003a). Massage treatment for back pain. *BMJ* 326: 562–563.

Ernst E (2003b). The safety of massage therapy. *Rheumatology* 42: 1101–1106.

Ernst E, Cassileth BR (1998). The prevalence of complementary/alternative medicine in cancer: a systematic review. *Cancer* 83: 777–782.

Ernst E, Huntley A (1996). Tea tree oil: a systematic review of randomised clinical trials. *Eur J Clin Pharmacol* 50: 443–447.

Ernst E, *et al.* (2001). *The Desktop Guide to Complementary and Alternative Medicine*. Edinburgh: Mosby.

ESCOP (European Scientific Cooperative on Phytotherapy) (1996–1999). *Monographs on the Medicinal Uses of Plant Drugs*, Fascicules 1 and 2 (1996), Fascicules 3, 4 and 5 (1997), Fascicule 6 (1999). Exeter: European Scientific Cooperative on Phytotherapy.

Evans B (1995). An audit into the effects of aromatherapy massage and the cancer patient in palliative and terminal care. *Complement Ther Med* 3: 239–241.

Evans F (1974). The power of a sugar pill. *Psychol Today* April.

Evans WC (1996). *Trease & Evans' Pharmacognosy*, 14th edn. London: WB Saunders.

Evening Standard (1998). Peppermint oil kills baby, 18 December.

Fakouri C, Jones P (1987). Relaxation rx: Slow stroke back rub. *J Gerontol Nurs* 13: 32–35.

Falk AA, *et al.* (1990). Uptake, distribution and elimination of alpha-pinene in man after exposure by inhalation. *Scand J Work Environ Health* 16: 372–378.

Falk-Filipsson A, *et al.* (1993). d-Limonene exposure to humans by inhalation: uptake, distribution, elimination, and effects on the pulmonary function. *J Toxic Environ Health* 38: 77–88.

Farnsworth NR (1975). Potential value of plants as sources of new antifertility agents I. *J Pharm Sci* 64: 535–598.

Farnsworth NR, Cordell GA (1976). A review of some biologically active compounds isolated from plants as reported in the 1974–1975 literature. *Lloydia* 39: 420–455.

Farnsworth NR, *et al.* (1985). Siberian ginseng (*Eleutherococcus senticosus*): current status as an adaptogen. In: *Economic and Medicinal Plant Research*, Vol 1, ed. Wagner H, *et al.* London: Academic Press, pp. 155–215.

Faust RA (1984). Chemical hazard information profile – Draft report. Dihydrosafrole, CAS No. 94-58-56. Office of Toxic Substances, US EPA, Washington, DC.

Felten DL, Felten SY (1987). Immune interactions with specific neural structures. *Brain Behav Immun* 1: 279–283.

Felten DL, *et al.* (1987). Central neural circuits involved in neural-immune interactions. In: Ader R, Felten DL and Cohen N, eds. *Psychoneuroimmunology*, 2nd edn. London: Academic Press, pp. 3–25.

Felter HW, Lloyd JU (1898). *King's American Dispensatory*, 18th edn. Sandy, OR: Eclectic Medical Publications.

Fenaroli G (1997). *Handbook of Flavour Ingredients*, 3rd edn, Vol 1. London: CRC Press.

Ferley JP, *et al.* (1989). Prophylactic aromatherapy for supervening infections in patients with chronic bronchitis. Statistical evaluation conducted in clinics against a placebo. *Phytother Res* 3: 97–100.

Fernie WT (1914). *Herbal Simples*. Bristol: John Wright.

Ferrell-Torry AT, Glick OJ (1993). The use of therapeutic massage as a nursing intervention to modify anxiety and the perception of cancer pain. *Cancer Nurs* 16: 93–101.

Ferry P, *et al.* (2002). Use of complementary therapies and non-prescribed medication in patients with Parkinson's disease. *Postgrad Med J* 78: 612–614.

Festing S (1989). *The Story of Lavender*. Surrey: Heritage in Sutton Leisure.

Fetrow CW, Avila JR (1999). *Professional's Handbook of Complementary and Alternative Medicines*. Springhouse: Springhouse Corporation.

Fidler P, *et al.* (1996). Prospective evaluation of a chamomile mouthwash for prevention of 5-FU-induced oral mucositis. *Cancer* 77: 522–525.

Field T (1995). Massage therapy for infants and children. *J Dev Behav Pediatr* 16: 105–111.

Field T, *et al.* (1986). Tactile/kinesthetic stimulation effect on preterm neonates. *Pediatrics* 77: 654–658.

Field T, *et al.* (1992). Massage reduced anxiety in child and adolescent psychiatric patients. *J Am Acad Child Adolesc Psychiatry* 31: 125–131.

Field T, *et al.* (1996). Massage therapy reduces anxiety and enhances EEG pattern of alertness and math patterns. *Int J Neurosci* 86: 197–205.

Field T, *et al.* (1997). Labor pain is reduced by massage therapy. *J Psychosom Obstet Gynaecol* 18: 286–291.

Figueiredo AC, *et al.* (1992). Composition of the essential oils from leaves and flowers of *Achillea millefolium* L. ssp. *millefolium*. *Flavour Fragrance J* 7: 219–222.

Figuereido AC, *et al.* (1995). Composition of the essential oil of *Lavandula pinnata* L. fi, var. *pinnata* grown on Madeira. *Flavour Fragrance J* 10: 93–96.

Final Report (1999a). Final report on the safety assessment of azulene. *Int J Toxicol* 18: 27–32.

Final Report (1999b). Final report on the safety assessment of bisabolol. *Int J Toxicol* 18: 33–40.

Final Report (2001a). Final report on the safety assessment of yarrow (*Achillea millefolium*) extract. *Int J Toxicol* 20: 79–84.

Final Report (2001b). Final report on the safety assessment of *Juniperus communis* extract, *Juniperus oxycedrus* extract, *Juniperus oxycedrus* Tar, *Juniperus phoenicea* extract, and *Juniperus virginiana* extract. *Int J Toxicol* 20 (suppl 2): 41–56.

Finkenrath K (1937). Schonheitsmittel als Krankheitursache. *Arztl Sachverst Ztg* 43: 193.

Fischer-Rizzi S (1990). *Complete Aromatherapy Handbook*. New York: Sterling Publishing.

Fischer-Rizzi S (1992). Dedicated to better births: Ups and downs. *Int J Aromather* 4: 10.

Fisher AA, *et al.* (1950). Toxicity of eugenol: Determination of LD50 on rats. *Proc Soc Exp Biol Med* 73: 148–151.

Flattery David Stophet, Schwartz Martin (1989). *Haoma and Harmaline. The Botanical Identity of the Indo-Iranian Sacred Hallucinogen 'Soma' and Its Legacy in Religion, Language and Middle Eastern Folklore*. Berkeley, CA: University of California Press.

Flemming K (2000). Review: Aromatherapy massage is associated with small, transient reductions in anxiety ... commentary on Cooke and Ernst (2000). *Evidence Based Nurs* 3: 118.

Florida Vet. Scene (1995). *Florida Veterinary Scene Newsletter* 4(5), May/June 1995.

Fluckiger F, Hanbury D (1885). *Pharmacographia – The History of the Principle*. London: FRS.

Forbes RJ (1955). Cosmetics and perfumes in antiquity. In: *Studies in Ancient Technology*, Vol III. Leiden: EJ Brill.

Ford RA (1990). Metabolic and kinetic criteria for assessment of reproductive hazard. In: Volans GF, Sis J, Sullivan FM and Turner P, eds. *Basic Science in Toxicology*. New York: Taylor and Francis, pp. 59–68.

Ford RA (1991). The toxicology and safety of fragrances. In: Muller PM and Lamparsky D, eds. *Perfumes, Art, Science and Technology*. New York: Elsevier, pp. 442–463.

Ford RA (1992). Studies of the quenching phenomenon. *Contact Dermatitis* 27: 60–1.

Ford RA, *et al.* (1990). 90-day dermal toxicity study and neurotoxicity evaluation of nitromusks in the albino rat. *Food Chem Toxicol* 28: 55–61.

Forsbeck M, Ros A-M (1979). Anaphylactoid reaction to celery. *Contact Dermatitis* 5: 191.

Fraj J, *et al.* (1990). *Aromathérapie exactement*. Paris: Roger Jollois.

Franchomme P, Penoel D (1990). *Aromathérapie exactement*. Paris: Roger Jollois.

Frank J (1973). *Persuasion and Healing*. New York: Schocken Books.

Franks A (1998). Contact allergy to anethole in toothpaste associated with loss of taste. *Contact Dermatitis* 38: 354–355.

Franzios G, *et al.* (1997). Insecticidal and genotoxic activities of mint essential oils. *J Agr Food Chem* 45: 2690–2694.

Fraser JL (1981). *The Medicine Men*. London: Thames/Methuen.

Freireich EJ (1975). In: *Cancer Chemotherapy: Fundamental Concepts and Recent Advances*. Chicago, IL: Year Book Medical Publishers.

Frey II WH (2002). Bypassing the blood–brain barrier to deliver therapeutic agents to the brain and spinal cord. *Drug Delivery Technol* 2: 46–49.

Friedman M, *et al.* (2002). Bactericidal activities of plant essential oils and some of their isolated constituents against *Campylobacter jejuni*, *Escherichia coli*, *Listeria monocytogenes* and *Salmonella enterica*. *J Food Protect* 65: 1545–1560.

Frosch PJ, *et al.*, eds (1998). *Fragrances: Beneficial and Adverse Effects*. Chichester: John Wiley.

Frosch PJ, *et al.* (1999). Lyral® is an important sensitizer in patients sensitive to fragrances. *Br J Dermatol* 141: 1076–1083.

Frosch PJ, *et al.* (2002a). Further important sensitizers in patients sensitive to fragrances: I. Reactivity to 14 frequently used chemicals. *Contact Dermatitis* 47: 78–85.

Frosch PJ, *et al.* (2002b). Further important sensitizers in patients sensitive to fragrances: II. Reactivity to essential oils. *Contact Dermatitis* 47: 279–287.

Fuchs N, *et al.* (1997). Systemic absorption of topically applied carvone: influence of massage technique. *J Soc Cosmet Chem* 48: 277–282.

Fujiwara R, *et al.* (1998). Effects of a long-term inhalation of fragrances on the stress-induced immunosuppression in mice. *Neuroimmunomodulation* 5: 318–322.

Fujiwara R, *et al.* (2002). Psychoneuroimmunological benefits of aromatherapy. *Int J Aromather* 12: 78–82.

Fukayama MY, *et al.* (1999). Subchronic inhalation studies of complex fragrance mixtures in rats and hamsters. *Toxicol Letters* 111: 175–187.

Fundaro A, Cassone MC (1980). Action of essential oils of chamomile, cinnamon, absinthium, mace and origanum on operant conditioning behaviour of the rat. *Boll Soc Ital Sper* 56: 2375–2380.

Furlan AD, *et al.* (2002). Massage for low back pain. *Cochrane Database Syst Rev* 2.

Furuhashi A, *et al.* (1994). Effects of AETT-induced neuronal ceroid lipofuscinosis on learning ability in rats. *Jpn J Psychiatry Neurol* 48: 645–653.

Futrell JM, Rietschel RL (1993). Spice allergy evaluated by results of patch tests. *Cutis* 52: 288–290.

Fyfe L, *et al.* (1997). Inhibition of *Listeria monocytogenes* and *Salmonella enteritidis* by combinations of plant oils and derivatives of benzoic acid: the development of synergistic antimicrobial combinations. *Int J Antimicrob Agents* 9: 195–199.

Gallardo PPR, *et al.* (1987). The antimicrobial activity of some spices on microorganisms of great interest to health. IV: Seeds, leaves and others. *Microbiol aliments Nutr* 5: 77–82.

Gambhir SS, *et al.* (1966). Studies on *Daucus carota*, Linn. Part I. Pharmacological studies with the water-soluble fraction of the alcoholic extract of the seeds: a preliminary report. *Indian J Med Res* 54: 178–187.

Gamez MJ, *et al.* (1987a). Hypoglycaemic activity in various species of the genus *Lavandula*. Part 1. *Lavandula stoechas* L. and *Lavandula multifida* L. *Pharmazie* 42: 706–707.

Gamez MJ, *et al.* (1987b). Hypoglycaemic activity in various species of the genus *Lavandula*. Part 2. *Lavandula dentata* and *Lavandula latifolia*. *Pharmazie* 43: 441–442.

Garcia-Bravo B, *et al.* (1997). Occupational contact dermatitis from anethole in food handlers. *Contact Dermatitis* 37: 38.

Garcia-Vallejo MC, *et al.* (1989). Essential oils of the Genus *Lavandula* L. in Spain. *Proc ICEOFF*, New Delhi, Vol 4, pp. 15–26.

Garg SC, Dengre SL (1986). Antibacterial activity of essential oil of *Tagetes erecta* Linn. *Hindustan Antibiotic Bull* 28: 27–29.

Garnett A, *et al.* (1994). Percutaneous absorption of benzyl acetate through rat skin in vitro. 3. A comparison with human skin. *Food Chem Toxicol* 32: 1061–1065.

Gattefossé M (1992). René-Maurice Gattefossé, The father of modern aromatherapy. *Int J Aromather* 4: 18–20.

Gattefossé RM (1928). *Formulaire du chimiste-Parfumeur et du Savonnier [Formulary of cosmetics]*. Paris: Librairie des Sciences.

Gattefossé RM (1937/1993). *Gattefosse's Aromatherapy* (edited by R Tisserand). Saffron Walden: CW Daniel Co.

Gattefossé RM (1952). *Formulary of Perfumery and of Cosmetology*. London: Leonard Hill.

Gatti G, Cajola R (1923a). L'Azione delle essenze sul systema nervoso. *Riv Ital Della Essenze e Profumi* 5: 133–135.

Gatti G, Cajola R (1923b). L'Azione terapeutica degli olii essenziali. *Riv Ital Della Essenze e Profumi* 5: 30–33.

Gatti G, Cajola R (1929). L'essenza di valeriana nella cura delle malattie nervose. *Riv Ital Della Essenze e Profumi* 2: 260–262.

Gedney JJ, *et al.* (2004). Sensory and affective pain discrimination after inhalation of essential oils. *Psychosom Med* 66: 599–606.

Geldof AA, *et al.* (1992). Estrogenic action of commonly used fragrant agent citral induces prostatic hyperplasia. *Urol Res* 20: 139–144.

Genders R (1972). *A History of Scent*. London: Hamish Hamilton.

Gerard J (1597). *The Herball or General History of Plants*. London: John North.

Gershbein LL (1977). Regeneration of rat liver in the presence of essential oils and their components. *Food Cosmet Toxicol* 15: 171–181.

Ghelardini C, *et al.* (1999). Local anaesthetic activity of the essential oil of *Lavandula angustifolia*. *Planta Med* 65: 700–703.

Giachetti D, *et al.* (1988). Pharmacological activity of essential oils on Oddi's sphincter. *Planta Med* 54: 389–392.

Gignoux M, Launoy G (1999). [Recent epidemiologic trends in cancer of the esophagus]. *Rev Prat* 49: 1154–1158.

Gilani AH, *et al.* (2000). Ethnopharmacological evaluation of the anticonvulsant, sedative and antispasmodic activities of *Lavandula stoechas* L. *J Ethnopharmacol* 71: 161–167.

Ginsburg F, Famaey JP (1987). A double-blind study of topical massage with rado-salil ointment in mechanical low back pain. *J Int Med Res* 15: 148–153.

Giri J, *et al.* (1984). Effect of ginger on serum cholesterol levels. *Indian J Nutr Diet* 21: 433–436.

Glowania HJ, *et al.* (1987). [Effect of chamomile on wound healing – a clinical double-blind study]. *Z Hautkr* 62: 1262, 1267–1271.

Goats GC (1994). Massage – the scientific basis of an ancient art: parts 1 and 2. *Br J Sports Med (UK)* 28: 149–152, 153–156.

Gobel H, *et al.* (1994). Effect of peppermint and eucalyptus oil preparations on neurophysiological and experimental algesimetric headache parameters. *Cephalagia* 14: 228–234.

Gobel H, *et al.* (1996). Effectiveness of *Oleum mentha piperitae* and paracetamol in therapy of headache of the tension type. *Nervenarzt* 67: 672–681.

Gogoi P, *et al.* (1997). Antifungal activity of the essential oil of *Litsea cubeba* Pers. *J Essent Oil Res* 9: 213–215.

Gold J, Cates W (1980). Herbal abortifacients. *JAMA* 243: 1365–1366.

Goldstone L (1999). From orthodox to complementary: the fall and rise of massage, with specific reference to orthopaedic and rheumatology nursing. *J Orthop Nurs* 3: 152–159.

Goldstone L (2000). Massage as an orthodox medical treatment, past and future. *Complement Ther Nurs Midwifery* 6: 169–175.

Gomes-Carneiro MR, *et al.* (1998). Mutagenicity testing ($\pm$)-camphor, 1,8-cineole, citral, citronellal, ($-$)-menthol and terpineol with the Salmonella/microsome assay. *Mutat Res* 416: 129–136.

Gómez Vázquez M, *et al.* (2002). Allergic contact eczema/dermatitis from cosmetics. *Allergy* 57: 268–269.

Goodrick-Clarke N (1990). *Paracelsus*. Northamptonshire: Crucible.

Goodwin J (1998). *Natural Babycare*. London: Ebury Press.

Gosselin RE, *et al.* (1976). *Clinical Toxicology of Commercial Products: Acute Poisoning*, 4th edn. Baltimore, MD: Williams and Wilkins.

Gould MN, *et al.* (1995). Regression of mammalian carcinomas. United States Patent No. 5 414 019.

Gower DB, Ruparelia BA (1993). Olfaction in humans with special reference to odorous 16-androstenes: their occurrence, perception and possible social, psychological and sexual impact. *J Endocrinol* 137: 167–187.

Grace Ulla-Maija (1996). *Aromatherapy for Practitioners*. Saffron Walden: CW Daniel Co.

Gracza L (1984). Molecular pharmacological investigation of medicinal plant substances. 2. Inhibition of acetylcholinesterase by monoterpene derivatives in vitro. *Z Naturforsch* 40C: 151–153.

Graham PH, *et al.* (2003). Inhalation aromatherapy during radiotherapy: results of a placebo-controlled double-blind randomized trial. *J Clin Oncol* 15: 2372–2376.

Grammer K, Jutte A (1997). Battle of odors: significance of pheromones for human reproduction. *Gynakol Geburtshilfliche Rundsch* 37: 150–153.

Grassmann J, *et al.* (2000). Antioxidant properties of essential oils. Possible explanations for their anti-inflammatory effects. *Arzneimittelforschung* 50: 135–139.

Gray LE Jr (1998). Xenoendocrine disrupters: laboratory studies on male reproductive effects. *Toxicol Lett* 102–103, 331–335.

Gray SG, Clair AA (2002). Influence of aromatherapy on medication administration to residential-care residents with dementia and behavioral challenges. *Am J Alzheimers Dis Other Demen* 17: 169–174.

Greenoak G (2000). Anti-inflammatory assay on 22 human subjects. Australian Photobiology Testing Facility, NSW.

Greig JE, *et al.* (1999). Allergic contact dermatitis following use of a tea tree oil hand-wash not due to tea tree oil. *Contact Dermatitis* 41: 354–355.

Grieve M (1937/1992). *A Modern Herbal*. London: Tiger Books International.

Grochulski VA, Borkowski B (1972). Influence of chamomile oil on experimental glomerulonephritis in rabbits. *Planta Med* 21: 289–292.

Groom, N (1992). *The Perfume Handbook*, 2nd edn. London: Chapman and Hall.

Grosjean N (1992). *Aromatherapy from Provence*. Saffron Walden: CW Daniel Co.

Gruncharov V (1973). Clinico-experimental study on the choleretic and cholagogic action of Bulgarian lavender oil. *Vutr Boles* 12: 90–96.

Guba R (2000). Toxicity myths: the actual risks of essential oil use. *Perfumer and Flavorist* 25: 10–28.

Guedes DN, *et al.* (2002). Muscarinic agonist properties involved in the hypotensive and vasorelaxant responses of rotundifolone in rats. *Planta Med* 700–704.

Guenther E (1948–1952). *The Essential Oils*, Vols I–VI. New York: Van Nostrand.

Guérin J-C, Réveillére H-P (1985). Antifungal activity of plant extracts used in therapy. II Study of 40 plant extracts against 9 fungi species. *Ann Pharm Fr* 43: 77–81.

Guerra P, *et al.* (1987). Contact dermatitis to geraniol in a leg ulcer. *Contact Dermatitis* 16: 298–299.

Guillemain J, *et al.* (1989). [Neurodepressive effects of the essential oil of *Lavandula angustifolia* Mill]. *Ann Pharm Fr* 47: 337–343.

Guin JD (1982). History, manufacture and cutaneous reaction to perfumes. In: Frost P, Horwitz SW, eds. *Principles of Cosmetics for the Dermatologist*. St. Louis: The CV Mosby Co.

Guin JD (1995). *Practical Contact Dermatitis*. New York: McGraw-Hill.

Guin JD, Berry VK (1980). Perfume sensitivity in adult females. *J Am Acad Dermatol* 3: 299–302.

Gujral S, *et al.* (1974). Effect of ginger (*Zingiber officinale* Roscoe) oleoresin on serum and hepatic cholesterol levels in cholesterol fed rats. *Nutr Rep Int* 17: 183–189.

Gunn JWC (1921). The carminative action of volatile oils. *J Pharmacol* 16: 39–47.

Gupta I, *et al.* (1997). Effects of *Boswellia serrata* gum resin in patients with ulcerative colitis. *Eur J Med Res* 2: 37–43.

Gupta I, *et al.* (1998). Effects of *Boswellia serrata* gum resin in patients with bronchial asthma: results of a double-blind, placebo-controlled, 6-week clinical study. *Eur J Med Res* 3: 511–514.

Guseinov DIa, *et al.* (1987). [Research on the chemical composition and aspects of the pharmacological action of the essential oil of Kochi thyme (*Thymus kotschyanus* Boiss)]. *Farmakol Toksikol* 50: 73–74.

Gutman SG, Somov BA (1968). Allergic reactions caused by components of perfumery preparations. *Vest Derm Verner* 42: 62.

Habersang S, *et al.* (1979). Pharmacological studies with compounds of chamomile IV. Studies on toxicity of (−)-α-bisabolol. *Planta Med* 37: 115–123.

Hadfield N (2001). The role of aromatherapy massage in reducing anxiety in patients with malignant brain tumours. *Int J Palliat Nurs* 7: 279–285.

Hagen EC, *et al.* (1961). Toxic properties of compounds related to safrole. *Toxicol Appl Pharmacol* 7: 18–24.

Haggard HW (1989). *The Doctor in History*. New York: Dorset Press.

Haginiwa J, *et al.* (1963). Pharmacological studies on crude drugs. VII Properties of the essential oil components of aromatics and their pharmacological effect on mouse intestine. *Yakugaku Zasshi* 83: 624–626.

Hajhashemi V, *et al.* (2000). Antispasmodic and antidiarrhoeal effect of *Satureja hortensis* L. essential oil. *J Ethnopharmacol* 71: 187–192.

Hajhashemi V, *et al.* (2002). Antinociceptive and anti-inflammatory effects of *Satureja hortensis* L. extracts and essential oil. *J Ethnopharmacol* 82: 83–87.

Hallstrom H, Thuvander A (1997). Toxicological evaluation of myristicin. *Nat Toxins* 5: 186–192.

Hammer KA, *et al.* (1996). Susceptibility of transient and commensal skin flora to the essential oil of *Melaleuca alternifolia* (tea tree oil). *Am J Infect Control* 24: 186–189.

Hammer KA, *et al.* (1997). In vitro susceptibility of *Malassezia furfur* to the essential oil of *Melaleuca alternifolia*. *J Med Vet Mycol* 35: 375–377.

Hammer KA, *et al.* (1998). In vitro activity of essential oils, in particular *Melaleuca alternifolia* (tea tree) oil and tea tree oil products, against *Candida* spp. *J Antimicrob Chemother* 42: 591–595.

Hammer KA, *et al.* (1999a). Antimicrobial activity of essential oils and other plant extracts. *J Appl Microbiol* 86: 985–990.

Hammer KA, *et al.* (1999b). In vitro susceptibilities of lactobacilli and organisms associated with bacterial vaginosis to *Melaleuca alternifolia* (tea tree) oil. *Antimicrob Agents Chemother* 43: 196.

Hammer KA, *et al.* (1999c). Influence of organic matter, cations and surfactants on the antimicrobial activity of *Melaleuca alternifolia* (tea tree) oil in vitro. *J Appl Microbiol* 86: 446–452.

Hammer KA, *et al.* (2000). *Melaleuca alternifolia* (tea tree) oil inhibits germ tube formation by *Candida albicans*. *Med Mycol* 38: 354–361.

Hammer KA, *et al.* (2003). In vitro activity of *Melaleuca alternifolia* (tea tree) oil against dermatophytes and other filamentous fungi. *J Antimicrob Chemother* 50: 195–199.

Harada M, *et al.* (1976). Pharmacological studies on Chinese cinnamon. III. Electroencephalographic studies of cinnamaldehyde in the rabbit. *Chem Pharm Bull (Tokyo)* 24: 1784–1788.

Harada M, *et al.* (1982). Pharmacological studies on Chinese cinnamon. V. Catecholamine releasing effect of cinnamaldehyde in dogs. *J Pharmacobiodyn* 5: 539–546.

Harada M, *et al.* (1984). Effect of Japanese angelica root and peony root on uterine contraction in the rabbit in situ. *J Pharmacobiodyn* 7: 304–311.

Harborne JB (1988). *Introduction to Ecological Biochemistry*, 3rd edn. London: Academic Press.

Hardy M, *et al.* (1995). Replacement of drug treatment for insomnia by ambient odour. *The Lancet* 346: 701.

Harkenthal M, *et al.* (1999). Comparative study on the in vitro antibacterial activity of Australian tea tree oil, cajuput oil, niaouli oil, manuka oil, kanuka oil, and eucalyptus oil. *Pharmazie* 54: 460–463.

Harmala P, *et al.* (1992a). A furanocoumarin from *Angelica archangelica*. *Planta Med* 58: 287–289.

Harmala P, *et al.* (1992b). Choice of solvent in the extraction of *Angelica archangelica* roots with reference to calcium blocking activity. *Planta Med* 58: 176–183.

Harris B, Lewis R (1994). Chamomile – part 1. *Int J Altern Complement Med* 1: 12.

Hart PH, *et al.* (2000). Terpinen-4-ol, the main component of the essential oil of *Melaleuca alternifolia* (tea tree oil), suppresses inflammatory mediator production by activated human monocytes. *Inflamm Res* 49: 619–626.

Hart SL, *et al.* (1994). Antinociceptive activity of monoterpenes in the mouse. *Can J Physiol Pharmacol* 72, 344.

Hartwig G (1996). Essential oils for prevention and treatment of decubitus ulcers. *Germany Offen* 19518836; *Chem Abstr* 126, 5, 65430e.

Hasenohrl RU, *et al.* (1996). Anxiolytic-like effect of combined extracts of *Zingiber officinale* and *Ginkgo biloba* in the elevated plus-maze. *Pharmacol Biochem Behav* 53: 271–275.

Hastings L, *et al.* (1991). Olfactory primary neurons as a route of entry for toxic agents into the CNS. *Neurotoxicology* 12: 707–714.

Hausen BM (1979). The sensitising capacity of Compositae plants. III. Test results and cross-reactions in Compositae-sensitive patients. *Dermatologica* 159: 1–11.

Hausen BM (1981). [Occupational contact allergy to feverfew *Tanacetum parthenium* (L.) Schultz-Bip, Asteraceae]. *Derm Beruf Umwelt* 29: 18–21.

Hausen BM (1996). A 6-year experience with compositae mix. *Am J Contact Dermat* 7: 94–99.

Hausen BM, Berger M (1989). The sensitizing capacity of coumarins. (III). *Contact Dermatitis* 201: 141–147.

Hausen BM, *et al.* (1984). The sensitizing capacity of Compositae plants. *Planta Med* 50: 229–234.

Hausen BM, *et al.* (1999). Degradation products of monoterpenes are the sensitizing agents in tea tree oil. *Am J Contact Dermat* 10: 68–77.

Hawkes C (2003). Olfaction in neurodegenerative disorder. *Mov Disord* 18: 364–372.

Hawkins DR, Ford RA (1999). Dermal absorption and disposition of musk ambrette, musk ketone and musk xylene in rats. *Toxicol Lett* 111: 95–103.

Hawthorn M, *et al.* (1988). The actions of peppermint oil and menthol on calcium channel dependent processes in intestinal, neuronal and cardiac preparations. *Alim Pharmacol Ther* 2: 101–118.

Hay IC, *et al.* (1998). Randomized trial of aromatherapy. Successful treatment for *Alopecia areata*. *Arch Dermatol* 134: 1349–1352.

Hayakawa R, *et al.* (1987). Airborne pigmented contact dermatitis due to musk ambrette in incense. *Contact Dermatitis* 16: 96–98.

Hayes J, Cox C (1999). Immediate effects of a five minute foot massage on patients in critical care. *Intensive Crit Care Nurs* 15: 77–82.

Hazelhoff B, *et al.* (1982). Antispasmodic effects of *Valeriana* compounds: an *in vivo* and *in vitro* study on the guinea-pig ileum. *Arch Int Pharmacodyn* 257: 274–287.

HEAL (Human Ecology Action League, Inc) (2005). http://members.aol.com/HEALNatnl/index.html (accessed June 2005).

Healey MA, Aslam M (1996). Aromatherapy: In: Evans WC, ed. *Trease & Evans' Pharmacognosy*, 14th edn. London: WB Saunders.

Heffer A (1894–5). Zur Pharmakologie de Safrole Gruppe. *Arch Exp Path Pharmacol* 35: 342–374.

Hendriks H, *et al.* (1985). Central nervous depressant activity of valerenic acid in the mouse. *Planta Med* 51: 28–31.

Hendriks SA, *et al.* (1999). Allergic contact dermatitis from the fragrance ingredient Lyral® in under-arm deodorant. *Contact Dermatitis* 41: 119.

Henry J, *et al.* (1994). Lavender for night sedation of people with dementia. *Int J Aromather* 5: 28–30.

Herrman EC, Kucera LS (1967). Antiviral substances in plants of the mint family (Labiatae). 2. Non-tannin polyphenol of *Melissa officinalis*. *Proc Soc Exp Biol Med* 124: 869–874.

Hertzka G, Strehlow W (1994). *Manuel de la Médicine de Saint Hildegarde*, 2nd edn. Monsurs: Edition Resiac.

Heuberger E, *et al.* (2001). Effects of chiral fragrances on human autonomic nervous system parameters and self-evaluation. *Chem Senses* 26: 281–292.

Hewitt PG, *et al.* (1993). Cutaneous retopical application of 4,4′-methylene-bis-(2-cloroaniline) and 4,4′-methylenedianiline to rat and human skin in vitro. In: Brain KR, *et al.*, eds. *Prediction of Percutaneous Penetration: Methods, Measurements and Modeling*, Vol 3b. Cardiff: STS, pp. 638–645.

Hicks G (1998). Aromatherapy as an adjunct to care in a mental health day hospital. *J Psychiatr Ment Health Nurs* 5: 317.

Highstein B, Zeligman I (1951). Nonthrombocytopenic purpura caused by mentholated cigarettes. *JAMA* 146: 816.

Hikino H (1985). Oriental medicinal plants. In: Wagner H, *et al.* eds. *Economic and Medicinal Plants*, Vol 1. London: Academic Press, pp. 69–70.

Hills JM, Aaronson PI (1991). The mechanism of action of peppermint oil on gastrointestinal smooth muscle. *Gastroenterology* 101: 55–65.

Hinou JB, *et al.* (1989). Antimicrobial activity screening of 32 common constituents of essential oils. *Pharmazie* 44: H4.

Hirsch A (1998). *Scentsational Sex: The Secret to Using Aroma for Arousal*. Boston, MA: Element.

Hof S, Ammon HPT (1989). Negative ionotropic action of rosemary oil, 1,8-cineole, and bornyl acetate. *Planta Med* 55: 106–107.

Hoffman C, Evans AC (1911). The use of spices as preservatives. *J Indian Eng Chem* 3: 835–838.

Hoffmeier JK (1983). Some Egyptian motifs related to warfare and enemies and their Old Testament counterparts. In: Hoffmeier JK, Melter ES, eds. *Egyptological Miscellanies: A Tribute to Professor Ronald J Williams*. Chicago: Ares.

Hof-Mussler S (1990). Atherische öle. *Dtsch Apoth Z* 130: 2407–2410.

Hohmann J, *et al.* (1999). Protective effects of the aerial parts of *Salvia officinalis*, *Melissa officinalis* and *Lavandula angustifolia* and their constituents against enzyme-dependent and enzyme-independent lipid peroxidation. *Planta Med* 65: 576–578.

Hold KM, *et al.* (2000). Alpha-thujone (the active component of absinthe): gamma-aminobutyric acid type A receptor modulation and metabolic detoxification. *Proc Natl Acad Sci USA* 97: 3826–3831.

Holm E, *et al.* (1974). Electrophysiologische analyse der einflusse von Terpinen auf das Gehirn der Katze. *Die Hielkunst* 87: 70–75.

Holm Y, *et al.* (1997). Enantiomeric composition of monoterpene hydrocarbons in n-hexane extracts of *Angelica archangelica* L. roots and seeds. *Flavour Fragrance J* 12: 397–400.

Holmes C, *et al.* (2002). Lavender oil as a treatment for agitated behaviour in severe dementia: a placebo controlled study. *Int J Geriatr Psychiatry* 17: 305–308.

Hölzl J, *et al.* (1986). Preparation of ^{14}C-spiro ethers by chamomile and their use by an investigation of absorption. *Planta Med* 52: 533.

Homberger F, Boger E (1968). The carcinogenicity of essential oils, flavours and spices: a review. *Cancer Res* 28: 2372–2374.

Homburger F, *et al.* (1971). Inhibition of murine sub-cutaneous and intravenous benzo(rst)pentaphene carcinogenesis by sweet orange oils and d-limonene. *Oncology* 25: 1–10.

Hong CZ, Shellock FG (1991). Effects of a topically applied counterirritant (Eucalyptamint) on cutaneous blood flow and on skin and muscle temperatures. A placebo-controlled study. *Am J Phys Med Rehabil* 70: 29–33.

Hongratanaworskit T, *et al.* (2000a). Effects of sandalwood oil and α-santalol on humans. 1. Inhalation. Poster presented at the International Essential Oil Symposium, Hamburg, 10–13 September.

Hongratanaworskit T, *et al.* (2000b). Effects of sandalwood oil and α-santalol on humans. 2. Percutaneous administration. Poster presented at the International Essential Oil Symposium, Hamburg, 10–13 September.

Honigsbaum F (1979). *The Division in British Medicine.* New York: St Martin's Press.

Horowitz DA (2000). Judgement (pursuant to stipulation). National Council Against Health Fraud, Inc, v. Aroma Vera, Inc, *et al.* Superior Court No. BC183903. 11 October.

Horowitz LF, *et al.* (1999). A genetic approach to trace neural circuits. *Proc Natl Acad Sci USA* 96: 3194–3199.

Hosoi J, Tsuchiya T (2000). Regulation of cutaneous allergic reaction by odorant inhalation. *J Invest Dermatol* 114: 541–544.

Houghton P (1994). Valerian. *Pharm J* 252: 95–96.

Huang MT, *et al.* (1994). Inhibition of skin tumorigenesis by rosemary and its constituents carnosol and ursolic acid. *Cancer Res* 54: 701–708.

Huntimer CM, Bean DW (2000). Delirium after ingestion of mentholatum. *Am J Psychiatry* 157: 483–484.

IFRA (1997). *IFRA Code of Practice.* Geneva: International Fragrance Association.

Igimi H, *et al.* (1974). Studies on the metabolism of D-limonene (*p*-mentha-1,8-diene). I. The absorption, distribution, and excretion of D-limonene in rats. *Xenobiotica* 4: 77–84.

Ikawati Z, *et al.* (2001). Screening of several Indonesian medicinal plants for their inhibitory effect on histamine release from RBL-2H3 cells. *J Ethnopharmacol* 75: 249–256.

Ikram M (1980). Medicinal plants as hypocholesterolemic agents. *J Pak Med Assoc* 30: 278–282.

Ilarionova M, *et al.* (1992). Cytotoxic effect on leukemic cells of the essential oils from rosemary, wild geranium and nettle and concrete of royal Bulgarian rose. *Anticancer Res* 12: 1915.

Ilmberger J, *et al.* (2001). The influence of essential oils on human attention: 1. Alertness. *Chem Senses* 26: 239–245.

Imai H, *et al.* (2001). Inhibition by the essential oils of peppermint and spearmint of the growth of pathogenic bacteria. *Microbios* 106 (Suppl 1): 31–39.

Imaseki I, Kitabatake Y (1962). Studies on effect of essential oils and their components on the isolated intestines of mice. *J Pharm Soc Jpn* 82: 1326–1328.

Inlander C, *et al.* (1988). *Medicine on Trial.* New York: Pantheon Books.

Innocenti G, *et al.* (1976). Investigations of the content of furocoumarins in *Apium graveolens* and in *Petroselinum sativum. Planta Med* 29: 165–170.

Inouye S, *et al.* (1983). Inhibitory effect of volatile components of plants on the proliferation of bacteria. *Bokin Bobai* 11: 609–615.

Inouye S, *et al.* (2001). Antibacterial activity of essential oils and their major constituents against respiratory tract pathogens by gaseous contact. *J Antimicrob Chemother* 47: 565–573.

Ironson G, *et al.* (1996). Massage therapy is associated with enhancement of the immune system's cytotoxic capacity. *Int J Neurosci* 84: 205–217.

Isaac O (1979). Pharmacological investigations with compounds of chamomile I. On the pharmacology of (–)-α-bisabolol and bisabolol oxides (review). *Planta Med* 35: 118–124.

Isaacs G (1983). Permanent local anaesthesia and anhidrosis after clove oil spillage. *Lancet* 16: 88.

Itai T, *et al.* (2000). Psychological effects of aromatherapy on chronic hemodialysis patients. *Psychiatry Clin Neurosci* 54: 393–397.

Ivancheva S, *et al.* (1992). Polyphenols from Bulgarian medicinal plants with anti-infectious activity. *Basic Life Sci* 59: 717–728.

Ivanic R, Savin K (1976). A comparative analysis of essential oils from several wild species of *Salvia. Planta Med* 30: 25–31.

Izzo AA, *et al.* (1996). Spasmolytic activity of medicinal plants used for the treatment of disorders involving smooth muscle. *Phytother Res* 10: S107–S108.

Jackson J (1987). *A Comprehensive Guide to Essential Oils and their Uses.* New York: Viking.

Jacobs MR, Hornfeldt CS (1994). Melaleuca oil poisoning. *J Toxicol Clin Toxicol* 32: 461–464.

Jacovlev V, *et al.* (1979). Pharmacological investigations with compounds of chamomile II. New investigations on the antiphlogistic effects of (–)-α-bisabolol and bisabolol oxides. *Planta Med* 35: 125–140.

Jaeger W, *et al.* (1996). Pharmokinetic studies of the fragrance compound 1,8-cineole in humans during inhalation. *Chem Senses* 21: 477–480.

Jager W, *et al.* (1992). Percutaneous absorption of lavender oil from a massage oil. *J Soc Cosmet Chem* 43: 49–54.

Jain SR, Kar A (1971). The antibacterial activity of some essential oils and their combinations. *Planta Med* 20: 118–123.

Jakovlev V, *et al.* (1983). Pharmacological investigations with compounds of chamomile VI. Investigations on the antiphlogistic effects of chamazulene and matricine [in German]. *Planta Med* 49: 67–73[RG1].

Jalsenjak V, *et al.* (1987). Microcapsules of sage oil: Essential oil content and antimicrobial activity. *Pharmazie* 42: 419–420.

James BM (1930). Dermatitis produced by compound tincture of benzoin. *J Med Soc New Jersey* 27: 596–597.

Janson T (1997). *Mundo Maya*. Guatemala: Editorial Artemis Editer.

Janssen MA, *et al.* (1987). Antimicrobial activities of essential oils: A 1976–1986 literature review on possible applications. *Pharmac Weekbl (Sci)* 9: 193–197.

Janssen MA, *et al.* (1988). Screening of some essential oils for their activities on dermatophytes. *Pharmac Weekbl (Sci)* 10: 277–280.

Janssens J, *et al.* (1990). Nutmeg oil: Identification and quantitation of its most active constituents as inhibitors of platelet aggregation. *J Ethnopharmacol* 29: 179–188.

Jay JM, Rivers GM (1984). Antimicrobial activity of some food flavouring compounds. *J Food Safety* 6: 129–139.

Jay M (1999). *Blue Tide*. New York: Autonomedia.

Jean FI, *et al.* (1991). Extraction au four micro-ondes des diverses plantes cultivées et spontanitées. *Riv Ital EPPOS (Numero Speciale)* 504–510.

Jeanfils J, *et al.* (1991). Antimicrobial activities of essential oils from different plant species. *Landbouwtijdschrift-Revue de l'Agriculture* 44: 1013–1019.

Jellinek Paul (1954). *The Practice of Modern Perfumery*. New York: Interscience.

Jellinek P (1956). *Die Psychologischen Grundlagen der Parfumerie*. Heidelberg: Alfred Hutig Verlag.

Jimenez J, *et al.* (1986). Hypoglycaemic activity of *Salvia lavandulifolia*. *Planta Med* 52: 260–262.

Jimenez J, *et al.* (1988). Hypotensive activity of *Thymus orospedanus* alcoholic extract. *Phytother Res* 2: 152–153.

Jirovetz L, *et al.* (1992). Analysis of fragrance compounds in blood samples of mice by gas chromatography, mass spectrometry, GC/FTIR and GC/AES after inhalation of sandalwood oil. *Biomed Chromatogr* 6: 133–134.

Johansen JD, *et al.* (1997). Fragrance allergic contact dermatitis and testing with commercially available fragrances. *J Eur Acad Dermatol Venereol* 9: 76.

Johansen JD, *et al.* (1998). Allergens in combination have a synergistic effect on the elicitation response: a study of fragrance-sensitized individuals. *Br J Dermatol* 139: 264–270.

Johansen JD, *et al.* (2000). Rash related to use of scented products. A questionnaire study in the Danish population. Is the problem increasing? *Contact Dermatitis* 42: 222–226.

Johansen JD, *et al.* (2002). Oak moss extracts in the diagnosis of fragrance contact allergy. *Contact Dermatitis* 46: 157–161.

Jones E (1998). Psychoneuroimmunology mind/body/ emotions and aromatherapy: A workshop. *Proceedings of the World of Aromatherapy II International Conference and Trade Show, St. Louis, Missouri, USA, September 25–28*. NAHA, pp. 137–144.

Jori A, Briatico G (1973). Effect of eucalyptol on microsomal activity of foetal and newborn rats. *Biochem Pharmacol* 22: 543–544.

Jori A, *et al.* (1969). Effect of essential oils on drug metabolism. *Biochem Pharmacol* 18: 2081–2085.

Joulain D (1993). Cryogenic vacuum trapping of scents from temperate and tropical flowers. In: Teramishu R, Buttery RG, Sugisawa H, eds. *Bioactive Volatile Compounds from Plants*. ACS Symposium Series 525. Washington DC: American Chemical Society, pp. 187–204.

Juergens UR, *et al.* (1998). The anti-inflammatory activity of L-menthol compared to mint oil in human monocytes *in vitro*: a novel perspective for its therapeutic use in inflammatory diseases. *Eur J Med Res* 3: 539–545.

Juven BJ, *et al.* (1994). Factors that interact with the antibacterial action of thyme essential oil and its active constituents. *Appl Bacteriol* 76: 626–631.

Kaaber K (2000). *Australian Sandalwood Oil, Acute Oral Toxicity and Acute Dermal Toxicity*. Denmark: Scantox.

Kaard B, Tostinbo O (1989). Increase of plasma beta endorphins in a connective tissue massage. *Gen Pharm* 20: 487–489.

Kaddu S, *et al.* (2001). Accidental bullous phototoxic reactions to bergamot aromatherapy oil. *J Am Acad Dermatol* 45: 458–461.

Kadir R, *et al.* (1991). Alpha-bisabolol, a possible safe penetration enhancer for dermal and transdermal therapeutics. *Int J Therapeut* 70: 87–94.

Kafferlein HU, *et al.* (1998). Musk xylene: analysis, occurrence, kinetics and toxicology. *Crit Rev Toxicol* 28: 431–476.

Kagawa D, *et al.* (2003). The sedative effects and mechanism of action of cedrol inhalation with behavioral pharmacological evaluation. *Planta Med* 69: 637–641.

Kaiser R, *et al.* (1975). Analysis of Buchu leaf oil. *J Agric Food Chem* 23: 943–950.

Kaliwal BB, Rao MA (1981). Inhibition of ovarian compensatory hypertrophy by carrot seed (*Daucus carota*) extract or estradiol-17β in hemi castrated albino rats. *Indian J Exp Biol* 19: 1058–1060.

Kallenborn R, *et al.* (1999). Gas chromatographic determination of synthetic musk compounds in Norwegian air samples. *J Chromatogr A* 846: 295–306.

Kant A, *et al.* (1986). The estrogenic efficacy of carrot (*Daucus carota*) seeds. *J Adv Zool* 7: 36–41.

Kar A, Jain SR (1971). Investigations on the antibacterial activity of some Indian indigenous aromatic plants. *Flavour Industry* February.

Karamat R, *et al.* (1992). Excitatory and sedative effects of essential oils on human reaction time performance. *Chem Senses* 17: 847.

Karita T (1996). Preparation of capsules, storage thin sheets, bag-type dosage forms for volatile drugs and topical administration of bag-type forms for treatment of skin diseases. *Japan Kokai Tokkyo Koho*, 96109137; *Chem. Abstr.*, 125, 8, 96069c.

Karlberg A-T (2003). Fragrance allergy: caused by oxidation of common fragrances: diagnosis and prevention. In: *Abstracts of the 14th International Congress of Contact Dermatitis, Seoul, Korea, September 2003.* Basel: Karger, p. 152.

Karlberg A-T, Dooms-Goossens A (1997). Contact allergy to oxidised d-limonene among dermatitis patients. *Contact Dermatitis* 36: 201–206.

Karlberg A-T, *et al.* (1994a). Hydroperoxides in oxidised d-limonene identified as potent contact allergens. *Arch Dermatol Res* 286: 97–103.

Karlberg A-T, *et al.* (1994b). Influence of an antioxidant on the formation of allergenic compounds during auto-oxidation of d-limonene. *Ann Occup Hyg* 38: 199–207.

Karnick CR (1994). *Pharmacopoeial Standards of Herbal Plants.* Delhi: Sri Satguru Publications. Vol 1, pp. 259–260; Vol 2, p. 83.

Karpouhtsis IE, *et al.* (1998). Insecticidal and genotoxic activities of oregano essential oils. *J Agric Food Chem* 46: 1111–1115.

Katona M, Egyud K (2001). [Increased sensitivity to balsams and fragrances among our patients.] *Orv Hetil* 142: 465–466.

Kauppinen TP, *et al.* (1986). Respiratory cancers and chemical exposure in the wood industry: a nested case-control study. *Br J Ind Med* 43: 84–90.

Kazanjian A, *et al.* (1999). A systematic review and appraisal of the scientific evidence on craniosacral therapy. *BCOHTA*, May.

Keane FM, *et al.* (2000). Occupational allergic contact dermatitis in two aromatherapists. *Contact Dermatitis* 43: 49–51.

Keil H (1947). Contact dermatitis due to oil of citronella. *J Investig Dermatol* 8: 327–334.

Keith HM, Starraky GW (1935). Experimental convulsions induced by the administration of thujone. A pharmacological study of the influence of the autonomic nervous system of these convulsions. *Neurol Psychiat* 34: 1022.

Kendal-Reed M (1990). Human infant olfaction responses to food odours measured by brain electrical activity mapping (BEAM). PhD thesis, Warwick University.

Kennedy DO, *et al.* (2002). Modulation of mood and cognitive performance following acute administration of *Melissa officinalis* (lemon balm). *Pharmacol Biochem Behav* 72: 953–964.

Kennett F (1975). *History of Perfume.* London: George G Harrap.

Kettel WG (1987). Allergy to *Matricaria chamomilla*. *Contact Dermatitis* 16: 50–51.

Keville K (1999). *Aromatherapy for Dummies.* California: IDG Books Worldwide.

Keville K, Green M (1995). *Aromatherapy: A Complete Guide to the Healing Art.* Fredom, CA: The Crossing Press.

Kilstoff K, Chenoweth L (1998). New approaches to health and well-being for dementia day-care clients, family carers and day-care staff. *Int J Nurs Pract* 4: 70–83.

Kim HM, Cho SH (1999). Lavender oil inhibits immediate-type allergic reaction in mice and rats. *J Pharm Pharmacol* 51: 221–226.

Kimber I, Basketter DA (1992). The murine local lymph node assay: a commentary on collaborative studies and new directions. *Food Chem Toxicol* 30: 165–169.

King JR (1988). Anxiety reducing effects of fragrances using electromyography. *Psychiatr Bull* Suppl 1: 58.

King JR (1994). Scientific status of aromatherapy. *Perspect Biol Med* 37: 409–415.

Kirk-Smith MD (1994). Comments on 'Has unconscious odour been demonstrated?' *Biol Psychol* 37: 269–273.

Kirk-Smith M (1995) Culture and olfactory communication. In: Gardner A, ed. *Ethological Roots of Culture*. Dordrecht: Kluwer, pp. 385–406.

Kirk-Smith M (1996a). Clinical evaluation: deciding what questions to ask. *Nurs Times* 92: 34–35.

Kirk-Smith M (1996b). Winning ways with research proposals and reports. *Nurs Times* 92: 36–39.

Kirk-Smith M (1997). Evaluating the psychological and pharmacological treatment effects of fragrance. In: *Proceedings of the Natural Oils Research Association Symposium, Boston, USA, November 1997*. Boston, MA: NORA.

Kirk-Smith MD, Booth DA (1980). Effect of androstenone on choice of location in others' presence. In: Van Der Starre H, ed. *Olfaction and Taste 7*. London: IRL Press, pp. 397–400.

Kirk-Smith MD, Booth DA (1987). Chemoreception in human behaviour: An analysis of the social effects of fragrances. *Chem Senses* 12: 159–166.

Kirk-Smith MD, Booth DA (1990). The effect of five odorants on mood and the judgement of others. In: MacDonald DW, Muller-Schwartz D, Natynzcuk S, eds. *Chemical Signals in Vertebrates*. Oxford: Oxford University Press, pp. 48–54.

Kirk-Smith MD, *et al.* (1983). Unconscious odour conditioning in human subjects. *Biol Psychol* 17: 221–231.

Kite SM, *et al.* (1998). Development of an aromatherapy service at a Cancer Centre. *Palliat Med* 12: 171–180.

Klarmann EG (1958). Perfume dermatitis. *Ann Allergy* 16: 425–434.

Klemm WR, *et al.* (1992). Topographical EEG maps of human responses to odors. *Chem Senses* 17: 347–361.

Kligman AM (1966a). The identification of contact allergens by human assay, III. The maximisation test. A procedure for screening and rating contact sensitizers. *J Invest Dermatol* 47: 393.

Kligman AM (1966b). The identification of human contact allergens by human exposure. *J Invest Dermatol* 47: 399.

Kligman A (1966, 1973, 1974). Reports to RIFM.

Kligman AM, Epstein W (1975). Updating the maximisation test for identifying contact allergens. *Contact Dermatitis* 1: 231.

Komori T, *et al.* (1995). Potential antidepressant effects of lemon odour in rats. *Eur Neuropsychopharmacol* 5: 477–480.

Kowalski LM (2002). Use of aromatherapy with hospice patients to decrease pain, anxiety, and depression and to promote an increased sense of well-being. *Am J Hosp Palliat Care* 19: 381–386.

Knasko SC (1992). Ambient odours effect on creativity, mood and perceived health. *Chem Senses* 17: 27–35.

Knasko SC (1993). Performance, mood and health during exposure to intermittent odours. *Arch Environ Health* 48: 3058.

Knasko SC, *et al.* (1990). Emotional state, physical well-being and performance in the presence of feigned ambient odour. *J Appl Soc Psychol* 20: 1345–1347.

Kneibel R, Burchard JM (1988). Zur Therapie depressiver Verstimmungen in der Praxis. *Z Allgemeinmed* 64: 689–696.

Knight TE, Hausen BM (1994). Melaleuca oil (tea tree oil) dermatitis. *J Am Acad Dermatol* 30: 423–427.

Knobloch K, *et al.* (1986). Action of terpenoids on energy metabolism. In: Brunke EJ, ed. *Progress in Essential Oil Research*. Berlin: Walter de Gruyther, p. 429.

Knobloch K, *et al.* (1988). Modes of action of essential oil components on whole cells of bacteria and fungi in plate tests. In: Schreier P, ed. *Bioflavour*. Berlin: Walter de Gruyther, pp. 287–299.

Kochi M, *et al.* (1980). Anti-tumour activity of benzaldehyde. *Cancer Treatment Rep* 64: 21–23.

Kohl L, *et al.* (2002). Allergic contact dermatitis from cosmetics: Retrospective analysis of 819 patch-tested patients. *Dermatology* 204: 334–337.

Kohn M (1999). Complementary therapies in cancer care. Macmillan Cancer Relief Report.

Kolodziej H, Kaiser O (1997). *Pelargonium sidoides* DC.-Neuste Erkenntnisse zum Verstandnis des

Phytotherapeutikums Umckaloabo. *Z Phytother* 19: 141–151.

Kolodziej H, *et al.* (1995). Arzneilich verwendete Pelargonien aus Sudafrika. *Dsch Apotheker Ztg* 135: 853–864.

Komori T, *et al.* (1995a). Potential antidepressant effects of lemon odor in rats. *Eur Neuropsychopharmacol* 5: 477–480.

Komori T, *et al.* (1995b). Effects of citrus fragrance on immune function and depressive states. *Neuroimmunomodulation* 2: 174–180.

Koren G (1993). Medications which can kill a toddler with one tablet or teaspoonful. *J Toxicol Clin Toxicol* 31: 407–413.

Kosta L (1999). *Fragrance and Health*. Atlanta, GA: Human Ecology Action League.

Kovar KA, *et al.* (1987). Blood levels of 1,8-cineole and locomotor activity of mice after inhalation and oral administration of rosemary oil. *Planta Med* 53: 315–318.

Kowalski Z, *et al.* (1962). *Medycyna Pr* 13: 69.

Kubota M, *et al.* (1992). Odor and emotion-effects of essential oils on contingent negative variation. In: *Proceedings of the 12th International Congress on Flavours, Fragrances and Essential Oils, Vienna, Austria, October 4–8*, pp. 456–461.

Kudrzycka-Bieloszabska FW, Glowniak K (1966). Pharmacodynamic properties of oleum chamomillae and oleum millefolii. *Diss Pharm Pharmacol* 18: 449–454.

Kumar P, *et al.* (1995). Inhalation challenge effects of perfume scent strips in patients with asthma. *Ann Allergy Asthma Immunol* 75: 429–433.

Kunta JR, *et al.* (1997). Effect of menthol and related terpenes on the percutaneous absorption of propranolol across excised hairless mouse skin. *J Pharmaceut Sci* 86: 1369–1373.

Kurita N, *et al.* (1979). Antifungal activity of molecular orbital energies of aldehyde compounds from oils of higher plants. *Agric Biol Chem* 43: 2365–2371.

Kurita N, *et al.* (1981). Antifungal activity of components of essential oils. *Agric Biol Chem* 45: 945–952.

Kyle L (1998). The use of aromatherapy in elder care. In: *Proceedings of the World of Aromatherapy II International Conference and Trade Show, St. Louis, Missouri, USA, September 25–28*, pp. 174–190.

LaBarre W (1989). *The Peyote Cult*. New Haven, CT: Yale University Press.

Labyak SE, Metzger BL (1997). The effects of effleurage backrub on the physiological components of relaxation: a meta-analysis. *Nurs Res* 46: 59–62.

Laffan G (1992). Chronic respiratory infection. *Int J Aromather* 4: 17.

Laffan G (1993). Pre-menstrual tension. *Int J Aromather* 5: 32.

Lahlou S, *et al.* (2002a). Cardiovascular effects of the essential oil of *Alpinia zerumbet* leaves and its main constituent, terpinen-4-ol, in rats: role of the autonomic nervous system. *Planta Med* 68: 1092–1096.

Lahlou S, *et al.* (2002b). Involvement of nitric oxide in the mediation of the hypotensive action of the essential oil of *Menthax villosain* in normotensive conscious rats. *Planta Med* 68: 694–699.

Lal R, *et al.* (1986). Antifertility effect of *Daucus carota* seeds in female albino rats. *Fitoterapia* 57: 243–246.

Lamey PJ, *et al.* (1990). Sensitivity reaction to the cinnamaldehyde component of toothpaste. *Br Dent J* 168: 115–118.

Larkin P, Castellano JC (1967). Laryngoscopic-findings in acute respiratory infections treated with and without a mentholated rub, In: Dost FH and Leiber B, eds. *Menthol and Menthol-containing External Remedies (Use, Mode of Effect and Tolerance in Children)*. Stuttgart: Georg Thieme Verlag, p. 108.

Larrondo JV, *et al.* (1995). Antimicrobial activity of essences from Labiatae. *Microbios* 82: 171–172.

Larsen W (1998). A study of new fragrance mixtures. *Am J Contact Dermat* 9: 202–206.

Launoy G, *et al.* (1997). Oesophageal cancer in France: potential importance of hot alcoholic drinks. *Int J Cancer* 71: 917–923.

Lautié R, Passebecq A (1979). *Aromatherapy: The Use of Plant Essences in Healing*. Wellingborough: Thorsons Publishers.

Lavy G (1987). Nutmeg intoxication in pregnancy. A case report. *J Reprod Med* 32: 63–64.

Lawless J (1992). *The Encyclopedia of Essential Oils*. Shaftesbury: Element Books.

Lawless J (1994). *Aromatherapy and the Mind*. London: Thorsons.

Lawrence BM (1976–2001). *Essential Oils*: 1976–1978 (published 1979); 1979–1980; 1981–1987 (published 1988); 1988–1991 (published 1992); 1994–1995 (published 1996); 1995–2000 (published 2001). Wheaton, IL: Allured Publishing.

Lawrence BM (1984). Major tropical spices – ginger (*Zingiber officinale* Rosc.). *Perfumer and Flavorist* 9: 1–40.

Lawrence BM (1985). A review of the world production of essential oils. *Perfumer and Flavorist* 10: 1–16.

Lawrence BM (1986). Essential oil production: A discussion of influencing factors. In: Parliament TH and Croteau R, eds. *Biogeneration of Aromas*. ACS Symposium Series 317. Washington, DC: American Chemical Society, pp. 363–369.

Lawrence BM (1992). Progress in essential oils. *Perfumer and Flavorist* 17: 46–49, 59–60.

Lawrence BM (1994). Progress in essential oils. *Perfumer and Flavorist* 19: 40–42.

Lawrence BM (1995). The isolation of aromatic materials from natural plant products. In: Tuley De Silva K, ed. *A Manual on the Essential Oil Industry*. Vienna: United Nations Industrial Development Organization, pp. 57–154.

Lawrence BM (2004). Progress in essential oils. *Perfumer and Flavorist* 29: 88–91.

Lazutka JR, *et al.* (2001). Genotoxicity of dill (*Anethum graveolens* L.), peppermint (*Mentha* x *piperita* L.) and pine (*Pinus sylvestris* L.) essential oils in human lymphocytes and *Drosophila melanogaster*. *Food Chem Toxicol* 39: 485–492.

Leach EH, Lloyd JPF (1956). Experimental ocular hypertension in animals. *Trans Ophthalmolog Soc UK* 76: 453–460.

Le Guérer A (1993). *Scent*. London: Chatto and Windus.

Lehrner J, *et al.* (2000). Ambient odor of orange in a dental office reduces anxiety and improves mood in female patients. *Physiol Behav* 71: 83–86.

Leight RS, *et al.* (1987). Method of causing reduction of physiological and/or subjective reactivity to stress in humans being subjected to stress conditions. US Patent No. 4 671 959, 9th June 1987.

Lermioglu F, *et al.* (1997). Evaluation of the long-term effects of oleum origani on the toxicity induced by administration of streptozotocin in rats. *J Pharm Pharmacol* 49: 1157–1161.

Le Roy R, *et al.* (1981). [Investigation of contact allergies in 100 cases of ulcus cruris (author's translation)]. *Derm Beruf Umwelt* 29: 168–170.

Leshchinskaia IaS, *et al.* (1983). [Effect of phytoncides on the dynamics of the cerebral circulation in flight controllers during their occupational activity]. *Kosm Biol Aviakosm Med* 17: 80–83.

Lessenger JE (2001). Occupational acute anaphylactic reaction to assault by perfume spray in the face. *J Am Board Fam Pract* 14: 137–140.

Letizia CS, *et al.* (2003a). Fragrance material review on linalool. *Food Chem Toxicol* 41: 943–964.

Letizia CS, *et al.* (2003b). Fragrance material review on linalyl acetate. *Food Chem Toxicol* 41: 965–976.

Leung AY (1980). *Encyclopedia of Common Natural Ingredients Used in Food, Drugs and Cosmetics*. New York: John Wiley.

Leung A, Foster S (1996). *Encyclopedia of Common Natural Ingredients Used in Foods, Drugs and Cosmetics*. New York: John Wiley, 1996.

Levine B (1984). Skin absorption. *J Anal Toxicol* 8: 239–241.

Lewis DA, *et al.* (1985). The anti-inflammatory activity of celery *Apium graveolens* L. (Fam. Umbelliferae). *Int J Crude Drug Res* 23: 27–32.

Liebel B, Ehrenstorfer S (1993). [Nitro musk compounds in milk.] *Gesundheitswesen* 55: 527–532.

Lindsay WR, *et al.* (2001). Effects of four therapy procedures on communication in people with profound intellectual disabilities. *J Appl Res Intellect Disabil* 14: 110–119.

Linnaeus C (1753). *Species Plantarum*. Stockholm.

Lis-Balchin M (1995). *Aroma Science: The Chemistry and Bioactivity of Essential Oils*. Surrey: Amberwood Publishing.

Lis-Balchin M (1997). Essential oils and 'aromatherapy': Their modern role in healing. *J R Soc Health* 117: 324–329.

Lis-Balchin M (1998a). Aromatherapy versus the internal intake of odours. *NORA Newsletter* 3: 17.

Lis-Balchin M (1998b) Aromatherapy for pain relief. *Pain Concern* Summer, 12–15. (Now available as a pamphlet from the organisation.)

Lis-Balchin M (1998c) *Shakespearian Aromatics*. Souvenir booklet from Chelsea Flower Show.

Lis-Balchin M (1999). Possible health and safety problems in the use of novel plant essential oils and extracts in aromatherapy. *J R Soc Promotion Health* 119: 240–243.

Lis-Balchin M, ed. (2002a). *Geranium* and *Pelargonium* Genera *Geranium* and *Pelargonium*: Medicinal and Aromatic Plants – Industrial Profiles. London: Taylor and Francis.

Lis-Balchin M, ed. (2002b). Genus *Lavandula*: Medicinal and Aromatic Plants – Industrial Profiles. London: Taylor and Francis.

Lis-Balchin M (2004a). Geranium. In: Peter KV, ed. *Handbook of Herbs and Spices*, Vol 2, pp. 162–178. CRC Press.

Lis-Balchin M (2004b). Lavender. In: Peter KV, ed. *Handbook of Herbs and Spices*, Vol 2, pp. 179–195. CRC Press.

Lis-Balchin M, Deans SG (1997). Bioactivity of selected plant essential oils against *Listeria monocytogenes. J Appl Microbiol* 82: 759–762.

Lis-Balchin M, Guittonneau G-G (1995). Preliminary investigations on the presence of alkaloids in the genus *Erodium* L'Herit. (Geraniaceae). *Acta Bot Gallica* 141: 31–35.

Lis-Balchin M, Hart S (1994). A pharmacological appraisal of the folk medicinal usage of *Pelargonium grossularioides* and *Erodium cicutarium* (Geraniaceae). *Herbs Spices Med Plants* 2: 41–48.

Lis-Balchin M, Hart S (1997a). Correlation of the chemical profiles of essential oil mixes with their relaxant or stimulant properties in man and smooth muscle preparations *in vitro.* In: Franz Ch, Mathé A, Buchbauer G, eds. *Proceedings of the 27th International Symp Essential Oils, Vienna, Austria, 8–11 September 1996.* Carol Stream, IL: Allured Publishing, pp. 24–28.

Lis-Balchin M, Hart S (1997b). The effect of essential oils on the uterus compared to that on other muscles. In: Franz Ch, Mathé A, Buchbauer G, eds. *Proceedings of the 27th International Symp Essential Oils, Vienna, Austria, 8–11 September 1996.* Carol Stream, IL: Allured Publishing, pp. 29–32.

Lis-Balchin M, Hart S (1997c). A preliminary study of the effect of essential oils on skeletal and smooth muscles *in vitro. J Ethnopharmacol* 58: 183–187.

Lis-Balchin M, Hart S (1998a). Studies on mode of action of essential oils of scented-leaf Pelargonium (Geraniaceae). *Phytother Res* 12: 215–217.

Lis-Balchin M, Hart S (1998b). An investigation of the actions of the essential oils of Manuka (*Leptospermum scoparium*) and Kanuka (*Kunzea ericoides*) Myrtaceae on guinea-pig smooth muscle. *J Pharm Pharmacol* 50: 809–811.

Lis-Balchin M, Hart S (1999a). Studies on the mode of action of the essential oil of lavender (*Lavandula angustifolia* Miller). *Phytother Res* 13: 540–542.

Lis-Balchin M, Hart S (1999b). Studies on mode of action of peppermint oil *Mentha x piperita* L. in the guinea-pig ileum *in vitro. Med Sci Res* 27: 307–309.

Lis-Balchin M, Hart S (2002). Correlation of the chemical profiles of the essential oil of *Pelargonium* (geranium oil) and others separately and in mixes, with their relaxant or stimulant properties in man and smooth muscle preparations *in vitro.* In: Lis-Balchin M, ed. *Geranium* and *Pelargonium* Genera *Geranium* and *Pelargonium*: Medicinal and Aromatic Plants – Industrial Profiles. London: Taylor and Francis, pp. 299–307.

Lis-Balchin M, Roth G (2000). Composition of the essential oils of *P. odoratissimum, P. exstipulatum* and *P. x fragrans* (Geraniaceae). *Flavour Fragrance J* 15: 391–394.

Lis-Balchin M, *et al.* (1996a). Comparison of the pharmacological and antimicrobial action of commercial plant essential oils. *J Herbs Spices Med Plants* 4: 69–86.

Lis-Balchin M, *et al.* (1996b). Bioactivity of commercial geranium oil from different sources. *J Essent Oil Res* 8: 281–290.

Lis-Balchin M, *et al.* (1996c). Bioactivity of the enantiomers of limonene. *Med Sci Res* 24: 309–310.

Lis-Balchin M, *et al.* (1996d). Bioactivity of New Zealand medicinal plant essential oils. In: Craker LE, Nolan L, Shetty K, eds. *Proceedings of the International Symposium on Medicinal and Aromatic Plants.* New York: Haworth Press, pp. 13–27.

Lis-Balchin M, *et al.* (1997a). Spasmolytic activity of the essential oils of scented *Pelargoniums* (Geraniaceae). *Phytother Res* 11: 583–584.

Lis-Balchin M, *et al.* (1997b). A study of the changes in the bioactivity of essential oils used singly and as mixtures in aromatherapy. *J Altern Complement Med* 3: 249–255.

Lis-Balchin M, *et al.* (1997c). A study of the variability of commercial peppermint oils using antimicrobial and pharmacological parameters. *Med Sci Res* 25: 151–152.

Lis-Balchin M, *et al.* (1998a). Relationship between the bioactivity and chemical composition of commercial plant essential oils. *Flavour Fragrance J* 13: 98–104.

Lis-Balchin M, *et al.* (1998b). Antimicrobial and antioxidant properties of 3 strains of *Origanum* and comparison with 10 antibiotics. In: *Proceedings of the 28th International Symposium on Essential Oils, Frankfurt, Germany, September 6–9.* ISEO.

Lis-Balchin M, *et al.* (1998c). Pharmacological and antimicrobial studies on different 'Tea tree' oils from Australia and New Zealand. In: *Proceedings of the 5th Annual Symposium on Complementary Healthcare, Exeter University, 10–12 December.* Exeter University.

Lis-Balchin M, *et al.* (1998d). Comparative antibacterial effects of novel *Pelargonium* essential oils and solvent extracts. *Letters Appl Microbiol* 27: 135–141.

Lis-Balchin M, *et al.* (1999). Differences in bioactivity between the enantiomers of α-pinene. *J Essent Oil Res* 11: 393–397.

Lis-Balchin M, *et al.* (2000). Pharmacological and antimicrobial studies on different tea tree oils (*Melaleuca alternifolia, Leptospermum scoparium* or Manuka and *Kunzea ericoides* or Kanuka), originating in Australia and New Zealand. *Phytother Res* 14: 623–629.

Lis-Balchin M, *et al.* (2001). Buchu (*Agathosma betulina* and *A. crenulata*, Rutaceae) essential oils: their pharmacological and antimicrobial activity. *J Pharm Pharmacol* 53: 579–582.

Lis-Balchin M, *et al.* (2002). Jasmine absolute (*Jasminum grandiflorum*, Oleaceae) and its mode of action on guinea-pig ileum *in vitro*. *Phytother Res* 16: 437–439.

Lis-Balchin M, *et al.* (2003). The comparative effect of novel pelargonium essential oils and their corresponding hydrosols as antimicrobial agents in a model food system. *Phytother Res* 17: 60–65.

Lisin G, *et al.* (1999). Antimicrobial activity of some essential oils. *Acta Hort. (ISHS)* 501: 283–288 (www.actahort.org/books/501/501_45.htm; accessed June 2005).

Lissak K (1962). Olfactory-induced sexual behaviour in female cats. In: *XXII International Congress on Physiological Science, Leiden*. pp. 653–656.

Liu JH, *et al.* (1997). Enteric-coated peppermint-oil capsules in the treatment of irritable bowel syndrome: a prospective, randomized trial. *J Gastroenterol* 32: 765–768.

Lo ACT, *et al.* (1995). Dong quai (*Angelica sinensis*) affects the pharmacodynamics but not the pharmaco kinetics of warfarin in rabbits. *Eur J Drug Metab Pharmacokinet* 20: 55–60.

Loret V (1887). Le kyphi, parfum sacre des anciens egyptiens. *J Asiatique* 10: 76–132.

Lorig TS (1989). Human EEG and odor response. *Prog Neurobiol* 33: 387–398.

Lorig TS (1994). EEG and ERP studies of low-level odor exposure in normal subjects. *Toxicol Industrial Health* 10.

Lorig TS, Roberts M (1990). Odor and cognitive alteration of the contingent negative alteration. *Chem Senses* 15: 537–545.

Louis M, Kowalski SD (2002). Use of aromatherapy with hospice patients to decrease pain, anxiety, and depression and to promote an increased sense of well-being. *Am J Hosp Palliat Care* 19: 381–386.

Loveless SE, *et al.* (1996). Further evaluation of the local lymph node assay in the final phase of an international collaborative trial. *Toxicology* 108: 141–152.

Lovell CR (1993). *Plants and the Skin*. Oxford: Blackwell Scientific.

Lowenstein L, Ballew DH (1958). Fatal acute haemolytic anaemia, thrombocytopenic purpura, nephrosis and hepatitis resulting from ingestion of a compound containing apiol. *Can Med Assoc J* 78: 195–198.

Lucas F, Sclafani A (1995). Carbohydrate-conditioned odor preferences in rats. *Behav Neurosci* 109: 446–454.

Luck G (1987). *Arcana Mundi*. England: Crucible.

Luck S, ed. (1999). *Science & Technology Encyclopedia*. London: Softback Preview.

Ludvigson HW, Rottmann TR (1989). Effects of ambient odors of lavender and cloves on cognition, memory, affect and mood. *Chem Senses* 14: 525–536.

Luke E (1962). Addiction to mentholated cigarettes. *Lancet* I: 110–111.

Lunder T, Kansky A (2000). Increase in contact allergy to fragrances: patch-test results 1989–1998. *Contact Dermatitis* 43: 107–109.

Lunny V (1997). *Aromatherapy. The Complete Guide to Aromatherapy for Natural Healing, Relaxation and Beauty*. London: Greenwich Editions.

Mabey R, ed. (1988). *The Complete New Herbal*. London: Elm Tree Books.

McDonald C (1975). *Medicine of the Maori*. Auckland: William Collins.

McEwan M (1994). The antifungal effects of plant essential oils and their production by transformed shoot culture. PhD thesis, Strathclyde Institute of Biomedical Sciences, University of Strathclyde, Glasgow.

McGeorge BC, Steele MC (1991). Allergic contact dermatitis of the nipple from Roman chamomile ointment. *Contact Dermatitis* 24: 139–140.

Macht DI, Ting GC (1921). Experimental inquiry into the sedative properties of some aromatic drugs and fumes. *J Pharmacol Exp Ther* 18: 361–372.

Mack RB (1997). Boldly they rode ... into the mouth of hell. Pennyroyal oil toxicity. *N C Med J* 58: 456–457.

MacMahon S, Kermode S (1998). A clinical trial of the effect of aromatherapy on motivational behaviour in a dementia care setting using a single subject design. *Aust J Holist Nurs* 5: 47–49.

MacNamara P (undated). Leaflet: Massage for Cancer Patients by Patricia MacNamara from the Wandsworth Cancer Support Centre, York Road, London SW11 3QE.

Mailhebiau P (1995). *Portraits in Oils*. Saffron Walden: CW Daniel Co.

Mak M, Del G (1994). *Aroma Therapy*. East Horsley: Amberwood Publishing.

Malhotra SC, Ahuja MMS (1971). Comparative hypolipidaemic effectiveness of gum guggulu (*Commiphora mukul*) fraction 'A', ethyl-*p*-chlorophenoxyisobutyrate and Ciba-13437-Su. *Indian J Med Res* 59: 1621–1632.

Malini T, *et al.* (1985). Effect of *Foeniculum vulgare* Mill. seed extract on the genital organs of male and female rats. *Indian J Physiol Pharmacol* 29: 21–26.

Malnic B, *et al.* (1999). Combinatorial receptor codes for odors. *Cell* 96: 713–723.

Malnic B, *et al.* (2004). The human olfactory receptor gene family. *Proc Natl Acad Sci USA* 101: 2584–2589.

Mankes RF, *et al.* (1983). Effects of various exposure levels of 2-phenylethanol on foetal development and survival in Long-Evans rats. *Toxicol Environ Health* 12: 235–244.

Manley CH (1993). Psychophysiological effect of odor. *Crit Rev Food Science Nutr* 33: 57–62.

Mann C, Staba EJ (1986). The chemistry, pharmacology, and commercial formulations of chamomile. In: Craker LE, Simon JE, eds. *Herbs, Spices, and Medicinal Plants*: *Recent Advances in Botany, Horticulture, and Pharmacology*, Vol 1. Arizona: Oryx Press, pp. 235–280.

Manniche L (1989). *An Ancient Egyptian Herbal*. London: British Museum Publications.

Manniche L (1999). *Sacred Luxuries. Fragrance, Aromatherapy and Cosmetics in Ancient Egypt*. London: Opus Publishing.

Margolin S (1970). Report to RIFM 1 July.

Martijena ID, *et al.* (1998) Anxiogenic-like and anti-depressant-like effects of the essential oil from *Tagetes minuta*. *Fitoterapia* LXIX: 155–160.

Martin G (1989). *Alternative Health – Aromatherapy*. London: Macdonald and Co.

Martindale (1982). *Martindale, The Extra Pharmacopoeia*, 28th edn (edited by JEF Reynolds). London: Pharmaceutical Press.

Martindale (1989). *Martindale, The Extra Pharmacopoeia*, 29th edn (edited by JEF Reynolds). London: Pharmaceutical Press.

Martindale (1993). *Martindale, The Extra Pharmacopoeia*, 30th edn (edited by JEF Reynolds). London: Pharmaceutical Press.

Martindale (1996). *Martindale, The Extra Pharmacopoeia*, 31st edn (edited by JEF Reynolds). London: Pharmaceutical Press.

Martindale (1999). *Martindale: The Complete Drug Reference*, 32nd edn (edited by K Parfitt). London: Pharmaceutical Press.

Martindale (2004). *Martindale: The Complete Drug Reference*, 34th edn (edited by S Sweetman). London: Pharmaceutical Press. Electronic version.

Martindale WH (1910). Essential oils in relation to their antiseptic powers as determined by their carbolic coefficients. *Perfumery Essent Oil Res* 1: 266–296.

Maruzella JC (1960). Antifungal activity of essential oils. *Soap Parfum Cosmet* 33: 835–837.

Maruzella JC, Henry A (1958). The *in vitro* antibacterial activity of essential oils and oil combinations *J Am Pharm Assoc* 47: 294–296.

Maruzella JC, Liguori L (1958). The *in vitro* antifungal activity of essential oils. *J Am Pharm Assoc* 47: 250–253.

Maruzella JC, Sicurella NA (1960). Antibacterial activity of essential oil vapours. *J Am Pharm Assoc* 49: 692–694.

Masago R, *et al.* (2000). Effects of inhalation of essential oils on EEG activity and sensory evaluation. *J Physiol Anthropol Appl Hum Sci* 19: 35–42.

Matsuda H, *et al.* (2000). Inhibitory mechanism of costunolide, a sesquiterpene lactone isolated from laurus nobilis, on blood-ethanol elevation in rats: involvement of inhibition of gastric emptying and increase in gastric juice secretion. *Alcohol Alcohol* 37: 121–127.

Matsunami H, Buck LB (1997). A multigene family encoding a diverse array of putative pheromone receptors in mammals. *Cell* 90: 775–784.

Maura A, *et al.* (1989). Negative evidence in vivo of DNA-damaging, mutagenic and chromosomal effects of eugenol. *Mutation Res* 227: 125–129.

Maury M (1989). *Marquerite Maury's Guide to Aromatherapy*. Saffron Walden: CW Daniel Co.

May B, *et al.* (1996). Efficacy of a fixed peppermint oil/caraway combination in non-ulcer dyspepsia. *Arzneimettelforsch* 146: 1149–1153.

Mazzanti G, *et al.* (1998). Spasmolytic action of the essential oil from *Hyssopus officinalis* L. var. *decumbens* and its major components. *Phytother Res* 12 (suppl): S92–S94.

Meador JP, *et al.* (1995). Bioaccumulation of polycyclic aromatic hydrocarbons by marine organisms. *Rev Environ Contam Toxicol* 143: 79–165.

Medical Economics (2000). *PDR for Herbal Medicine*, 2nd edn. Montvale, NJ: Medical Economics, pp. 880–881.

Meding B (1993). Skin symptoms among workers in a spice factory. *Contact Dermatitis* 29: 202–205.

Meek SS (1993). Effects of slow stroke back massage on relaxation in hospice clients. *Image J Nurs Sch* 25: 17–21.

Meeker HG, Linke HA (1988). The antibacterial action of eugenol, thyme oil, and related essential oils used in dentistry. *Compendium* 9: 32, 34–5, 38 passim.

Mehta S, *et al.* (1998). Use of essential oil to promote induction of anaesthesia in children. *Anaesthesia* 53: 711.

Mele A (1952). Acute fatal poisoning with chenopodium oil. *Folia Med* 35: 955–963.

Melegari M, *et al.* (1988). Chemical characteristics and pharmacological properties of the essential oils of *Anthemis nobilis*. *Fitoterapia* 59: 449–455.

Menard E (1961). Les dermatoses profesionelles. *Concours Med* 83: 4308–4311.

Meyer Fr, Meyer E (1959). Percutaneous absorption of essential oils and their constituents *Arzneimittel-Forsch* 9: 516.

Meynadier JM, *et al.* (1986). [Clinical forms of skin manifestations in allergy to perfume.] *Ann Dermatol Venereol* 113: 31–41.

Michie CA, Cooper E (1991). Frankincense and myrrh as remedies in children. *J R Soc Med* 84: 602–605.

Middleton A, *et al.* (1979). Effects of monocyclic terpenes on hepatic S-3-hydroxy-3-methylglutaryl-coenzyme A reductase in vivo. *Biochem Soc Trans* 7: 407–408.

Mihail RC (1992). Oral leukoplakia caused by cinnamon food allergy. *J Otolaryngol* 21: 366–367.

Millenson JR (1995). *Mind Matters: Psychological Medicine in Holistic Practice*. Seattle, WA: Eastland Press.

Millet Y (1980). Experimental study of the toxic convulsant properties of commercial preparations of essences of sage and hyssop. *Electroencephal Clin Neurophysiol* 49: 102P.

Millet Y, *et al.* (1981). Toxicity studies of some essential plant oils. Clinical and experimental study. *Clin Toxicol* 18: 1485–1498.

Millqvist E, Lowhagen O (1996). Placebo-controlled challenges with perfume in patients with asthma-like symptoms. *Allergy* 51: 434–439.

Millqvist E, *et al.* (1999). Provocations with perfume in the eyes induce airway symptoms in patients with sensory hyperreactivity. *Allergy* 54: 495–499.

Minski R, Bowles EJ (2002). Letter to editor. *Int J Aromather* 12: 225–226.

Miraldi E (1999). Comparison of the essential oils from ten *Foeniculum vulgare* Miller samples of fruits of different origin. *Flavour Fragrance J* 14: 379–382.

Miraldi E, *et al.* (2001). Quality control of aromatic drugs reported in European Pharmacopoeia, 3rd edn. *Il Farmaco* 56: 365–371.

Mitchell JC, Dupuis G (1971). Allergic contact dermatitis from sesquiterpenoids of the Compositae family of plants. *Br J Dermatol* 84: 139–150.

Mitchell J, Rook A (1979). *Botanical Dermatology – Plants and Plant Products Injurious to the Skin*. Vancouver: Greengrass.

Mitchell KA, *et al.* (1998). Pigment chemistry and colour of *Pelargonium* flowers. *Phytochemistry* 47, 355–361.

Mitchell S (1993a). Aromatherapy's effectiveness in disorders associated with dementia. *Int J Aromather* 5: 20–24.

Mitchell S (1993b). Dementia: aromatherapy's effectiveness in disorders associated with dementia. *Int J Aromather* 3: 20–23.

Moghimi HR, *et al.* (1998). Enhancement by terpenes of 5-fluorouracil permeation through the stratum corneum: model solvent approach. *J Pharm Pharmacol* 50: 955–964.

Mohsin A, *et al.* (1989). Analgesic, antipyretic activity and phytochemical screening of some plants used in traditional Arab system of medicine. *Fitoterapia* 60: 174.

Mojay G (1996). *Aromatherapy for Healing the Spirit*. New York: Henry Holt.

Moleyar V, Narasimham P (1986). Antifungal activity of some essential oil components. *Food Microbiol* 3: 331–336.

Monographs on the Medicinal Uses of Plant Drugs, Fascicules 1 and 2 (1996), Fascicules 3, 4 and 5 (1997), Fascicule 6 (1999). Exeter: European Scientific Cooperative on Phytotherapy.

Monzon RB, *et al.* (1994). Larvicidal potential of five Philippine plants against *Aedes aegypti* (Linnaeus) and *Culex quinquefasciatus* (Say). *Southeast Asian J Trop Med Public Health* 25: 755–759.

Moorthy B, *et al.* (1991). Destruction of rat liver microsomal cytochrome P-450 in vitro by a monoterpene ketone, pulegone – a hepatotoxin. *Ind J Chem* 30: 138–146.

Moreira MR, *et al.* (2001). Effects of terpineol on the compound action potential of the rat sciatic nerve. *Braz J Med Biol Res* 34: 1337–1340.

Moretti MDL, *et al.* (1997). A study of anti-inflammatory and peripheral analgesic action of *Salvia sclarea* oil and its main components. *J Essent Oil Res* 9: 199–204.

Morice AH, *et al.* (1994). Effect of inhaled menthol on citric acid induced cough in normal subjects. *Thorax* 49: 1024–1026.

Morris JA, *et al.* (1979). Antimicrobial activity of aroma chemicals and essential oils. *J Am Oil Chem Soc* 56: 595–603.

Morris N (2002a). Detecting concentration differences in aromatic oils. *Percept Mot Skills* 95: 767–768.

Morris N (2002b). The effects of lavender (*Lavandula angustifolium*) baths on psychological well-being: two exploratory randomised control trials. *Complement Ther Med* 10: 223–228.

Morris N, *et al.* (1995). Anxiety reduction by aromatherapy: anxiolytic effects of inhalation of geranium and rosemary. *Int J Aromatherapy* 7: 33–39.

Mortimer PS, *et al.* (1990). The measurement of skin lymph flow by isotope clearance – reliability, reproducibility, injection dynamics, and the effect of massage. *J Invest Dermatol* 95: 766–682.

Morton CA, *et al.* (1995). Contact sensitivity to menthol and peppermint in patients with intra-oral symptoms. *Contact Dermatitis* 32: 281–284.

Moss M, *et al.* (2003). Aromas of rosemary and lavender essential oils differentially affect cognition and mood in healthy adults. *Int J Neurosci* 113: 15–38.

Motomura N, *et al.* (2001). Reduction of mental stress with lavender odorant. *Percept Mot Skills* 93: 713–718.

Moyler DA (1993). Extraction of essential oils with carbon dioxide. *Flavour Fragrance J* 8: 235–247.

Müller J, *et al.* (1984). *The H&R Book of Perfume*. London: Johnson Publications.

Muller S, *et al.* (1996). Occurrence of nitro and non-nitro benzeoid musk compounds in human adipose tissue. *Chemosphere* 33.

Munro IC, *et al.* (1996). Correlation of structural class with no-observed-effect levels: A proposal for establishing a threshold of concern. *Food Cosmet Toxicol* 34: 829–867.

Naef R, Morris AF (1992). Lavender–lavandin – a comparison. *Riv Ital EPPOS* 3 (special issue): 365.

Nagai M, *et al.* (2000). Pleasant odors attenuate the blood pressure increase during rhythmic handgrip in humans. *Neurosci Lett* 289: 227–229.

Naigre R, *et al.* (1996). Comparison of antimicrobial properties of monoterpenes and their carbonylated products. *Planta Med* 62: 275–277.

Nair B (2001a). Final report on the safety assessment of *Mentha piperita* (peppermint) oil, *Mentha piperita* (peppermint) leaf extract, *Mentha piperita* (peppermint) leaf, and *Mentha piperita* (peppermint) leaf water. *Int J Toxicol* 20 (Suppl 3): 61–73.

Nair B (2001b). Final report on the safety assessment of benzyl alcohol, benzoic acid, and sodium benzoate. *Int J Toxicol* 20 (Suppl 3): 23–50.

Nakamatsu Y (1995). Brain stimulants containing terpenes. *Japan Kokai Tokkyo Koho*, 95, 258113; *Chem Abstr* 124 (2): 15522z.

Nakayama H (1974). Perfume allergy and cosmetic dermatitis. *Jap J Dermatol* 84: 659–667.

Nakayama H (1998). Fragrance hypersensitivity and its control. In: Frosch PJ, Johansen JD, White IR eds. *Fragrances: Beneficial and Adverse Affects*. Berlin: Springer Verlag, pp. 83–91.

Nakayama H, *et al.* (1976). Pigmented cosmetic dermatitis. *Int J Dermatol* 15: 673–675.

Nakayama *et al.* (1984). Pigmented cosmetic dermatitis. *Int J Dermatol* 23: 299–305.

Nakayama H, *et al.* (1996). *Allergen Controlled System*. Tokyo: Kanehara Shuppan, pp. 1–42.

Narayana MR, *et al.* (1986). Geranium cultivation in India: potentials and prospects. *Pafai J* 8: 25–29.

Nasel C, *et al.* (1994). Functional imaging of effects of fragrances on the human brain after prolonged inhalation. *Chem Senses* 19: 359–364.

Nash P, *et al.* (1986). Peppermint oil does not relieve the pain of irritable bowel syndrome. *Br J Clin Pract* 40: 292–293.

Navarro V, *et al.* (1996). Antimicrobial evaluation of some plants used in Mexican traditional medicine for the treatment of infectious diseases. *J Ethnopharmacol* 53: 143–147.

Naves J-R, *et al.* (1961). Études sur les matières végétales volatiles CLXXIV (1). Présence de tétrahydropyrannes dans l'huile essentielle de géranium. *Bull Soc Chim France* 645–647.

Naves J-R, *et al.* (1963). Études sur les matières végétales volatiles CLXXXVI (1). Présence d'acétonyl-2-méthyl-4-tétrahydropyranne dans l'huile essentielle de géranium. *Bull Soc Chim France* 1608–1611.

Needleman J (1985). *The Way of the Physician*. San Francisco, CA: Harper and Row.

Neill J (1884). *New Zealand Family Herb Doctor*. Dunedin: Miller, Dick and Co.

Nelson NJ (1997). Scents or nonsense: Aromatherapy's benefits still subject to debate. *J Natl Cancer Inst* 89: 1334–1336.

Nelson RRS (1997). In vitro activities of five plant essential oils against methicillin resistant *Staphylococcus aureus* and vancomycin-resistant *Enterococcus faecium*. *J Antimicrob Chemother* 40: 305–306.

Nenoff P, *et al.* (1996). Antifungal activity of the essential oil of *Melaleuca alternifolia* (tea tree oil) against pathogenic fungi in vitro. *Skin Pharmacol* 9(6): 388–394.

Neuhaus-Carlisle K, *et al.* (1993). Calcium channel blocking activity of essential oils from *Petroselinum crispum*, *Apium graveolens* and isolated phenylpropane constituents. *Pharm Pharmacol Lett* 3: 77.

Neuhaus-Carlisle K, *et al.* (1997). Screening of plant extracts and plant constituents for calcium-channel blocking activity. *Phytomedicine* 4: 67–69.

Newall CA, *et al.* (1996). *Herbal Medicines. A Guide for Healthcare Professionals*. London: Pharmaceutical Press.

Newberne P, *et al.* (1999). The FEMA GRAS assessment of trans-anethole used as a flavouring substance. *Food Chem Toxicol* 37: 789–811.

NIEHS. http://ntp-server.niehs.nih.gov/Main_Pages/Chem-HS.html

Nielsen NH, *et al.* (2001). Allergic contact sensitization in an adult Danish population: Two cross-sectional surveys eight years apart (The Copenhagen Allergy Study). *Acta Dermato-Venereol* 81: 31–34.

Nijssen LM, Maarse H (1986). Volatile compounds in black currant products. *Flavour Fragrance J* 1: 143–148.

Nikolaevskii UV, *et al.* (1990). Effect of essential oils on the course of experimental atherosclerosis. *Patol Fiziol Eksp Ter* Sep–Oct: 52–53.

Nishino T, *et al.* (1997). Nasal inhalation of l-menthol reduces respiratory discomfort associated breathing. *Am J Respir Crit Care Med* 156: 309–313.

Nishioka M (1997). Contact cheilitis due to peppermint oil and menthol in toothpaste. *Environ Dermatol* 4: 43–47.

Nogueira, AC, *et al.* (1995). Study on the embryofetotoxicity of citral in the rat. *Toxicology* 96: 105–113.

NTP Reports (2000). TR-491 Toxicology and Carcinogenesis Studies of Methyleugenol (CAS NO. 93-15-2). in F344/N Rats and B6C3F1 Mice (Gavage Studies). National Toxicological Program, Dept. Health and Human Services. www.ncbi.nlm.nih.gov/entrez/eutils/ elink.fcgi?

Nunn JF (1997). *Ancient Egyptian Medicine*. London: British Museum Press.

Ognyanov I (1985). Bulgarian Zdravetz oil. *Perfumer and Flavorist* 10: 38–44.

Ohashi S, *et al.* (1997). *Perfumer and Flavorist* 22: 1–5.

Ohloff G (1978). Importance of minor components in flavors and fragrances. *Perfumer and Flavorist* 3: 10–22.

Ohloff G (1994). Rose oil. In: *Scent and Fragrances*. Berlin: Springer-Verlag, pp. 154–158.

Ollevant NA, *et al.* (1999). How big is a drop? A volumetric assay of essential oils. *J Clin Nurs* 8: 299–304.

Olowe SA, Ransome-Kuti O (1980). The risk of jaundice in glucose-6-phosphate dehydrogenase deficient babies exposed to menthol. *Acta Paediatr Scand* 69: 341–345.

Olsen RW (2000). Absinthe and gamma-aminobutyric acid receptors. *Proc Natl Acad Sci USA* 97: 4417–4418.

O'Mullane NM, *et al.* (1982). Adverse CNS effects of menthol-containing olbas oil. *The Lancet* 111: 1121.

Oosthuizen LD (1983). The taxonomic value of trichomes in *Pelargonium* L'Hérit (Geraniaceae). *J S Afr Bot* 49: 221–242.

Opdyke DLJ (1974). Aldehyde quenching. Monographs on fragrance raw materials. *Food Cosmet Toxicol*.

Opdyke DL (1977). Safety testing of fragrances: problems and implications. *Clin Toxicol* 10: 61–77.

Opie J, *et al.* (1999). The efficacy of psychosocial approaches to behaviour disorders in dementia: a systematic literature review. *Aust NZ J Psychiatry* 33: 789–799.

Opper L (1939). Pathologic picture of thujone: comparison with pathologic picture of human epilepsy. *Arch Neurol Psychiat* 41: 460.

Ostad SN, *et al.* (2001). The effect of fennel essential oil on uterine contraction as a model for dysmenorrhea, pharmacology and toxicology study. *J Ethnopharmacol* 76: 299–304.

Ott Jonathan (1993). *Pharmacotheon.* Kennewick, WA: Natural Products Co.

Pages N, *et al.* (1989). Teratological evaluation of *Juniperus sabina* essential oil in mice. *Planta Med* 55: 144–146.

Pages N, *et al.* (1990). Essential oils and their potential teratogenic properties: The case of *Eucalyptus globulus* essential oil – preliminary study on mice. *Plantes Med Phytother* 24: 21–26.

Pages N, *et al.* (1992). Potential teratogenicity in mice of the essential oil of *Salvia lavandulifolia* Vahl. Study of a fraction rich in sabinyl acetate. *Phytother Res* 6: 80–83.

Palmer R (1993). In bad odour: smell and its significance in medicine from antiquity to the seventeenth century. In: Byrum WF, Porter Roy, eds. *Medicine and the Five Senses.* Cambridge: Cambridge University Press.

Panizzi L, *et al.* (1993). Composition and antimicrobial properties of essential oils of four Mediterranean Lamiaceae. *J Ethnopharmacol* 39: 167–170.

Pappas GP, *et al.* (2000). The respiratory effects of volatile organic compounds. *Int J Occup Environ Health* 6: 1–8.

Pappe L (1868). *Florae Capensis Medicae, Prodromus,* 3rd edn. Cape Town: W Brittain.

Paster N, *et al.* (1995). Antifungal activity of oregano and thyme essential oils applied as fumigants against fungi attacking stored grain. *J Food Protect* 58: 81–85.

Patoir A, *et al.* (1936). Le Role Abortif de L'apiol. *Paris Medical* 12 December.

Paton WDM (1954). The response of the guinea-pig ileum to electrical stimulation by coaxial electrodes. *J Physiol (Lond)* 127: 40–41.

Paton WDM (1957). The action of morphine and related substances on contraction and on acetylcholine output of coaxially stimulated guinea-pig ileum. *Br J Pharmacol* 12: 119–127.

Pattnaik S, *et al.* (1995a). Characterization of resistance to essential oils in a strain of *Pseudomonas aeruginosa* (VR-6). *Microbios* 81: 29–31.

Pattnaik S, *et al.* (1995b). Antibacterial activity of essential oils from *Cymbopogon*: Inter- and intra-specific differences. *Microbios* 84: 239–245.

Pattnaik S, *et al.* (1996). Antibacterial and antifungal activity of ten essential oils in vitro. *Microbios* 86: 237–246.

Pattnaik S, *et al.* (1998). Effect of essential oils on the viability and morphology of *Escherichia coli* (SP-11). *Microbios* 84: 195–199.

Patton DW, *et al.* (1985). Oro-facial granulomatosis: a possible allergic basis. *Br J Oral Maxillofac Surg* 23: 235–242.

Pauli A, Knobloch K (1987). Inhibitory effects of essential oil components on growth of food-contaminating fungi. *Z Lebensmitt Untersuch Forsch* 185: 10–13.

Pauli G, *et al.* (1985). Celery sensitivity: clinical and immunological correlations with pollen allergy. *Clin Allergy* 15: 273–279.

Peana A, *et al.* (1994). A study on choleretic activity of *Salvia desoleana* essential oil. *Planta Med* 60: 478–479.

Peana AT, *et al.* (2002). Anti-inflammatory activity of linalool and linalyl acetate constituents of essential oils. *Phytomedicine* 9: 721–726.

Peana AT, *et al.* (2003). (−)-Linalool produces antinociception in two experimental models of pain. *Eur J Pharmacol* 460: 37–41.

Peana AT, *et al.* (2004). Profile of spinal and supraspinal antinociception of (–)-linalool. *Eur J Pharmacol* 485: 165–174.

Pedro LG, *et al.* (1992). Composition of the essential oil of *Geranium robertianum* L. *Flavour Fragrance J* 7: 223–226.

Peirce W (1961). Tumour-promotion by lime oil in the mouse forestomach. *Nature* 189: 497–498.

Pelczar MJ, *et al.* (1988). Control of microorganisms by physical agents. In: *Microbiology.* New York: McGraw-Hill, pp. 469–509.

Pélissier Y, *et al.* (1994). A chemical, bacteriological, toxicological and clinical study of the essential oil of *Lippia multiflora* [Verbenaceae]. *J Essential Oil Res* 6: 623–630.

Pellerin R (1991). Supercritical fluid extraction of natural raw materials for the flavor and fragrance industry. *Perfumer Flavorist* 16: 37–39.

Pena EF (1962). *Melaleuca alternifolia* oil. Its use for trichomonal vaginitis and other vaginal infections. *Obstet Gynaecol* 19: 793–795.

Pénoel D (1991a). *Médecine Aromatique, Médecine Planétaire*. Limoges: Roger Jollois.

Pénoel D (1991b). *Cf. les travaux de J.-A. Giralt-Gonzalez*. Limoges: Roger Jollois.

Pénoel D (1998). *A Natural Home Health Care using Essential Oils*. Hurricane, UT: Essential Science Publishing.

Perazzo FF, et al. (2003). Central properties of the essential oil and the crude ethanol extract from aerial parts of *Artemisia annua* L. *Pharmacol Res* 48: 497–502.

Perry EK, et al. (1998). Medicinal plants and Alzheimer's disease. *J Altern Complement Med* 4: 419–428.

Perry EK, et al. (1999). Medicinal plants and Alzheimer's disease: from ethnobotany to phytotherapy. *J Pharm Pharmacol* 51: 527–534.

Perry N, et al. (1996). European herbs with cholinergic activities: potential in dementia therapy. *Int J Geriat Psychiat* 11: 1063–1069.

Perry NB, et al. (1997a). Essential oils from New Zealand manuka and kanuka: chemotaxonomy of *Leptospermum*. *Phytochemistry* 44: 1485–1494.

Perry NB, et al. (1997b). Essential oils from New Zealand manuka and kanuka: chemotaxonomy of *Kunzea*. *Phytochemistry* 45: 1606–1612.

Perry NS, et al. (2000). In-vitro inhibition of human erythrocyte acetylcholinesterase by *Salvia lavandulaefolia* essential oil and constituent terpenes. *J Pharm Pharmacol* 52: 895–902.

Perry NS, et al. (2001). In-vitro activity of *S. lavandulaefolia* (Spanish sage) relevant to treatment of Alzheimer's disease. *J Pharm Pharmacol* 53: 1347–1356.

Perry NS, et al. (2002). *Salvia lavandulaefolia* essential oil inhibits cholinesterase in vivo. *Phytomedicine* 9: 48–51.

Perry NSL, et al. (2003). Salvia for dementia therapy: review of pharmacological activity and pilot tolerability clinical trial. *Pharmacol Biochem Behav* 75: 651–659.

Perry PA, et al. (1990). Cinnamon oil abuse by adolescents. *Vet Hum Toxicol* 32: 162–164.

Petkov V (1979). Plants with hypotensive, antiatheromatous and coronarodilatating action. *Am J Chin Med* 7: 197–236.

Philip G (1998). *Science and Technology Encyclopedia*. London: George Philip.

Piesse SGW (1855). *The Art of Perfumery*. London: Longman, Brown, Green.

Pilapil VR (1989). Toxic manifestations of cinnamon oil ingestion in a child. *Clin Pediatr (Phila)* 28: 276.

Pilcher JD, Mauer RT (1918). The action of female remedies on the intact uteri of mammals. *Surg Gynaecol Obstet* 97–99.

Pilcher JD, et al. (1916). The action of so-called female remedies on the excised uterus of the guinea-pig. *Arch Intern Med* 18: 557–583.

Pinch G (1994). *Magic in Ancient Egypt*. London: British Museum Press.

Pittler MH, Ernst E (1998). Peppermint oil for irritable bowel syndrome: a critical review and meta-analysis. *Am J Gastroenterol* 93: 1131–1135.

Plant OH (1920). The effect of carminative volatile oils on the muscular movements of the intestine. *J Pharmacol Exp Ther* 16: 311–325.

Plant OH, Miller GH (1926). Effects of carminative volatile oils on the muscular activity of the stomach and colon. *J Pharmacol Exp Ther* 27: 149–164.

Polack JS (1840). *Manners and Customs of the New Zealanders*, 2 Vols. London: Madden and Co.

Porter NG, Wilkins AL (1999). Chemical, physical and antimicrobial properties of essential oils of *Leptospermum scoparium* and *Kunzea ericoides*. *Phytochemistry* 50: 407–415.

Porter NG, et al. (1998). Variability in essential oil chemistry and plant morphology within a *Leptospermum scoparium* population. *NZ J Bot* 36: 125–133.

Posthumus MA, et al. (1996). Chemical composition of the essential oils of *Agathosma betulina*, *A. crenulata* and an *A. betulina x crenulata* hybrid (buchu). *J Essent Oil Res* 8: 223–228.

Pourgholami MH, et al. (1999). The fruit essential oil of pimpinella anisum exerts anticonvulsant effects in mice. *J Ethnopharmacol* 66: 211–215.

Prakasa Rao EVS, et al. (1984). Micronutrient studies in geranium (*Pelargonium graveolens* l'Hérit.) and davana (*Artemisia pallens* Wall.). *Indian Perfumer* 28: 88–90.

Prakasa Rao EVS, et al. (1986). Effect of nitrogen fertilizer on geranium (*Pelargonium graveolens* L'Hérit ex. Ait.), cowpea and blackgram grown in sole cropping and intercropping systems. *Int J Trop Agric* 4: 341–345.

Prakasa Rao EVS, et al. (1988). Effect of plant spacings and nitrogen levels on herb and essential oil yields and nutrient uptake in geranium (*Pelargonium graveolens* L'Hérit. ex Ait.). *Int J Trop Agric* 6: 95–101.

Prakash AO (1984). Biological evaluation of some medicinal plant extracts for contraceptive efficacy. *Contracept Deliv Syst* 5: 9.

Prakash AO (1986). Potentialities of some indigenous plants for antifertility activity. *Int J Crude Drug Res* 24: 19–24.

Prakash AO, *et al.* (1985). Anti-implantation activity of some indigenous plants in rats. *Acta Eur Fertil* 16: 441–448.

Pribble JP, *et al.* (1988). Poisoning. In: *Applied Therapeutics*. Vancouver: Applied Therapeutics.

Price S (1973). *Aromatherapy for Common Ailments*. New York: Simon and Schuster.

Price S (1983). *Practical Aromatherapy*. Wellingborough: Thorsons.

Price S (1993). *Aromatherapy Workbook*. London: Thorsons.

Price S, Price L (1999). *Aromatherapy for Health Professionals*, 2nd edn. London: Churchill Livingstone.

Proust M (1981). *Remembrance of Things Past*, Vol 1. New York: Random House.

Pybus D, Sell C (1999). *The Chemistry of Fragrances*. London: RSC Paperbacks.

Quale JM, *et al.* (1996). In vitro activity of *Cinnamomum zeylanicum* against azole resistant and sensitive *Candida* species and a pilot study of cinnamon for oral candidiasis. *Am J Chin Med* 24: 103–109.

Quilici S, *et al.* (1992). Les insects ravageurs. In: *Le Géranium Rosat á la Réunion*. CA Hauts. Saint-Denis (Réunion Island): Graphica, pp. 79–90.

Quinhua Z (1993). China's perfumery industry picks up. *Perfumer and Flavorist* 18: 47–48.

Raffa KF, Berryman AA (1987). Interacting selective pressures in conifer-bark beetle systems: a basis for reciprocal adaptations? *American Naturalist* 129: 234–262.

Raharivelomanana PJ, *et al.* (1989). Study of the antimicrobial action of various essential oils extracted from Malagasy plants. II: Lauraceae. *Arch Inst Pasteur Madagascar* 56: 261–271.

Rai MK, *et al.* (1999). In vitro susceptibility of opportunistic *Fusarium* spp. to essential oils. *Mycoses* 42: 97–101.

Raman A, *et al.* (1995). Antimicrobial effects of tea-tree oil and its major components on *Staphylococcus aureus*, *S. epidermidis* and *Propionibacterium acnes*. *Lett Appl Microbiol* 21: 242–245.

Randerath K, *et al.* (1993). Flavour constituents in cola drinks induce hepatic DNA adducts in adult and fetal mice. *Biochem Biophys Res Commun* 192: 61–68.

Rao VS, *et al.* (1990). Effect of myrcene on nociception in mice. *J Pharm Pharmacol* 42: 877–878.

Rastogi SC, *et al.* (1999). Contents of fragrance allergens in children's cosmetics and cosmetic-toys. *Contact Dermatitis* 41: 84–88.

Rätsch C (1992). *The Dictionary of Sacred and Magical Plants*. Dorset: Prism Press.

Ravid U, *et al.* (1992). Determination of the enantiomeric composition of citronellol in essential oils by chiral GC analysis on a modified γ-cyclodextrin phase. *Flavour Fragrance J* 7: 235–238.

Re L, *et al.* (2000). Linalool modifies the nicotinic receptor–ion channel kinetics at the mouse neuromuscular junction. *Pharmacol Res* 42: 177–182.

Recsan Z, *et al.* (1997). Effect of essential oils on the lipids of the retina in the ageing rat: A possible therapeutic use. *J Essent Oil Res* 9: 53–56.

Redd W, Manne S (1991). Fragrance reduces patient anxiety during stressful medical procedures. *Focus on Fragrance* Summer: 1.

Redd WH, *et al.* (1994). Fragrance administration to reduce anxiety during MR imaging. *J Magn Reson Imaging* 4: 623–626.

Reddy AC, Lokesch B (1992). Studies of spice principles as antioxidants in the inhibition of lipid peroxidation of rat liver microsomes. *Mol Cell Biochem* 111: 117–124.

Reddy BS, *et al.* (1997). Chemoprevention of colon carcinogenesis by dietary perillyl alcohol. *Cancer Res* 57: 420–425.

Redgrove HS (1920). *Bygone Beliefs*. London: William Rider and Sons.

Reichling J, *et al.* (1991). Studies on the biological activities of rare phenylpropanoids of the genus *Pimpinella*. *J Nat Prod* 54: 1416–1418.

Reiter M, Brandt W (1985). Relaxant effects on tracheal and ileal smooth muscles of the guinea-pig. *Arzneim-Forsch Drug Res* 35: 408–414.

Riechelmann H, *et al.* (1997). Response of human ciliated respiratory cells to a mixture of menthol, eucalyptus oil and pine needle oil. *Arzneimittelforschung* 47: 1035–1039.

Riedel E, *et al.* (1982). Inhibition of γ-aminobutyric acid catabolism by valerenic acid derivatives. *Planta Med* 48: 219–220.

Riedel J, *et al.* (1999). Haemoglobin binding of a musk xylene metabolite in man. *Xenobiotica* 29: 573–582.

RIFM (2003). Toxicologic and dermatologic assessment of linalool and related esters when used as fragrance ingredients. *Food Chem Toxicol* 41: 919–1027.

Rimkus GG (1999). Polycyclic musk fragrances in the aquatic environment. *Toxicol Lett* 111: 37–56.

Rimkus GG, Wolf M (1996). Polycyclic musk fragrances in human adipose tissue and human milk. *Chemosphere* 33: 2033–2043.

Rimmel E (1865). *The Book of Perfumes*. London: Chapman and Hall.

Rios JL, *et al.* (1987). Antimicrobial activity of selected plants employed in the Spanish Mediterranean area. *J Ethnopharmacol* 21: 139–152.

Rios JL, *et al.* (1988). Screening methods for natural products with antibacterial activity: A review of the literature. *J Ethnopharmacol* 23: 127–149.

Rippon Mandy (1993). Infertility and stress. *Int J Aromather* 5: 33.

Roberts A, Williams JM (1992). The effect of olfactory stimulation on fluency, vividness of imagery and associated mood: a preliminary study. *Br J Med Psychol* 65: 197–199.

Robinson M, Robinson R (1932). A survey of anthocyanins. Part II. *Biochem. J* 26: 1647–1664.

Rochefort C, *et al.* (2002). Enriched odor exposure increases the number of newborn neurons in the adult olfactory bulb and improves odor memory. *J Neurosci* 22: 2679–2689.

Roe F (1959). Oil of sweet orange: a possible role in carcinogenesis. *Br J Cancer* 13: 92–93.

Roe F, Peirce W (1960). Tumour promotion by citrus oils. *J Natl Cancer Inst* 24: 1389–1403.

Roffey SJ, *et al.* (1990). Hepatic peroxisomal and microsomal enzyme induction by citral and linalool in rats. *Food Chem Toxicol* 28: 403–408.

Rogers S (1990). *Tired or Toxic*. New York: Prestige Publishing.

Romaguera C, *et al.* (1986). Geraniol dermatitis. *Contact Dermatitis* 14: 185–186.

Romaguera C, Vilplana J (2000). Occupational contact dermatitis from ylang-ylang oil. *Contact Dermatitis* 43: 251.

Romine IJ, *et al.* (1999). Lavender aromatherapy in recovery from exercise. *Percept Motor Skills* 88: 756–758.

Rompelberg CJM, *et al.* (1993). Effects of the naturally occurring alkenylbenzenes eugenol and trans-anethole on drug-metabolising enzymes in the rat liver. *Food Chem Toxicol* 31: 637–645.

Rook A (1961). Plant dermatitis-botanical aspects. *Trans St. John's Dermatol Soc* 46: 41–47.

Roos G, *et al.* (1997). Isolation, identification and screening for COX-1 and 5-LO inhibition of coumarins from *Angelica archangelica*. *Pharm Pharmacol Lett* 7: 157–160.

Rose HJ (1959). *A Handbook of Greek Mythology*. New York: EP Dutton.

Rose J (1992a). *The Aromatherapy Book*. Berkeley, CA: North Atlantic Books.

Rose J (1992b). *Herbal Studies Course*. San Francisco, CA: Jeanne Rose.

Rose J, *et al.* (1993). Water-borne pathogens: assessing the health risks. *Health Environment Digest* 7(3): 1–3.

Rose JE, Behm FM (1994). Inhalation of vapour from black pepper extract reduces smoking withdrawal symptoms. *Drug Alcohol Depend* 34: 225–229.

Rossi T, *et al.* (1988). Sedative, anti-inflammatory and anti-diuretic effects induced in rats by essential oils of varieties of *Anthemis nobilis*: a comparative study. *Pharmacol Res Commun* 20 (Suppl 5): 71–74.

Rotton J, *et al.* (1978). Air pollution and interpersonal attraction. *J Appl Soc Psychol* 8: 57–71.

Roulier G (1990). *Les Huiles Essentielles pour votre Santé*. Dangles: St-Jean-de-Braye.

Rovesti P, Colombo E (1973). Aromatherapy and aerosols. *Soap Parfum Cosmet* 46: 475–477.

Rudzki E, Rebandel P (1998). Positive patch test with Kamillosan in a patient with hypersensitivity to camomile. *Contact Dermatitis* 38: 164.

Rudzki E, *et al.* (1976). Sensitivity to 35 essential oils. *Contact Dermatitis* 2: 196–200.

Ryman D (1984). *The Aromatherapy Handbook*. Saffron Waldon: CW Daniel Co.

Ryman D (1986). *Using Essential Oils for Health and Beauty*. London: Century Hutchinson.

Ryman D (1991). *Aromatherapy. The Encyclopedia of Plants and Oils and How they Help You*. London: Piatkus.

Sadraei H, *et al.* (2003). Relaxant effect of essential oil of *Melissa officinalis* and citral on rat ileum contractions. *Fitoterapia* 74: 445–452.

Saeki Y (2000). The effect of foot-bath with or without the essential oil of lavender on the autonomic nervous system: a randomised trial. *Complement Ther Med* 8: 2–7.

Saeki Y (2001). Physiological effects of inhaling fragrances. *Int J Aromather* 11: 18–25.

Saeki Y, *et al.* (1989). Antimicrobial action of natural substances on oral bacteria. *Bull Tokyo Dent Coll* 30: 129–135.

Safayhi H, *et al.* (1994). Chamazulene: an antioxidant-type inhibitor of leukotriene B4 formation. *Planta Med* 60: 410–413.

Safford RJ, *et al.* (1990). Immediate contact reactions to chemicals in the fragrance mix and a study of the quenching action of eugenol. *Br J Dermatol* 123: 595–606.

Sahraei H, *et al.* (2002). The effects of fruit essential oil of the *Pimpinella anisum* on acquisition and expression of morphine induced conditioned place preference in mice. *J Ethnopharmacol* 80: 43–47.

Sainte-Laudy J, *et al.* (1997). [Bioclinical interest in the assay of leukotrienes in four cases of sensitization to trophallergens.] *Allerg Immunol (Paris)* 29: 152, 155–156, 159.

Saleh MM, *et al.* (1996). Volatile oil of Egyptian sweet fennel and its effect on isolated smooth muscles. *Pharm Pharmacol Lett* 6: 6–7.

Sam M, *et al.* (2001). Neuropharmacology. Odorants may arouse instinctive behaviours. *Nature* 412: 142.

Samson Julia (1985). *Nefertiti and Cleopatra.* London: The Rubicon Press.

Sanchez-Perez J, Garcia-Diez A (1999). Occupational allergic contact dermatitis from eugenol, oil of cinnamon and oil of cloves in a physiotherapist. *Contact Dermatitis* 41: 346–347.

Sandbank M, *et al.* (1988). Sebaceous gland hyperplasia following topical application of citral: an ultrastructural study. *Am J Dermatopathol* 10: 415–418.

Sanders C, *et al.* (2002). EEG asymmetry responses to lavender and rosemary aromas in adults and infants. *Int J Neurosci* 12: 1305–1320.

Sanderson H, *et al.* (1991). Aromatherapy and massage for people with learning difficulties. Hands on Publishing and Training, Birmingham.

Sano A, *et al.* (1998). Influence of cedar essence on spontaneous activity and sleep of rats and human daytime nap. *Psychiatry Clin Neurosci* 52: 133–135.

Santos FA, Rao VS (2000). Antiinflammatory and antinociceptive effects of 1,8-cineole a terpenoid oxide present in many plant essential oils. *Phytother Res* 14: 240–244.

Santos FA, Rao VS (2001). 1,8-Cineol, a food flavouring agent, prevents ethanol-induced gastric injury in rats. *Digest Dis Sci* 46: 331–337.

Sato S, *et al.* (1998). The inhibitory effect of funoran and eucalyptus extract-containing chewing gum on plaque formation. *J Oral Sci* 40: 115–117.

Sax NI, Lewis RJ (1989). *Dangerous Properties of Industrial Materials*, 7th edn, Vol III. New York: Van Nostrand Reinhold, p. 2388.

Sayyah M, *et al.* (2002). Anticonvulsant activity of the leaf essential oil of *Laurus nobilis* against pentylenetetrazole- and maximal electroshock-induced seizures. *Phytomedicine* 9: 212–216.

Scafidi FA, *et al.* (1993). Factors that predict which preterm infants benefit most from massage therapy. *J Dev Behav Pediatr* 14: 176–180.

Scardamaglia L, *et al.* (2003). Compound tincture of benzoin: A common contact allergen? *Australas J Dermatol* 44: 180.

Schaller M, Korting HC (1995). Allergic airborne contact dermatitis from essential oils used in aromatherapy. *Clin Exp Dermatol* 20: 143–145.

Scheinman PL (1996). Allergic contact dermatitis to fragrance. *Am J Cont Dermatol* 7: 65–76.

Schiffman SS (1991). Taste and smell losses with age. *Contemp Nutr* 16.

Schiffman S (1992). Aging and the sense of smell: potential benefits of fragrance enhancement. In: van Toller S and Dodd GH, eds. *Fragrance: The Psychology and Biology of Perfume*. New York: Chapman and Hall.

Schiffman SS, Siebert JM (1991). New frontiers in fragrance use. *Cosmet Toiletries* 106: 39–45.

Schiffman SS, *et al.* (1995). Pleasant odors improve mood of men as well as women at mid-life. In: Gilbert A, ed. *Compendium of Olfactory Research*. Dubuque, Iowa: Kendall/Hunt Publishing Co., pp. 97–103.

Schilcher H (1984). Essential oils – effects and side effects. *Dtsch Apoth Z* 124: 1433–1442.

Schilcher H, Leuschner F (1997). The potential nephrotoxic effects of essential juniper oil. *Arzneimittelforschung* 47: 855–858.

Schleidt M, *et al.* (1988). Pleasure and disgust: memories and associations of pleasant and unpleasant odours in Germany and Japan. *Chem Senses* 13: 279–293.

Schleuter DP (1978). Airway response to hair spray in normal subjects and subjects with hyperactive airways. *Chest* 75: 544–547.

Schnaubelt K (1986). *Aromatherapy Course*, 2nd edn. San Raphel: Kurt Schnaubelt.

Schnaubelt K (1995). *Advanced Aromatherapy – The Science of Essential Oils Therapy*. Rochester, Vermont: Healing Arts Press.

Schnaubelt K (1998). The FDA and other demons. *Aromatic Thymes* 5: 14–15.

Schnaubelt K (1999). *Medical Aromatherapy – Healing with Essential Oils*. Berkeley, CA: Frog Ltd.

Schreck CE, Leonhardt BA (1991). Efficacy assessment of Quwenling, a mosquito repellent from China. *J Am Mosq Control Assoc* 7: 433–436.

Schultes RE, Raffauf RF (1992). *Vine of the Soul*. Arizona: Synergetic Press.

Schultz V, *et al.* (1997). Clinical trials with phyto-psychopharmacological agents. *Phytomedicine* 346: 701.

Schultz V, *et al.* (1998). *Rational Phytotherapy*, 3rd edn. Berlin: Springer-Verlag, pp. 146–147.

Schultze W, *et al.* (1994). Differentiation of true lemon balm oil (*Melissa officinalis* L.) from adulterations by chirospecific GC analysis of citronellal and isotope ratio mass spectrometry. Paper presented at the 25th International Symposium on Essential Oils, Grasse, France, 5–7 September.

Schumann Antelme R, Rossini S (2001). *Sacred Sexuality in Ancient Egypt*. Vermont: Inner Traditions International.

Scolnik M, *et al.* (1994). Immediate vasoactive effect of citral on the adolescent rat ventral prostate. *Prostate* 25: 1–9.

SEAC (2000). Quenching: fact or fiction. *Contact Dermatitis* 43: 253–258.

Seawright A (1993). Tea tree oil: comment. *Med J Aust* 159: 831.

Sekizawa J, Shibamoto T (1982). Genotoxicity of safrole-related chemicals in microbial test systems. *Mutat Res* 101: 127–140.

Sellar W (1992). *The Directory of Essential Oils*, revised ed. Saffron Walden: CW Daniel Co.

Serkedjieva J (1995). Inhibition of influenza virus protein synthesis by a plant preparation from *Geranium sanguineum* L. *Acta Virol* 39: 5–10.

Servadio C, *et al.* (1986). Early stages of the pathogenesis of rat ventral prostate hyperplasia induced by citral. *Eur Urol* 12: 195–200.

Shaparenko BA, *et al.* (1979). On use of medicinal plants for treatment of patients with chronic suppurative otitis. *Zh Ushn Gorl Bolezn* 39: 48–51.

Shapiro AK (1959). The placebo effect in the history of medical treatment: Implications for psychiatry. *Am J Psychiatry* 116: 298–304.

Shapiro S, *et al.* (1994). The antimicrobial activity of essential oils and essential oil components towards oral bacteria. *Oral Microbiol Immunol* 9: 202–204.

Sharma JN, *et al.* (1994). Suppressive effects of eugenol and ginger oil on arthritic rats. *Pharmacology* 49: 314–318.

Sharma M, Shukla S (1977). Hypoglycaemic effect of ginger. *J Res Ind Med Yoga Homoeopath* 12: 127–130.

Shavit Y (1987). Stress-related immune modulation in animals: Opiates and endogenous opioid peptides. In: Ader R, Felten DL, Cohen N, eds. *Psychoneuroimmunology*, 2nd edn. London: Academic Press, pp. 789–806.

Shaw G, *et al.* (1991). Stress management for irritable bowel syndrome. *Digestion* 50: 36–42.

Shawe K (1998). Frankincense and myrrh – incense gum-oleoresins. In: *Purdue International Training Program in Essential Oils*. Purdue International.

Shelef LA (1984). Antimicrobial effects of spices. *J Food Safety* 6: 29–44.

Shemesh A, Mayo WL (1991). Australian tea tree oil: a natural antiseptic and fungicidal agent. *Aust J Pharm* 72: 802–803.

Sheppard-Hanger S (1995). *The Aromatherapy Practitioner Reference Manual*. Florida: Atlantic Institute of Aromatherapy.

Sheppard-Hanger S, Burfield T (1999). What is sensitisation? *Scensitivity* 9: 6–7.

Sheppard-Hanger S, Stokes T (1999). Aromatherapy, psychotherapy. *Aromatic Thymes* 6: 17–23.

Sherif A, *et al.* (1987). Drugs, insecticides and other agents from *Artemisia*. *Medical Hypotheses* 23: 187–193.

Shim C, Williams MH Jr. (1986). Effect of odors in asthma. *Am J Med* 80: 18–22.

Shipochliev T (1968). Pharmacological investigation into several essential oils. First communication. Effect on the smooth musculature. *Vet Med Nauki* 5: 63–69.

Shipochliev T (1981). Extracts from a group of medicinal plants enhancing the uterine tonus. *Vet Med Nauki* 18: 94–98.

Shoji Y, *et al.* Enhancement of anti-herpetic activity of antisense phosphorothioate oligonucleotides 5′ modified with geraniol. *J Drug Target* 5: 261–273.

Shrivastav P, *et al.* (1988). Suppression of puerperal lactation using jasmine flowers (*Jasminum sambac*). *Aust NZ J Obstet Gynaecol* 28: 68–71.

Shulman KR, Jones GE (1996). The effectiveness of massage therapy intervention on reducing anxiety in the workplace. *J Appl Behav Sci* 32: 160–173.

Sieben S, *et al.* (2001). Characterization of T cell responses to fragrances. *Toxicol Appl Pharmacol* 172: 172–178.

Silva Brum LF, *et al.* (2001a). Effects of linalool on [3H] MK801 and [3H] muscimol binding in mouse cortical membranes. *Phytother Res* 15: 422–425.

Silva Brum LF, *et al.* (2001b). Effects of linalool on glutamate release and uptake in mouse cortical synaptosomes. *Neurochem Res* 26: 191–194.

Simmonds SJ (1997). Whitefly toxins. *Pharmac J* 259: 481.

Simon JE (1990). Essential oils and culinary herbs. In: Janick J, Simon JE (eds) *Advances in New Crops*. Portland, OR: Timber Press, pp. 472–483.

Simon JE, Quinn J (1988). Characterization of essential oil of parsley. *J Agric Food Chem* 36: 467–472.

Simon JE, *et al.* (1984). *Herbs – An Indexed Bibliography, 1971–80*. Oxford: Elsevier.

Simpson D (1998). Buchu – South Africa's amazing herbal remedy. *Scott Med J* 43: 189–191.

Singh GB, Atal CK (1986). Pharmacology of an extract of salai guggal ex-*Boswellia serrata*, a new non-steroidal anti-inflammatory agent. *Agents Actions* 18: 407–412.

Sinha KK, *et al.* (1993). The effect of clove and cinnamon oils on growth of and aflatoxin production by *A. flavus*. *Lett Appl Microbiol* 16: 114–117.

Siurin SA (1997). [Effects of essential oil on lipid peroxidation and lipid metabolism in patients with chronic bronchitis.] *Klin Med* (*Mosk*) 75: 43–45.

Skoeld M, *et al.* (2002a). Sensitization studies on the fragrance chemical linalool, with respect to autooxidation. Abstract. *Contact Dermatitis* 46 (suppl 4): 20.

Skoeld M, *et al.* (2002b). Studies on the autooxidation and sensitizing capacity of the fragrance chemical linalool, identifying a linalool hydroperoxide. *Contact Dermatitis* 46: 267–272.

Skoula M, *et al.* (1996). Essential oil variation of *Lavandula stoechas* L. ssp. *stoechas* growing wild in Crete (Greece). *Biochem System Ecol* 24: 255–260.

Smallwood J, *et al.* (2001). Aromatherapy and behaviour disturbances in dementia: a randomized controlled trial. *Int J Geriatr Psychiatry* 16: 1010–1013.

Smith A, Margolis G (1954). Camphor poisoning. *Am J Pathol* 30: 857–869.

Smith LL, *et al.* (1994). The effects of athletic massage on delayed onset muscle soreness, creatine kinase, and neutrophil count: A preliminary report. *J Orthop Sports Phys Ther* 19: 93–99.

Smith MC, *et al.* (1999). Benefits of massage therapy for hospitalized patients: a descriptive and qualitative evaluation. *Altern Ther Health Med* 5: 64–71.

Smith R, Asjes E (1989). Cancer of the liver. *Int J Aromather* 1: 26.

Smith-Palmer A, *et al.* (1998). Antimicrobial properties of plant essential oils and essences against five important food-borne pathogens. *Lett Appl Microbiol* 26: 118–122.

Smith-Palmer A, *et al.* (2004). Influence of subinhibitory concentrations of plant essential oils on the production of enterotoxins A and B and α-toxin by *Staphylococcus aureus*. *J Med Microbiol* 53: 1023–1027.

Snow AL, *et al.* (2004). A controlled trial of aromatherapy for agitation in nursing home patients with dementia. *J Alt Complem Med* 10: 431–437.

Soden K, *et al.* (2004). A randomized controlled trial of aromatherapy massage in a hospice setting. *Palliat Med* 18: 87–92.

Soliman KM, Badeaa RI (2002). Effect of oil extracted from some medicinal plants on different mycotoxigenic fungi. *Food Chem Toxicol* 40: 1669–1675.

Somal N, *et al.* (1994). Susceptibility of *Helicobacter pylori* to the antibacterial activity of Manuka honey. *J R Soc Med* 87: 9–11.

Somerville KW, *et al.* (1984). Delayed release peppermint oil capsules (Colpermin) for the spastic colon syndrome – a pharmaco-kinetic study. *Br J Clin Pharm* 18: 638–640.

Somerville KW, *et al.* (1985). Stones in the common bile duct: experience with medical dissolution therapy. *Postgrad Med J* 61: 313–316.

Soulimani R, *et al.* (1991). Neurotropic action of the hydroalcoholic extract of *Melissa officinalis* in the mouse. *Planta Med* 57: 105–109.

Southwell IA (1988). Australian tea tree: oil of melaleuca, terpinen-4-ol type. *Chem Austr* 11: 400–402.

Southwell IA (1997). Skin irritancy of tea tree oil. *J Essent Oil Res* 9: 47–52.

Sow AI, *et al.* (1995). Antibacterial activity of essential oils from mint in Senegal. *Dakar Med* 40: 193–195.

Sparks T (1985). Cinnamon oil burn. *West J Med* 142: 835.

Spencer DG Jr, *et al.* (1988). Behavioral and physiological detection of classically-conditioned blood pressure reduction. *Psychopharmacology (Berl)* 95: 25–28.

Spencer PS, *et al.* (1979). Neurotoxic fragrance produces ceroid and myelin disease. *Science* 204: 633–635.

Spencer PS, *et al.* (1984). Neurotoxic properties of musk ambrette. *Toxicol Appl Pharmacol* 75: 571–575.

Spott DA, Shelley WB (1970). Exanthema due to contact allergen (benzoin) absorbed through skin. *JAMA* 214: 1881–1882.

Srivastava KC (1989). Effect of onion and ginger consumption on platelet thromboxane production in humans. *Prostaglandins Leukot Essent Fatty Acids* 35: 183–185.

Stafford HA (1961). Distribution of tartaric acid in the Geraniaceae. *Am J Bot* 48: 699–701.

Stager J, *et al.* (1991). Spice allergy in celery-sensitive patients. *Allergy* 46: 475–478.

Stahl E (1973). *Drug Analysis by Chromatography and Microscopy*. Ann Arbor, MI: Ann Arbor Science.

Stammati A, *et al.* (1999). Toxicity of selected plant volatiles in microbial and mammalian short-term assays. *Food Chem Toxicol* 37: 813–823.

Stampf JL, *et al.* (1982). The sensitising capacity of helenin and two of its main constituents the sesquiterpene lactones alantolactone and isoalantolactone: a comparison of epicutaneous and intradermal sensitising methods in different strains of guinea pig. *Contact Dermatitis* 8: 16–24.

Steen EB (1971). *Dictionary of Biology*. New York: Barnes and Noble.

Steinberg P, *et al.* (1999). Acute hepatotoxicity of the polycyclic musk 7-acetyl-1,1,3,4,4,6-hexamethyl-1,2,3,4-tetrahydronaphthaline (AHTN). *Toxicol Lett* 111: 151–160.

Steinmetz MD, *et al.* (1987). Actions of essential oils of rosemary and certain of its constituents (eucalyptol and camphor) on the cerebral cortex of the rat in vitro. *J Toxicol Clin Exp* 7: 259–271.

Sternberg RJ (1993). *The Psychologist's Companion: A Guide to Scientific Writing for Students and Researchers*, 3rd edn. Cambridge: Cambridge University Press.

Stevens K (1991). How safe are perfumes? *AEHA Quarterly* XIII.

Stevenson CS (1937). Oil of wintergreen (methyl salicylate) poisoning. Report of three cases, one with autopsy, and a review of the literature. *Am J Med Sci* 193: 772–788.

Stevenson C (1994). The psychophysiological effects of aromatherapy massage following cardiac surgery. *Comp Ther Med*, 2: 27–35.

Stevinson C, Ernst E (2000). Valerian for insomnia: a systematic review of randomised clinical trials. *Sleep Med* 1: 91–99.

Sticher O (1977). Plant mono-, di- and sesquiterpenoids with pharmacological or therapeutical activity. In: Wagner H and Wolf P, eds. *New Natural Products and Plant Drugs with Pharmacological, Biological or Therapeutic Activity*. Berlin: Springer-Verlag.

Stoddart DM (1990). *The Scented Ape*. Cambridge: Cambridge University Press.

Streicher C (1998). Aroma chemistry to aroma physiology: How aromatic molecules aid in various body systems. In: *Proceedings of the World of Aromatherapy II International Conference and Trade Show, St. Louis, Missouri, USA, September 25–28*. NAHA, pp. 209–218.

Subiza J, *et al.* (1989). Anaphylactic reaction after the ingestion of chamomile tea: a study of cross-reactivity with other composite pollens. *J Allergy Clin Immunol* 84: 353–358.

Suganda AG, *et al.* (1983). [Inhibitory effects of some crude and semi-purified extracts of indigenous French plants on the multiplication of human herpesvirus 1 and poliovirus 2 in cell culture.] *J Nat Prod* 46: 626–632.

Sugawara Y, *et al.* (1999). Alteration of perceived fragrance of essential oils in relation to type of work: a simple screening test for efficacy of aroma. *Chem Senses* 24: 415–421.

Sugawara Y, *et al.* (2000). Odor distinctiveness between enantiomers of linalool: difference in perception and responses elicited by sensory test and forehead surface potential wave measurement. *Chem Senses* 25: 77–84.

Sugiura M, *et al.* (2000). Results of patch testing with lavender oil in Japan. *Contact Dermatitis* 43: 157–160.

Sullivan JB Jr, *et al.* (1979). Pennyroyal oil poisoning and hepatotoxicity. *JAMA* 242: 2873–2874.

Sullivan JB Jr, *et al.* (1995). Spatial patterning and information coding in the olfactory system. *Curr Opin Genet Devel* 5: 516–523.

Sunshine W, *et al.* (1996). Fibromyalgia benefits from massage therapy and transcutaneous electrical stimulation. *J Clin Rheumatol* 12: 18–22.

Surburg H, *et al.* (1993). Volatile compounds from flowers. Analytical and olfactory aspects. In: Teramishu R, Buttery RG, Sugisawa H, eds. *Bioactive Volatile Compounds from Plants.* ACS Symposium Series 525. Washington DC: American Chemical Society, pp. 168–186.

Surh Y-J, *et al.* (1998). Chemoprotective properties of some pungent ingredients present in red pepper and ginger. *Mutat Res* 402: 259–267.

Sweet R (1820–1830). *Geraniaceae the natural order of Gerania,* 5 vols. London: J Ridgway.

Sysoev NP, Lanina SI (1990). The results of sanitary chemical research into denture base materials coated with components from essential oil plants. *Stomatologiia* July–Aug: 59–61.

Szelenyi I, *et al.* (1979). Pharmacological experiments with compounds of chamomile III. Experimental studies of the ulcerprotective effect of chamomile. *Planta Med* 35: 218–227.

Tabak M, *et al.* (1996). In vitro inhibition of *Helicobacter pylori* by extracts of thyme. *J Appl Bacteriol* 80: 667–672.

Taddei I, *et al.* (1988). Spasmolytic activity of peppermint, sage and rosemary essences and their major constituents. *Fitoterapia* 59: 463–468.

Takayama K, Nagai T (1994). Limonene and related compounds as potential skin penetration promoters. *Drug Devel Ind Pharm* 20: 677–684.

Tantaoui-Elaraki A, Beraoud L (1994). Inhibition of growth and aflatoxin production in *Aspergillus parasiticus* by essential oils of selected plant materials. *J Environ Pathol Toxicol Oncol* 13: 67–72.

Taran DD, *et al.* (1989). [The wound-healing properties of the essential oils of yarrow and Yakut wormwood and khamazulen in napalm burns.] *Voen Med Zh* 8: 50–52.

Taroeno BJ, *et al.* (1989). Anthelmintic activities of some hydrocarbons and oxygenated compounds in the essential oil of *Zingiber purpureum. Planta Med* 55: 105.

Tasev T, *et al.* (1969). [Neurophysical effect of Bulgarian essential oils from rose, lavender and geranium.] *Folia Med (Plovdiv)* 11: 307–317.

Tate S (1997). Peppermint oil: a treatment for post-operative nausea. *J Adv Nurs* 26: 543–549.

Tateo F (1989). Composition and quality of super-critical CO_2 extracted cinnamon. *J Essent Oil Res* 1: 165–168.

Taylor BA, *et al.* (1983). Inhibitory effect of peppermint oil on gastrointestinal smooth muscle. *Gut* 24: A992.

Taylor BA, *et al.* (1985). Calcium antagonist activity of menthol on gastrointestinal smooth muscle. *Br J Clin Pharmacol* 20: 293P–294P.

Teisseire P (1987). Industrial quality control of essential oils by capillary GC. In: Sandra P and Bicchi C, eds. *Capillary Gas Chromatography in Essential Oil Analysis.* Heidelberg: Huethig, pp. 215–258.

Temesvari E, *et al.* (2002). Multicentre study of fragrance allergy in Hungary. Immediate and late type reactions. *Contact Dermatitis* 46: 325–330.

Teng CM, *et al.* (1988). Inhibition of platelet aggregation by apigenin from *Apium graveolens. Asia Pac J Pharmacol* 1: 85–89.

Teuscher E, *et al.* (1989). Components of essential oils as membrane-active compounds. *Planta Med* 55: 660.

Teuscher E, *et al.* (1990). Untersuchungen zum wirkungsmechanismus atherischer Ole. *Z Phytother* 11: 87–92.

Thacharodi D, Rao DP (1994). Transdermal absorption of nifedipine from microemulsions of lipophilic skin penetration enhancers. *Int J Pharm* 111: 235–240.

The International School of Aromatherapy (1993). *A Safety Guide on the use of Essential Oils.* London: Natural by Nature Oils.

Theophrastus (1916/1926). *Enquiry into Plants,* Vols 1 and 2, translated by AF Hort. Cambridge, MA: Harvard University Press.

Thomas JG (1962). Peppermint fibrillation, *The Lancet* I: 222.

Thorgrimsen L, *et al.* (2003). Aroma therapy for dementia. *Cochrane Database Syst Rev* 3.

Thorup I, *et al.* (1983). Short term toxicity study in rats dosed with pulegone and menthol. *Toxicol Lett* 19: 207–210.

Throop P (1994). *Hildegard von Bingen's Physica.* Rochester, Vermont: Healing Arts Press.

Tibballs J (1995). Clinical effects and management of eucalyptus oil ingestion in infants and young children. *Med J Aust* 163: 177–180.

Tildesley NT, *et al.* (2003). *Salvia lavandulaefolia* (Spanish Sage) enhances memory in healthy young volunteers. *Pharmacol Biochem Behav* 75: 669–674.

Tisserand R (1977). *The Art of Aromatherapy*. Saffron Walden: CW Daniel Co.

Tisserand R, Balacs T (1995). *Essential Oil Safety – A Guide for Health Care Professionals*. Edinburgh: Churchill Livingstone.

Tobyn G (1997). *Culpeper's Medicine: A Practice of Holistic Medicine*. Shaftesbury: Element Books.

Todorov S, *et al.* (1984). Experimental pharmacological study of three species from genus *Salvia*. *Acta Physiol Pharmacol Bulg* 10: 13–20.

Tong MM, *et al.* (1992). Tea tree oil in the treatment of tinea pedis. *Aust J Dermatol* 33: 145–149.

Torii S, *et al.* (1988). Contingent negative variation and the psychological effects of odor. In: Toller S and Dodd GH, eds. *Perfumery: The Psychology and Biology of Fragrance*. New York: Chapman and Hall.

Torrado S, *et al.* (1995). Effect of dissolution profile and (–)-alpha-bisabolol on the gastrotoxicity of acetylsalicylic acid. *Pharmazie* 50: 141–143.

Toulemonde B, Beauverd D (1984). Contribution a l'étude d'une camomille sauvage du Maroc: huile essentielle d'Ormenis mixta. *Parf Cosmet Aromes* 60: 65–67.

Toulon J, *et al.* (1983). [Malignant arterial hypertension induced by the ingestion of 'alcohol-free aniseed drink'.] *Presse Med* 12: 1171–1172.

Trabut Dr. (1920). L'eucalyptus et le Diabète. *Bull Gen Therap* 429–430.

Trevelyan J (1996). A true complement. *Nurs Times* 92: 42–43.

Triebs W (1956). *Die Atherischen Öle*. Berlin: Akademie-Verlag.

Trigg JK (1996). Evaluation of a eucalyptus-based repellent against *Culicoides impunctatus* (Diptera: Ceratopogonidae) in Scotland. *J Am Mosq Control Assoc* 12: 329–330.

Trono D, *et al.* (1983). [Pseudo-Conn's syndrome due to intoxication with nonalcoholic pastis.] *Schweiz Med Wochenschr* 113: 1092–1095.

Truitt EB, *et al.* (1961). Pharmacology of myristicin. A contribution to the psychopharmacology of nutmeg. *J Neuropsychiat* 2: 205.

Tsuchiya T, *et al.* (1991). Effects of olfactory stimulation on the sleep time induced by pentobarbital administration in mice. *Brain Res Bull* 26: 397–401.

Tsuchiya T, *et al.* (1992). Effects of olfactory stimulation with jasmine and its component chemicals on the duration of pentobarbital-induced sleep in mice. *Life Sci* 50: 1097–1102.

Tubaro A, *et al.* (1984). Evaluation of anti-inflammatory activity of a chamomile extract after topical application. *Planta Med* 50: 359.

Tucker AO (1981). The correct name for Lavandin and its cultivars Labiatae. *Baileya* 21: 131–133.

Tucker AO (1981). Which is the true oregano? *Horticulture* 59(7): 57–59.

Tucker AO, Lawrence BM (1987). Botanical nomenclature of commercial sources of essential oils, concretes and absolutes. In: Craker LE and Simon JE, eds. *Herbs, Spices and Medicinal Plants: Recent Advances in Botany, Horticulture and Pharmacology*. Phoenix, AZ: Oryx Press, pp. 183–220.

Turner G, Collins E (1975). Fetal effects of regular salicylate ingestion in pregnancy. *Lancet* 2: 338–339.

Turner JA, *et al.* (1994). The importance of placebo effects in pain treatment and research. *JAMA* 271: 1609–1914.

Tyler V (1993). *The Honest Herbal*, 3rd edn. New York: Pharmaceutical Products Press.

Tyler V (1996). Lecture for International Training in Essential Oils: Advanced Studies Course held at Purdue University, Indiana, USA.

Ueda S, *et al.* (1982). Inhibition of microorganisms by spice extracts and flavouring compounds. *Nippon Shokuhin Kogyo Gakkaishi* 29: 111–116.

Uedo N, *et al.* (1999). Inhibition by D-limonene of gastric carcinogenesis induced by *N*-methyl-*N′*-nitro-N-nitroguanidine in Wistar rats. *Cancer Lett* 137: 131–136.

Uehleke H, Brinkschulte-Freitas M (1979). Oral toxicity of an essential oil from myrtle and adaptive liver stimulation. *Toxicology* 12: 335–342.

Ultee A, *et al.* (1998). Bactericidal activity of carvacrol towards the food-borne pathogen *Bacillus cereus*. *J Appl Microbiol* 85: 211–218.

Ultee A, *et al.* (1999). Mechanisms of action of carvacrol on the food-borne pathogen *Bacillus cereus*. *Appl Environ Microbiol* 65: 4606–4610.

Umezu T (1999). Anticonflict effects of plant-derived essential oils. *Pharmacol Biochem Behav* 64: 35–40.

Umezu T (2000). Behavioral effects of plant-derived essential oils in the Geller types conflict test in mice. *Jpn J Pharmacol* 83: 150–153.

Umezu T, *et al.* (2001). Ambulation-promoting effect of peppermint oil and identification of its active constituents. *Pharmacol Biochem Behav* 69: 383–390.

Umezu T, *et al.* (2002). Anticonflict effects of rose oil and identification of its active constituents. *Life Sci* 72: 91–102.

Unterman A (1991). *Dictionary of Jewish Lore & Legend*. London: Thames and Hudson.

Upton R, ed. (1999). *American Herbal Pharmacopoeia and Therapeutic Compendium. Valerian root. Valeriana officinalis. Analytical, Quality Control, and Therapeutic Monograph*. Santa Cruz: American Herbal Pharmacopoeia.

Uragoda CG (1984). Asthma and other symptoms in cinnamon workers. *Br J Ind Med* 41: 224–227.

Urba SG (1996). Nonpharmacologic pain management in terminal care. *Clin Geriatr Med* 12: 301–311.

Urbach E, Kral F (1937). Lichtschutz durch Kombination von Vitamin C und Bergamotol. *Klin Wochnschr* 16: 960.

Urbach F, Forbes PD (1972). Report to RIFM, 22 September.

Valette G (1945). Sur la penetration transcutanée des huiles essentielles et de leurs constituants chimiques. *Soc Biol* 904–906.

Valette MC (1946–7). Penetration transcutée des essences. *Parfumerie Moderne* 39: 64–66.

Valnet J (1964). *Aromathérapie. Traitement des Maladies par les Essences des Plantes*, 10th edn. Paris: Maloine.

Valnet J (1982). *The Practice of Aromatherapy*. Saffron Walden: CW Daniel Co.

Van Den Broucke CO, Lernli JA (1981). Pharmacological and chemical investigation of thyme liquid extracts. *Planta Med* 41: 129–135.

Van Den Broucke CO (1983). The therapeutic value of *Thymus* species. *Fitoterapia* 4: 171–174.

Van Der Walt JJA, Demarne JE (1988). *Pelargonium graveolens* and *P. radens*: a comparison of their morphology and essential oils. *S Afr J Bot* 54: 617–622.

Van Der Walt JJA, *et al.* (1990). Delimitation of *Pelargonium* sect. *Glaucophyllum* (Geraniaceae). *Plant Syst Evol* 171: 15–26.

Van Der Walt JJA, *et al.* (1997). A biosystematic study of *Pelargonium* section *Ligularia*: 3. Reappraisal of section *Jenkinsonia*, *S Afr J Bot* 63: 4–21.

Van Toller S, Dodd GH (1991). *Perfumery: The Psychology and Biology of Fragrance*. New York: Chapman and Hall.

Van Toller S, *et al.* (1985). *Ageing and the Sense of Smell*. Springfield, IL: Charles C Thomas.

Van Toller S, *et al.* (1993). An analysis of spontaneous human cortical EEG activity to odours. *Chem Senses* 18: 1–16.

Veal L (1996). The potential effectiveness of essential oils as a treatment for headlice, *Pediculus humanus capitis*. *Complement Ther Nurs Midwifery* 2: 97–101.

Veien NK, *et al.* (1985). Reduction of intake of balsams in patients sensitive to balsam of Peru. *Contact Dermatitis* 12: 270–273.

Veien NK, *et al.* (1996). Can oral challenge with balsam of Peru predict possible benefit from a low-balsam diet? *Am J Contact Dermat* 7: 84–87.

Verlet N (1992). Geranium Bourbon: quel avenir? *Parf Cosmet Aromes* 108: 49–51.

Vernet-Maury E, *et al.* (1999). Basic emotions induced by odorants: a new approach based on autonomic pattern results. *J Auton Nerv Syst* 75: 176–183.

Vernin G, *et al.* (1983). Etude des huiles essentielles par GC-SM-banque specma: essences de geranium. *Parf Cosmet Aromes* 52: 51–61.

Viana GS, *et al.* (2000). Antinociceptive effect of the essential oil from *Cymbopogon citratus* in mice. *J Ethnopharmacol* 70: 323–327.

Vickers A (1996). *Massage and Aromatherapy*. London: Chapman and Hall.

Vilaplana J, Romaguera C (2000). Allergic contact dermatitis due to eucalyptol in an anti-inflammatory cream. *Contact Dermatitis* 43: 118.

Vilaplana J, Romaguera C (2002).Contact dermatitis from the essential oil of tangerine in fragrance. *Contact Dermatitis* 46: 108.

Villar D, *et al.* (1994). Toxicity of melaleuca oil and related essential oils applied topically on dogs and cats. *Vet Hum Toxicol* 36: 139–142.

Vinci L (1980). *Incense: Its Ritual Significance, Use and Preparation*. Northamptonshire: Aquarian Press.

Vogel G (1992). Clinical uses and advantages of low doses of benzodiazepines hypnotics. *J Clin Psychiat* 53: 19–22.

Vokou D, *et al.* (1993). Effects of aromatic plants on potato storage: sprout suppression and antimicrobial activity. *Agric Ecosyst Environ* 47: 223–225.

von Burg R (1995). Toxicology update. *J Appl Toxicol* 15: 495–499.

von Skamlik EV (1959). Uber die Giftigkeit und Vertraglichkeit von atherischen Olen. *Pharmazie* 14: 435–445.

Vuorela H, *et al.* (1990). Extraction of the volatile oil in chamomile flowerheads using supercritical carbon dioxide. *Flavour Fragrance J* 5: 81–84.

Vuorela H, *et al.* (1997). Calcium channel blocking activity: screening methods for plant derived compounds. *Phytomedicine* 4: 167–181.

Wabner D (1994). How pure are our oils? In: *Proceedings from the 1994 Aromatherapy Symposium – Essential Oils, Health and Medicine, New York.*

Wagner H (1985). In: *Economic and Medicinal Plant Research*, Vol 1. London: Academic Press.

Wagner H, Bladt S (1975). Coumarine aus südafrikanischen *Pelargonium*-arten. *Phytochemistry* 14: 2061–2064.

Wagner H, Sprinkmeyer L (1973). Uber die pharmakologische wirkung von Melissengeis. *Dtsch Apoth Z* 113: 1159–1166.

Wagner H, Wolff P, eds (1977). *New Natural Products and Plant Drugs with Pharmacological, Biological or Therapeutical Activity.* Berlin: Springer Verlag.

Wake G, *et al.* (2000). CNS acetylcholine receptor activity in European medicinal plants traditionally used to improve failing memory. *J Ethnopharmacology* 69: 105–114.

Wakelin SH, *et al.* (1998). Allergic contact dermatitis from d-limonene in a laboratory technician. *Contact Dermatitis* 38: 164–165.

Walsh D (1996). Using aromatherapy in the management of psoriasis. *Nurs Stand* 11: 53–56.

Walsh LJ, Longstaff J (1987). The antimicrobial effects of an essential oil on selected oral pathogens. *Periodontology* 8: 11–15.

Walters DS, *et al.* (1988). Geranium defensive agents. III. Structural determination and biosynthetic considerations of anacardic acids of geranium. *J Chem Ecol* 14: 743–751.

Wan J, *et al.* (1998). The effect of essential oils of basil on the growth of *Aeromonas hydrophila* and *Pseudomonas fluorescens. J Appl Microbiol* 84: 152–158.

Warin RP, Smith RJ (1982). Chronic urticaria investigations with patch and challenge tests. *Contact Dermatitis* 8: 117–121.

Warm JS, Dember WN (1999). Effect of fragrances on vigilance, performance and stress. *Perfumer Flavorist* 15: 15–18.

Warren C, Warrenburg S (1993). Mood benefits of fragrance. *Perfumer Flavorist* 18: 9–16.

Warren CB, *et al.* (1999). *Jacobson's Organ.* London: The Penguin Press.

Watson L (1999). *Jacobson's Organ.* London: Penguin.

Watt JM, Breyer-Brandwijk MG (1962). *The Medicinal Plants of Southern Africa.* Edinburgh: Livingstone.

Wattenberg LW, *et al.* (1989). Inhibition of N-nitrosodiethylamine carcinogenesis in mice by naturally occurring organosulfur compounds and monoterpenes. *Cancer Res* 49: 2689–2692.

Watts K (1993). Pregnancy and birth. *Int J Aromather* 5: 33.

Watts M (1997). *The Aromatherapy Practitioners Manual*, obtainable from the author, see http://www.aromamedical.com/ (accessed May 2005).

Webb NJ, Pitt WR (1993). Eucalyptus oil poisoning in childhood: 41 cases in south-east Queensland. *J Paediatr Child Health* 29: 368–371.

Webster's (1938). *Webster's New International Dictionary of the English Language*, 2nd edn. Unabridged. Springfield, MA: G&C Merriam Co.

Webster's (1994). *Webster's Encyclopedic Unabridged Dictionary of the English Language.* New York: Gramercy Books.

Wedeck HE (1994). *Dictionary of Aphrodisiacs.* London: Bracken Books.

Weibel H, Hansen J (1989). Interaction of cinnamaldehyde (a sensitizer in fragrance) with protein. *Contact Dermatitis* 20: 161–166.

Weibel H, *et al.* (1989). Cross-sensitization patterns in guinea pigs between cinnamaldehyde, cinnamyl alcohol and cinnamic acid. *Acta Dermatol Venereol* 69: 302–307.

Weil AT (1965). Nutmeg as a narcotic. *Econ Bot* 17: 194.

Weil A (1983). *Health and Healing.* Boston, MA: Houghton Mifflin.

Weintraub M (1992). Shiatsu, Swedish muscle massage and trigger point suppression in spinal pain syndrome. *Am J Pain Manage* 2: 74–78.

Weisboro SD, *et al.* (1997). Poison on line – acute renal failure caused by oil of wormwood purchased through the Internet. *N Engl J Med* 337: 825–827.

Weiss EA (1997). *Essential Oil Crops.* Oxford: CAB International.

Weiss J, Catalano P (1973). Camphorated oil intoxication during pregnancy. *Pediatrics* 52: 713–714.

Welsh C (1997). Touch with oils: A pertinent part of holistic hospice care. *Am J Hospice Palliat Care* Jan/Feb: 42–44.

Weston S, *et al.* (1997). Evaluation of essential oils and some of their component terpenoids as pediculicides for the treatment of human lice. *J Pharm Pharmacol* 49: 120–132.

Westra WH, *et al.* (1998). Squamous cell carcinoma of the tongue associated with cinnamon gum use: a case report. *Head Neck* 20: 430–431.

Westwood C (1991). *Aromatherapy. A Guide for Home Use.* Dorset: Amberwood Publishing.

Weyers W (1989). Skin absorption of volatile oils. Pharmokinetics. *Pharm Unserer Z* 18: 82–86.

Weyers W, *et al.* (2000). The 21st century – time for a reliable method for diagnosis in clinical dermatology. *Arch Dermatol* 136: 103–105.

Which? (2001). Essential oils. *Health Which?* February: 17–19.

White J (1991). Cancer. *Int J Aromather* 3: 21.

Whysner J, Williams GM (1996). D-limonene mechanistic data and risk assessment: Absolute species-specific toxicity, enhanced cell proliferation, and tumor promotion. *Pharmacol Therap* 71: 127–136.

Wichtl M, ed. (1994). *Herbal Drugs and Phytopharmaceuticals*, translated by NG Bisset. Stuttgart: MedPharm.

Wiebe E (2000). A randomized trial of aromatherapy to reduce anxiety before abortion. *Eff Clin Pract* 3: 166–169.

Wiesenfeld E (1999). *Aroma Profiles of Various Lavandula Species.* South Hackensack, NJ: Noville. http://www.sisweb.com.referenc/applnote/noville. htm (accessed 2005).

Wiesinger GF, *et al.* (1997). Benefit and costs of passive modalities in back pain outpatients: a descriptive study. *Eur J Phys Med Rehabil* 7: 182–186.

Wilbert J (1991). Does pharmacology corroborate the nicotine therapy and practices of South American shamanism? *J Ethnopharmacol* 32: 179–186.

Wilcock A, *et al.* (2004). Does aromatherapy massage benefit patients with cancer attending a specialist palliative care day centre? *Palliat Med* 18: 287–290.

Wilde P (1994). Interview. *Int J Aromather* 6: 3–7.

Wilkenfeld IR (1994). *Prescription Environments: Solutions to the Sick Building Syndrome.* video. Available from: www.chebucto.ns.ca/Education/CASLE/scentseem.html (accessed 14 May 2005).

Wilken-Jensen K (1967). Investigations on children inunctioned with a mentholated ointment from allergologic viewpoint. In: Dost FH and Leiber B, eds. *Menthol and Menthol-containing External Remedies (Use, Mode of Effect and Tolerance in Children).* Stuttgart: Georg Thieme Verlag, p. 154.

Wilkinson S (1995). Aromatherapy and massage in palliative care. *Int J Palliat Care* 1: 21–30.

Wilkinson SM (2003). Evaluating the efficacy of massage in cancer care. *BMJ* 326: 562–563.

Wilkinson S, *et al.* (1999). An evaluation of aromatherapy massage in palliative care. *Palliat Med* 13: 409–417.

Williams AC (2003). *Transdermal and Topical Drug Delivery.* London: Pharmaceutical Press, p. 101.

Williams AC, Barry BW (1989). Essential oils as novel skin penetration enhancers. *Int J Pharm* 57: R7–R9.

Williams AC, Barry BW (1991). Terpenes and the lipid protein partitioning theory of skin penetration enhancement. *Pharmaceut Res* 8: 17–24.

Williams CA, *et al.* (1997). Chrysin and other leaf exudate flavonoids in the genus *Pelargonium.* *Phytochemistry* 46: 1349–1353.

Williams CA, *et al.* (2000). The application of leaf phenolic evidence for systematic studies within the genus *Pelargonium* (Geraniaceae). *Biochem Syst Ecol* 28: 119–132.

Williams DG (1996). *The Chemistry of Essential Oils.* Weymouth: Micelle Press.

Williams LR (1998). Clonal production of tea tree oil high in terpinen-4-ol for use in formulations for the treatment of thrush. *Complement Ther Nurs Midwifery* 4: 133–136.

Willix DJ, *et al.* (1992). A comparison of the sensitivity of wound-infecting species of bacteria to the antibacterial activity of manuka honey and other honey. *J Appl Bacteriol* 73: 388–394.

Wilson FP (1925). *The Plague Pamphlets of Thomas Dekker.* Oxford: Clarendon Press.

Wölbling RH, Leonhardt K (1994). Local therapy of herpes simplex with dried extract from *Melissa officinalis.* *Phytomedicine* 1: 25–31.

Woldemariam TZ, *et al.* (1997). Whitefly toxins. *Pharm J* 259: 481.

Woodward M, ed. (1994). *Gerard's Herbal*. London: Studio Editions.

Woolfson A, Hewitt D (1992). Intensive aromacare. *Int J Aromather* 4: 12–13.

Wordsworth Editions (1999). *The Wordsworth Encyclopedia of World Religions*. Ware, Herts: Wordsworth Editions.

Worwood V (1986). *Aromantics*. London: Pan Books.

Worwood V (1991). *The Fragrant Pharmacy*. London: Bantam Books.

Worwood V (1996). *The Fragrant Mind*. London: Doubleday.

Worwood V (1998). *The Fragrant Heavens. The Spiritual Dimension of Fragrance and Aromatherapy*. Novato, CA: New World Library.

Wren RC (1988). *Potter's New Cyclopedia of Botanical Drugs and Preparations*, revised by Williamson EW and Evans FJ. Saffron Walden: CW Daniel.

Wuthrich B, Dietschi R (1985). [The celery-carrot-mugwort-condiment syndrome: skin test and RAST results.] *Schweiz Med Wochenschr* 115: 258–264.

Yagyu T (1994). Neurophysiological findings on the effects of fragrance: lavender and jasmine. *Integr Psychiatry* 10: 62–67.

Yamada K, *et al.* (1994). Anticonvulsive effects of inhaling lavender oil vapour. *Biol Pharm Bull* 17: 359–360.

Yamada K, *et al.* (1996). Effect of inhalation of chamomile oil vapour on plasma ACTH level in ovariectomized-rat under restriction stress. *Biol Pharm Bull* 19: 1244–1246.

Yamaguchi H (1990). Effect of odor on heart rate in the psychophysiological effects of odor. In: Indo M, ed. *Aromachology*. Koryo, p. 168.

Yamahara J, *et al.* (1985). Cholagogic effect of ginger and its active constituents. *J Ethnopharmacol* 13: 217–225.

Yamahara J, *et al.* (1994). Herbal extracts containing d-borneol for treatment of periodontal diseases. *Japan Kokai Tokkyo Koho*, 94 247864; *Chem. Abstr* 122, 2, 17180u.

Yamasaki K, *et al.* (1998). Anti-HIV-1 activity of herbs in Labiatae. *Biol Pharm Bull* 21: 829–833.

Yeo TC, *et al.* (1994). Massive haematoma from digital massage in an anticoagulant patient: a case report. *Singapore Med J* 35: 319–320.

Youdim KA, Deans SG (2000). Effect of thyme oil and thymol dietary supplementation on the antioxidant status and fatty acid composition of the ageing rat brain. *Br J Nutr* 83: 87–93.

Youdim KA, *et al.* (1999). The antioxidant effectiveness of thyme oil, α-tocopherol and ascorbyl palmitate on evening primrose oil oxidation. *J Essent Oil Res* 11: 643–648.

Young AR, *et al.* (1990). Phototumorigenesis studies of 5-methoxypsoralen in bergamot oil: evaluation and modification of risk of human use in an albino mouse skin model. *J Phytochem Photobiol* 7: 231–250.

Yourick JJ, Bronaugh RL (1997). Percutaneous absorption and metabolism of coumarin in human and rat skin. *J Appl Toxicol* 17: 153–158.

Yousef RT, Tawil GG (1980). Antimicrobial activity of volatile oils. *Pharmazie* 35: 698–701.

Zanker KS, *et al.* (1980). Evaluation of surfactant-like effects of commonly used remedies for colds. *Respiration* 39: 150–157.

Zanolla R, *et al.* (1984). Evaluation of the results of three different methods of postmastectomy lymphedema treatment. *J Surg Oncol* 26: 210–213.

Zarno V (1994). Candidiasis: a holistic view. *Int J Aromatherapy* 6(2): 20–23.

Zarzuelo *et al.* (1987). Spasmolytic activity of *Thymus membranaceus* essential oil. *Phytother Res* 1: 114.

Zarzuelo A, *et al.* (1989). Spasmolytic action of the essential oil of *Thymus longiflorus* Boiss in rats. *Phytother Res* 3: 36–37.

Zaynoun ST, *et al.* (1977). A study of bergamot and its importance as a phototoxic agent. II. Factors which effect the phototoxic reaction induced by bergamot oil and psoralen derivates. *Contact Dermatitis* 3: 225–239.

Zaynoun S, *et al.* (1985). The bergapten content of garden parsley and its significance in causing cutaneous photosensitization. *Clin Exp Dermatol* 10: 328–331.

Zgorniak-Nowosielska I, *et al.* (1989). A study on the antiviral action of a polyphenolic complex isolated from the medicinal plant *Geranium sanguineum* L. VIII Inhibitory effect on the reproduction of herpes simplex virus type 1. *Acta Microbiol Bulg* 24: 3–8.

Zhao K, Singh J (1999). In vitro percutaneous absorption enhancement of propranolol hydrochloride through porcine epidermis by terpenes/ethanol. *J Controlled Release* 62: 359–366.

Zheng G-G, *et al.* (1992). Anethofuran, carvone, limonene: Potential cancer-chemopreventative agents from dill weed oil and caraway oil. *Planta Med* 58: 338–341.

Zibrowski EM, *et al.* (1998). Fast wave activity in the rat rhinencephalon: elicitation by the odors of phytochemicals, organic solvents, and a rodent predator. *Brain Res* 800: 207–215.

Zielinska-Jenczylik J, *et al.* (1984). Effect of plant extracts on the *in vitro* interferon synthesis. *Arch Immunol Ther Exp* 32: 577.

Zobel AM, Brown SA (1991). Dermatitis-inducing psoralens on the surface of seven medicinal plant species. *J Toxicol Cutan Ocul Toxicol* 10: 223–231.

Zondek B, Bergman E (1938). Phenol methyl esters as estrogenic agents. *Biochem J* 32: 641–645.

Zou Z, *et al.* (2001). Genetic tracing reveals a stereotyped sensory map in the olfactory cortex. *Nature* 414: 173–179.

Appendix 1

Bioactivity of commercial essential oils: antibacterial and antifungal activities

Essential oil	Antibacterial activity (no. affected)		Antifungal activity*		
	25 Different bacteria	20 Listeria monocytogenes varieties	Aspergillus niger	A. ochraceus	Fusarium culmorum
Angelica root	23	20	0	16	−18
Aniseed	6	0	83	82	69
Basil	15	20	94	76	71
Bay	25	20	95	80	69
Bergamot	23	20	13	31	34
Bergamot FCF	22	20	70	30	89
Cajeput	21	19	−12	30	−1
Camphor	25	20	95	96	0
Cardamom	14	15	89	19	40
Carrot	3	0	7	0	24
Cassia	23	20	87	89	54
Cedarwood, Atlas	2	0	0	0	0
Cedarwood, Chinese	3	0	6	7	4
Cedarwood, Texas	3	0	6	7	5
Cedarwood, Virginia	4	0	8	17	14
Celery	17–25	19	13–25	35–48	31–36
Chamomile (6)	2–14	0–11	−1–63	5–56	−18–75
Clary sage	11–18	9–15	72–92	91–96	67–69
Clove bud	23	20	95	94	73
Clove leaf	24	20	93	94	73
Cinnamon leaf	24	20	95	94	73
Cumin	22	18	91	92	67
Dill	20	11	95	90	88
Eucalyptus (3)	10–21	6–20	0–87	24–61	−18–78
Fennel	6	0	95	78	66
Frankincence	24	18	7	65	28
Geranium (16)	8–18	3–16	0–94	12–95	40–86
Ho wood	23	15	73	93	81
Lavender (7)	13–23	0–18	57–93	29–90	31–89
Lemongrass	18	20	90	83	63
Lemon	8	3	4	22	0
Litsea cubeba	16–18	18–19	87–94	80–90	40–64

(Continued)

Essential oil	Antibacterial activity (no. affected)		Antifungal activity*		
	25 Different bacteria	20 Listeria monocytogenes varieties	Aspergillus niger	A. ochraceus	Fusarium culmorum
Marjoram (4)	23–25	15–20	16–84	8–79	26–48
Melissa	22	9	89	73	60
Myrrh	6	6	0	21	4
Myrtle	22	17	10	3	15
Niaouli	24	19	85	79	46
Neroli	20–22	11–19	66–86	43–90	63–71
Nutmeg	18–19	0–12	46–88	41–86	20–72
Myrtle	22	17	10	3	15
Orange	19	10	0	34	84
Palmarosa (2)	21–23	17–18	73–92	55–79	55–78
Patchouli	6	15	6	29	27
Peppermint (20)	15–22	13–20	80–98	70–93	47–85
Petitgrain	21	16	61	69	78
Pimento berry	25	20	96	82	65
Pine needle	19	18	11	18	16
Ravensara aromatica	20	16	27	35	−12
Rosewood	24	12	72	63	71
Rosemary	21	16	12	14	0
Sage, Dalmatian	16	6	0	53	33
Tea tree	24	20	85	91	76
Thyme (9)	14–25	6–20	91–96	61–92	75–86
Verbena	18	20	86	85	61

Antibacterial activity (left column) against 25 different bacteria tested and against 20 strains of *L. monocytogenes* (right column); numbers represent zones of inhibition in mm. Zero numbers indicate that the inhibition zone was less than 4 mm of the original 'well' where the essential oil was applied. Each test was done in triplicate. The larger the number, the greater the antimicrobial activity.

*Antifungal activity: calculated from the decrease in dry weights of the fungi treated with 1 μL essential oil compared with controls after 10 days. Each test was done in triplicate. Numbers approaching 100 indicate high antimicrobial activity.

Data from: Lis-Balchin *et al.* (1996a) (reproduced with the permission of the Haworth Press Inc); (1998a) (Copyright Society of Chemical Industry. Reproduced with permission. Permission is granted by John Wiley & Sons Ltd on behalf of the SCI).

List of bacteria:

Acinetobacter calcoaceticus
Aeromonas hydrophila
Alcaligenes faecalis
Bacillus subtilis
Beneckea natriegens
Brevibacterium linens
Brochothrix thermosphacta
Citrobacter freundii
Clostridium sporogenes
Enterobacter aerogenes
Erwinia carotovora
Escherichia coli
Flavobacterium suaveolens

Klebsiella pneumoniae
Lactobacillus plantarum
Leuconostoc cremoris
Micrococcus luteus
Moraxella sp.
Proteus vulgaris
Pseudomonas aeruginosa
Salmonella pullorum
Serratia marcescens
Staphylococcus aureus
Staphylococcus faecalis
Yersinia enterocolitica

L. monocytogenes varieties and sources:

L3 (frozen meal)
L5 (frozen meal)
L54 (raw chicken)
L55 (milk product)
L61 (raw chicken)
L63 (margarine)
L66 (raw chicken)
L67 (margarine)
L71 (kabanos)
L74 (margarine)

L81 (pork sausage)
L82 (cauliflower)
L84 (carrots)
L86 (cooked chicken)
L90 (gateau)
L93 (diced steak)
L100 (vegetables)
L105 (pate)
L130 (?)
L131 (boiled egg)

Appendix 2

Pharmacological properties of some commercial essential oils on electrically stimulated smooth muscle of guinea-pig ileum *in vitro*

Essential oil	Spasmogenic (contraction)	Spasmolytic (relaxation)
Aloysia	xxx	x
Angelica root	xxx	–
Aniseed	xx	x
Basil	x	x
Bay	x	xxx
Bergamot	x	x
Cajuput	x	x
Chamomiles		
Roman	xx	xx
German	–	x
Moroccan	x	x
Camphor	xxx	–
Cardamom	–	x
Carrot	–	x
Cassia	–	x
Cedarwood		
Atlas	–	x
Chinese	–	x
Texas	–	x
Virginian	–	x
Celery	xxx	–
Clove, bud, leaf	–	x
Cinnamon, leaf, bark	–	x
Cumin	xx	x
Dill	xxx	x
Eucalyptus		
globulus	–	x
radiata	–	xx
citriodora	–	xxx
Fennel	xxx	–
Frankincense	xxx	–
Geranium	–	xxx
Kanuka	xxx	x
Ho wood	–	x

(Continued)

Essential oil	Spasmogenic (contraction)	Spasmolytic (relaxation)
Lavender[a]		
Bulgarian	x	x
English	x	x
French	x	x
Lavandin	–	x
Lavender, spike	–	xxx
Lemongrass	–	x
Lemon	xxx	–
Litsea cubeba	–	x
Manuka	–	xxx
Marjoram	–	x
Melissa	–	xx
Myrrh	–	xx
Myrtle	xx	x
Niaouli	–	xx
Neroli	–	xx
Nutmeg	xxx	–
Orange	xxx	–
Palmarosa	–	xx
Parsley	xx	x
Patchouli	–	xxx
Peppermint	–	xx
Petitgrain	xx	xx
Pimento berry	–	xx
Pineneedle	xx	x
Ravensara aromatica	–	x
Rosewood	–	xx
Rosemary	xxx	–
Sage		
Clary	xx	x
Dalmatian	–	xx
Sweet cicely	xx	–
Tarragon	–	xx
Tea tree	xx	xx
Thyme (red/sweet)	–	xx
Valerian	–	xxxx
Verbena	xx	–
Wormwood	–	xx

All essential oils were used at the same concentration (4×10^{-6} g/mL) diluted in methanol. There was a dose-related increase in the contraction as well as relaxation with higher concentrations.

[a] Variable, depending on supplier, but usually labelled *L. angustifolia*.

x denotes low activity; xx denotes medium activity; xxx denotes high activity; – denotes no activity.

Methodology: Segments of ileum (2 cm) from a guinea-pig are mounted in an organ bath (25 mL) containing Krebs solution maintained at 37°C and gassed continually with 95% oxygen in carbon dioxide. The preparation is placed under a tension of 1 g and contractions recorded through an isometric force transducer connected to a pen recorder or Mac-Lab. The method of Paton (1954) is used to stimulate nerves within the wall of the intestine. Two platinum electrodes, attached to a stimulator, are placed on either side of the intestine and a square wave (width, 0.5 ms) delivered every 10 s (0.1 Hz) at an appropriate voltage (about 50 V) produces a regular and reproducible contraction of the intestine. The addition of an extract with spasmogenic activity during field stimulation is recognised as a rise in the baseline and/or an increase in the size of the electrically induced contraction. A reduction in the size of the contraction indicates spasmolytic activity.

Data from: Lis-Balchin *et al.* (1996a) (reproduced with the permission of the Haworth Press Inc), (1996c), (1999); Lis-Balchin and Hart (1998a) (Copyright Society of Chemical Industry. Reproduced with permission. Permission is granted by John Wiley & Sons Ltd on behalf of the SCI), (1998b), (1999a) (Copyright Society of Chemical Industry. Reproduced with permission. Permission is granted by John Wiley & Sons Ltd on behalf of the SCI), (1999b), (2000), (2001a,b).

Appendix 3

Pharmacological effect of selected essential oils on rat uterus compared with that on the guinea-pig ileum *in vitro*

Essential oil	Effect	
	Rat uterus	*Guinea-pig ileum*
Angelica	R	S
Camphor	R	S
Chamomile, Roman	R	S/R
Chamomile, German	R	R
Celery	R	S
Dill	R	S/r
Fennel	R	S
Frankincense	R	S
Geranium	R	R
Kanuka	R	S/R
Lavender, French	R	s/R
Lemon	R	S
Manuka	R	R
Nutmeg	R	S
Orange	R	S
Parsley	R	S/R
Peppermint	R	R
Pine needle	R	S/r
Rosemary	R	S/r
Thyme	R	R
Valerian	R	R

R (uterus) = reduction in size (force) of spontaneous contraction.

S (ileum) = spasmogenic action; s = smaller spasmolysis.

R/r (ileum) = spasmolytic action (i.e. reduction in response of tissue to electrical stimulation), r = smaller reduction.

All essential oils were used at the same concentration in the ileum and uterus (4×10^{-6} g/mL). The essential oils were diluted in methanol and only a maximum of 0.2 mL was applied to a 25 mL organ bath, at which concentration no solvent effect was apparent. There was a dose-related increase in the contraction as well as relaxation in both tissues.

Experiments on the uterus of the rat: the uterus is mounted in an organ bath containing Krebs solution maintained at 37°C and gassed continually with 95% oxygen in carbon dioxide. Activity of the tissue is monitored with an isometric force transducer connected to a pen recorder. Uterine tissue may be quiescent but usually exhibits regular contractions and relaxations, after a short period of equilibration, depending on the oestrus cycle of the rat. The ability of an essential oil to increase or decrease the overall activity of the uterus is readily demonstrated.

Data from: Lis-Balchin *et al.* (1996a) (reproduced with the permission of the Haworth Press Inc); Lis-Balchin and Hart (1997b).

Appendix 4

Pharmacological effect of components on rat uterus compared with that on guinea-pig ileum *in vitro*

Component	Effect	
	Rat uterus	*Guinea-pig ileum*
2-Carene	R	R/S
(−)-Carvone	R	R
(+)-Carvone	R	R
1,8-Cineole	R	S
para-Cymene	R	S
Farnesol	R	R
Fenchone	R	R
Geraniol	R	R
Limonene	R	S
Linalool	R	R
Linalyl acetate	R	R
Menthol	R	R
Myrcene	R	S
Nerol	R	R
α-Pinene	R	S
Sabinene	R	S
Terpinen-4-ol	R	R
α-Terpineol	R	R
α-Terpinene	R	S
γ-Terpinene	R	S/R

R (uterus) = reduction in size (force) of spontaneous contraction.

S (ileum) = spasmogenic action.

R/r (ileum) = spasmolytic action (i.e. reduction in response of tissue to electrical stimulation).

All components were used at the same concentration in the ileum and uterus (4×10^{-6} g/mL). The components were diluted in methanol and only a maximum of 0.2 mL was applied to a 25 mL organ bath, at which concentration no solvent effect was apparent. There was a dose-related increase in the contraction as well as relaxation in both tissues.

See methodology in Appendices 2 and 3.

Data from: Lis-Balchin *et al.* (1996a) (reproduced with the permission of the Haworth Press Inc); Lis-Balchin and Hart (1997b).

Appendix 5

Pharmacological effects of blends of essential oils on rat uterus compared with that on guinea-pig ileum *in vitro*

Blend	*Effect*	
	Rat uterus	*Guinea-pig ileum*
Angelica 1: Nutmeg 1: Roman chamomile 1	R + S**	R/S
Angelica 1: Nutmeg 1: Dill 1	R + S*	S/R
Basil 1: Bergamot 1: Clary sage 1: Jasmine 1	R	S/R
Clove bud 1: Caraway 1: Celery 1	R	S/R
Caraway 1: Aniseed 1: Cassia 1	R	S/R
Cinnamon 1: Coriander 1: Rosewood 1	R	S/R
Chamomile, Roman 1: Dill 1: Angelica 1	R + S**	S/R
Dill 1: Aniseed 1: Rosemary 1: Angelica 1	R + S*	S/R
Dill 1: Orange 1: Kanuka 1	R	S/r
Frankincense 1: Geranium 1: Bergamot 2	R	S/R
Frankincense 2: Ylang Ylang 1: Geranium 1	R	R
Frankinsence 1: Rose 1: Clary sage 1	R	S/R
Kanuka 1: Lavender 1: Frankincense 1	R	R
Marjoram 1: Jasmine 1: Palmarosa 1	R	R
Orange 2: Nutmeg 1: Dill 1	R	S/R
Rose Abs. 1: Geranium 2: Lavender 1	R	R/S
Valerian 1: Dill 1: Rosemary 1	R	R
Ylang ylang 1: Marjoram 1: Thyme 1	R	R

R (uterus) = reduction in size (force) of spontaneous contraction.
S (ileum) = spasmogenic action.
R/r (ileum) = spasmolytic action (i.e. reduction in response of tissue to electrical stimulation).
S* = Increase in rate/force of spontaneous contraction after wash-out.
S** = Increase in rate/force of spontaneous contractions, even without wash-out, following initial spasmolytic action.
All essential oils were used at the same concentration in the ileum and uterus (4×10^{-6} g/mL). The numbers after the essential oils indicate the parts (by volume) used in the blend and the essential oils in the mixes were therefore diluted by each other. The essential oils were diluted in methanol and only a maximum of 0.2 mL was applied to a 25 mL organ bath, at which concentration no solvent effect was apparent. There was a dose-related increase in the contraction as well as relaxation in both tissues.
Data from: Lis-Balchin and Hart (1997a,b), (2002a, ch.25) (reproduced with the permission of Taylor and Francis).

Appendix 6

Correlation between 1,8-cineole content of commercial essential oils and bioactivity

Essential oil	1,8-cineole (%)	Antibacterial activity (no. affected)		Antifungal activity*			Antioxidant activity***
		25 Different bacteria*	20 Listeria monocytogenes varieties**	Aspergillus niger	A. ochraceus	Fusarium culmorum	
E. globulus[a]	90.8	14	6	2	24	−18	0
E. radiata[b]	84.0	21	20	0	35	36	0
Cajeput[c]	69.3	21	19	27	35	−12	13.4+
Ravensara[d]	65.6	20	16	−12	30	−1	0
Niaouli[e]	57.6	24	19	85	79	46	7.6+
Rosemary	49.9	21	16	12	14	0	0
Camphor	47.9	25	16	95	96	0	0
Tea tree[f]	7.1	24	20	85	91	76	0
E. citriodora[g]	0.6	10	20	87	61	78	0

[a] *Eucalyptus globulus* (Myrtaceae).
[b] *Eucalyptus radiata* (Myrtaceae).
[c] *Melaleuca cajeputi* (Myrtaceae).
[d] *Ravensara aromatica* (Lauraceae).
[e] *Melaleuca quinquenervia* (Myrtaceae).
[f] *Melaleuca alternifolia* (Myrtaceae).
[g] *Eucalyptus citriodora* (Myrtaceae).
* Twenty-five different bacteria as listed in Appendix 1.
** Twenty *L. monocytogenes* varieties as in Appendix 1.
*** Antioxidant activity: zones of inhibition of carotene remaining after exposure to 100 μL of essential oil.
Data from: Lis-Balchin *et al.* (1996a) (reproduced with the permission of the Haworth Press Inc), (1998a) (Copyright Society of Chemical Industry. Reproduced with permission. Permission is granted by John Wiley & Sons Ltd on behalf of the SCI).

Appendix 7

Comparison of the antibacterial and antifungal properties of selected essential oils

Angelica root oil, frankincense, cajuput, rosemary and bergamot	Strongly antibacterial, but with no antifungal activity (and in fact can promote fungal growth)
Aniseed oil and fennel	No antibacterial activity, but strongly antifungal
Celery	Much lower antifungal activity than its moderate to good antibacterial activity
Orange	Good antibacterial effect but is not antifungal for *Aspergillus* species
Lemon oil	Virtually no activity
Chamomiles	Almost completely non-active (Roman and German) but one sample of Moroccan chamomile showed some antimicrobial activity against both bacteria and fungi
Patchouli, myrrh and carrot oils	Inactive
Cedarwood (Atlas, Chinese, Texas and Virginia)	Virtually inactive against both bacteria and fungi
Clary sage	Activity against 11 out of 25 bacteria for one sample and 18 for another; whilst antifungal activity was high for both
Ravensara aromatica	Good antibacterial action but poor antifungal action
Pine needle and myrtle	Good antibacterial action but poor antifungal action
Eucalyptus (i.e. *E. globulus* and *E. radiata*)	Strong antibacterial activity but *E. citriodora* is almost inactive in comparison, therefore one cannot generalise about eucalyptus. However the activity against fungi is opposite to the antibacterial effect and is negatively correlated to the concentration of eucalyptol (1,8-cineole), i.e. the greater the content, the lower the antifungal activity: *E. globulus* and *E. radiata* are poorly antifungal, if not promoting growth: *E. citriodora* is relatively good as an antifungal agent
Bay, tea tree, clove bud and leaf, cassia, cinnamon, cumin, and marjoram	Both strongly antibacterial and strongly antifungal
Thyme containing thymol and carvacrol	Strongly antibacterial and antifungal
Sweet thyme with geraniol and geranyl acetate	Relatively poor antibacterially, though still very good against fungi
Spanish marjoram	Poor against fungi, though its activity against bacteria was excellent: the chemical composition (by GC) did not show great changes compared with other marjorams, which were excellent against both, suggesting some adulteration perhaps
Verbena, lemongrass and *Litsea cubeba*	Good antimicrobial agents and moderately effective against fungi

Adapted from Lis-Balchin *et al.* (1996a, 1998a).

Appendix 8

Mode of adulteration of the most commonly used essential oils

Essential oil	Natural oils	Components plant/synthetic	Unnaturals
Bergamot	Bitter orange, lime Linalool, limonene	Linalyl acetate Citral, terpinyl acetate	Diethylphthalate[a]
Clary sage	Lavender, lavandin, *Mentha citrata*	Linalool, linalyl acetate (from lavender or lavandin oils/synthetic)	
Frankincense		Mostly synthetic, e.g. α-pinene/others	
Geranium	Bourbon type substitute Chinese geranium oil	Citronellol, geraniol epi-γ-eudesmol, linalool citronellyl and geranyl formate, menthone, isomenthone	
Jasmine	Ylang ylang	(Ylang ylang fractions), indole, cinnamaldehyde, linalool, eugenol, *cis*-jasmone, farnesene, benzyl benzoate, benzyl acetate	
Lavender	Lavandin	(Fractions of ho leaf, rosewood), linalool, linalyl acetate	
Lemon	Distilled, vacuum distilled or concentrated lemon oil, orange	Limonene, citral, dipentene	(Antioxidants: BHT and BHA prolong shelf-life)
Melissa	Lemongrass, lemon, verbena, citronella	Citronellal, citral, neral, geranial, nerol, nerolidol	
Neroli	Petitgrain, bergamot, bitter orange	Linalool, linalyl acetate, nerol, nerolidol, phenylethyl alcohol, decanal, nonalal, isojasmone	
Rose	Palmarosa, geranium	Citronellol, geraniol, linalool, nerol, phenylethyl, alcohol	

(Continued)

Essential oil	Natural oils	Components plant/synthetic	Unnaturals
Sandalwood	Cedarwood, amyris, araucaria, castor	Sandela, sandalore, copaibal	Odourless organic solvents: liquid paraffin, glyceryl acetate, diethylphthalate (DEP), benzyl benzoate, benzyl alcohol, dipropylglycol (DPG)
Ylang ylang Extra	Cananga, gurjun balsam[b] Peru balsam, copaiba, lesser grades of ylang ylang	Vanillin *p*-Cresyl methyl ether, methyl benzoate, geraniol, isoeugenol, isosafrole, benzyl alcohol, benzyl benzoate, benzyl propionate, cinnamate, anisyl acetate, anisyl alcohol	

[a] Could be used in all essential oils. This is a diluent, rather than a contaminant of plastic containers, as only glass or metal containers are used.
[b] Gas chromatographic analysis can easily detect this by the presence of α-gurjunene; most samples contain some of this adulterant.
Adapted from Lawrence (1995); Baser (1995); Lawrence (1976–2001); Burfield (2003); see also Chapter 4.

Appendix 9

Drop volume versus weight of certain essential oils/absolutes

	No. of drops per g	Weight per drop (mg)
Aqua destillata	20	50
Alcohol absolutus	39	26
Oleum foeniculi	44	23
Oleum lini	48	21
Oleum menthae piperitae	53	19
Oleum ricini	45	22
Oleum terebinthinae	54	19
Tinctura benzoes	60	17
Oleum citri	51	20
Tinctura myrrhae	60	17
Tinctura valerianae	56	18

Because the size of a drop depends on the nature of the liquid there will be a large difference in the weight of a drop of essential oil where viscosity is taken into account. For example, the weight per drop of benzoin and myrrh tinctures are perhaps very odd if one compares this to the present day commercial tinctures, which are very thick in consistency and difficult to flow out of the dropper, especially in cold temperatures. This is due to the pharmacists' prescribed tinctures, which are very much more diluted than those obtained as aromatherapy products and the diluent used by them is alcohol.

Data from: Netherlands Pharmacopoeia (section VI).

Appendix 10

Weight of one drop of essential oils using the droppers provided with the bottles

	Weight of one drop (mg)
Rosewood (Natural by Nature Oils)	24.0
Rosewood (Pure Essential Oil QP)	19.7
Rosewood (Amphora Aromatics)	18.1
Rosewood (Butterbur and Sage)	5.8
Rose Attar (Butterbur and Sage)	34.9
Rose Absolute (Butterbur and Sage)	29.6
Bergamot (Natural by Nature Oils)	26.5
Bergamot (Baldwins)	30.4
Bergamot (Tisserand)	8.4
Bergamot (Italian)	10.7
Bergamot FCF (Butterbur and Sage)	18.6
Ylang Ylang (Boots)	24.3
Ylang Ylang extra (Butterbur and Sage)	34.3
Cananga Odorata (Butterbur and Sage)	31.0
Peru Balsam Resinoid (Butterbur and Sage)	19.7
Valerian Oil (Butterbur and Sage)	32.8
Sandalwood (Baldwins)	24.9
Safeways Olive Oil, 5 mL (using a laboratory pipette)	3625.8

Data given from a selection collected by students at South Bank University, London, 1999. Each value is a mean of three readings.

Note: The droppers can differ in different bottles of essential oils, etc. especially from different suppliers.

Appendix 11

Comparison of the actual effect of essential oils on guinea-pig ileum *in vitro* and the predicted effects using chemical composition and aromatherapists' predictions

	Actual effect on ileal tissue	*Chemical prediction*	*Aromatherapists' prediction*
Bergamot	s/R	S/R	S/R
Black pepper	S/r	S/r	S/r
Chamomile, German	R	R	R
Chamomile, Roman	S/R and s/R	S/R	R
Camphor	S	S	S
Clary sage	S and S/r	R	r
Dillweed	S/r	s/R	r
Eucalyptus globulus	R	S	S
Frankincense	S	S	R
Geranium, Bourbon	R	R	R
Ginger	R	s/R	s/r
Juniper	R	S	S
Lavender	R and s/R	R	R
Lemongrass	R	R	S/r
Manuka	R	R	R
Neroli	R	s/R	S/r
Nutmeg	S	S	r
Petitgrain	S/r	R	S/R
Rosemary	S/r	S/r	S
Rosewood	R	R	R
Sandalwood	R	R	r
Spikenard	R	R	r
Tea tree	R and s/R	s/R	s/r
Valerian	R	R	R
Vetivert	R	R	R
Ylang ylang	R	R	r

S (ileum) = spasmogenic action, i.e. contraction.

R/r (ileum) = spasmolytic action, i.e. reduction in response of tissue to electrical stimulation or relaxation.

All essential oils were used at the same concentration in the ileum and uterus (4×10^{-6} g/mL).

The essential oils were diluted in methanol and only a maximum of 0.2 mL was applied to a 25 mL organ bath, at which concentration no solvent effect was apparent. There was a dose-related increase in the contraction as well as relaxation.

Data from: Lis-Balchin and Hart (1997a,b); Lis-Balchin (2002a, ch.25).

Appendix 12

Comparison of the actual effect of essential oil blends on guinea-pig ileum and the predicted effects using chemical composition and aromatherapists' predictions

Blend	Actual effect on ileum	Effects predicted	
		Aromatherapist	Chemical effect
1. Orange 2: Nutmeg 1: Dill 1	S	S	s/R
2. Lemongrass 1: Juniper 1: Rosemary 2	S	S	R
3. Frankincense 1: Rose absolute 1: Clary sage 2	R/S	R/S	s/R
4. *Eucalyptus glob.* 1: Black pepper 1: Ginger 1	S	S	s/R
5. Ginger 1: Tea tree 1: Rosemary 2	S	S/R	S/R
6. Frankincense 2: Ylang ylang 1: Geranium 1	R/S	S/R	R
7. Frankincense 1: Geranium 1: Bergamot 2	S/R	S/R	S/R
8. Chamomile Roman 1: Lavender 1: Geranium 1	R/S	s/R	S/R
9. Frankincense 1: Mandarin 2: Scotch Pine 1	S/R	S	S/R
10. Chamomile Roman 1: Valerian 1: Rose abs. 1	R/S	s/R	R
11. Ylang ylang 1: Marjoram 1: Thyme red 1	R	s/R	R
12. Petitgrain 1: Melissa 1: Sage Dalmatian 1	s/r	R	R
13. Kanuka 1: Lavender 1: Frankincense 1	S/r	?R	R
14. Manuka 1: Lavender 1: Frankincense 1	s/R	?S	R
15. Fennel 1: Orange 1: Bergamot 1	S/r	S/R	S/R
16. Basil 1: Bergamot 1: Clary sage 1: Jasmine 1	S	s/R	S/R

S = Spasmogenic; s = small spasmogenic effect; R = Relaxant; r = small relaxant effect; ? = unsure. Numbers after the essential oil denote parts by volume in the blend.
The aromatherapists' predictions were not based on the use of any of these mixtures, as these were devised by the author. The predictions were therefore solely based on the possible effects of each essential oil in the mixture.
Data from: Lis-Balchin and Hart (1997a,b); Lis-Balchin (2002a, ch.25).

Appendix 13

The predicted effect (percentage of components at the retention times shown) of essential oils on guinea-pig ileum *in vitro*

Essential oil	Retention time (minutes)					Effect
	>10	11–15	16–20	21–30	30+	
1	–	85	2	–	7	R
2	41	5	49	–	–	S/R
3	85	1	–	6	–	S
4	78	22	1	14	–	S/r
5	86	2	2	1	–	S
6	44	45	–	5	–	S/R
7	37	47	8	4	–	S/R
8	4	90	–	2	–	R
9	9	56	12	15	–	s/R
10	–	–	–	58	37	R
11	98	–	–	–	–	S
12	99	–	–	–	–	S
13	–	–	–	71	19	R
14	22	69	–	–	–	S/R
15	10	26	4	41	6	s/R
16	10	39	36	9	–	s/R
17	78	9	3	5	–	S

S = Spasmogenic; s = small spasmogenic effect.
R = Relaxant; r = small relaxant effect.
The numbers denote the same essential oil mixtures as shown in Appendix 12.
Gas chromatography (GC) conditions: A Shimadzu GC8A instrument was used with an OV 101 capillary column 50 m × 0.32 mm internal diameter. The injection and detector temperature was 230°C and the instrument was programmed from 100 to 250°C at 4°C/min using helium.

The percentage of all the components was calculated in each selected retention time interval of under 10 min, 11–15 min, 16–20 min, 21–30 min and 30+ min. The main components present in each retention time interval were also determined.

Appendix 14

Psychological and physiological effects of odours: comparison of sedative and stimulant essential oils as determined by using different parameters by different researchers

Essential oil	Reference numbers	
	Sedative	*Stimulant*
Aniseed		5a,5c,5e
Angelica	5b,5c	5a
Basil	5a,5b,5c	1,2,3,4,5a
Bergamot	2,3,5a	5a
Cassia	5c	
Chamomile	1,2,3,5a,5b,5c	5a
Cinnamon	5a,5b,5c	
Clove	5a,5b,5c	2,3
Dill	1	5a
Eucalyptus (globulus?)	5a	1
Fennel		5a,5c,5e
Frankincense		5a
Geranium	2,3,5a	2,3
Ginger	5b,5c	
Jasmine	5a	1,2,4,9
Lavender	1,2,4,5a,8,11	5a,6
Lemon	1,2,3	5a,7
Lemongrass	5a	3
Marjoram	1,2,3,5a	
Melissa	1,5a,5b,5c,8	
Myrrh	5a	
Neroli	4,5a	2,3
Nutmeg	5b	5a,5c
Orange	5b	5a,5c,5e
Patchouli	5a	2,3,4
Pepper	5b	5c
Peppermint	5a,5c,5d	1,2,3,9
Pine		3,5a,8
Rose	5a,7	2,3

(Continued)

413

Essential oil	Reference numbers		
	Sedative		Stimulant
Rosewood	2,3,5a		2,3
Rosemary	1,4,5a,5d		8,11,5d
Sage	3,5a,5c,5d		3,5d
Sandalwood	1,2,3,4,5a		
Spearmint	5a		1
Thyme	5a,5c		1
Valerian	1,3,5a		3,8
Verbena			5a
Ylang ylang	5a		1,2,3,4

References:

1. Contingent negative variation (CNV) studies in humans (Kubota *et al.*, 1992).
2. CNV studies in humans (Torii *et al.*, 1988).
3. CNV studies in humans (Manley, 1993).
4. Motility of mice (Jager *et al.*, 1992; Buchbauer *et al.*, 1993a).
5a. Smooth muscle *in vitro* (Lis-Balchin *et al.*, 1996a,c, 1999c; Lis-Balchin and Hart, 1998a,b, 1999a,b; 2000, 2001a,b).
5b. Smooth muscle *in vitro* (Brandt, 1988).
5c. Smooth muscle *in vitro* (Reiter and Brandt, 1985).
5d. Smooth muscle *in vitro* (Taddei *et al.*, 1988).
5e. Smooth muscle *in vitro* (Hof-Mussler, 1990).
6. Decision times in humans (Karamat *et al.*, 1992).
7. Heart rate in humans (Yamaguchi, 1990).
8. Motility in mice (Kovar *et al.*, 1987).
9. Memory, mood in humans (Ludvigson and Rottmann, 1989).
10. Sleep in humans (Badia, 1991).
11. Mood, EEG in humans (Diego *et al.*, 1998).

Appendix 15

Comparison of sedative and stimulant components as determined by using different parameters by different researchers

Component	Sedative	Stimulant
Anethol		5c
Benzyldehyde	4	
Borneol	5a,5d	
Camphor	5a,5d	
2-Carene	5a	5a
Caryophyllene	5a,5b,5c	
Carvone (+) and (−)	5a	
1,8-Cineole		5a,8
Cinnamaldehyde	5c	5c
Citral (cis-, trans-)	5a,5b,5c	
Citronellal	4,5a,5b,5c	
Citronellol	5a,5c	
p-Cymene		5a
Eugenol	5a,5b,5c	
Farnesol	5a	
Fenchone		5a
Guaiadiene	5a	
Geraniol	5a,5c	
Heliotropin	9	
Limonene	5c,5d	5a,5c,5d
Linalool	4,5a,5b,5c	
Linalyl acetate	5a,5d	5d
Menthol	5a,5d	
Menthone	5a,5d	
Myrcene	5a	5a
Nerol	5a,5c	
Phenylethylacetate	5a	
α-, β-Pinene	5a,5d	5a,5d
Sabinene	5a	5a

(Continued)

Component	Sedative	Stimulant
α-Terpineol	4	
α-Terpinene	5a	5a
γ-Terpinene	5a	5a
Thujone	5a	

References:

1. CNV studies in humans (Kubota *et al.*, 1992).
2. CNV studies in humans (Torii *et al.*, 1988).
3. CNV studies in humans (Manley, 1993).
4. Motility of mice (Jager *et al.*, 1992; Buchbauer *et al.*, 1993a).
5a. Smooth muscle *in vitro* (Lis-Balchin *et al.*, 1996a,c, 1999c; Lis-Balchin and Hart, 1998a,b, 1999a,b; 2000, 2001a,b).
5b. Smooth muscle *in vitro* (Brandt, 1988).
5c. Smooth muscle *in vitro* (Reiter and Brandt, 1985).
5d. Smooth muscle *in vitro* (Taddei *et al.*, 1988).
5e. Smooth muscle *in vitro* (Hof-Mussler, 1990).
6. Decision times in humans (Karamat *et al.*, 1992).
7. Heart rate in humans (Yamaguchi, 1990).
8. Motility in mice (Kovar *et al.*, 1987).
9. Memory, mood in humans (Ludvigson and Rottmann, 1989).
10. Sleep in humans (Badia, 1991).
11. Mood, EEG in humans (Diego *et al.*, 1998).

Appendix 16

Some techniques used for psychophysiological measurements in humans

Technique	Reference
Heart rate	Yamaguchi, 1990; Schwartz *et al.*, 1988; Warren and Warrenberg, 1993
Blood pressure	Warren and Warrenberg, 1993; Schwartz *et al.*, 1988
Skin potentials	Warren and Warrenberg, 1993
EEG	van Toller, 1996; Diego *et al.*, 1998
CNV	Torii *et al.*, 1988; Lorig and Roberts, 1990; Kubota *et al.*, 1992; Manley, 1993
BEAM	Kendal-Reed, 1990; van Toller *et al.*, 1993
Cognition, memory, mood	Ludvigson and Rottman, 1989
Creativity, mood, perceived health	Knasko, 1992
Mood changes	Warren and Warrenberg, 1993
Cerebral blood flow	Nasel *et al.*, 1994
Vigilance tasks	Warm and Dember, 1990; Knasko *et al.*, 1990
Anxiety	Redd and Manne, 1991; Redd *et al.*, 1994
Retrieval of memories	Ehrlichman and Halpern, 1988
Decision times	Karamat *et al.*, 1992
Sleep	Badia, 1991

EEG, electroencephalogram; CNV, contingent negative variation; BEAM, brain electrical activity mapping.

Appendix 17

Evidence for transfer of components of essential oils into blood/brain when applied to skin, orally or by inhalation

Reference	Essential oil administered	Components found in blood/brain
Jager *et al.* (1992)	Lavender (massage)	Linalool, linalyl acetate (blood)
Buchbauer *et al.* (1992)	Limeblossom and benzyl alcohol (inhalation) Benzaldehyde (inhalation) Passiflora and 2-phenylethanol (inhalation)	Benzyl alcohol (blood) Benzaldehyde (blood) 2-Phenylethanol (blood)
Kovar *et al.* (1987)	Rosemary (oral and inhalation)	1,8-Cineole (blood)
Buchbauer *et al.* (1993b)	Benzaldehyde (inhalation) Carvone (inhalation)	Benzaldehyde (blood) Carvone (brain)
Fuchs *et al.* (1997)	Carvone (massage)	Carvone (blood)

Appendix 18

'Absorption' of essential oils from the animal skin, i.e. rate of disappearance

Time	Essential oil/component
Under 20 min	Terebinth, thyme, eucalyptus, α-pinene, eucalyptol
20–40 min	Bergamot, citron, anise, eugenol, linalool, anethole, linalyl acetate, geranyl acetate, methylnonyl ketone
40–60 min	Citronella, pine, lavender, geranium, cinnamon (cannelle), methyl salicylate
60–80 min	Cinnamaldehyde, citronellal
Over 80 min	Mint, rue, coriander, geraniol, citral

Data from Valette (1946–7).

Appendix 19

Common uses of essential oils

Food industry (general)	Cheeses, puddings, gelatine desserts, rennet desserts, sauerkraut, mince meat, prepared cake mixes, soups, meats and vegetables, pie-fillers, sweets, confectionary, chocolate, pickles
Household products	Deodorants, furniture polishes, room sprays, starches, detergents, floor polishes and waxes, soaps, cleaners
Ice cream industry	Ice cream, sherbets, mixes
Insecticide industry	Disinfectants, insecticides, repellents, attractants, sprays
Meat industry	Sausages, frankfurters, prepared meats
Paint industry	Paints, casein and bituminous paints, enamels, lacquers, varnish and varnish removers, rubber paints
Paper and printing	Carbon paper, crayons, drinking cups, tapes, labels, bags, inks, printing paper
Perfumery and cosmetics	Baby products, bath preparations, body deodorants, colognes, creams, depilatories, eye-shadow, facial masks, hair products, incense, lipsticks, lotions, manicure preparations, talcum powders, face powders, shaving preparations, suntan preparations, toilet water, etc.
Petroleum and chemical industry	Grease deodorants, lubricating oils, solvents, polishes, waxes, aroma-chemicals
Pharmaceutical industry	Cough drops, elixirs, germicides, hospital sprays, inhalants, laxatives, liniments, medicinal preps, ointments, patent medicines, tonics, vitamin flavours, flu remedies
Preserve industry	Jams, marmalades, jellies
Soap industry	Cleaning powders, household soaps, shampoos, toilet soaps
Soft drinks industry	Carbonated drinks, colas, syrups, ginger ales, soft drink powders
Alcoholic drinks	Absinth, and most odorous liqueurs and shorts
Textile processing industry	Artificial leather and fabric coatings, dyes, linoleum and floor covering, textile chemicals, water-proofing agents, textile oils
Tobacco industry	Cigarette flavours, cigars, chewing tobacco, snuff
Veterinary supplies	Cattle sprays, deodorants, pet shampoos, pet soaps, insect powders, veterinary medicines and ointments, bird attractants
Miscellaneous uses	Embalming fluids, candles, alcohol denaturing compounds

Data from: Lis-Balchin, unpublished South Bank University BSc (Hons)/Dip HE Health Studies degree notes.

Appendix 20

Miscellaneous functions of essential oils according to pharmacopoeias

Cinnamon	Dental medicine Germicidal additive to toothpastes Carminative Antidiarrhoeal Inhalant for colds
Clove bud and leaf	Dentistry: local anaesthetic for toothache Sealant (germicidal/anaesthetic) for dental cavities, temporary fillings Counterirritant Carminative Food preservative (patented) Air disinfectant (patented) External use for degenerative bone, inflammation of joints, bursitis, sinusitis (patented)
Cajuput, camphor, *Eucalyptus globulus*	Rubefacient Decongestant Inhalant
Chamomile (German)	Anti-inflammatory
Dill, fennel, ginger	Carminative, especially for children
Juniper	Carminative Diuretic (not in renal disease)
Lemon	D-Limonene in preparation for dissolving gallstones
Nutmeg	Carminative Antidiarrhoeal Rubefacient ? Inhibits prostaglandin synthesis, therefore prevent coronaries Soothing effect on humans and decrease in blood pressure (patented)
Peppermint	Dyspepsia Bronchitis Irritable bowel syndrome
Thyme	Mouthwash, gargle bactericidal ingredient Cough linctus Elixir for whooping cough and bronchitis Rubefacient, counterirritant

Data from: *British Pharmacopoeia* 1998, 2001.

Appendix 21

Established uses of essential oils/components: conventional rather than complementary or alternative uses

External application	Internal application (including inhalation and oral)
Hyperaemic	Expectorant
Anti-inflammatory	Appetite stimulating
Antiseptic/disinfectant	Carminative
Deodorising	Antiseptic/disinfectant
Insecticidal/insect repellent	Choleretic/cholekinetic/sedative

Hyperaemic effects (externally)

- Increase local blood circulation, by primary irritation (visible as redness of skin)
- Influence local organs below skin
- Primary irritation sets free mediators in body, e.g. bradykinin, which cause vasodilation (cf. cardiac ointments for angina pectoris)

Hyperaemic effects are useful in:

- Rheumatic disease of joints
- Lumbago
- Neuritis
- Sciatica
- Shoulder aches
- Sports injuries, e.g. sprains

Examples of essential oils and components with hyperaemic effects include:

- *Eucalyptus* (*globulus*, *radiata*) – 1,8-cineole
- Gaultheria – methyl salicylate
- Rosemary – 1,8-cineole
- Turpentine (rectified)- α-, β-pinenes, δ-3-carene
- Camphor
- Numerous sprain/muscular rubs such as Deep Heat, Boot's Embrocation, etc.

Anti-inflammatory effects (externally)

- Due to skin irritation, setting free or binding endogenous substances
- Antimicrobial action, also an important aspect of inflammation
- Better circulation due to irritation also important as local inflammation can start due to circulatory disturbances caused by contraction of arterioles

Examples of essential oils and components with anti-inflammatory effects include:

- Chamomile (German), *Chamomila matricaria* – matricine, chamazulene, (−)-α-bisabolol (Note: Experiments have shown that synthetic bisabolol is lower in activity due to its different enantiomeric form, as in the case of limonene and α-pinene enantiomers. Also the (+)-α-bisabolol from *Populus balsamifera* was less active – thus supporting enantiomeric variation)
- Yarrow – chamazulene

Expectorating effects

- Due possibly to secretolytic and secretomotoric effect rather than bronchospasmolytic effect as inhaled or

Adapted from *British Pharmacopoeia* (1998); Newall *et al.* (1996); Trease and Evans (1996); Hof-Mussler (1990); Sticher (1977); Tisserand and Balacs (1996); Lis-Balchin (1995, 1997); Lis-Balchin *et al.* (1996a,c); Lis-Balchin and Hart (1999b).

systemically resorbed essential oils arrive at bronchi, where most are exhaled by lungs

- Increased secretion will occur either way due to a direct action on the tracheal and bronchial mucous membrane (NB: A real antitussive effect is not shown)

Examples of essential oils and components that have expectorating effects include:

- Aniseed
- Eucalyptus
- Fennel
- Pine needle
- Turpentine
- Thyme
- Wild thyme
- Camphor
- Menthol
- Peppermint
- Sage
- Cinnamon

Stimulation of secretion of digestive glands

Mainly alcoholic extracts of crude drugs (herbs, etc.) are used for this purpose and not essential oils *per se*.

- Stomachic effect – e.g. anise, angelica, peppermint, cinnamon
- Gallbladder (cholekinetic) – e.g. curcuma, caraway, lavender, peppermint
- Bile secretion increase (choleretic) – e.g. peppermint, menthol, borneol, camphor, 1,8-cineole, α-, β-pinenes, menthone

- Carminative effect – due possibly to a number of factors, such as:
  - local irritation of gastric mucosa
  - reflectoric stimulation of secretion of gastric cells thereby improving digestion
  - spasmolytic effect and relief of flatulence
  - antiseptic effect (on bacteria, etc.)
- Cholagogic effect – e.g. anise, basil, fennel, chamomile, coriander, caraway, peppermint (Note: Fennel and anise were spasmogenic on guinea-pig ileum rather than spasmolytic. This is in contrast to earlier work often quoted (Die Atherische Öle, 1950), where essential oils were given as an aqueous suspension.)

Diuretics

Buchu (diosphenol) and juniper (terpinen-4-ol) (Note: Probably act simply through irritation of kidneys.)

References

Sticher (1977); Hof-Mussler (1990); Lis-Balchin (1995, 1997); Tisserand and Balacs (1995); Lis-Balchin *et al.* (1996a,c); Newall *et al.* (1996); Trease and Evans (1996); British Pharmacopoeia (1998); Lis-Balchin and Hart (1999b).

Appendix 22

RIFM toxicological monographs

Most of these were by Opdyke, DLJ.

Angelica root oil, RIFM monograph (1975) *Food Cosmet Toxicol* 13, Supplement-Special issue II, 713–714

Angelica seed oil, RIFM monograph (1974) *Food Cosmet Toxicol* 12, Supplement-Special issue I, 821

Anise oil, RIFM monograph (1973) *Food Cosmet Toxicol* 11(5): 865–866

Basil oil, sweet, RIFM monograph (1973) *Food Cosmet Toxicol* 11(5): 867–868

Bay oil, RIFM monograph (1973) *Food Cosmet Toxicol* 11(5): 869–870

Benzoin resinoid, RIFM monograph (1973) *Food Cosmet Toxicol* 11(5): 871–872

Bergamot oil expressed, RIFM monograph (1973) *Food Cosmet Toxicol* 11(6): 1031–1033

Black pepper oil, RIFM monograph (1976) *Food Cosmet Toxicol* 16, Supplement-Special Issue IV, 651–652

Bois de Rose oil, RIFM monograph (1978) *Food Cosmet Toxicol* 16, Supplement-Special Issue IV, 653–654

Cajeput oil, RIFM monograph (1976) *Food Cosmet Toxicol* 14, Supplement-Special Issue III, 701

Carrot seed oil, RIFM monograph (1976) *Food Cosmet Toxicol* 14, Supplement-Special Issue III, 705–706

Cassia oil, RIFM monograph (1975) *Food Cosmet Toxicol* 13(1): 109–110

Cedarwood oil, Atlas, RIFM monograph (1976) *Food Cosmet Toxicol* 14, Supplement-Special Issue III, 709

Cedarwood oil, Texas, RIFM monograph (1976) *Food Cosmet Toxicol* 14, Supplement-Special Issue III, 711–712

Celery seed oil, RIFM monograph (1974) *Food Cosmet Toxicol* 12, Supplement-Special Issue I, 849–850

Chamomile oil, German, RIFM monograph (1974) *Food Cosmet Toxicol* 12, Supplement-12, Special Issue I, 851–852

Chamomile oil, Roman, RIFM monograph (1974) *Food Cosmet Toxicol* 12, Supplement-Special Issue I, 853

Cinnamon bark oil, RIFM monograph (1975) *Food Cosmet Toxicol* 13(1): 111–112

Cinnamon leaf oil, Ceylon, RIFM monograph (1975) *Food Cosmet Toxicol* 13, Supplement-Special Issue II, 749

Citronella oil, RIFM monograph (1973) *Food Cosmet Toxicol* 11(6): 1066–1068

Clary sage oil, Russian, RIFM monograph (1982) *Food Cosmet Toxicol* 20, Supplement-Special Issue VI, 823–824

Clary sage, French, RIFM monograph (1974) *Food Cosmet Toxicol* 12, Supplement 12, Special Issue I, 865–866

Clove bud oil, RIFM monograph (1975) *Food Cosmet Toxicol* 13, Supplement-Special Issue II, 762–763

Clove leaf oil, RIFM monograph (1978) *Food Cosmet Toxicol* 16, Supplement-Special Issue IV, 695

Clove stem oil, RIFM monograph (1975) *Food Cosmet Toxicol* 13, Supplement-Special Issue II, 765–767

Cornmint oil, RIFM monograph (1975) *Food Cosmet Toxicol* 13, Supplement-Special Issue II, 771–772

Cubeb oil, RIFM monograph (1976) *Food Cosmet Toxicol* 14, Supplement-Special Issue III, 729–730

Cypress oil, RIFM monograph (1978) *Food Cosmet Toxicol* 16, Supplement-Special Issue IV, 699

Dill weed oil, RIFM monograph (1976) *Food Cosmet Toxicol* 14, Supplement-Special Issue III, 747–748

Eucalyptus citriodora, RIFM monograph (1988) *Food Chem Toxicol* 26, Supplement-Special Issue VII, 323

Eucalyptus oil, RIFM monograph (1975) *Food Cosmet Toxicol* 13(1): 107–108

Fennel oil, sweet, RIFM monograph (1974) *Food Cosmet Toxicol* 12, Supplement-Special Issue I, 879–880

Galbanum oil, RIFM monograph (1978) *Food Cosmet Toxicol* 16, Supplement-Special Issue IV, 765–766

Geranium oil (Bourbon), RIFM monograph (1974) *Food Cosmet Toxicol* 12, Supplement-Special Issue I, 883–884

Geranium oil, Moroccan, RIFM monograph (1975) *Food Cosmet Toxicol* 13(4): 452

Geranium oil, Algerian, RIFM monograph (1976) *Food Cosmet Toxicol* 14, Supplement-Special Issue III, 781–782

Ginger oil, RIFM monograph (1974) *Food Cosmet Toxicol* 12, Supplement-Special Issue I, 901–902

Helichrysum oil, RIFM monograph (1978) *Food Cosmet Toxicol* 16, Supplement-Special Issue IV, 769–770

Ho leaf oil, RIFM monograph (1974) *Food Cosmet Toxicol* 12, Supplement-Special issue I, 917

Hyacinth absolute, RIFM monograph (1976) *Food Cosmet Toxicol* 14, Supplement-Special Issue III, 795

Hyssop oil, RIFM monograph (1978) *Food Cosmet Toxicol* 16, Supplement-Special Issue IV, 783–784

Jasmine absolute, RIFM monograph (1976) *Food Cosmet Toxicol* 14(4): 331

Jonquil absolute, RIFM monograph (1983) *Food Chem Toxicol* 21(6): 861

Juniper berry oil, RIFM monograph (1976) *Food Cosmet Toxicol* 14(4): 333

Laurel leaf oil, RIFM monograph (1976) *Food Cosmet Toxicol* 14(4): 337–338

Lavandin absolute, RIFM monograph (1988) *Food Chem Toxicol* 30, Supplement-Special Issue VIII, 65

Lavandin oil, RIFM monograph (1976) *Food Cosmet Toxicol* 14(5): 447

Lavender absolute, RIFM monograph (1976) *Food Cosmet Toxicol* 14(5): 449

Lavender oil, RIFM monograph (1976) *Food Cosmet Toxicol* 14(5): 451

Lavender oil, Spike, RIFM monograph (1976) *Food Cosmet Toxicol* 14(5): 453

Lemon oil distilled, RIFM monograph (1974) *Food Cosmet Toxicol* 12(5/6): 727

Lemon oil expressed, RIFM monograph (1974) *Food Cosmet Toxicol* 12(5/6): 725–726

Lemongrass oil, East Indian, RIFM monograph (1976) *Food Cosmet Toxicol* 14(5): 455

Lemongrass oil, West Indian, RIFM monograph (1976) *Food Cosmet Toxicol* 14(5): 457

Litsea cubeba oil, RIFM monograph (1982) *Food Cosmet Toxicol* 20, Supplement-Special Issue VI, 731–732

Marjoram oil, Spanish, RIFM monograph (1976) *Food Cosmet Toxicol* 14(5): 467

Marjoram oil, sweet, RIFM monograph (1976) *Food Cosmet Toxicol* 14(5): 469

Mentha citrata, RIFM monograph (1988) *Food Chem Toxicol* 30, Supplement-Special Issue VIII, 73

Myrrh absolute, RIFM monograph (1988) *Food Chem Toxicol* 30, Supplement-Special Issue VIII, 91

Myrrh oil, RIFM monograph (1976) *Food Cosmet Toxicol* 14(6): 621

Myrtle oil, RIFM monograph (1983) *Food Chem Toxicol* 21(6): 869–870

Narcissus absolute, RIFM monograph (1978) *Food Cosmet Toxicol* 16, Supplement-Special Issue IV, 827

Neroli absolute, RIFM monograph (1982) *Food Cosmet Toxicol* 20, Supplement-Special Issue VI, 785

Neroli oil, RIFM monograph (1976) *Food Cosmet Toxicol* 14, Special Issue III, 813–814

Nutmeg oil, RIFM monograph (1976) *Food Cosmet Toxicol* 14(6): 631–633

Olibanum absolute, RIFM monograph (1978) *Food Cosmet Toxicol* 16, Supplement-Special Issue IV, 835

Olibanum gum, RIFM monograph (1978) *Food Cosmet Toxicol* 16, Supplement-Special Issue IV, 837

Orange oil, sweet, expressed, RIFM monograph (1974) *Food Cosmet Toxicol* 12(5/6): 733–734

Oregano oil, RIFM monograph (1974) *Food Cosmet Toxicol* 12, Supplement-Special Issue I, 945–946

Palmarosa oil, RIFM monograph (1974) *Food Cosmet Toxicol* 12, Supplement-Special Issue I, 947

Parsley seed oil. RIFM monograph (1975) *Food Cosmet Toxicol* 13: 897–898

Patchouli oil, RIFM monograph (1982) *Food Cosmet Toxicol* 20, Supplement, Special Issue VI, 791–793

Pennyroyal oil, RIFM monograph (1974) *Food Cosmet Toxicol* 12, Supplement-Special Issue I, 949–950

Peru balsam oil, RIFM monograph (1974) *Food Cosmet Toxicol* 12, Supplement-Special Issue I, 953–954

Peru balsam, RIFM monograph (1974) *Food Cosmet Toxicol* 12, Supplement-Special Issue I, 951–952

Petitgrain oil, lemon, RIFM monograph (1978) *Food Cosmet Toxicol* 16, Supplement-Special Issue IV, 807

Petitgrain, bigarade oil, RIFM monograph (1988) *Food Chem Toxicol* 30, Supplement-Special Issue VIII, 101

Petitgrain, Paraquay, RIFM monograph (1982) *Food Cosmet Toxicol* 20, Supplement-Special Issue VI, 801–802

Pinus sylvestris, RIFM monograph (1976) *Food Cosmet Toxicol* 14, Supplement-Special Issue III, 845–846

Rose absolute, French, RIFM monograph (1975) *Food Cosmet Toxicol* 13, Supplement-Special Issue II, 911–912

Rose oil, Bulgarian, RIFM monograph (1974) *Food Cosmet Toxicol* 12, Special Issue I, 979–980

Rose oil, Moroccan, RIFM monograph (1974) *Food Cosmet Toxicol* 12, Supplement-Special Issue I, 981–982

Rose oil, Turkish, RIFM monograph (1975) *Food Cosmet Toxicol* 13, Supplement-Special Issue II, 913

Rosemary oil, RIFM monograph (1974) *Food Cosmet Toxicol* 12, Supplement-Special Issue I, 977–978

Sage oil, Dalmatian, RIFM monograph (1974) *Food Cosmet Toxicol* 12, Supplement-Special Issue I, 987–988

Sage oil, Spanish, RIFM monograph (1976) *Food Cosmet Toxicol* 14, Supplement-Special Issue III, 857–858

Sandalwood oil, East Indian, RIFM monograph (1974) *Food Cosmet Toxicol* 12, Supplement-Special Issue I, 989–990

Savory oil, summer, RIFM monograph (1976) *Food Cosmet Toxicol* 14, Supplement-Special Issue III, 859–860

Spearmint oil, RIFM monograph (1978) *Food Cosmet Toxicol* 16, Supplement-Special Issue IV, 871–872

Star anise oil, RIFM monograph (1975) *Food Cosmet Toxicol* 13, Supplement-Special Issue II, 715–716

Tagetes oil, RIFM monograph (1982) *Food Cosmet Toxicol* 20, Supplement-Special Issue VI, 829–830

Tansy oil, RIFM monograph (1976) *Food Cosmet Toxicol* 14, Supplement-Special Issue III, 869–870

Tea tree oil, RIFM monograph (1988) *Food Chem Toxicol* 26, Supplement-Special Issue VII, 407

Thyme oil, red, RIFM monograph (1974) *Food Cosmet Toxicol* 12, Supplement-Special Issue I, 1003–1004

Vanilla tincture, RIFM monograph (1982) *Food Cosmet Toxicol* 20, Supplement-Special Issue VI, 849–850

Verbena absolute, RIFM monograph (1988) *Food Chem Toxicol* 30, Supplement-Special Issue VIII, 135

Verbena oil, RIFM monograph (1988) *Food Chem Toxicol* 30, Supplement-Special Issue VIII, 137–138

Vetiver oil, RIFM monograph (1974) *Food Cosmet Toxicol* 12, Special Issue I, 1013

Violet leaf absolute, RIFM monograph (1976) *Food Cosmet Toxicol* 14, Supplement-Special Issue III, 747–748

Virginian cedarwood oil, RIFM monograph (1974) *Food Cosmet Toxicol* 12, Supplement-Special Issue I, 845–846

Ylang Ylang oil, RIFM monograph (1974) *Food Cosmet Toxicol* 12, Supplement-Special Issue I, 1015–1016

Appendix 23

RIFM recommended limit for safe use of essential oils

	RIFM %
1. Aniseed	
a. *Pimpinella anisum*	2
b. *Star anise, Illicium verum*	2
2. Angelica, *Angelica archangelica*	0.78 phototoxic
3. Basil, *sweet, Ocimum basilicum*	4
4. Bay, *Laurus nobilis*	2
5. Benzoin resinoid, *Styrax benzoin*	3
6. Bergamot oil, *Citrus bergamia*	0.4 phototoxic (expressed) 20 rectified
7. Buchu, *Agathosma betulina*	NFST
8. Cajuput, *Melaleuca leucadendron* L.	4
9. Camphor *Cinnamomum camphora* (L.) Nees & Ebermeier	white 20
10. Carrot seed, *Daucus carota*	4
11. Cassia, *Cinnamomum cassia* Bl.	(sensitiser) 0.2
12. Cedarwood oil	
a. Virginia *Juniperus virginiana* L.	1
b. Texas, *J. mexicana* Spring	
c. Atlas, *Cedrus atlantica* Manetti	8
13. Celery seed, *Apium graveolens*	4
14. Chamomile, Roman, *Anthemis nobilis*	4
15. Chamomile, German, *Matricaria recutica*	4
16. Cinnamon bark oil, *Cinnamomum zeylanicum* Nees	1; leaf 10
17. Citronella, *Cymbopogon nardus* (Rendel)	1
18. Clary sage oil, *Salvia sclarea* L.	8
19. Clove oil, *Eugenia caryophyllata* Thumb., *Syzygium aromaticum*	bud 4; leaf 2; stem 4
20. Cornmint, *Mentha arvensis* var. *piperascens* Holmes	8
21. Cubeb, *Piper cubeba* L.	8
22. Cypress oil, *Cupressus sempervirens*	4
23. Dill, *Anethum graveolens* L.	4
24. Elecampane, *Inula helenium*	0.1 Elecampane oil
25. Eucalyptus oils	
a. *Eucalyptus globulus* Labill.	10
b. *E. radiata* R.T. Baker	
c. *E. citriodora* Hooker	10
26. Fennel	
a. Sweet, *Foeniculum vulgare* Miller subsp. *capillaceum* (Galib.) Holmboe	seed 4
b. Bitter, var. *vulgare* Miller	seed 4
27. Frankincense (olibanum), *Boswellia carterii* Birdw.	abs 3; oil 8 tentative

(Continued)

	RIFM %
28. Geranium, *Pelargonium* species, e.g. cv Rose	10
29. Ginger oil, *Zingiber officinale* Roscoe	4
30. Ho leaf, *Cinnamomum camphora* L. Nees & Eberneier	10
31. Hyssop oil, *Hyssopus officinalis*	4
32. Jasmine absolute, *Jasminum grandiflorum* L.	3
33. Juniper berry, *Juniperus communis* L.	8
34. Kanuka, *Kunzea ericoides*	NFST
35. Lavender oil, *Lavandula angustifolia* P. Miller	abs 3; oil 15
a. Lavandin, *L. angustifolia* × *L. latifolia* (L.) Medikus	abs 3; oil 4
36. Lemon oil, *Citrus limonum* (L.) Burm. F.	dist. 10; expressed (phototoxic) 2
37. Lemon balm, *Melissa officinalis* L.	uncertain NFST
38. Lemongrass oil, *Cymbopogon citratus* L./flexuosus (Nees) Stapf.	4
39. *Litsea cubeba* L.	8
40. Manuka, *Leptospermum scoparium*	NFST
41. Marjoram oil, *Origanum marjorana*	4
42. Myrrh oil, *Commiphora myrrha* (Nees) Engler	abs 3; oil 8
43. Myrtle, *Myrtus communis*	4
44. Neroli oil, *Citrus aurantium* L.	abs 3; oil 4
45. Nutmeg, *Myristica fragrans* Houtt.	2; mace oil 10
46. Orange	
a. Sweet, *Citrus sinensis* (L.) Osbeck, expressed	10
b. Bitter C. *aurantium* L. subsp. *amara,* expressed	1.4 phototoxic
47. Palmarosa, *Cymbopogon martini* Stapf.	8
48. Parsley, *Petroselinum sativum*	herb and seed 2
49. Patchouli, *Pogestemon cablin* (Blanco) Benth.	10
50. Pepper, black, *Piper nigrum*	4
51. Peppermint oil, *Mentha piperita* L. (see also spearmint and cornmint)	4 tentative
52. Peru balsam, *Myroxylon pereirae*	balsam: do not use; oil 8
53. Petitgrain, *Citrus aurantium* L. subsp. *amara*	bigarade 8; lemon 10
54. Pine oil, *Pinus sylvestris* L.	>10 mmol/L peroxide per litre (sensitiser)
55. Rose oil, *Rosa centifolia* L. Rose otto, *Rosa damascena* Mill.	abs and oil 2
56. Rosemary oil, *Rosmarinus officinalis* L.	10
57. Rosewood, *Aniba roseodora* var. *amazonica* Ducke (Bois de Rose)	10
58. Sage	
a. Dalmatian, *Salvia officinalis* L.	8
b. Spanish, *Salvia lavandulaefolia* Vahl.	8
59. Sandalwood oil, East Indian, *Santalum album*	10
60. Savory oil, *Satureia montana*	*S. hortensis* 0.5
61. Spearmint, *Mentha spicata* L.	4
62. Spike lavender, *Lavandula latifolia* Vill.	Oil 8
63. Tea tree oil, *Melaleuca alternjfolia* (Maiden & Betche) Cheel	1
64. Thyme oil	
a. *Thymus vulgaris* L.	red 8, tentative
b. *T. serphyllum*	8
65. Valerian root oil, *Valeriana officinalis*	Safety testing oral but not dermal
66. Vanilla, *Vanilla plantifolia*	tincture 3
67. Wintergreen oil, *Gaultheria procumbens*	not to use
68. Yarrow, *Achillea ligusticum*	4 tentative NFST
69. Ylang ylang, *Cananga odorata* Hook. f. et Thomson	10; also Cananga 10

(Continued)

Essential oils and balsams used rarely (most will just be mentioned in the chapters; a few described in more detail in the text)

	RIFM %
Cardamom, *Ellateria cardamomum*	4
Coriander, *Coriandrum sativum*	4
Davana, *Artemisia pallens*	4
Eriocephalus, *Eriocephalus punctulatus*	uncertain NFST
Fir needle	
Canadian, *Abies balsamea*	10
Siberian, *Abies sibirica*	1
Galbanum, *Ferula galbaniflua*	oil 4; resin 5
Labdanum/cyste, *Cistus ladaniferus*	abs. 3; oil 8
Layana, *Artemisia afra*	2
Opoponax absolute, *Opoponax chironium*	8
Spikenard, *Nardostachys jatamansi*	0 tentative NFST
Storax resinoid, *Styrax officinalis*	4
Tagetes, *Tagetes minuta*	0.05%
Tansy, *Tanacetum vulgare*	4
Tolu balsam, *Myroxylon balsamum*	2
Tonka absolute, *Dipteryx odorata*	3
Verbena oil, *Lippia citriodora*	0.25

NFST = No formal scientific testing.

Appendix 24

Hazards and toxicity: CHIP

Hazard symbols

Xn	Harmful	**Hazard:** harmful to one's health by inhalation, ingestion or skin penetration; recurring or lengthy exposure to these substances may result in irreversible damage **Caution:** Avoid contact with the human body, including inhalation of vapours and in case of malaise consult a doctor
Xi	Irritant	**Hazard:** May have an irritant effect on skin, eyes and respiratory organs **Caution:** do not breathe vapours and avoid contact with skin and eyes
T	Toxic	**Hazard:** Very hazardous to health by inhalation, ingestion or skin contact and may even lead to death; recurring or lengthy exposure to these substances may result in irreversible damage **Caution:** Avoid contact with the human body, and in case of malaise immediately consult a doctor
Other symbols		Explosive, oxidising, extremely or highly flammable, corrosive, irritant and dangerous for the environment

Risk phrases

Examples

R10	Flammable	Angelicas, camphor (white), caraway, carrot seed, chamomile (Roman), cumin, cypress, elemi, galbanum, garlic, grapefruit, helichrysum, hop, horseradish, juniper berry, laurel leaf, lavender (spike), lemon, lime (distilled/expressed), mace, mandarin, marjoram, yarrow, mustard, myrtle, neroli, niaouli, nutmeg, onion, orange, olibanum, pepper, pine needles, rosemary, sages, savin, tagetes, tangerine, tea tree, thymes
R21	Harmful in contact with skin	Cassia, cinnamon bark, clove leaf, origanum, parsley seed, Tonka, wormseed
R22	Harmful if swallowed	*Artemisia vulgaris*, basils, bay, buchu, cedar leaf, clove leaf, cornmint, tarragon, hyssop, myrrh, origanum, parsley seed, tansy, wintergreen, wormseed and wormwood
R42/43	May cause sensitisation by inhalation and skin contact	Peru balsam

Safety phrases

Examples

| S53 | Avoid exposure; obtain special instructions before use | Sassafras |
| S36 | Wear suitable protective clothing | Tolu balsam |

Transport

Examples: ADR/SDR transport implies road transport. Others for rail, air, sea freight. A number 1–10 is given according to hazard classification.

Appendix 25

Aspiration hazards (R65)

This aspiration hazard (R65) labelling is a requirement for essential oils. The R65 relates to the potential to cause lung damage after swallowing. It is based on the inherent low viscosity of materials containing more than 10% of aliphatic, alicylic and aromatic hydrocarbons. Requirements for R65 labelling came in on 31 May 1988.

Many essential oils have more than 10% of hydrocarbons. Here is a small selection:

Essential oil	Total hydrocarbon content %
Angelica	95
Bay	30
Bergamot	65
Cajuput	40
Carrot seed	60
Cascarilla	30
Cedarwood	60
Celery	80
Cistus	10
Copaiba balsam + oil	90
Chamomile	15
Citronella Ceylon	15
Clove leaf	15
Clove stem	15
Costus	30
Cubeb	70
Cumin	50
Cypress	70
Dill	35
Elemi	70
Estragon (tarragon)	20
Eucalyptus citriodora	20
Fennel	20
Lime expressed	90
Lime distilled	90
Lovage root and stem	20
Mace	90
Mandarin	8
Marjorams sweet	20
Mastic	90
Myrrh	70
Myrtle	50

(Continued)

Essential oil	Total hydrocarbon content %
Neroli	40
Niaioli	15
Nutmeg	85
Olibanum	90
Orange	97
Origanum	25
Parsley herb/seed	40
Parsnip	50
Patchouli	60
Pepper	95
Pepper oleoresin	20
Pimento leaf	25
Pine needle	95

The UK Health and Safety Executive's *Approved Guide to the Classification and Labelling of Substances and Preparations Dangerous for Supply – Guidance regulations* (3rd edn) sets out criteria for the R65 classification.

Appendix 26

Safety data: CHIP symbols explained in detail

Abbreviation	Hazard	Description of hazard
Physicochemical		
E	Explosive	Chemicals that explode
O	Oxidising	Chemicals that react exothermically with other chemicals
F+	Extremely flammable	Chemicals that have an extremely low flash point and boiling point, and gases that catch fire in contact with air
F	Highly flammable	Chemicals that may catch fire in contact with air, only need brief contact with an ignition source, have a very low flash point or evolve highly flammable gases in contact with water
Health		
T+	Very toxic	Chemicals that at very low levels cause damage to health
T	Toxic	Chemicals that at low levels cause damage to health
Carc Cat 1	Category 1 carcinogens	Chemicals that may cause cancer or increase its incidence
Carc Cat 2	Category 2 carcinogens	
Carc Cat 3	Category 3 carcinogens	
Muta Cat 1	Category 1 mutagens	Chemicals that induce heritable genetic defects or increase their incidence
Muta Cat 2	Category 2 mutagens	
Muta Cat 3	Category 3 mutagens	
Repr Cat 1	Category 1 reproductive toxins	Chemicals that produce or increase the incidence of non-heritable effects in progeny and/or an impairment in reproductive functions or capacity
Repr Cat 2	Category 2 reproductive toxins	
Repr Cat 3	Category 3 reproductive toxins	
Xn	Harmful	Chemicals that may cause damage to health
C	Corrosive	Chemicals that may destroy living tissue on contact
Xi	Irritant	Chemicals that may cause inflammation to the skin or other mucous membranes
Environmental		
N	Dangerous for the environment	Chemicals that may present an immediate or delayed danger to one or more components of the environment

Risk phrases

R1	Explosive when dry
R2	Risk of explosion by shock, friction, fire or other sources of ignition
R3	Extreme risk of explosion by shock, friction, fire or other sources of ignition
R4	Forms very sensitive explosive metallic compounds
R5	Heating may cause an explosion
R6	Explosive with or without contact with air
R7	May cause fire
R8	Contact with combustible material may cause fire
R9	Explosive when mixed with combustible material
R10	Flammable
R11	Highly flammable
R12	Extremely flammable
R14	Reacts violently with water
R14/15	Reacts violently with water, liberating extremely flammable gases
R15	Contact with water liberates extremely flammable gases
R15/29	Contact with water liberates toxic, extremely flammable gases
R16	Explosive when mixed with oxidising substances
R17	Spontaneously flammable in air
R18	In use, may form flammable/explosive vapour-air mixture
R19	May form explosive peroxides
R20	Harmful by inhalation
R20/21	Harmful by inhalation and in contact with skin
R20/21/22	Harmful by inhalation, in contact with skin and if swallowed
R20/22	Harmful by inhalation and if swallowed
R21	Harmful in contact with skin
R21/22	Harmful in contact with skin and if swallowed
R22	Harmful if swallowed
R23	Toxic by inhalation
R23/24	Toxic by inhalation and in contact with skin
R23/24/25	Toxic by inhalation, in contact with skin and if swallowed
R23/25	Toxic by inhalation and if swallowed
R24	Toxic in contact with skin
R24/25	Toxic in contact with skin and if swallowed
R25	Toxic if swallowed
R26	Very toxic by inhalation
R26/27	Very toxic by inhalation and in contact with skin
R26/27/28	Very toxic by inhalation, in contact with skin and if swallowed
R26/28	Very toxic by inhalation and if swallowed
R27	Very toxic in contact with skin
R27/28	Very toxic in contact with skin and if swallowed
R28	Very toxic if swallowed
R30	Can become highly flammable in use
R31	Contact with acids liberates toxic gas
R32	Contact with acids liberates very toxic gas
R33	Danger of cumulative effects
R34	Causes burns
R35	Causes severe burns
R36	Irritating to eyes

(Continued)

R36/37	Irritating to eyes and respiratory system
R36/37/38	Irritating to eyes, respiratory system and skin
R36/38	Irritating to eyes and skin
R37	Irritating to respiratory system
R37/38	Irritating to respiratory system and skin
R38	Irritating to skin
R39	Danger of very serious irreversible effects
R39/23	Toxic: danger of very serious irreversible effects through inhalation
R39/23/24	Toxic: danger of very serious irreversible effects through inhalation and in contact with skin
R39/23/24/25	Toxic: danger of very serious irreversible effects through inhalation, in contact with skin and if swallowed
R39/23/25	Toxic: danger of very serious irreversible effects through inhalation and if swallowed
R39/24	Toxic: danger of very serious irreversible effects in contact with skin
R39/24/25	Toxic: danger of very serious irreversible effects in contact with skin and if swallowed
R39/25	Toxic: danger of very serious irreversible effects if swallowed
R39/26	Very toxic: danger of very serious irreversible effects through inhalation
R39/26/27	Very toxic: danger of very serious irreversible effects through inhalation and in contact with skin
R39/26/27/28	Very toxic: danger of very serious irreversible effects through inhalation, in contact with skin and if swallowed
R39/26/28	Very toxic: danger of very serious irreversible effects through inhalation and if swallowed
R39/27	Very toxic: danger of very serious irreversible effects in contact with skin
R39/27/28	Very toxic: danger of very serious irreversible effects in contact with skin and if swallowed
R39/28	Very toxic: danger of very serious irreversible effects if swallowed
R40	Limited evidence of a carcinogenic effect
R40/20	Harmful: possible risk of irreversible effects through inhalation
R40/20/21	Harmful: possible risk of irreversible effects through inhalation and in contact with skin
R40/20/21/22	Harmful: possible risk of irreversible effects through inhalation, in contact with skin and if swallowed
R40/20/22	Harmful: possible risk of irreversible effects through inhalation and if swallowed
R40/21	Harmful: possible risk of irreversible effects in contact with skin
R40/21/22	Harmful: possible risk of irreversible effects in contact with skin and if swallowed
R40/22	Harmful: possible risk of irreversible effects if swallowed
R41	Risk of serious damage to eyes
R42	May cause sensitisation by inhalation
R43	May cause sensitisation by skin contact
R42/43	May cause sensitisation by inhalation and skin contact
R44	Risk of explosion if heated under confinement
R45	May cause cancer
R46	May cause heritable genetic damage
R48	Danger of serious damage to health by prolonged exposure
R48/20	Harmful: danger of serious damage to health by prolonged exposure through inhalation
R48/20/21	Harmful: danger of serious damage to health by prolonged exposure through inhalation and in contact with skin
R48/20/21/22	Harmful: danger of serious damage to health by prolonged exposure through inhalation, in contact with skin and if swallowed
R48/20/22	Harmful: danger of serious damage to health by prolonged exposure through inhalation and if swallowed
R48/21	Harmful: danger of serious damage to health by prolonged exposure in contact with skin

(Continued)

R48/21/22	Harmful: danger of serious damage to health by prolonged exposure in contact with skin and if swallowed
R48/22	Harmful: danger of serious damage to health by prolonged exposure if swallowed
R48/23	Toxic: danger of serious damage to health by prolonged exposure through inhalation
R48/23/24	Toxic: danger of serious damage to health by prolonged exposure through inhalation and in contact with skin
R48/23/24/25	Toxic: danger of serious damage to health by prolonged exposure through inhalation, in contact with skin and if swallowed
R48/23/25	Toxic: danger of serious damage to health by prolonged exposure through inhalation and if swallowed
R48/24	Toxic: danger of serious damage to health by prolonged exposure in contact with skin
R48/24/25	Toxic: danger of serious damage to health by prolonged exposure in contact with skin and if swallowed
R48/25	Toxic: danger of serious damage to health by prolonged exposure if swallowed
R49	May cause cancer by inhalation
R50	Very toxic to aquatic organisms
R50/53	Very toxic to aquatic organisms, may cause long-term adverse effects in the aquatic environment
R51	Toxic to aquatic organisms
R51/53	Toxic to aquatic organisms, may cause long-term adverse effects in the aquatic environment
R52	Harmful to aquatic organisms
R52/53	Harmful to aquatic organisms, may cause long-term adverse effects in the aquatic environment
R53	May cause long-term adverse effects in the aquatic environment
R54	Toxic to flora
R55	Toxic to fauna
R56	Toxic to soil organisms
R57	Toxic to bees
R58	May cause long-term adverse effects in the environment
R59	Dangerous for the ozone layer
R60	May impair fertility
R61	May cause harm to the unborn child
R62	Possible risk of impaired fertility
R63	Possible risk of harm to the unborn child
R64	May cause harm to breast-fed babies
R65	Harmful: may cause lung damage if swallowed
R66	Repeated exposure may cause skin dryness or cracking
R67	Vapours may cause drowsiness and dizziness
R68	Possible risk of irreversible effects

Safety phrases

S1	Keep locked up
S(1/2)	Keep locked up and out of the reach of children
S2	Keep out of the reach of children
S3	Keep in a cool place
S3/7	Keep container tightly closed in a cool place
S3/7/9	Keep container tightly closed in a cool, well-ventilated place

(Continued)

S3/9/14	Keep in a cool, well-ventilated place away from … (incompatible materials to be indicated by the manufacturer)
S3/9/14/49	Keep only in the original container in a cool, well-ventilated place away from … (incompatible materials to be indicated by the manufacturer)
S3/9/49	Keep only in the original container in a cool, well-ventilated place
S3/14	Keep in a cool place away from … (incompatible materials to be indicated by the manufacturer)
S4	Keep away from living quarters
S5	Keep contents under … (appropriate liquid to be specified by the manufacturer)
S6	Keep under … (inert gas to be specified by the manufacturer)
S7	Keep container tightly closed
S7/8	Keep container tightly closed and dry
S7/9	Keep container tightly closed and in a well-ventilated place
S7/47	Keep container tightly closed and at temperature not exceeding … °C (to be specified by the manufacturer)
S8	Keep container dry
S9	Keep container in a well-ventilated place
S12	Do not keep the container sealed
S13	Keep away from food, drink and animal feeding stuffs
S14	Keep away from … (incompatible materials to be indicated by the manufacturer)
S15	Keep away from heat
S16	Keep away from sources of ignition – No smoking
S17	Keep away from combustible material
S18	Handle and open container with care
S20	When using do not eat or drink
S20/21	When using do not eat, drink or smoke
S21	When using do not smoke
S22	Do not breathe dust
S23	Do not breathe gas/fumes/vapour/spray (appropriate wording to be specified by the manufacturer)
S24	Avoid contact with skin
S24/25	Avoid contact with skin and eyes
S25	Avoid contact with eyes
S26	In case of contact with eyes, rinse immediately with plenty of water and seek medical advice
S27	Take off immediately all contaminated clothing
S27/28	After contact with skin, take off immediately all contaminated clothing, and wash immediately with plenty of … (to be specified by the manufacturer)
S28	After contact with skin, wash immediately with plenty of … (to be specified by the manufacturer)
S29	Do not empty into drains
S29/35	Do not empty into drains; dispose of this material and its container in a safe way
S29/56	Do not empty into drains, dispose of this material and its container at hazardous or special waste collection point
S30	Never add water to this product
S33	Take precautionary measures against static discharges
S35	This material and its container must be disposed of in a safe way
S36	Wear suitable protective clothing
S36/37	Wear suitable protective clothing and gloves
S36/37/39	Wear suitable protective clothing, gloves and eye/face protection
S36/39	Wear suitable protective clothing and eye/face protection
S37	Wear suitable gloves

(Continued)

S37/39	Wear suitable gloves and eye/face protection
S38	In case of insufficient ventilation wear suitable respiratory equipment
S39	Wear eye/face protection
S40	To clean the floor and all objects contaminated by this material use ... (to be specified by the manufacturer)
S41	In case of fire and/or explosion do not breathe fumes
S42	During fumigation/spraying wear suitable respiratory equipment (appropriate wording to be specified by the manufacturer)
S43	In case of fire use ... (indicate in the space the precise type of fire-fighting equipment. If water increases the risk add – Never use water)
S45	In case of accident or if you feel unwell seek medical advice immediately (show the label where possible)
S46	If swallowed, seek medical advice immediately and show this container or label
S47	Keep at temperature not exceeding ... °C (to be specified by the manufacturer)
S47/49	Keep only in the original container at temperature not exceeding ... °C (to be specified by the manufacturer)
S48	Keep wet with ... (appropriate material to be specified by the manufacturer)
S49	Keep only in the original container
S50	Do not mix with ... (to be specified by the manufacturer)
S51	Use only in well-ventilated areas
S52	Not recommended for interior use on large surface areas
S53	Avoid exposure – obtain special instructions before use
S56	Dispose of this material and its container at hazardous or special waste collection point
S57	Use appropriate containment to avoid environmental contamination
S59	Refer to manufacturer/supplier for information on recovery/recycling
S60	This material and its container must be disposed of as hazardous waste
S61	Avoid release to the environment. Refer to special instructions/safety data sheet
S62	If swallowed, do not induce vomiting: seek medical advice immediately and show this container or label
S63	In case of accident by inhalation: remove casualty to fresh air and keep at rest
S64	If swallowed, rinse mouth with water (only if the person is conscious)

Data from the HSE list of symbols, abbreviations, risk and safety phrases. Crown copyright material is reproduced with the permission of the controller of HMSO and the Queen's Printer for Scotland.

Appendix 27

New 7th Amendment: European Parliament 2002

To Annex III – Part 1 (Directive 76/768/EEC)

This regards the conditions of use and the warnings which must be printed on the label of essential oils containing these components. The following components must be indicated in the list of ingredients and the warning given that: can cause an allergic reaction:

- Anisyl alcohol (CAS 105-13-5)
- Benzyl alcohol (CAS 100-51-6)
- Benzyl benzoate (CAS 120-51-4)
- Benzyl cinnamate (CAS 103-41-3)
- Benzyl salicylate (CAS 118-68-1)
- Cinnamal (CAS 104-55-2)
- Cinnamyl alcohol (CAS 104-54-1)
- Citral (CAS 5392-40-5)
- Citronellol (CAS 106-22-9)
- Coumarin (CAS 91-64-5)
- Eugenol (CAS 97-53-0)
- Farnesol (CAS 4602-84-0)
- Gerianol (CAS 106-24-1)
- Hydroxycitronellal (CAS 107-75-5)
- Isoeugenol (CAS 97-54-1)
- D-Limonene (CAS 5989-27-5)
- Linalool (CAS 78-70-6)
- Oakmoss and treemoss extract

This will make it very difficult for perfumers but also aromatherapists, as some of the components occur in essential oils that are considered to be very gentle (e.g. geranium, clary sage and lavender oil).

EC regulations 2002 (CHIP) governing geranium EOs major components – given here as there is frequent adulteration with these synthetic components, all of which are allergens:

D-Limonene, CAS no. 5989-27-5; EEC no. 227-813-5; Hazard symbol: Xn N; Risk phrase: R10, 38, 43, 50/53; H/C: 100%; Safety phrase: S24, 37, 60, 61.

L-Limonene, CAS no. 5989-54-8; EEC no. 228-813-5; Hazard symbol: Xn N; Risk phrase: R10, 38, 43, 50/53; H/C: 100%; Safety phrase: S24, 37, 60, 61.

Linalool, CAS no. 78-70-6; EEC no. 201-134-4; Hazard symbol: none; Risk phrase: none; H/C: none; Safety phrase: none.

Citral, CAS no. 5392-40-5; EEC no. 226-394-6; Hazard symbol: Xi; Risk phrase: R38, 43; H/C: none; Safety phrase: S24/25, 37.

Citronellol, CAS no. 106-22-9; EEC no. 203-375-0; Hazard symbol: Xi N; Risk phrase: R38, 43, 51/53; H/C: none; Safety phrase: S24, 37, 61.

Geraniol, CAS no. 106-24-1; EEC no. 203-377-1; Hazard symbol: Xi; Risk phrase: R38, 43; H/C: none; Safety phrase: S24, 37.

The presence of these substances must be indicated in the list of ingredients when its concentration exceeds 0.001% in leave-on products and 0.01% in rinse-off products.

Reference: maximum levels of fragrance allergens in aromatic natural raw materials. European Parliament and Council Directive 76/768/EEC on Cosmetic Products, 7th Amendment 2002.

Appendix 28

Sensitisers and their essential oil sources

From the European Cosmetic, Toiletry and Perfumery Association (COLIPA) list, these 16 'ingredients' occur in the vast majority of essential oils

Sensitisers	Examples of sources
Anisyl alcohol	Vanilla absolute (esp. Tahiti)
Benzyl alcohol	Ylang ylang, styrax, Peru balsam
Benzyl benzoate	Cassia, cinnamon, jasmine absolute, tolu, ylang ylang
Benzyl cinnamate	Benzoin, immortelle, Peru oil, Tolu balsam
Benzyl salicylate	Ylang ylang, cananga
Cinnamic aldehyde (Cinnamal)	Cinnamon bark oil, cassia, tolu
Cinnamyl alcohol	Cassia, cinnamon, styrax oils/oleoresins
Citral	Bergamot, orange, lemon, lime, lemongrass, *Litsea cubeba*
Citronellol	Citronella, geranium, rose, melissa
Coumarin	Cinnamon, hay, lavender absolute, myrtle, Tonka bean oil, deer tongue absolute, melilot absolute, cassia oil
Eugenol	Bay, cinnamon leaf, clove, pimento, basil, and rose oils
Farnesol	Ambrette, cananga, neroli, palmarosa, rose, ylang ylang
Geraniol	Carrot, citronella, geranium, palmarosa
Isoeugenol	Clove, origanum, nutmeg, pimento, ylang ylang
Limonene	A vast majority of the oils listed, especially citrus (e.g. grapefruit) and *Helichrysum* and caraway
Linalool	A vast majority essential oils (e.g. rosewood, *Mentha citrata*)

Appendix 29

Harmful and sensitising oils (EFFA-IOFI-IFRA)

Xn (harmful)

Artemisia vulgaris
Basils
Bay
Birch, sweet
Buchu
Calamus
Caraway
Cassia
Cedar leaf
Chenopodium (wormseed)
Cinnamon bark
Clove leaf
Cornmint
Costus
Estragon (Tarragon)
Hyssop
Myrrh
Origanum
Parsley herb
Pennyroyal
Tansy
Tea tree
Thuja (cedar leaf)
Tonka bean
Turpentine
Wintergreen
Wormseed (*Chenopodium*)
Wormwood (*Artemisia*)

Xi (irritant)

Litsea cubeba
Melissa
Oakmoss
Opoponax resin
Parsley seed
Peru balsam
Styrax oil/resin
Tagetes
Thymes
Tree moss
Verbena

T (toxic)

Mustard
Sassafras
Savory, summer

Appendix 30

List of banned oils/restricted oils: IFRA list

Carcinogenic and controlled drugs	*Saffrole and those containing it at over 1%* Nutmeg Brown camphor Ylang ylang Wormseed *Methyl chavicol-containing oils (possible carcinogens)* Basil Tarragon Fennel
Severely restricted	Calamus oil (*Acorus calamus*) *Citral-containing oils* *Backhousia citriodora* Lemongrass *Litsea cubeba* Melissa (should be used with quencher according to IFRA: lemongrass with citrus terpenes, 80:20)
Sensitisers banned by IFRA	Costus root oil, absolute, concrete Elecampane oil Verbena oil, absolute Fig leaf absolute Peru balsam
Restricted by IFRA	Cinnamon bark Cassia Oakmoss extracts Treemoss extracts Fennel Opoponax extracts Styrax Verbena absolute Pinaceae extracts Peru balsam Tagetes
Phototoxic/sensitisers	Citrus oils Bergamot Orange Lemon Grapefruit Lime Tangerine, etc.

(*Continued*)

	Rue
	Fig leaf absolute
	Tagetes
	Angelica root
	Celery
Irritants	Clove bud
	Pimento
	Cornmint
	Peppermint
	Cassia
	Savory
	Clove leaf
	Thyme
	Orange (folded × 10)
Severe irritants	Garlic
	Massoia
	Horseradish
	Mustard
Neurotoxicants	Hyssop
	Camphor
	Cedarleaf
	Tansy
Hepatotoxicants	(*Due to pulegone; menthofuran*)
	Pennyroyal oils *(Mentha pulegium, Hedeoma pulegioides)*
	Buchu *(Agathosma crenulata)*
	Spearmint
	Catnip
	Peppermint
	Cornmint
	Anethole-containing
	Aniseed
	Star anise (+ methyl chavicol)
Teratogens	*Juniperus sabina* (savin)
	Spanish lavender *(Salvia lavandulifolia)*
Salicism-causing (methyl salicylate toxicity)	Wintergreen
	Sweet birch
Other essential oils and resins that are dangerous	Benzoin resinoid and oil

Appendix 31

Toxic or dangerous essential oils versus their usage as food additives

Specified substance	Standard permitted proportion	Permitted proportion in particular food
β-Asarone (Calamus)	0.1 mg/kg	(a) Alcoholic drinks = 1 mg/kg (b) Seasonings in snacks = 1 mg/kg
Coumarin (Bergamot)	2 mg/kg	(a) Chewing gum = 50 mg/kg (b) Alcoholic drinks = 10 mg/kg (c) Caramel confectionery = 10 mg/kg
Pulegone (Pennyroyal)	25 mg/kg	(a) Mint confectionery = 350 mg/kg (b) Mint/spearmint drink = 250 mg/kg (c) Other drinks = 100 mg/kg
Safrole (Sassafras)	1 mg/kg	(a) Food with mace, nutmeg or isosafrole both = 15 mg/kg (b) Alcoholic drinks with more than 25% alcohol v/v = 5 mg/kg (c) Other drinks = 2 mg/kg
Thujone α- or β-	0.5 mg/kg	(a) Bitters = 35 mg/kg (b) Food (not drinks) containing sage = 25 mg/kg (c) Alcoholic drinks with more than 25% v/v alcohol = 10 mg/kg (d) Other alcoholic drinks = 5 mg/kg

Data from: UK Flavourings in Food Regulations (1992). 1971 Flavourings in Food Regulations 1992, www.foodstandards.gov.uk/food industry/regulation/foodlawguidebranch/.

Appendix 32

Guide for non-scientists on making a judgement on the scientific merit of published papers on clinical studies and other research

Scientific journals vary greatly in their scientific merit and therefore the quality of the publications and the peer reviewers consulted. There is a general format, but each journal has its own 'Instructions to authors', as there are large or sometimes subtle variations in the format for each individual journal. The manuscript may be rejected simply on the grounds of non-conformity with these rules and not even read/sent out to referees. The present author has personally reviewed hundreds of papers for a wide variety of international journals over 30 years, so has had experience of many papers which are rejected by a 'good' journal, and which later appeared in another journal of a much lower standard. Most nursing journals, unfortunately, do not set the same scientific standards as the truly scientific journals.

Introduction

This should contain information as to what exactly (or as precisely as possible) is the problem: How common is it? What are the current methods of treating this problem and why could it be made better using aromatherapy? What is the proposed method of aromatherapy to be applied and is it with/without conventional therapy? The introduction should not use anecdotal 'evidence' for the clinical usage of essential oils, but statements made must be supported by relevant references from peer-reviewed papers/ books. If a given essential oil is to be used as a stress reliever, for example, it is pointless to give references concerning its antimicrobial activity *in vitro*.

Methodology

Fullest details of methodology are required, as any peer-reviewed study must be able to provide enough data to be repeated by others. This needs to be checked for accuracy by a scientist working in the same field – a referee.

Sample

A description of the sample chosen is required and perhaps reasons why it was chosen. Note: are the numbers likely to provide statistical significance? Numbers less than ten are definitely not to be relied on, although several papers have been published with four people in the study. There is therefore a scientific reason for not accepting single-case studies as being very meaningful. Other important information concerns the age, the sex of the clients in all groups (experimental/controls) and also how the clients were allocated to each group (randomisation?). Many papers have severe scientific drawbacks in this area. For example, one study in an intensive care unit cited an age range of 2–85 years and required verbal responses to many questions (see Chapter 8).

Intervention

This requires detail of exactly what was done to the clients? What essential oils were used: their exact name, source, including where purchased or who provided them plus any reference numbers, how were they extracted, etc. (essential oils can vary tremendously from batch to batch, but even more from one supplier to another).

Gas chromatography (GC) or gas chromatography/ mass spectrometry (GC/MS) data of the essential oils used (with main component concentrations) and details of apparatus and conditions used are also essential to confirm the essential oil chemistry and therefore make it possible to do the same study again, if necessary. Details of how the essential oil was diluted and the percentage in a specific solvent/carrier oil is imperative, as this can make very large differences in physiological/biochemical, microbiological and other studies.

Measures

It should be made clear how the experiment was assessed. What measurements were taken? What particular assessment packages were used, with references. Any statistical analysis should be very clearly stated, as non-statistical effects can be totally disregarded. Trends can only be assumed if very large numbers are used in the studies – which happens very rarely.

Design of experiment

Good solid design principles (which may be very simple) are looked for. Eradication of any bias/psychological factors should be confirmed at the start and included in the final appraisal. Details of planned outcome for positive/negative evaluation are of merit.

Procedure

Details of exactly how the study was conducted should be included. For example, at what intervals were the aromatherapy treatments applied? For how long was the therapy given? Where was the massage applied (if relevant), e.g. the whole body, hands, feet; and how was it conducted (e.g. gentle effleurage?). Was the massage always confined to the same area? This is extremely important and is one of the factors which causes scientific concern in some of the clinical studies (see Chapter 8).

How many people performed the massage (or other treatment)? Was it always done by the same person? Were the groups of experimental/control clients treated at the same time and by the same person?

Results

Clear tabulated results are always better to understand, and usually indicate a good paper. Who assessed the results on the clients? Who analysed the outcomes? How was this assessed scientifically?

Statistically significant differences between groups must be clearly shown and described. Results showing significance of $P > 0.05$ are acceptable: this indicates a probability of the results occurring by chance as 1 in 20. Any higher P-values should not be offered as significant. P-values of >0.01 and 0.001 are definitely significant, showing a 1 in 100 and 1 in 1000 probability respectively. Results that are not statistically significant should not be used later as indicating a trend, or for showing some change.

Graphs can also be useful in illustrating changes and may show them more clearly. They should not duplicate the tables, as this often indicates shortage of data.

Discussion

The authors' interpretation of results must be given clearly and then followed by details of the relevance of the results to past scientific publications. Their relevance to aromatherapy generally should then be stated.

Possible problems encountered should be outlined, with some ideas as to how these could be dealt with in future. For example, was there a chance that the illness was in remission? Was there any other cause for the improvement noted (especially if the aromatherapy was a complementary measure and other conventional therapy was given as well)? Was the observer/client biased in any way, even unintentionally? This question of bias is very important regarding CAM publications: there can be a bias by the provider of the therapy if the same person is involved in the assessment of the results; secondly, there could be a very positive bias by the client receiving the treatment if asked by the provider about the benefits of the therapy, as the client may simply be reluctant to cause offence by being negative.

Lastly, mention should be made of any further studies that are pending or should be instigated as a result of some unanswered questions in the present studies.

Conclusion

This should contain a brief summary of results and possible follow-ups and should be similar to the heading, and also in line with the original introduction. Results that were statistically insignificant should be clearly separated from the significant ones and not lumped together.

Bibliography/references

Scientific references relevant to the topic of the paper should make up the greater part of the references. Only a peer-reviewed book such as Tisserand and Balacs (1995) can be treated as a scientific reference. Non-scientific references from aromatherapy books and journals can then be included in moderation.

Appendix 33

Some aromatherapy-related organisations

AMA	American Medical Association	
COLIPA	The European Cosmetic, Toiletry and Perfumery Association	
CTFA	The Cosmetic Toiletry and Fragrance Association (USA)	
EFFA	European Flavours and Fragrance Association	Represents the interests of its member associations to the authorities and professional bodies of the European Union. It works with member states and their scientific advisers to establish a workable legislative framework and generally works and cooperates with associations in other countries (e.g. US and Japan) and the International Organization of the Flavour Industry (IOFI). Member states have their own national trade associations, e.g. in the UK, BEMA (British Essence Manufacturers Association).
FDA	Food and Drug Administration (USA)	
FEMA	Flavor and Extract Manufacturers Association	FEMA/RIFM and also the FMA (Food Manufacturing Association) produce Fragrance and Flavor Data Sheets, including many on essential oils.
IFEAT	International Federation of Essential Oil and Aroma Trades	
IFRA	International Fragrance Research Association	Receives and considers recommendations and produces guidelines for the individual fragrance ingredients for its members in the fragrance industry.
RIFM	Research Institute for Fragrance Manufacturers	Set up by the American Fragrance Manufacturers Association. RIFM collects, produces and publishes data on fragrance materials, including essential oils. RIFM makes a risk assessment from all the data and provides safety recommendations for the use of individual components used in fragrances.

Index

Abbreviations are as listed on page xv
Page numbers in **bold** refer to monographs, please refer to individual monographs for more information

memory
  odour and, 60, 63, 66
  performance
    lemon balm/melissa essential
      oil, 229
    rosemary oil, 298
    sage oil, 303
menstrual cycle
  myrrh oil, 250
  parsley oil, 269
  sage oil, 306
  thyme oil, 329
mentally ill patients, clinical
    trials, 99
Mentha arvensis, 174
Mentha spicata, 312
Mentha spp., 275
Mentha viridis, 312
menthofuran, 276
mentholated cigarettes, 277
menthone, antibacterial effects, 51
metabolism, essential oils, 50
metal ring, 18
methicillin-resistant
    Staphylococcus aureus
    (MRSA), 55
methyl salicylate, 336
Mexican oregano, 245
microbial contamination, 86
milfoil, 338
mimosa absolute, 349
mineral oil, essential oil dilution,
    26
minimum bactericidal
    concentration (MBC), tea
    tree oil, 52
minimum inhibitory concentration
    (MIC), tea tree oil, 52
mint oil, anti-inflammatory
    effects, 55
mints, 276, 313
  see also individual mints
mint tea, 278
misconceptions about essential
    oils, 75
Mitcham mint *see* peppermint oil
modification, 39
monograph guide, 105–107
monoterpenes, 48
mood
  fragrance effect on, 4
  odour and, 67

Moroccan chamomile, 151
mothers, odours, 62
motion sickness, ginger oil, 204
mouth ulcer treatment, myrrh oil,
    249
mucous membrane irritants
  cinnamon oil, 163
  thyme oil, 327
muguet, mood effects, 67
multiple sclerosis, 101–102
'mummy liquor', 11–12
muscle soreness, delayed onset,
    massage, 25
musculoskeletal system, massage,
    24
musk, 13
  behaviour, 62
  history, 64
  synthetic, toxicity, 81–82
musk ambrette, 81
musk xylene, 81–82
myalgia, peppermint oil, 276
Myristica fragrans, 256
myristicin content
  nutmeg oil, 256
  parsley oil, 268
Myroxylon balsamum, 40, 282
myrrh, 8, 64
myrrh oil, **248**
myrtle oil, **251**
Myrtus communis, 251

narcissus absolute, 349
narcotic effects
  heavy florals, 347
  nutmeg oil, 256
  orange oil, 261
narrow-leaved paperback tea tree
    see tea tree oil
National Institute of
    Occupational Safety and
    Health (NIOSH), 78
nausea, clinical studies, 98
neroli oil, **253**
Neuragen, 200
neuralgia, peppermint oil, 276
neuropharmacology, 56
neurotoxicity, 81, 84–85
  hyssop oil, 84–85, 208
NOELs (no-observed-adverse-
    effect levels), 78
nurses, safety concerns, 90

nutmeg
  extraction, 36
  toxicity, 83
nutmeg oil, **256**

Ocimum basilicum, 117
Ocotea pretiosa (sassafras oil),
    83, 90
odorants
  differentiation between, 61–62
  incense, 9
  opioids and, 73
odours
  adaptation, 70
  brain receptors, 60–62
  consumers and, 63
  dosages, 70
  methods of capture, 35
  perception, 61–62
  placebo effect, 72–73
  primary, 62
  putrid, 65
  sedative *vs.* stimulant essential
    oils, 413–414
  sleep, 71
olbas oil, 278
olfaction, 59–74
  adaptation, 70
  neurophysiology, 60–62
  physiological responses, 67–73
  see also psychological effects
olfactory nerve, 61
olfactory neuron, 60
olfactory protection, aromatic
    history, 12
olfactory receptor protein, 62
olibanum *see* frankincense
onions, 11
opioids, odorants and, 73
opoponax, 8–9
Opoponax chironium, 8–9
oral contact urticaria, 148
oral intake, 19, 27–28
  conventional use, 27–28
  dangerous practices, 88
  oil contraindications, 87
  safety issues, 27
  transfer of components, 418
oral lesions, 161–162
orange oil, 253, **260**, 286
  excluded components, 1
  yield/cost, 38